# Principles of Pain Management

# Principles of Pain Management

Editor: Emerson Haynes

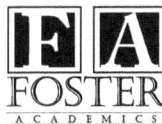

FA
FOSTER
ACADEMICS

www.fosteracademics.com

www.fosteracademics.com

FA
FOSTER
ACADEMICS

**Cataloging-in-Publication Data**

Principles of pain management / edited by Emerson Haynes.
    p. cm.
Includes bibliographical references and index.
ISBN 978-1-63242-829-5
1. Pain--Treatment. 2. Pain medicine. I. Haynes, Emerson.
RB127 .P75 2019
617.9--dc23

Foster Academics,
118-35 Queens Blvd., Suite 400,
Forest Hills, NY 11375, USA

ISBN 978-1-63242-829-5 (Hardback)

# Contents

# Preface

Pain management is a branch of medicine that is involved in the provision of a better quality of life to individuals with chronic pain by easing their suffering. Pain resolves when the underlying pathology has been treated or the trauma is healed. However, chronic pain requires long-term pain management. Some of the treatment approaches to chronic pain are prescription pain medicine, interventional procedures, physical exercise and therapy, psychological therapy, etc. Various interventional procedures such as epidural steroid injections, spinal cord stimulators, neurolytic blocks, etc. may be used for chronic pain. Most of the topics introduced in this book cover new pain management techniques and their applications. It includes some of the vital pieces of work being conducted across the world, on various topics related to pain management. It attempts to assist those with a goal of delving into this field.

The information shared in this book is based on empirical researches made by veterans in this field of study. The elaborative information provided in this book will help the readers further their scope of knowledge leading to advancements in this field.

Finally, I would like to thank my fellow researchers who gave constructive feedback and my family members who supported me at every step of my research.

Editor

# Gaps in Understanding Mechanism and Lack of Treatments: Potential Use of a Nonhuman Primate Model of Oxaliplatin-Induced Neuropathic Pain

**Aldric Hama⑩,[1] Takahiro Natsume,[1] Shin'ya Ogawa,[1] Noriyuki Higo,[2] Ikuo Hayashi,[3] and Hiroyuki Takamatsu[1]**

[1]*Hamamatsu Pharma Research, Inc., Hamamatsu, Shizuoka 431-2103, Japan*
[2]*Human Informatics Research Institute, National Institute of Advanced Industrial Science and Technology (AIST), Tsukuba, Ibaraki 305-8568, Japan*
[3]*Hamamatsu Pharma Research USA, Inc., San Diego, CA 92122, USA*

Correspondence should be addressed to Aldric Hama; aldric-hama@hpharma.jp

Academic Editor: Ulises Coffeen

The antineoplastic agent oxaliplatin induces an acute hypersensitivity evoked by cold that has been suggested to be due to sensitized central and peripheral neurons. Rodent-based preclinical studies have suggested numerous treatments for the alleviation of oxaliplatin-induced neuropathic pain, but few have demonstrated robust clinical efficacy. One issue is that current understanding of the pathophysiology of oxaliplatin-induced neuropathic pain is primarily based on rodent models, which might not entirely recapitulate the clinical pathophysiology. In addition, there is currently no objective physiological marker for pain that could be utilized to objectively indicate treatment efficacy. Nonhuman primates are phylogenetically and neuroanatomically similar to humans; thus, disease mechanism in nonhuman primates could reflect that of clinical oxaliplatin-induced neuropathy. Cold-activated pain-related brain areas in oxaliplatin-treated macaques were attenuated with duloxetine, the only drug that has demonstrated clinical efficacy for chemotherapy-induced neuropathic pain. By contrast, drugs that have not demonstrated clinical efficacy in oxaliplatin-induced neuropathic pain did not reduce brain activation. Thus, a nonhuman primate model could greatly enhance understanding of clinical pathophysiology beyond what has been obtained with rodent models and, furthermore, brain activation could serve as an objective marker of pain and therapeutic efficacy.

## 1. Introduction

A common complication arising from anticancer pharmacotherapy is peripheral sensory neuropathy. Symptoms of peripheral neuropathy include tingling or pins-and-needles dysesthesia and pain, beginning in the distal feet and hands and spreading proximally in a stocking/glove type distribution [1, 2]. The symptoms of chemotherapy-induced peripheral neuropathy are strikingly similar to other peripheral sensory neuropathies such as painful diabetic neuropathy [3]. The general incidence of peripheral neuropathy in chemotherapy patients is estimated to be about 48%, and around 40–60% of patients experience symptoms which persist long after termination of chemotherapy [4]. The incidence of neuropathy during treatment and after termination of treatment depends on factors such as total dosage, overall duration of chemotherapy and preexisting medical conditions, as well as the particular class of chemotherapeutic [5, 6]. Severe cases of chemotherapy-induced peripheral neuropathy may necessitate dose reduction or termination of potentially life-extending treatment [7–10]. Thus, treatments that ameliorate peripheral neuropathy during the course of treatment as well as prophylactic treatments that prevent the onset of symptoms are much sought-after and goals of vigorous ongoing research.

## 2. Oxaliplatin-Induced Neuropathic Pain

It has been estimated that 81–91% of patients experience a peripheral neuropathy within hours or days of treatment, lasting for up to a week, with the organoplatinum chemotherapeutic oxaliplatin [11, 12]. Unique to oxaliplatin and other platinum-based chemotherapeutics, neuropathic pain is provoked by cold. A clinical study reported that 89% of patients experienced acute "moderate/severe symptoms" evoked by cold and discomfort swallowing "cold items" during the first treatment cycle with a standard dose of oxaliplatin (85 mg/m$^2$, or a human equivalent dose of 2.3 mg/kg, every two weeks) [2, 5, 13]. (One treatment cycle is two weeks in duration.) The study also reported that symptoms peaked three days following treatment and subsided, though full recovery was not obtained by the next treatment cycle. On subsequent treatment cycles, similar time course profiles were obtained, with symptoms tending to worsen with subsequent treatments. The incidence of persistent peripheral neuropathy increased by the third treatment cycle and by the ninth cycle, half of all patients reported dysesthesia, characterized by pain in the absence of stimulation, which persisted for over 14 days following treatment [14, 15]. Within the first three months following the final oxaliplatin treatment, symptoms tended to worsen rather than improve. Eighteen months following the end of treatment, sensory neuropathy tended to improve; however, complete resolution was not observed [5]. Persistent peripheral neuropathy was observed in 60% of patients two years after the final treatment [5].

As noted earlier, a unique symptom of oxaliplatin-induced neurotoxicity is cold-evoked pain. The early, acute hypersensitivity to cold and the persistent neuropathic symptoms long after treatment termination suggest pathophysiological changes to the peripheral and central nervous systems. For example, by the third treatment cycle, cold temperatures (5–20°C) that were perceived as somewhat noxious before the start of oxaliplatin treatment are now perceived as painful ("cold hyperalgesia") following oxaliplatin treatment [16]. Noxious heat (42–48°C) that was mildly painful is now perceived as excruciating ("heat hyperalgesia") following oxaliplatin treatment. By contrast, no change in responsiveness to either non-noxious or noxious mechanical stimulation was observed during the oxaliplatin treatment period. Nearly all patients (96%) in the study by Attal et al. reported sensory neuropathy after each treatment cycle. The emergence of heat and cold hyperalgesia suggests dysfunction in small-diameter unmyelinated C-fiber and myelinated A$\delta$ primary afferent nociceptors, respectively. Attal et al. [16] also noted a gradual loss of myelinated, large-diameter A$\beta$ primary afferents, as indicated by a loss of vibration sensitivity. The loss of large-diameter primary afferents could have a role in the development of hyperalgesia and dysesthesia as the loss of these fibers reduces peripherally mediated inhibition of noxious cutaneous signaling to the spinal cord dorsal horn [10, 16, 17]. Nonetheless, a nonspecific loss of sensory nerve function suggests a generalized oxaliplatin-induced neurotoxicity.

## 3. Changes from Normal Pain Perception to Injury-Induced Pain

In humans, an intact pain-perception system is necessary in order to acquire information of the external environmental and body functional status. Diminished sensitivity to acute pain perception could lead to self-injury, as seen, for example, in patients with congenital insensitivity to pain [18]. At the same time, pain and hypersensitivity to cutaneous stimuli that persists well beyond tissue injury recovery are nonadaptive and suggest a dysfunctional nervous system. Thus, the main goals of pain research are identifying and targeting mechanisms that sustain chronic pain while at the same time preserving normal pain perception.

Painful cutaneous or deep tissue stimulation from the periphery reaches spinal cord dorsal horn neurons via primary afferent neurons (a separate group of primary afferent neurons innervate viscera [19]). Noxious sensation crosses a synapse between central terminals of primary afferent neurons and spinal dorsal horn sensory neurons via a number of excitatory neurotransmitters that activate their respective receptor [20, 21]. Dorsal horn neurons send noxious signals supraspinally to subcortical nuclei involved in the sensory-discriminatory aspects of pain perception, such as the thalamus, which, in turn, sends projections to cortical nuclei such as somatosensory cortex, informing the organism of the somatotopic origin of the noxious stimulus and pain intensity. Noxious sensations are also sent to nuclei involved with the affective-motivational aspects of pain, such as the insula, cingulate cortex, amygdala, and hippocampus, giving pain its aversive quality [22–24].

By contrast, pain associated with injury or neurotoxicity is characterized by significant changes to the somatosensory system wherein central neurons show increased basal activity. Neurons are said to be "sensitized," wherein neurons now respond to stimulation that previously did not evoke responses and show greatly increased responses to normal or intense stimulation [20]. These neural responses are suggested to be the physiological basis of "allodynia," the perception of non-noxious stimulation as painful, and "hyperalgesia," an enhanced responsiveness to painful stimulation.

Mediating these pathophysiological changes are injury-associated changes in the expression of membrane-associated proteins and intracellular messenger systems [20]. (Numerous changes in glia phenotype in response to peripheral injury are also observed thereby amplifying changes in neural functioning [20].) Changes to neural phenotype may become permanent and lead to dramatic changes in function, which in turn further alters phenotype. This feed-forward cycle is believed to be the basis of the chronicity of the chronic pain state.

While changes to somatosensation suggest central sensitization, demonstrating that particular pain-related molecular entities in the human brain are directly responsible for clinical "allodynia" or "hyperalgesia" requires observation in and experimentation with human tissue. Alternatively, nonhuman animal models are used to observe and measure these changes [25, 26]. In fact, findings from rodent models serve as the cornerstone for the theoretical construct called "sensitization" and issues related to findings in rodent models of oxaliplatin-induced neuropathic pain and their clinical relevance will be raised later in this review.

## 4. A Nonhuman Primate Model of Oxaliplatin-Induced Neuropathic Pain

*4.1. The Nonhuman Primate as a Preclinical Species.* Nonhuman animal models are crucial in understanding biological processes in the healthy and diseased state. Nonhuman animal models that reflect the diseased state may be further used to develop diagnostic methods and therapeutics [27]. Rodents are the primary preclinical species and findings in these models, in general, drive clinical studies of novel therapeutics. While rodents as a species have a number of benefits, such as physiological and anatomical homogeneity and amenability to genetic manipulation, there are significant genetic and anatomical differences between rodents and humans, including a number of functional differences in pain-related molecules [28, 29]. By contrast, nonhuman primates are phylogenetically closer to humans than rodents and share a number of neuroanatomical and neurophysiological similarities with humans [27, 30]. The parallels between humans and nonhuman primates are particular striking in neurological disorders such as Alzheimer's disease, spinal cord injury, and Parkinson's disease [30–32]. Given the neurological similarity and capacity for emotional behaviors reminiscent of that of humans, ethical concerns accompany the use of nonhuman primates in basic science and drug discovery programs. The use of any nonhuman animal should be justified from scientific and welfare perspectives. Alternatives to the use of animals, including nonhuman primates, should be investigated. A careful cost/benefit analysis for each study utilizing nonhuman animals should be performed, such that significant human benefit is derived from the use of the fewest possible number of nonhuman animals. In the case of disorders, including pain, where alternatives are not available or inappropriate, it is crucial to perform studies with nonhuman primates. As will be described later, there is currently low confidence in the rodent models of oxaliplatin-induced neuropathic pain [33]. Thus, nonhuman primates are an appropriate species. Given that there are currently no approved therapeutics for oxaliplatin-induced neuropathic pain, a positive finding of efficacy from a novel therapeutic in a nonhuman primate model would be a significant step toward developing a life-enhancing treatment.

*4.2. Noninvasive Visualization of Central Sensitization in Oxaliplatin-Induced Neuropathic Pain.* Previous methods that have visualized central sensitization in nonhuman animals have utilized invasive *in vivo* techniques such as extracellular recording of neurons. A limited number of clinical studies demonstrating central sensitization in chronic pain patients have also utilized extracellular recordings [34–36]. Because of the technical difficulties, finding appropriate patients, the lack of neural responses in neurologically

healthy subjects for comparison purposes, and limited opportunity for pharmacological manipulation, less invasive methods are utilized to visualize *in vivo* neural activity. Functional magnetic resonance imaging (fMRI) allows for noninvasive observation of brain activation. In addition, possible changes in activation over time and following pharmacotherapy may be observed within the same subject [37]. Ideally, changes in brain activity or connectivity between brain nuclei involved in pain processing should correlate with changes in behavioral outcomes. Brain imaging, then, could be used both as an objective marker of pain, itself a subjective experience, and as an indicator of analgesic efficacy of treatments [38]. A limitation of data obtained by fMRI is that brain activity is inferred, in that fMRI measures changes in blood oxygenation due to neural activity. Thus, physiological parameters, beyond neural activity, which may change blood flow and blood oxygenation, are carefully monitored. One other limitation of fMRI is that the molecular mechanism mediating observed changes in brain activity can only, at the moment, be inferred—from findings in nonhuman animals.

A number of clinical fMRI studies of chronic pain patients have shown significant changes from "resting" brain activity following peripheral stimulation [39, 40]. In patients with chemotherapy-induced peripheral neuropathy, activation of cortical areas in response to heat applied to a neuropathic region has been noted, which differs from heat response in healthy subjects [41]. A positive correlation was observed between brain activation in response to heat stimulation and total neuropathy score, which incorporates a number of observed signs and symptoms of peripheral neuropathy, but not specifically neuropathic pain.

A similar fMRI study on the effect of cold sensation on brain activation in oxaliplatin-induced neuropathic pain has yet to be reported, but brain activation in oxaliplatin-treated nonhuman primates has been recently reported using fMRI [42]. Oxaliplatin treatment in cynomolgus macaques leads to a significant hypersensitivity to 10°C cold, beginning three days after intravenous oxaliplatin infusion (two-hour i.v. infusion 5 mg/kg; human equivalent dose of 1.6 mg/kg [13, 43]) (Figure 1(a)). Furthermore, treatment with the serotonergic-norepinephrine reuptake inhibitor duloxetine (p.o. 30 mg/kg; human equivalent dose approximately 10 mg/kg [13]) ameliorated cold hypersensitivity. By contrast, the anticonvulsant pregabalin (p.o. 30 mg/kg) and the opioid/serotonergic-norepinephrine reuptake inhibitor tramadol (p.o. 30 mg/kg) did not alter cold hypersensitivity (Figure 1(b)). The lack of efficacy of pregabalin and tramadol in the macaque model contrasts with robust efficacy observed in rodent models of oxaliplatin-induced neuropathic pain [33, 43–45]. The limited macaque pharmacological data parallel findings from randomized, placebo-controlled clinical trials, in that duloxetine showed significant efficacy in chemotherapy-induced peripheral neuropathic pain [46], whereas pregabalin did not [47]. There are no reports of tramadol efficacy for oxaliplatin-induced neuropathic pain in a randomized, placebo-controlled clinical trial, but the macaque result would predict a lack of efficacy. The limited convergence between

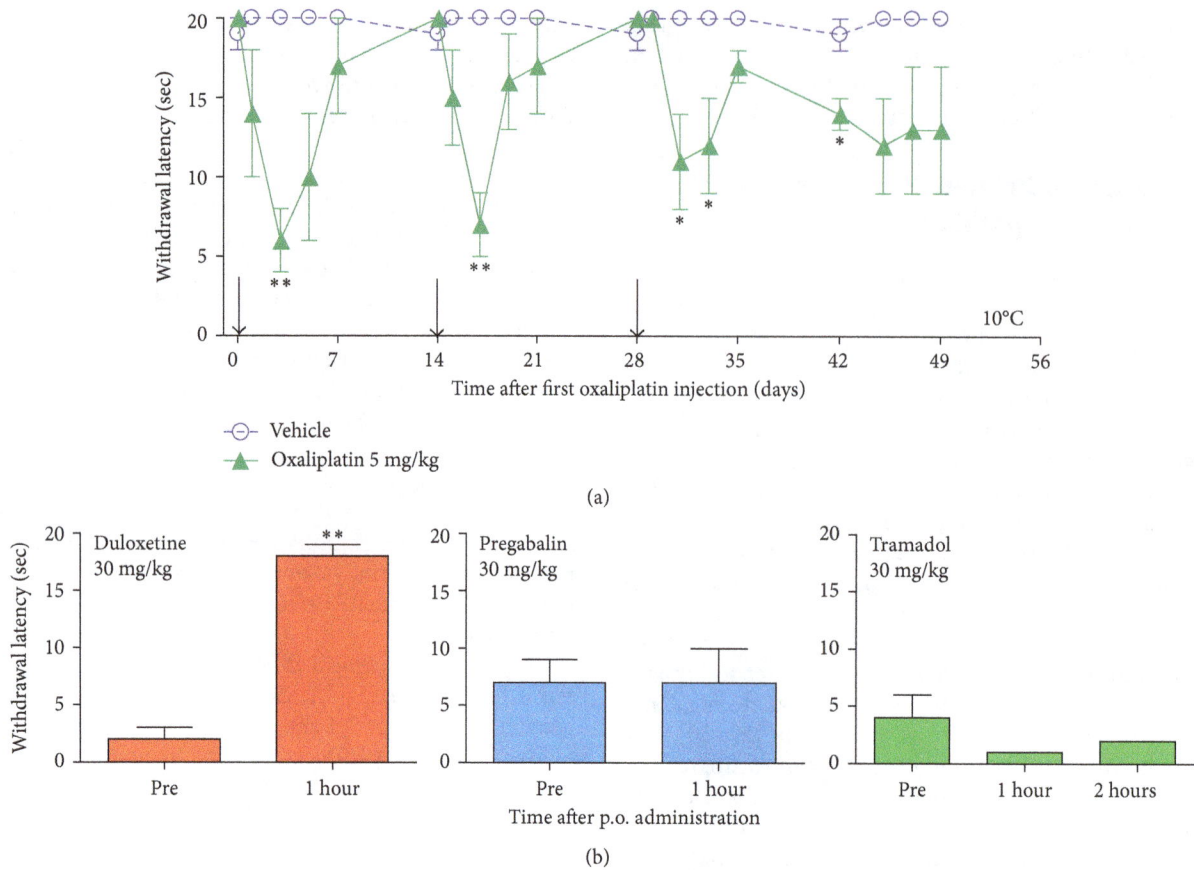

(a)

(b)

FIGURE 1: Cold hypersensitivity over time in oxaliplatin-treated macaques. To assess changes to temperature sensitivity, the tail withdrawal test was used [43]. Following habituation to chair restraint, baseline responses of awake cynomolgus macaques to 10°C cold water were measured. The distal 10 cm of the tail was cleaned and immersed in a cold water bath. The amount of time (in seconds) between tail immersion and withdrawal from the water was recorded and reported as the withdrawal latency. A maximum immersion time of 20 sec. was utilized. Prior to oxaliplatin treatment, the withdrawal latency to cold water was 20 sec. (a) Significant sensitivity to cold (10°C) was observed following oxaliplatin treatment. Following baseline assessment, macaques were treated with oxaliplatin (i.v. 5 mg/kg, 2 hr. infusion; ▲). Three days after oxaliplatin treatment (↓), the mean withdrawal latency was significantly decreased compared to the pretreatment latency, indicating cold hypersensitivity. Hypersensitivity to cold dissipated over time—by seven days after oxaliplatin treatment, the response to cold was similar to that prior to oxaliplatin treatment. Subsequent oxaliplatin treatments evoked an acute hypersensitivity to cold beginning three days after treatment. By contrast, vehicle treatment (i.v. glucose 5% in water; ○) did not significantly affect response to cold. Data presented as mean ± S.E.M. Vehicle, $n = 3$. Oxaliplatin, $n = 5$-6. $^*p < 0.05$, $^{**}p < 0.01$ versus baseline (day "0"). (b) Pharmacological modulation of oxaliplatin-induced neuropathic pain in macaques. Tail withdrawal latencies were measured three days after oxaliplatin treatment. Macaques were tested one hour after treatment (one and two hours after tramadol treatment) [43]. The antidepressant drug duloxetine (p.o. 30 mg/kg) reversed hypersensitivity to cold. By contrast, the anticonvulsant drug pregabalin (p.o. 30 mg/kg) and the opioid/serotonin-norepinephrine reuptake inhibitor tramadol (p.o. 30 mg/kg) did not. Data presented as mean ± S.E.M. $n = 4$/duloxetine, $n = 4$/pregabalin, $n = 3$/tramadol. $^{**}p < 0.01$ versus pretreatment ("Pre"), paired $t$-test. Slightly modified from [43].

the rodent models and the macaque model, and by extension clinical oxaliplatin-induced neuropathic pain, should be of concern to those who are trying to elaborate mechanism and to those who are developing treatments based on mechanisms derived from rodents.

Brain activation was visualized in sedated oxaliplatin-treated cynomolgus macaques with a 3T Philips Ingenia MRI system. Temperature stimuli were applied to the tail with either a cold (10°C) or warm (37°C) gel pack. Brain activity was acquired before and after oxaliplatin treatment. Before oxaliplatin treatment, 10°C evoked activation in brain areas involved with sensation, such as primary somatosensory cortex, and areas involved with movement, such as areas PE/PG of parietal cortex. These brain areas were also found

to be activated following innocuous cold stimulation in humans [48]. Following oxaliplatin treatment, significant cold-evoked activation was observed in secondary somatosensory cortex and insula (Figure 2). Activation of these areas in healthy humans is observed with noxious cold [49]. The insula has been identified as being involved in processing both the sensory-discriminative and affective-discriminative aspects of pain [48]. This observation is based on the findings that connections between the insula and other brain areas mediate somatosensation and affect-motivation [48]. Stimulus-evoked activation of the insula has been observed in other neuropathic pain states, suggesting a potential "universal" brain mechanism across neuropathic pain states [50–52]. The sensitivity of the

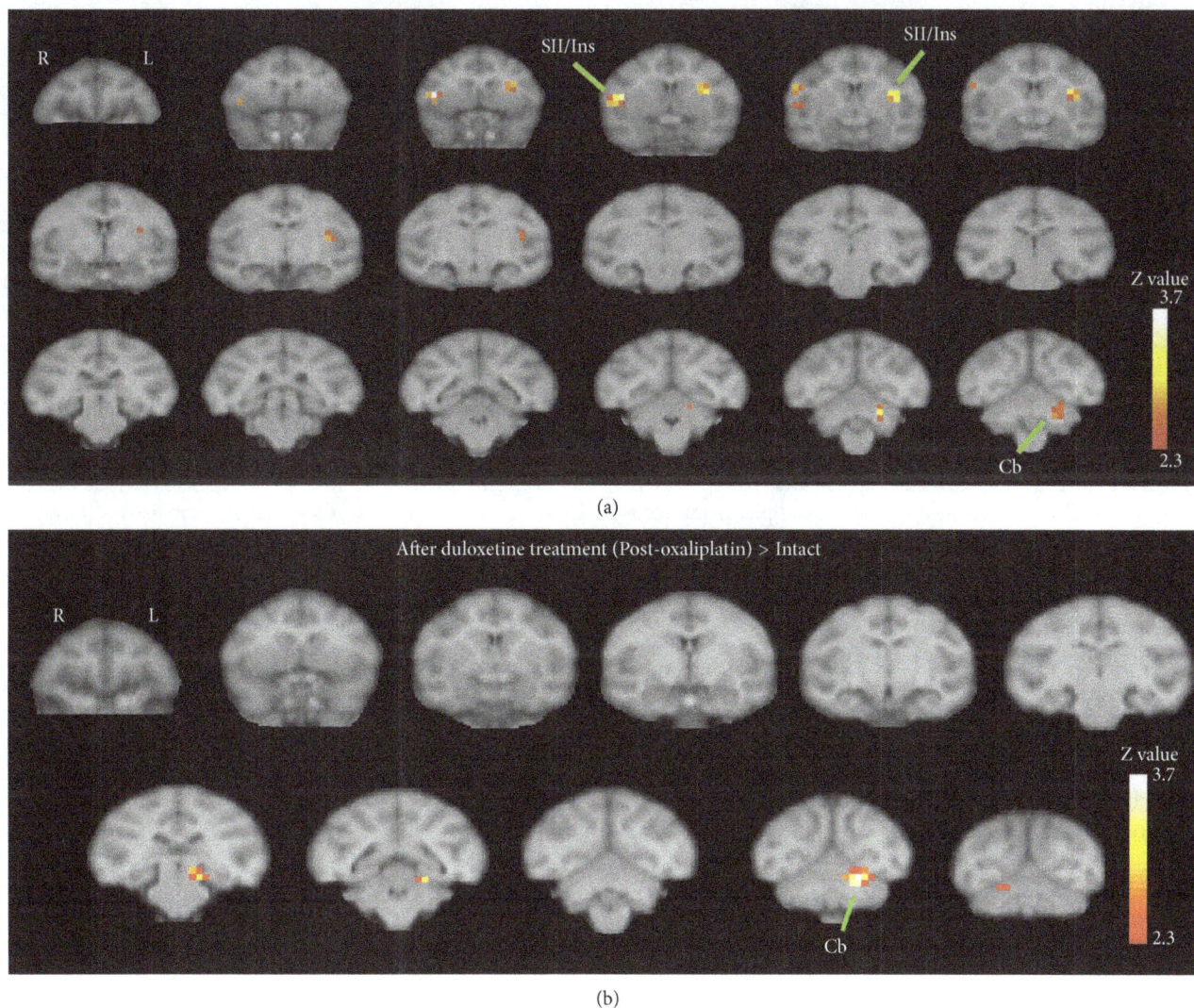

FIGURE 2: Cold stimulation evokes brain activation in oxaliplatin-treated macaques, which is attenuated with duloxetine. Before and three days after oxaliplatin treatment, brain activation was visualized with a 3.0 T Philips Healthcare MRI system in propofol-sedated macaques [42]. Alternating temperatures (cold, 10°C and neutral, 37°C) were applied to the tail for 30 sec. each with a 30 sec. interval without stimulation. (a) Cold stimulation in oxaliplatin-treated macaques activated secondary somatosensory cortex (SII) and insula (Ins). Activation in the left cerebellum (Cb) following cold stimulation was also observed. Contrast was defined as (10°C stimulation −37°C stimulation after oxaliplatin treatment)–(10°C stimulation −37°C stimulation before oxaliplatin treatment; "intact"). Peak voxels $Z$ values greater than 3.0 were $p < 0.001$ (uncorrected for multiple comparisons, one-tailed). Coronal sections of oxaliplatin-treated macaques averaged from four macaques. Sections arranged from rostral (upper left) to caudal (lower right) and spaced 2 mm apart. R, right; L, left. (b) Duloxetine suppressed cold-induced activation in SII and Ins in oxaliplatin-treated macaques. However, activation in Cb was still present following duloxetine treatment. Three days after oxaliplatin treatment, macaques were dosed with duloxetine (p.o. 30 mg/kg) and cold-evoked brain activation was measured one hour following duloxetine treatment. The effect of duloxetine treatment on cold-evoked brain activation in oxaliplatin-treated macaques ("after duloxetine treatment (Post-oxaliplatin)") was compared to cold-evoked brain activation before oxaliplatin treatment ("intact"). No significant activation in SII and Ins was observed following duloxetine treatment ($p > 0.05$). Thus, the lack of activity in SII and Ins following duloxetine administration in oxaliplatin-treated macaques was similar to that of macaques prior to oxaliplatin treatment. (An additional analysis was performed comparing cold-evoked SII and Ins activation after and before duloxetine treatment in oxaliplatin-treated macaques (data not shown, [42]). Activation in SII and Ins following duloxetine treatment was significantly suppressed—the difference in peak voxels, between after and before duloxetine treatment, was $p < 0.001$. See [42] for details.) Coronal sections of oxaliplatin-treated macaques averaged from four macaques. Sections arranged from rostral (upper left) to caudal (lower right) and spaced 4 mm apart. R, right; L, left. Data previously published in [42].

insula, and secondary somatosensory cortex, to pharmacological modulation in oxaliplatin-induced neuropathic pain has yet to be clinically examined.

In the oxaliplatin-treated macaques, duloxetine significantly reduced cold-evoked activation in secondary somatosensory cortex and insula, whereas pregabalin, used in the management of a number of painful peripheral neuropathies, did not [53]. These findings suggest a mechanism for duloxetine's clinical efficacy in chemotherapy-induced neuropathic pain and suggest that targeting these areas in humans could lead to analgesia [38, 42].

Furthermore, the macaque findings suggest the utility of brain activation as an objective index of drug efficacy. At the same time, drugs that did not alleviate clinical oxaliplatin-induced neuropathic pain (there are a number of these [54, 55]) could be evaluated in the current macaque model in order to pharmacologically confirm the importance of secondary somatosensory cortex and insula in mediating oxaliplatin-induced neuropathic pain.

The lack of efficacy with pregabalin suggests that oxaliplatin-induced neuropathic pain is mechanistically distinct from other painful peripheral neuropathies. Perhaps pregabalin's target, the $\alpha2\delta$ subunit of the voltage-gated calcium channel, is absent in the case of oxaliplatin-induced neuropathic pain but present in other neuropathic pains that are responsive to pregabalin. In any event, the differential responding between rodents and macaques suggests further investigation as to why this is the case and may have significant bearing on the mechanism of clinical oxaliplatin-induced neuropathic pain.

It would be interesting to compare and contrast brain areas activated with cold between rodents and macaques with oxaliplatin-induced neuropathic pain. Thus far, fMRI has not been utilized as a method of observing brain activation in oxaliplatin-treated rodents.

*4.3. What Is the Extent of Peripheral Nerve Involvement in Oxaliplatin-Induced Neuropathic Pain?* The neurotoxicity associated with oxaliplatin is primarily of peripheral sensory nerves. In cerebrospinal fluid (CSF), the concentration of oxaliplatin is about 1.6% of that found in plasma, indicating extremely limited penetration of oxaliplatin of the blood-brain barrier [56]. Thus, sensitization of peripheral nerves could be as important (or more so) as sensitization of CNS neurons in mediating oxaliplatin-induced neuropathic pain. Targets expressed on peripheral nerves are advantageous in that potential therapeutics do not need to cross the blood-brain barrier and could also have the potential of demonstrating fewer psychomotor effects compared to centrally acting drugs. However, the exact contribution of peripheral nerves to clinical oxaliplatin-induced neuropathic pain is not entirely clear, and what has been described is largely based on rodent models.

Significant levels of oxaliplatin have been measured in rat dorsal root ganglion (DRG) neurons, as DRG neurons lie outside of the blood-brain barrier [25, 57, 58]. As per its mechanism of action in tumors, platinum binds to peripheral nerve nuclear and mitochondrial DNA and proteins, forming adducts and thereby inhibiting DNA replication and transcription [59, 60]. Details of a putative pathway between decreased gene transcription and neural functioning are lacking, but the pathway could involve changes in the expression of membrane-associated proteins, such as ion channels, related to propagation of action potentials.

As a consequence of changes in mitochondrial DNA transcription, cellular metabolism is decreased, reactive oxygen species are formed and cytosolic ion concentrations are altered. Changes to cellular metabolism are suggested morphologically as abnormally shaped or swollen mitochondria in peripheral nerves from oxaliplatin-treated rats [57, 61, 62]. Further inhibition of cellular metabolism induces proteins involved in apoptosis and eventual death of DRG neurons [57, 58, 62]. At $33.2\,\mu M$, 20–40% of rat DRG neurons *in vitro* were viable after a 24-hr incubation in oxaliplatin [59]. A similar lethality was observed in rat DRG neurons incubated for 48 hrs in $12.6\,\mu M$ oxaliplatin [63]. The *in vitro* findings suggest marked nerve degeneration as a consequence of oxaliplatin exposure and that this pathology is somehow expressed as pain. It should be noted that the clinically attained plasma levels of oxaliplatin is in the range of $3.8–12.1\,\mu M$, lower than the *in vitro* concentrations that have been utilized in most studies utilizing rat tissues [64].

While the *in vitro* findings suggest significant neurotoxicity, to the point of cell death, loss of DRG neurons was not observed in oxaliplatin-treated mice dosed over a period of nine weeks [65]. Prior to euthanasia, these mice demonstrated robust hind paw mechanical hypersensitivity. (The presence of cold hypersensitivity following nine weeks of oxaliplatin treatment was not mentioned.) Also, in rats, no loss of DRG neurons or sensory nerve axonal degeneration was reported 31 days after the last oxaliplatin treatment [62]. At this time point, oxaliplatin-treated rats showed significant hind paw "cold allodynia" as well as "mechano-hyperalgesia," and "mechano-allodynia". (Note that persistent mechano-hyperalgesia or mechanical-allodynia has not been demonstrated in oxaliplatin-treated patients [10, 16].) In oxaliplatin-treated patients with "mild to moderate" neuropathy, DRG observed using magnetic resonance neurography (MRN) demonstrated hypertrophy, suggesting increased metabolic activation rather than cell atrophy and death [66, 67]. Peripheral nerve cross-sectional volumes were unchanged in these patients, indicating an absence of axonal damage or a loss of DRG neurons.

There appears to be no consensus between the clinical MRN findings, *in vivo* rodent findings and *in vitro* rat DRG neuron findings. Perhaps longer treatment periods and higher doses of oxaliplatin *in vivo* will lead to significant cell death and nerve fiber loss. Nonetheless, the findings thus far do not suggest that peripheral nerve loss is necessary for the emergence of oxaliplatin-induced neuropathic pain. If the rodent model is to have any construct or predictive validity [68], it would be important to confirm that mechanisms described in rats are also present in humans. However, given limitations concerning access to human tissue and studies on patients, the nonhuman primate model, combined with *in vivo* imaging, could be used to explore the involvement of peripheral neurotoxicity in oxaliplatin-induced neuropathic pain.

*4.4. Other Possible Therapeutic Targets: Voltage-Gated Sodium Channels?* In addition to oxaliplatin's indirect disruptive effect on neural metabolism, oxaliplatin appears to directly affect peripheral nerve function [57]. A direct effect is suggested by the observation that within hours, oxaliplatin applied to rat cutaneous nerves via intraplantar injection into the hind paw leads to robust, short-duration mechanical and cold allodynia. The rapid onset of pain has been suggested to be due to a direct effect of oxaliplatin on voltage-gated $Na^+$ channels expressed on peripheral nerves [69–71]. While a number of *in vitro* studies in rat tissue support this hypothesis, as in the *in vitro* neurotoxicity studies described earlier, concentrations of oxaliplatin used were well above clinical therapeutic levels. Nonetheless, oxaliplatin's effect was limited to peripherally expressed $Na^+$ channels—no changes in $K^+$ channel activity and $Na^+$ channels expressed in brain slices were noted [71].

The *in vitro* and *in vivo* findings appear to indicate that attenuating prolonged activation of $Na^+$ channels by blocking them could lead to pain relief. Pretreatment of rat peripheral nerves with carbamazepine ($1,000\,\mu M$), an anticonvulsant drug that blocks voltage-gated $Na^+$ channels, prevented the onset of oxaliplatin-induced changes in $Na^+$ conductance [71, 72]. Similarly, carbamazepine ($300\,\mu M$) prevented oxaliplatin-induced changes in $Na^+$ conductance in mouse peripheral nerve-tissue preparations [73]. Whether these findings can be directly translatable to the clinical situation is not at all clear, as the therapeutic serum concentration of carbamazepine is $34–51\,\mu M$ [74].

In a rat model of oxaliplatin-induced neuropathic pain, systemic carbamazepine (i.p. 30 mg/kg, or a human equivalent dose of 4.8 mg/kg) significantly ameliorated hypersensitivity to cold [75]. In contrast to the *in vivo* preclinical rat finding, however, clinical findings of carbamazepine efficacy are equivocal. In a nonblinded, nonrandomized study, carbamazepine treatment prior to the first dose of oxaliplatin prevented the emergence of "neurotoxicity,"—pain was not directly assessed in this trial [76]. Three other pre-oxaliplatin, prophylactic studies did not confirm a potential protective effect of carbamazepine [74, 77, 78]. Furthermore, in the case of the open-label study by Wilson et al. [74], seven out of 12 patients reported "adverse effects" with carbamazepine treatment. In the phase II study by von Delius et al. [77], the effect of carbamazepine on either pain or abnormal cold sensation was not specifically evaluated.

The nonrobust efficacy of carbamazepine observed in clinical oxaliplatin-induced neuropathic pain could, in part, be related to its modest affinity for $Na^+$ channels. Other drugs with greater affinity for $Na^+$ channels could be used to determine whether peripherally expressed $Na^+$ channels are in fact involved in oxaliplatin-induced neuropathic pain [79, 80]. One potent $Na^+$ channel blocker that has shown sustained analgesia long after treatment termination is tetrodotoxin, a neurotoxin isolated from puffer fish. In cancer pain patients, analgesia was observed for a mean of 57 days following a four-day treatment trial of intramuscular tetrodotoxin ($20\,\mu g$ BID) [81, 82].

The *in vivo* findings based on the rodent models, while encouraging, have not predicted successful clinical outcomes with $Na^+$ channel-blocking drugs. Perhaps testing in the macaque model will clarify whether it is in fact worthwhile to advance this class of therapeutics to large clinical trials for oxaliplatin-induced neuropathic pain.

*4.5. Other Possible Therapeutic Targets: Transient Receptor Potential Ankyrin-1 (TRPA1) and Transient Receptor Potential Melastatin-8 (TRPM8)?* The transient receptor potential (TRP) channels form a family of 28 cation-permeable channels, some of which are responsive to temperature and naturally occurring ligands. Because many of these channels are expressed in DRG neurons, it is likely that they have some role in the initiation and maintenance of peripheral neuropathies [83]. Of particular interest in the context of oxaliplatin-induced cold hypersensitivity are two TRP channels activated at cool ($\leq25°C$; TRPM8) and cold ($\leq17°C$; TRPA1) temperatures [83]. Findings in rodent oxaliplatin-induced neuropathic pain models show upregulation of TRPA1 and TRPM8 in DRG neurons, and mice lacking TRPM8 channels do not demonstrate cold hypersensitivity following oxaliplatin treatment [84]. Oxaliplatin-induced cold hypersensitivity is alleviated with most, but not all [84], TRPM8 and TRPA1 channel blockers [85]. Thus, the findings in rodent models suggest that these peripherally expressed channels could be targeted to develop therapeutics for oxaliplatin-induced neuropathic pain.

While much has been reported on the role of TRPA1 in cold sensation and its potential role in neuropathic pain, it is not entirely clear whether this target will be useful for the treatment of clinical cold hypersensitivity. Cold activates the rat and mouse TRPA1 channel, but cold does not appear to activate human and macaque TRPA1 [28]. Similar species differences in other receptor functioning and physiological processes have been described elsewhere, underscoring the need of evaluating potential pain-related targets in the relevant species where possible [86, 87]. With regard to TRPA1, Chen et al. [28] suggested that "nonhuman primates should serve as a surrogate species for TRPA1 drug development." A potential issue Chen noted in utilizing nonhuman primates as a model species is that there are a "limited number of monkey disease models available," but currently, this may no longer be an issue [43, 88–90].

A potential analgesic effect of blocking human TRPM8 channels was assessed with the TRPM8 antagonist PF-05105679 in the cold pressor test [91]. In the cold pressor test, subjects immerse their hands or forelimbs in cold water (between 1 and 7°C) for up to two minutes. Subjects report the first instance of pain (pain threshold) and withdraw from the water when the cold becomes too painful to continue (pain tolerance). Alternatively, subjects score their pain (from 0 to 10, 0 being no pain and 10 being the worst possible pain) over time during hand immersion in cold water (the cold pressor test is similar to that of the cold withdrawal test in the macaques (Figure 1) [43].) PF-05105679 was as equianalgesic as the opioid analgesic oxycodone [91]. Peak efficacy apparently matched the peak plasma concentration of PF-05105679. An adverse effect at higher doses was sensations of perioral heat and heat experienced on parts of the upper body. Whether this adverse effect was in fact mediated by TRPM8 is currently unknown. Interestingly, while TRPM8 is known to regulate body temperature—blocking TRPM8 reduced body temperature in rats—no significant change in core body temperature was observed in healthy subjects treated with PF-05105679. There are a number of other TRPM8 antagonists that have yet to be tested in humans [92].

Whether similar adverse effects are observed with TRPM8 antagonists from other chemical series have yet to be determined. Testing in nonhuman primates could uncover species-specific TRPM8 functioning, such as temperature regulation, as observed with the TRPV1 channel.

An orally bioavailable TRPM8 antagonist developed by RaQualia, RQ-00434739, demonstrated efficacy in a rodent and nonhuman primate model of oxaliplatin-induced cold hypersensitivity [93]. The compound inhibited *in vitro* responses to TRPM8 agonists menthol and icilin at nanomolar concentrations in both rat and human TRPM8 channels. A significant antinociceptive effect was observed at 10 mg/kg of RQ-00434739 on acetone-evoked pain-related behavior in oxaliplatin-treated rats [94]. Likewise, significant antinociception was observed on oxaliplatin-induced cold hypersensitivity in nonhuman primates with 10 mg/kg of RQ-00434739 [93]. The effects of blocking TRPM8 on cold-evoked brain activation and body temperature have yet to be evaluated. The finding of antinociception with TRPM8 blockade in both rat and macaque models suggests a similar role of the rat and nonhuman primate (and, thus, human) TRPM8 channel in mediating oxaliplatin-induced cold hypersensitivity [95]. Perhaps there are other molecular targets that demonstrate similar functions across species. However, as observed so far with the limited number of analgesics tested in both rats and macaques, interspecies similarity may be few and far between.

## 5. Conclusion

There is a growing recognition that there are significant differences between species of the functioning of a number of molecular target and a need to evaluate therapeutics destined for clinical study in the appropriate disease model. There is also the recognition that nonsubjective, quantifiable indicators of biological activity for both preclinical nonhuman animals and patients, "biomarkers," are needed. Biomarkers, such as *in vivo* brain activation, could be used to select patients and serve as an indicator of target engagement by the therapeutic, thereby serving as a secondary measure of clinical efficacy. Indeed, it appears that the use of biomarkers enhances the "probability of success" of drug development programs [96]. The current review pointed out several potential avenues for the development of novel therapeutics for a condition that has no US FDA-approved treatments. However, it is hoped that the reader will also come to the realization that the current developmental approach focused exclusively on rodent models leaves much to be desired. Macaques as a preclinical model species are challenging in terms of care and handling. However, given the critical need to elaborate disease mechanism and test potential therapeutics in a species that shares genetic similarity with humans, it is hoped that there will be more interest in developing methodologies and infrastructure necessary for the use of nonhuman primates for basic science and drug development.

## Acknowledgments

The authors thank the HPR Animal Care Group for expert technical support and animal care. Noriyuki Higo supported by the Japan Society for the Promotion of Science (JSPS) KAKENHI Grants nos. 25351004 and 16K01489.

## References

[1] R. Heide, H. Bostock, L. Ventzel et al., "Axonal excitability changes and acute symptoms of oxaliplatin treatment: in vivo evidence for slowed sodium channel inactivation," *Clinical Neurophysiology*, vol. 129, no. 3, pp. 694–706, 2017.

[2] D. R. Pachman, R. Qin, D. K. Seisler et al., "Clinical course of oxaliplatin-induced neuropathy: results from the randomized phase III trial N08CB (Alliance)," *Journal of Clinical Oncology*, vol. 33, no. 30, pp. 3416–3422, 2015.

[3] A. Hartemann, N. Attal, D. Bouhassira et al., "Painful diabetic neuropathy: diagnosis and management," *Diabetes and Metabolism*, vol. 37, no. 5, pp. 377–388, 2011.

[4] M. Cascella, "Chemotherapy-induced peripheral neuropathy: limitations in current prophylactic strategies and directions for future research," *Current Medical Research and Opinion*, vol. 33, no. 6, pp. 981–984, 2017.

[5] S. B. Park, D. Goldstein, A. V. Krishnan et al., "Chemotherapy-induced peripheral neurotoxicity: a critical analysis," *CA: A Cancer Journal for Clinicians*, vol. 63, no. 6, pp. 419–437, 2013.

[6] M. Ewertz, C. Qvortrup, and L. Eckhoff, "Chemotherapy-induced peripheral neuropathy in patients treated with taxanes and platinum derivatives," *Acta Oncologica*, vol. 54, no. 5, pp. 587–591, 2015.

[7] W. Grisold, G. Cavaletti, and A. J. Windebank, "Peripheral neuropathies from chemotherapeutics and targeted agents: diagnosis, treatment, and prevention," *Neuro-Oncology*, vol. 14, no. 4, p. iv45, 2012.

[8] A. A. Argyriou, A. P. Kyritsis, T. Makatsoris, and H. Kalofonos, "Chemotherapy-induced peripheral neuropathy in adults: a comprehensive update of the literature," *Cancer Management and Research*, vol. 6, pp. 135–147, 2014.

[9] N. C. Miltenburg and W. Boogerd, "Chemotherapy-induced neuropathy: a comprehensive survey," *Cancer Treatment Reviews*, vol. 40, no. 7, pp. 872–882, 2014.

[10] M. de Carvalho Barbosa, A. K. Kosturakis, C. Eng et al., "A quantitative sensory analysis of peripheral neuropathy in colorectal cancer and its exacerbation by oxaliplatin chemotherapy," *Cancer Research*, vol. 74, no. 21, pp. 5955–5962, 2014.

[11] K. Yin, K. Zimmermann, I. Vetter, and R. J. Lewis, "Therapeutic opportunities for targeting cold pain pathways," *Biochemical Pharmacology*, vol. 93, no. 2, pp. 125–140, 2015.

[12] H. Starobova and I. Vetter, "Pathophysiology of chemotherapy-induced peripheral neuropathy," *Frontiers in Molecular Neuroscience*, vol. 10, p. 174, 2017.

[13] Food and Drug Administration, *Guidance for Industry: Estimating the Maximum Safe Starting Dose in Initial Clinical Trials for Therapeutics in Adult Healthy Volunteers*, US Department of Health and Human Services, Food and Drug Administration, Center for Drug Evaluation and Research (CDER), Rockville, MD, USA, 2005.

[14] L. M. Alejandro, C. E. Behrendt, K. Chen, H. Openshaw, and S. Shibata, "Predicting acute and persistent neuropathy associated with oxaliplatin," *American Journal of Clinical Oncology*, vol. 36, no. 4, pp. 331–337, 2013.

[15] G. D. Leonard, M. A. Wright, M. G. Quinn et al., "Survey of oxaliplatin-associated neurotoxicity using an interview-based questionnaire in patients with metastatic colorectal cancer," *BMC Cancer*, vol. 5, no. 1, p. 116, 2005.

[16] N. Attal, D. Bouhassira, M. Gautron et al., "Thermal hyperalgesia as a marker of oxaliplatin neurotoxicity: a prospective quantified sensory assessment study," *Pain*, vol. 144, no. 3, pp. 245–252, 2009.

[17] R. Baron, G. Haendler, and H. Schulte, "Afferent large fiber polyneuropathy predicts the development of postherpetic neuralgia," *Pain*, vol. 73, no. 2, pp. 231–238, 1997.

[18] A. E. Golshani, A. A. Kamdar, S. C. Spence, and N. Beckmann, "Congenital indifference to pain: an illustrated case report and literature review," *Journal of Radiology Case Reports*, vol. 8, no. 8, pp. 16–23, 2014.

[19] N. J. Spencer, V. Zagorodnyuk, S. J. Brookes, and T. Hibberd, "Spinal afferent nerve endings in visceral organs: recent advances," *American Journal of Physiology Gastrointestinal and Liver Physiology*, vol. 311, no. 6, pp. G1056–G1063, 2016.

[20] M. J. Millan, "The induction of pain: an integrative review," *Progress in Neurobiology*, vol. 57, no. 1, pp. 1–164, 1999.

[21] A. I. Basbaum and T. N. Jessell, "Pain," in *Principles of Neural Science*, E. R. Kandel, Ed., pp. 530–553, McGraw Hill, New York, NY, USA, 5th edition, 2013.

[22] C. Lu, T. Yang, H. Zhao et al., "Insular cortex is critical for the perception, modulation, and chronification of pain," *Neuroscience Bulletin*, vol. 32, no. 2, pp. 191–201, 2016.

[23] C. E. Wilcox, A. R. Mayer, T. M. Teshiba et al., "The subjective experience of pain: an FMRI study of percept-related models and functional connectivity," *Pain Medicine*, vol. 16, no. 11, pp. 2121–2133, 2015.

[24] M. G. Liu and J. Chen, "Roles of the hippocampal formation in pain information processing," *Neuroscience Bulletin*, vol. 25, no. 5, pp. 237–266, 2009.

[25] A. S. Jaggi and N. Singh, "Mechanisms in cancer-chemotherapeutic drugs-induced peripheral neuropathy," *Toxicology*, vol. 291, no. 1–3, pp. 1–9, 2012.

[26] N. Authier, D. Balayssac, F. Marchand et al., "Animal models of chemotherapy-evoked painful peripheral neuropathies," *Neurotherapeutics*, vol. 6, no. 4, pp. 620–629, 2009.

[27] J. M. Verdier, I. Acquatella, C. Lautier et al., "Lessons from the analysis of nonhuman primates for understanding human aging and neurodegenerative diseases," *Frontiers in Neuroscience*, vol. 9, p. 64, 2015.

[28] J. Chen, D. Kang, J. Xu et al., "Species differences and molecular determinant of TRPA1 cold sensitivity," *Nature Communications*, vol. 4, p. 2501, 2013.

[29] C. Han, M. Estacion, J. Huang et al., "Human Na(v)1.8: enhanced persistent and ramp currents contribute to distinct firing properties of human DRG neurons," *Journal of Neurophysiology*, vol. 113, no. 9, pp. 3172–3185, 2015.

[30] J. P. Capitanio and M. E. Emborg, "Contributions of nonhuman primates to neuroscience research," *The Lancet*, vol. 371, no. 9618, pp. 1126–1135, 2008.

[31] L. Teo, J. V. Rosenfeld, and J. A. Bourne, "Models of CNS injury in the nonhuman primate: a new era for treatment strategies," *Translational Neuroscience*, vol. 3, no. 2, pp. 181–195, 2012.

[32] G. Courtine, M. B. Bunge, J. W. Fawcett et al., "Can experiments in nonhuman primates expedite the translation of treatments for spinal cord injury in humans?," *Nature Medicine*, vol. 13, no. 5, pp. 561–566, 2007.

[33] A. Hama and H. Takamatsu, "Chemotherapy-induced peripheral neuropathic pain and rodent models," *CNS and Neurological Disorders Drug Targets*, vol. 15, no. 1, pp. 7–19, 2016.

[34] K. D. Davis, Z. H. Kiss, R. R. Tasker, and J. O. Dostrovsky, "Thalamic stimulation-evoked sensations in chronic pain patients and in nonpain (movement disorder) patients," *Journal of Neurophysiology*, vol. 75, no. 3, pp. 1026–1037, 1996.

[35] J. L. Parker, D. M. Karantonis, P. S. Single, M. Obradovic, and M. J. Cousins, "Compound action potentials recorded in the human spinal cord during neurostimulation for pain relief," *Pain*, vol. 153, no. 3, pp. 593–601, 2012.

[36] S. Falci, L. Best, R. Bayles, D. Lammertse, and C. Starnes, "Dorsal root entry zone microcoagulation for spinal cord injury-related central pain: operative intramedullary electrophysiological guidance and clinical outcome," *Journal of Neurosurgery*, vol. 97, no. 2, pp. 193–200, 2002.

[37] J. Upadhyay, J. Anderson, A. J. Schwarz et al., "Imaging drugs with and without clinical analgesic efficacy," *Neuropsychopharmacology*, vol. 36, no. 13, pp. 2659–2673, 2011.

[38] S. M. Smith, R. H. Dworkin, D. C. Turk et al., "The potential role of sensory testing, skin biopsy, and functional brain imaging as biomarkers in chronic pain clinical trials: IMMPACT considerations," *Journal of Pain*, vol. 18, no. 7, pp. 757–777, 2017.

[39] M. C. Reddan and T. D. Wager, "Modeling pain using fMRI: from regions to biomarkers," *Neuroscience Bulletin*, vol. 34, no. 1, pp. 208–215, 2018.

[40] U. Friebel, S. B. Eickhoff, and M. Lotze, "Coordinate-based meta-analysis of experimentally induced and chronic persistent neuropathic pain," *Neuroimage*, vol. 58, no. 4, pp. 1070–1080, 2011.

[41] E. G. Boland, D. Selvarajah, M. Hunter et al., "Central pain processing in chronic chemotherapy-induced peripheral neuropathy: a functional magnetic resonance imaging study," *PLoS One*, vol. 9, no. 5, article e96474, 2014.

[42] K. Nagasaka, K. Yamanaka, S. Ogawa, H. Takamatsu, and N. Higo, "Brain activity changes in a macaque model of oxaliplatin-induced neuropathic cold hypersensitivity," *Scientific Reports*, vol. 7, no. 1, p. 4305, 2017.

[43] Y. Shidahara, S. Ogawa, M. Nakamura et al., "Pharmacological comparison of a nonhuman primate and a rat model of oxaliplatin-induced neuropathic cold hypersensitivity," *Pharmacology Research and Perspectives*, vol. 4, no. 1, p. e00216, 2016.

[44] B. Ling, F. Coudore, L. Decalonne, A. Eschalier, and N. Authier, "Comparative antiallodynic activity of morphine, pregabalin and lidocaine in a rat model of neuropathic pain produced by one oxaliplatin injection," *Neuropharmacology*, vol. 55, no. 5, pp. 724–728, 2008.

[45] M. Zhao, S. Nakamura, T. Miyake et al., "Pharmacological characterization of standard analgesics on oxaliplatin-induced acute cold hypersensitivity in mice," *Journal of Pharmacological Sciences*, vol. 124, no. 4, pp. 514–517, 2014.

[46] E. M. Smith, H. Pang, C. Cirrincione et al., "Effect of duloxetine on pain, function, and quality of life among patients with chemotherapy-induced painful peripheral neuropathy: a randomized clinical trial," *Journal of the American Medical Association*, vol. 309, no. 13, pp. 1359–1367, 2013.

[47] D. C. de Andrade, M. Jacobsen Teixeira, R. Galhardoni et al., "Pregabalin for the prevention of oxaliplatin-induced painful

neuropathy: a randomized, double-blind trial," *Oncologist*, vol. 22, no. 10, pp. 1154–e1105, 2017.

[48] E. Peltz, F. Seifert, R. DeCol, A. Dörfler, S. Schwab, and C. Maihöfner, "Functional connectivity of the human insular cortex during noxious and innocuous thermal stimulation," *Neuroimage*, vol. 54, no. 2, pp. 1324–1335, 2011.

[49] L. M. Chen, "Cortical representation of pain and touch: evidence from combined functional neuroimaging and electrophysiology in non-human primates," *Neuroscience Bulletin*, vol. 34, no. 1, pp. 165–177, 2018.

[50] V. Wanigasekera, K. Wartolowska, J. P. Huggins et al., "Disambiguating pharmacological mechanisms from placebo in neuropathic pain using functional neuroimaging," *British Journal of Anaesthesia*, vol. 120, no. 2, pp. 299–307, 2018.

[51] F. Seifert and C. Maihofner, "Central mechanisms of experimental and chronic neuropathic pain: findings from functional imaging studies," *Cellular and Molecular Life Sciences*, vol. 66, no. 3, pp. 375–390, 2009.

[52] R. Peyron, "Functional brain imaging: what has it brought to our understanding of neuropathic pain? A special focus on allodynic pain mechanisms," *Pain*, vol. 157, no. 1, pp. S67–S71, 2016.

[53] T. Natsume, S. Ogawa, Y. Awaga et al., "Brain activation in a nonhuman primate model of oxaliplatin-induced peripheral neuropathy: suppression with duloxetine," in *Proceedings of the 11th Annual Pain and Migraine Therapeutics Summit*, Arrowhead Publishers, San Diego, CA, USA, October 2017.

[54] D. L. Hershman, C. Lacchetti, R. H. Dworkin et al., "Prevention and management of chemotherapy-induced peripheral neuropathy in survivors of adult cancers: American Society of Clinical Oncology clinical practice guideline," *Journal of Clinical Oncology*, vol. 32, no. 18, pp. 1941–1967, 2014.

[55] N. Majithia, S. M. Temkin, K. J. Ruddy, A. S. Beutler, D. L. Hershman, and C. L. Loprinzi, "National Cancer Institute-supported chemotherapy-induced peripheral neuropathy trials: outcomes and lessons," *Supportive Care in Cancer*, vol. 24, no. 3, pp. 1439–1447, 2016.

[56] S. S. Jacobs, E. Fox, C. Dennie et al., "Plasma and cerebrospinal fluid pharmacokinetics of intravenous oxaliplatin, cisplatin, and carboplatin in nonhuman primates," *Clinical Cancer Research*, vol. 11, no. 4, pp. 1669–1674, 2005.

[57] A. Canta, E. Pozzi, and V. A. Carozzi, "Mitochondrial dysfunction in chemotherapy-induced peripheral neuropathy (CIPN)," *Toxics*, vol. 3, no. 2, pp. 198–223, 2015.

[58] N. Kerckhove, A. Collin, S. Conde, C. Chaleteix, D. Pezet, and D. Balayssac, "Long-term effects, pathophysiological mechanisms, and risk factors of chemotherapy-induced peripheral neuropathies: a comprehensive literature review," *Frontiers in Pharmacology*, vol. 8, p. 86, 2017.

[59] L. E. Ta, L. Espeset, J. Podratz, and A. J. Windebank, "Neurotoxicity of oxaliplatin and cisplatin for dorsal root ganglion neurons correlates with platinum-DNA binding," *Neurotoxicology*, vol. 27, no. 6, pp. 992–1002, 2006.

[60] M. J. McKeage, T. Hsu, D. Screnci et al., "Nucleolar damage correlates with neurotoxicity induced by different platinum drugs," *British Journal of Cancer*, vol. 85, no. 8, pp. 1219–1225, 2001.

[61] H. Zheng, W. H. Xiao, and G. J. Bennett, "Functional deficits in peripheral nerve mitochondria in rats with paclitaxel- and oxaliplatin-evoked painful peripheral neuropathy," *Experimental Neurology*, vol. 232, no. 2, pp. 154–161, 2011.

[62] W. H. Xiao, H. Zheng, and G. J. Bennett, "Characterization of oxaliplatin-induced chronic painful peripheral neuropathy in

[63] U. Anand, W. R. Otto, and P. Anand, "Sensitization of capsaicin and icilin responses in oxaliplatin treated adult rat DRG neurons," *Molecular Pain*, vol. 6, p. 82, 2010.

[64] M. A. Graham, G. F. Lockwood, D. Greenslade et al., "Clinical pharmacokinetics of oxaliplatin: a critical review," *Clinical Cancer Research*, vol. 6, pp. 1205–1218, 2000.

[65] S. Toyama, N. Shimoyama, Y. Ishida, T. Koyasu, H. H. Szeto, and M. Shimoyama, "Characterization of acute and chronic neuropathies induced by oxaliplatin in mice and differential effects of a novel mitochondria-targeted antioxidant on the neuropathies," *Anesthesiology*, vol. 120, no. 2, pp. 459–473, 2014.

[66] G. Cavaletti, G. Tredici, M. G. Petruccioli et al., "Effects of different schedules of oxaliplatin treatment on the peripheral nervous system of the rat," *European Journal of Cancer*, vol. 37, no. 18, pp. 2457–2463, 2001.

[67] L. Apostolidis, D. Schwarz, A. Xia et al., "Dorsal root ganglia hypertrophy as in vivo correlate of oxaliplatin-induced polyneuropathy," *PLoS One*, vol. 12, no. 8, article e0183845, 2017.

[68] M. A. Geyer and A. Markou, "Animal models of psychiatric disorders," in *Psychopharmacology: The Fourth Generation of Progress*, F. E. Bloom and D. J. Kupfer, Eds., pp. 787–798, Raven Press, New York, NY, USA, 1995.

[69] E. K. Joseph, X. Chen, O. Bogen, and J. D. Levine, "Oxaliplatin acts on IB4-positive nociceptors to induce an oxidative stress-dependent acute painful peripheral neuropathy," *Journal of Pain*, vol. 9, no. 5, pp. 463–472, 2008.

[70] J. R. Deuis, Y. L. Lim, S. Rodrigues de Sousa et al., "Analgesic effects of clinically used compounds in novel mouse models of polyneuropathy induced by oxaliplatin and cisplatin," *Neuro-Oncology*, vol. 16, no. 10, pp. 1324–1332, 2014.

[71] H. Adelsberger, S. Quasthoff, J. Grosskreutz, A. Lepier, F. Eckel, and C. Lersch, "The chemotherapeutic oxaliplatin alters voltage-gated Na(+) channel kinetics on rat sensory neurons," *European Journal of Pharmacology*, vol. 406, no. 1, pp. 25–32, 2000.

[72] C. P. Taylor and L. S. Narasimhan, "Sodium channels and therapy of central nervous system diseases," *Advances in Pharmacology*, vol. 39, pp. 47–98, 1997.

[73] R. G. Webster, K. L. Brain, R. H. Wilson, J. L. Grem, and A. Vincent, "Oxaliplatin induces hyperexcitability at motor and autonomic neuromuscular junctions through effects on voltage-gated sodium channels," *British Journal of Pharmacology*, vol. 146, no. 7, pp. 1027–1039, 2005.

[74] R. H. Wilson, T. Lehky, R. R. Thomas et al., "Acute oxaliplatin-induced peripheral nerve hyperexcitability," *Journal of Clinical Oncology*, vol. 20, no. 16, pp. 1767–1774, 2002.

[75] B. Ling, N. Authier, D. Balayssac et al., "Behavioral and pharmacological description of oxaliplatin-induced painful neuropathy in rat," *Pain*, vol. 128, no. 3, pp. 225–234, 2007.

[76] C. Lersch, R. Schmelz, F. Eckel et al., "Prevention of oxaliplatin-induced peripheral sensory neuropathy by carbamazepine in patients with advanced colorectal cancer," *Clinical Colorectal Cancer*, vol. 2, no. 1, pp. 54–58, 2002.

[77] S. von Delius, F. Eckel, S. Wagenpfeil et al., "Carbamazepine for prevention of oxaliplatin-related neurotoxicity in patients with advanced colorectal cancer: final results of a randomised, controlled, multicenter phase II study," *Investigational New Drugs*, vol. 25, no. 2, pp. 173–180, 2007.

[78] T. J. Lehky, G. D. Leonard, R. H. Wilson, J. L. Grem, and M. K. Floeter, "Oxaliplatin-induced neurotoxicity: acute

Gaps in Understanding Mechanism and Lack of Treatments: Potential Use of a Nonhuman Primate...

11

hyperexcitability and chronic neuropathy," *Muscle and Nerve*, vol. 29, no. 3, pp. 387–392, 2004.

[79] S. A. S. van den Heuvel, S. E. I. van der Wal, L. A. Smedes et al., "Intravenous lidocaine: old-school drug, new purpose-reduction of intractable pain in patients with chemotherapy induced peripheral neuropathy," *Pain Research and Management*, vol. 2017, Article ID 8053474, 9 pages, 2017.

[80] R. Baron, M. Allegri, G. Correa-Illanes et al., "The 5% lidocaine-medicated plaster: its inclusion in international treatment guidelines for treating localized neuropathic pain, and clinical evidence supporting its use," *Pain Therapeutics*, vol. 5, no. 2, pp. 149–169, 2016.

[81] N. A. Hagen, L. Cantin, J. Constant et al., "Tetrodotoxin for moderate to severe cancer-related pain: a multicentre, randomized, double-blind, placebo-controlled, parallel-design trial," *Pain Research and Management*, vol. 2017, Article ID 7212713, 7 pages, 2017.

[82] J. M. Chung and K. Chung, "Sodium channels and neuropathic pain," in *Pathological Pain: From Molecular to Clinical Aspects*, D. J. Chadwick and J. Goode, Eds., vol. 261, pp. 19–27, John Wiley & Sons, Chichester, UK, 2004.

[83] M. Naziroglu and N. Braidy, "Thermo-sensitive TRP channels: novel targets for treating chemotherapy-induced peripheral pain," *Frontiers in Physiology*, vol. 8, p. 1040, 2017.

[84] W. M. Knowlton, R. L. Daniels, R. Palkar, D. D. McCoy, and D. D. McKemy, "Pharmacological blockade of TRPM8 ion channels alters cold and cold pain responses in mice," *PLoS One*, vol. 6, no. 9, article e25894, 2011.

[85] T. Nakagawa and S. Kaneko, "Roles of transient receptor potential ankyrin 1 in oxaliplatin-induced peripheral neuropathy," *Biological and Pharmaceutical Bulletin*, vol. 40, no. 7, pp. 947–953, 2017.

[86] A. Dhopeshwarkar and K. Mackie, "CB2 Cannabinoid receptors as a therapeutic target-what does the future hold?," *Molecular Pharmacology*, vol. 86, no. 4, pp. 430–437, 2014.

[87] P. G. Blanchard and V. Luu-The, "Differential androgen and estrogen substrates specificity in the mouse and primates type 12 17beta-hydroxysteroid dehydrogenase," *Journal of Endocrinology*, vol. 194, no. 2, pp. 449–455, 2007.

[88] S. Ogawa, Y. Awaga, M. Takashima, A. Hama, A. Matsuda, and H. Takamatsu, "Antinociceptive effect of clinical analgesics in a nonhuman primate model of knee osteoarthritis," *European Journal of Pharmacology*, vol. 786, pp. 179–185, 2016.

[89] S. Ogawa, Y. Awaga, M. Takashima, A. Hama, A. Matsuda, and H. Takamatsu, "Knee osteoarthritis pain following medial meniscectomy in the nonhuman primate," *Osteoarthritis and Cartilage*, vol. 24, no. 7, pp. 1190–1199, 2016.

[90] J. Chen and D. H. Hackos, "TRPA1 as a drug target-promise and challenges," *Naunyn-Schmiedeberg's Archives of Pharmacology*, vol. 388, no. 4, pp. 451–463, 2015.

[91] W. J. Winchester, K. Gore, S. Glatt et al., "Inhibition of TRPM8 channels reduces pain in the cold pressor test in humans," *Journal of Pharmacology and Experimental Therapeutics*, vol. 351, no. 2, pp. 259–269, 2014.

[92] A. D. Weyer and S. G. Lehto, "Development of TRPM8 antagonists to treat chronic pain and migraine," *Pharmaceuticals*, vol. 10, no. 4, p. 37, 2017.

[93] H. Ohshiro, A. Fujiuchi, A. Yamada et al., "In vitro and in vivo characterization of RQ-00434739, a novel orally active and selective trpm8 antagonist for the treatment of oxaliplatin-induced peripheral neuropathic pain," in *Proceedings of the 16th World Congress on Pain*, Yokohama, Japan, September 2016.

[94] M. Sakurai, N. Egashira, T. Kawashiri, T. Yano, H. Ikesue, and R. Oishi, "Oxaliplatin-induced neuropathy in the rat: involvement of oxalate in cold hyperalgesia but not mechanical allodynia," *Pain*, vol. 147, no. 1, pp. 165–174, 2009.

[95] D. J. Storey, L. A. Colvin, M. J. Mackean et al., "Reversal of dose-limiting carboplatin-induced peripheral neuropathy with TRPM8 activator, menthol, enables further effective chemotherapy delivery," *Journal of Pain and Symptom Management*, vol. 39, no. 6, pp. e2–e4, 2010.

[96] C. H. Wong, K. W. Siah, and A. W. Lo, "Estimation of clinical trial success rates and related parameters," *Biostatistics*, 2018, In press.

# An Interdisciplinary Pain Rehabilitation Program for Veterans with Chronic Pain: Description and Initial Evaluation of Outcomes

Nidhi S. Anamkath ⓘ,[1,2] Sarah A. Palyo,[1,2] Sara C. Jacobs,[1,2] Alain Lartigue,[1,2] Kathryn Schopmeyer,[1] and Irina A. Strigo ⓘ[1,2]

[1]*Department of Veterans Affairs, San Francisco VA Healthcare System, 4150 Clement Street, San Francisco, CA, USA*
[2]*University of California, San Francisco, CA, USA*

Correspondence should be addressed to Irina A. Strigo; irina.strigo@ucsf.edu

Academic Editor: Anna Maria Aloisi

*Objective*. Chronic pain conditions are prominent among Veterans. To leverage the biopsychosocial model of pain and comprehensively serve Veterans with chronic pain, the San Francisco Veterans Affairs Healthcare System has implemented the interdisciplinary pain rehabilitation program (IPRP). This study aims to (1) understand initial changes in treatment outcomes following IPRP, (2) investigate relationships between psychological factors and pain outcomes, and (3) explore whether changes in psychological factors predict changes in pain outcomes. *Methods*. A retrospective study evaluated relationships between clinical pain outcomes (pain intensity, pain disability, and opioid use) and psychological factors (depressive symptoms, catastrophizing, and "acceptable" level of pain) and changes in these outcomes following treatment. Multiple regression analysis explored whether changes in psychological variables significantly predicted changes in pain disability. *Results*. Catastrophizing and depressive symptoms were positively related to pain disability, while "acceptable" level of pain was idiosyncratically related to pain intensity. Pain disability and psychological variables showed significant changes in their expected directions. Regression analysis indicated that only changes in depressive symptoms significantly predicted changes in pain disability. *Conclusion*. Our results are consistent with evidence-based clinical practice guidelines for the management of chronic pain in Veterans. Further investigation of interdisciplinary treatment programs in Veterans is warranted.

## 1. Introduction

Chronic pain is a highly prevalent condition estimated to affect over 50% of Veterans who receive care through the Veterans Health Administration (VHA) [1, 2]. In addition, an investigation by Nahin [3] found that Veterans not only have high rates of pain but also generally report more pain than non-Veterans and have increased rates of severe pain. There is a large body of evidence showing that pain is associated with a plethora of deleterious consequences, including affective distress, long-term opioid use, greater utilization of healthcare services, and significant financial distress for patients and society [1, 4, 5]. More concerning is that the incidence of persistent pain in Veterans seems to be growing and standalone treatments, such as medication, physical therapy, or Cognitive-Behavioral Therapy may not be adequate for all patients [2, 5, 6]. To this end, the VHA has implemented a National Pain Management Strategy calling for integrated treatment to specifically improve pain management for Veterans nationwide [7, 8].

Pain is a multifaceted experience affected by genetic and biological vulnerabilities, as well as by psychosocial factors [9]. Thus, treatments that use a biopsychosocial model in the treatment of chronic pain have been recommended and have demonstrated good clinical outcomes [9–12]. Specifically, integrated biopsychosocial treatments are designed to facilitate functional restoration by addressing not only physiological processes of pain but also the cognitive appraisals and emotional reactions which may exacerbate the pain experience [13, 14]. One such psychological process known to affect the pain experience is pain catastrophizing, which is a multidimensional construct reflecting a collection of negative cognitions one has about experienced or anticipated pain [15]. Pain catastrophizing has shown to be a robust predictor of pain-related outcomes such as analgesic use and disability [15, 16]. Likewise, depression is another important psychological process, which has a dramatic negative effect on the pain experience [13, 17, 18]. A review of the comorbidity between depression and pain by Bair et al. [19] indicates that those with depression experience more intense pain for longer periods of time. Additionally, experimental investigations repeatedly show that individuals with depression have increased emotional reactivity to experimentally induced pain compared to never depressed controls [13, 17]. These results reinforce abnormal emotional processing in response to pain in those with depression, which therefore may exacerbate the pain experience for these individuals [20]. Of note, although often positively correlated, depression and catastrophizing have been shown to uniquely contribute to the pain experience, and thus, these two psychosocial facets should be examined separately [21–23]. Finally, one's perceived "acceptable" level of pain may also contribute to the pain experience. Clinically, "acceptable" level of pain is often assessed as a means of understanding patients' expectations for their pain care. Expectations regarding pain treatment and outcomes may drive motivations, adherence, and coping behaviors, thereby affecting overall treatment outcomes [24–26]. As such, it is crucial to understand how changes in one's expectation for what is an "acceptable level of pain" affect clinical pain outcomes.

The evidenced interplay between physiological, emotional, and cognitive aspects of pain warrants that these various components be addressed through treatment. Thus, the VHA has implemented interdisciplinary pain rehabilitation programs informed by the biopsychosocial model of pain to better address these different aspects of Veterans' pain experience [8]. Within the San Francisco Veterans Affairs Healthcare System (SFVAHCS), one such program, the Intensive Pain Rehabilitation Program (IPRP), was implemented in 2012 to address the increasing pain rehabilitation needs of Veterans. IPRP consists of several treatment components including the following: Acceptance and Commitment Therapy, Cognitive-Behavioral Therapy, physical therapy, pain education, and pharmacy counseling. One goal of the program has been to specifically address cognitive and emotional factors that may impact clinical pain outcomes such as pain intensity, pain-related disability, and current opioid medication use in Veterans with chronic, noncancer pain. Prior meta-analyses, which included studies mostly examining non-Veterans populations, have shown psychological interventions to be successful in reducing pain intensity, physical disability, and pain behaviors in individuals with chronic, musculoskeletal, noncancer pain [27, 28]. Several factors, such as decreased cognitive distortions and increased psychological flexibility, have been identified as potential mechanisms by which these treatment

changes occur [29, 30]. However, there is a dearth of literature examining the relationship between cognitive and emotional psychological factors and clinical pain outcomes, particularly in Veterans receiving the highest, or "tertiary," level of integrated pain rehabilitation. Such a treatment may be best suited to address the complex nature of the pain experience, especially in the veteran population, which has been shown to report more pain than the non-Veterans population [3]. Thus, to expand upon the current literature conducted primarily in the non-Veterans population, further investigation of treatment outcomes specifically in Veterans who attend an integrated pain rehabilitation program, such as IPRP, is warranted.

The present observational study had three goals. The first was to examine the relationship between clinical pain outcomes (pain intensity, pain-related disability, and opioid medication use) and cognitive and emotional psychological factors (subjective "acceptable" pain level, pain catastrophizing, and depressive symptoms) in Veterans undergoing a 12-week intensive interdisciplinary treatment at both baseline and follow-up. The second goal was to examine whether there were statistically significant changes in clinical pain outcomes, as well as in cognitive and emotional variables following treatment. The third goal was to explore changes in which psychological factors best predicted changes in clinical pain outcomes. An evolving understanding of the relationships between these factors in a veteran sample undergoing such integrated rehabilitation may further inform treatment development, assessments, and protocols.

## 2. Methods

Study procedures were approved by the SFVAHCS and University of California San Francisco Institutional Review Boards. Patient data were gathered from the Intensive Pain Rehabilitation Program (IPRP), which is an intensive and interdisciplinary treatment program designed for patients receiving care through the SFVAHCS who suffer from functionally impairing chronic, noncancer pain conditions. Inclusion in the program requires a referral from a clinician within the Veterans Affairs Healthcare System and an IPRP team-based evaluation to determine an individual's fit for the program. The patients in this sample attended the program three half-days a week for twelve weeks and were provided with education and self-management skills to facilitate practice at home. Skills were designed to help patients meet functional goals. All patients received the following components as part of the program: physical therapy (PT), CBT, Acceptance and Commitment Therapy (ACT), pain education (PEd), and pharmacy counseling (PharmC). PT included instructions on gentle movements, novel movement strategies, and self-applied massage techniques designed to increase body awareness, recover ease of movement, and re-engage in daily physical activities without causing a significant increase in pain. CBT focused on introduction of skills such as activity pacing, activity scheduling, relaxation training, and cognitive restructuring. Distraction was de-emphasized to be consistent with ACT, which focuses on participants developing mindfulness skills, being present-focused, and engaging in valued activities. PEd provided participants with education about chronic pain, including neurophysiology and neuroplasticity concepts, as well as healthy lifestyle choices as they relate to living with chronic pain. PharmC included education about the balancing risk and benefits of pain medications through group classes and individualized counseling with optimization of pain medication regimens when appropriate. Of note, opioid use reduction was not an explicit treatment goal of IPRP; however, IPRP supported the reduction of opioid medication as a patient-initiated goal or if a provider identified safety concerns.

As part of their clinical care, patients completed pre- and posttreatment measures. Data for this study were retrospectively examined from the clinical data collected by the program. Of the 55 patients who enrolled in the 3-day/week IPRP program between December 2012 and May 2015, individuals were excluded from data analysis if (1) they dropped out, (2) they completed the program but had not completed posttreatment questionnaires, (3) more than 15% of a questionnaire was missing either pre- or posttreatment (4) they were not Veterans, or (5) they were re-enrolled in the program (only the first enrollment was included in analyses to control for repetition effects). The final sample included 35 participants.

## 2.1. Measures

### 2.1.1. Demographic and Clinical Data.
Patients self-reported clinical and demographic information both pre- and posttreatment. Information included age, sex, race, years of education completed, duration of pain, and identified pain sites. Additionally, average or "usual" pain intensity (during the past week) and "acceptable" pain level were reported using a numeric rating scale (0–10). Of note, "acceptable" level of pain refers to an anticipated pain score with which a patient would be comfortable rather than acceptance of their pain condition. Here, it is a measure of patients' expectations regarding treatment.

### 2.1.2. Pain Disability.
The Pain Disability Questionnaire (PDQ) [31] is a 15-item measure of pain-related disability. Each item is rated from 0 to 10 with higher scores indicating greater pain-related disability. The measure is divided into two subscales. The first is the functional status component which reflects general functioning; the second is the psychosocial component. Scores on the PDQ are broken down to categorize pain disability as mild/moderate (0–70), severe (71–100), or extreme (101–150) [32].

### 2.1.3. Pain Catastrophizing.
The Pain Catastrophizing Scale (PCS) [15] is a 13-item self-report measure comprising three subscales used to assess an individual's negative cognitions (rumination, magnification, and hopelessness) about actual or anticipated pain. Items are rated using a 5-point Likert scale (0 = not at all and 4 = all the time). The PCS is a widely used measure of pain cognitions amongst a variety of chronic pain populations and has been shown to have good internal consistency [15, 33].

### 2.1.4. Depression.
The Patient Health Questionnaire (PHQ9) [34] is a nine-item self-report measure of depressive symptoms. Questions correspond to diagnostic criteria from the *Diagnostic and Statistical Manual of Mental Disorders*, 4th edition. Each item is rated from 0 to 3 (0 = not at all and 3 = nearly every day). Scores are broken down into five categories: minimal depression (0–4); mild depression (5–9); moderate depression (10–14); moderately severe depression (15–19); and severe depression (20–27). The questionnaire has been shown to be reliable and has good sensitivity and specificity [34, 35].

### 2.1.5. Pharmacy Data.
A pharmacist collected information on the number and type of medications that patients were taking specifically for their pain. Medication types included opioids, antidepressants, anticonvulsants, muscle relaxants, nonsteroidal anti-inflammatory drugs (NSAIDS), topical agents, and a category for other miscellaneous pain relievers. In addition, morphine daily equivalent doses (MEDD) were calculated for each patient as a measure of opioid medication use.

### 2.1.6. Treatment Satisfaction.
Five questions from the Pain Outcomes Questionnaire [36] which reflect treatment satisfaction (TxSat) were asked posttreatment. Each question asks participants to rate their satisfaction of the care they received on a scale from 0 to 10 (0 = no satisfaction and 10 = complete satisfaction). The questions ask patients to rate their satisfaction with the overall treatment, staff (personality and competence), and treatment schedule, as well as whether they would recommend the treatment. Rating of individual components of the program was not administered to this cohort but is being implemented currently.

### 2.2. Data Analysis.
All statistical analyses were performed using IBM SPSS Statistics Version 24 (IBM, Chicago, IL). Parametric tests were used for all analyses. Demographic information and descriptive statistics for all outcome measures have been provided. Pretreatment correlations and posttreatment Pearson's correlations were investigated amongst variables (usual pain, acceptable pain, PDQ, PCS, PHQ9, MEDD, and TxSat). To assess differences in pre- and posttreatment scores for outcome variables, paired $t$-tests were performed. For all analyses, $p < 0.05$ was considered significant.

Lastly, due to the interdisciplinary nature of the IPRP which aimed to improve cognitive and emotional symptoms associated with chronic pain, we wanted to explore changes in what emotional and cognitive symptoms best predicted changes in pain outcomes in our study. Hence, a multiple linear regression model was conducted for pre-post changes in pain-related disability as a pain outcome and acceptable level of pain, PHQ9, and PCS as psychosocial predictors.

TABLE 1: Veteran sample characteristics ($n = 35$).

| | Pretreatment | Posttreatment |
|---|---|---|
| Demographic | | |
| Mean age in years (SD) | 56.2 (7.9) | — |
| Male sex, $n$ (%) | 25 (71%) | — |
| Caucasian race, $n$ (%) | 22 (62.9%) | — |
| Mean pain duration (SD), $n = 33^{\#}$ | 18.70 (13.20) | |
| Mean number of pain sites (SD) | 7.89 (4.40) | 6.94 (4.26) |
| Reported pain sites, $f$ (%) | | |
| Leg | 26 (74.29%) | 26 (74.29%) |
| Low back | 32 (91.43%) | 30 (85.71%) |
| Mid-back | 22 (62.86%) | 18 (51.43%) |
| Upper back | 17 (48.57%) | 12 (34.29%) |
| Head | 12 (34.29%) | 9 (25.71%) |
| Neck | 25 (71.43%) | 20 (57.14%) |
| Shoulder | 19 (54.29%) | 20 (57.14%) |
| Buttocks | 19 (54.29%) | 12 (34.29%) |
| Foot | 15 (42.86%) | 16 (45.71%) |
| Jaw | 10 (28.57%) | 7 (20.00%) |
| Chest | 6 (17.14%) | 3 (8.57%) |
| Abdomen | 7 (20.00%) | 4 (11.43%) |
| Arm/hand | 17 (48.57%) | 13 (37.14%) |
| Fingers | 14 (40.00%) | 10 (28.57%) |
| Toes | 12 (34.29%) | 7 (20.00%) |
| Face | 4 (11.43%) | 2 (5.71%) |
| Genitals | 6 (17.14%) | 5 (14.29%) |
| Others | 8 (22.86%) | 8 (22.86%) |
| Medications, $f$ (%) | | |
| Opioids | 26 (74.29%) | 25 (71.43%) |
| Antidepressants | 16 (45.71%) | 18 (51.43%) |
| Anticonvulsants | 17 (48.57%) | 17 (48.57%) |
| Muscle relaxants | 14 (40.00%) | 16 (45.71%) |
| NSAID | 13 (37.14%) | 15 (42.86%) |
| Topical agents | 20 (57.14%) | 22 (62.86%) |
| Others | 8 (22.86%) | 8 (22.86%) |
| Clinical pain outcomes, mean (SD) | | |
| Usual pain$^{\&}$ | 6.40 (1.94) | 5.76 (1.69), $n = 34^{\#}$ |
| PDQ | 103.14 (23.01) | 87.77 (24.40) |
| MEDD | 69.68 (100.88), $n = 34^{\#}$ | 62.32 (91.90), $n = 34^{\#}$ |
| Psychological outcomes, mean (SD) | | |
| PHQ9 | 14.29 (6.23), $n = 34^{\#}$ | 9.89 (5.50) |
| PCS | 23.78 (12.21), $n = 32^{\#}$ | 13.85 (8.46), $n = 33^{\#}$ |
| Acceptable pain$^{\&}$ | 2.63 (1.50), $n = 32^{\#}$ | 3.76 (1.50), $n = 34^{\#}$ |
| Others | | |
| Treatment satisfaction | — | 46.06 (5.99) |

SD = standard deviation; NSAID = nonsteroidal anti-inflammatory drugs; PHQ9 = Patient Health Questionnaire; PCS = Pain Catastrophizing Scale; PDQ = Pain Disability Questionnaire; MEDD = morphine equivalent daily dose; $^{\&}$numeric rating scale from 0 (no pain) to 10 (worst pain imaginable). $^{\#}$The number of patients is lower than the total number of patients ($n = 35$).

Associations among individual demographic factors (age and sex) and outcomes were tested before running each regression to identify potential covariates. These predictors were chosen based on the components of the program that are meant to target cognitive and emotional symptoms of chronic pain.

## 3. Results

*3.1. Veteran Sample Characteristics.* Individuals in this sample were primarily male (71%) and Caucasian (62.9%). The mean age was 56.2 years (SD = 7.9). Means and standard deviations for pre- and posttreatment variables are

presented in Table 1. As can be seen in Table 1, on average, patients' self-reported scores at baseline (or pretreatment self-reported scores) indicated moderate depression and extreme disability. Average pain duration (in years) and number of pain sites reported were 18.7 (SD = 13.2) and 7.9 (SD = 4.4), respectively. Table 1 also depicts sample characteristics for medication use, which showed that majority of these patients were receiving opioids.

*3.2. Bivariate Associations.* Pre- and posttreatment bivariate correlations are depicted in Tables 2 and 3, respectively. Usual pain was significantly correlated with the acceptable

Table 2: Pretreatment correlations.

| Variable | 1 | 2 | 3 | 4 | 5 | 6 |
|---|---|---|---|---|---|---|
| (1) Usual pain$^\&$ | — | 0.39* | 0.20 | 0.08 | 0.39* | −0.08 |
| (2) Acceptable pain$^\&$ | | — | 0.03 | −0.07 | 0.26 | −0.08 |
| (3) PHQ | | | — | 0.54** | 0.64** | 0.15 |
| (4) PCS | | | | — | 0.51** | 0.10 |
| (5) PDQ | | | | | — | 0.25 |
| (6) MEDD | | | | | | — |

PHQ9 = Patient Health Questionnaire; PCS = Pain Catastrophizing Scale; PDQ = Pain Disability Questionnaire; MEDD = morphine equivalent daily dose; $^\&$numeric rating scale from 0 (no pain) to 10 (worst pain imaginable); *correlation is significant at the 0.05 level (2-tailed); **correlation is significant at the 0.01 level (2-tailed).

Table 3: Posttreatment correlations.

| Variable | 1 | 2 | 3 | 4 | 5 | 6 |
|---|---|---|---|---|---|---|
| (1) Usual pain$^\&$ | — | 0.34 | 0.21 | 0.29 | 0.36* | −0.17 |
| (2) Acceptable pain$^\&$ | | — | −0.18 | −0.14 | 0.01 | 0.05 |
| (3) PHQ | | | — | 0.45** | 0.50** | 0.31 |
| (4) PCS | | | | — | 0.34 | −0.08 |
| (5) PDQ | | | | | — | 0.20 |
| (6) MEDD | | | | | | — |

PHQ9 = Patient Health Questionnaire; PCS = Pain Catastrophizing Scale; PDQ = Pain Disability Questionnaire; MEDD = morphine equivalent daily dose; $^\&$numeric rating scale from 0 (no pain) to 10 (worst pain imaginable); *correlation is significant at the 0.05 level (2-tailed); **correlation is significant at the 0.01 level (2-tailed).

Table 4: Examination of changes in pre- and posttreatment measures.

| | $t$ | df | Significance (2-tailed) |
|---|---|---|---|
| Usual pain$^\&$ | 1.77 | 33 | 0.09 |
| Acceptable pain$^\&$ | −4.87* | 31 | 0.00 |
| PHQ9 | 4.47* | 33 | 0.00 |
| PCS | 4.75* | 29 | 0.00 |
| PDQ | 4.38* | 34 | 0.00 |
| MEDD | 1.88 | 33 | 0.07 |

PHQ9 = Patient Health Questionnaire; PCS = Pain Catastrophizing Scale; PDQ = Pain Disability Questionnaire; MEDD = morphine equivalent daily dose; $^\&$numeric rating scale from 0 (no pain) to 10 (worst pain imaginable); *correlation is significant at the 0.05 level (2-tailed).

level of pain only at baseline ($r = 0.39$, $p < 0.05$) but not with PCS or PHQ at neither pre- nor posttreatment. PDQ was significantly correlated with PHQ ($r = 0.64$, $p < 0.01$) and PCS ($r = 0.51$, $p < 0.01$) but was not significantly related to the acceptable level pain. Posttreatment correlations between PDQ and PCS remained positive, but only the relationship to PDQ and PHQ remained significant ($r = 0.50$, $p < 0.01$). MEDD did not significantly relate to any of the psychological outcomes both pre- and posttreatment in our sample.

*3.3. Comparison of Pre- and Posttreatment Outcomes.* Paired *t*-tests for pre- and posttreatment values from completed self-report measures are presented in Table 4. Results indicate significant decreases in all variable scores except for "acceptable pain levels," which significantly increased, as

Table 5: Linear regression analysis predicting pre-post PDQ.

| | Coefficients | $t$ | Significance |
|---|---|---|---|
| ΔPHQ9 | 0.45 | 2.90 | 0.00 |
| ΔAcceptable pain$^\&$ | −0.03 | −0.21 | 0.84 |
| ΔPCS | 0.18 | 1.11 | 0.28 |

[a]Standardized coefficients are shown; stepwise linear regression models with changes in pain disability (PDQ) as dependent variables and three pre-post predicting factors: depression (PHQ9), acceptable level of pain, and pain catastrophizing (PCS); PHQ9 = Patient Health Questionnaire; PCS = Pain Catastrophizing Scale; PDQ = Pain Disability Questionnaire; $^\&$numeric rating scale from 0 (no pain) to 10 (worst pain imaginable).

expected. Conversely, no significant changes were observed for pain intensity (usual pain) or for daily morphine equivalent dose (although tendencies were noted).

*3.4. Exploratory Regression Analyses.* The results of exploratory stepwise linear regression analysis with changes in pain disability (PDQ) as a dependent variable and changes in three predicting factors (depression, acceptable level of pain, and catastrophizing) are shown in Table 5. Improved pain disability scores (PDQ) were significantly predicted by improvements in depression scores, whereby changes in PHQ9 explained most of the changes in pain-related disability; adding acceptable levels of pain and/or catastrophizing did not improve the model.

## 4. Discussion

The present study retrospectively examines a sample of Veterans enrolled in interdisciplinary pain rehabilitation with the goal of exploring (1) the relationships between cognitive and emotional psychological variables and clinical pain outcomes, (2) changes in these psychological variables and outcomes following interdisciplinary treatment, and (3) whether changes in psychological variables predict changes in clinical pain outcomes. Expanding upon the existing literature, which has primarily evaluated interdisciplinary pain rehabilitation in the non-Veterans population, our findings indicate distinct relationships between pain-related clinical outcomes and the assessed psychological processes. Additionally, we found that the 12-week interdisciplinary pain rehabilitation program shows promise in improving pain-related psychological factors and pain-related disability in a mixed sample of extremely disabled, moderately depressed Veterans with severe chronic pain in multiple body sites. Lowering depressive symptoms may predict improvements in disability, and given the limited non-pharmacological options available to Veterans with such disability, these promising findings merit further examination.

We found several associations between clinical pain outcomes (i.e., self-reported pain intensity, pain-related disability, and opioid medication use) and the evaluated psychological measures, suggesting that pain-related clinical outcomes may be differentially influenced by the underlying cognitions and emotion. Specifically, pain intensity was significantly and positively associated with subjective acceptable pain level but not with pain catastrophizing or depressive symptom severity at both pre- and posttreatment. In contrast, pretreatment pain-related disability was positively related to depressive symptoms severity and pain catastrophizing but not with subjective acceptable level of pain. Such idiosyncratic relationships between the pain-related clinical outcomes and psychological features may have important implications for treatment planning based on a patient's specific goals. As an example, IPRP may choose to focus on functional restoration for a patient and use behavioral interventions (i.e., CBT and/or ACT) to target depressive symptom severity and pain catastrophizing, as these psychological processes were distinctly related to pain-related disability and therefore have the potential to impact pain-related debilitation if reduced. Targeting underlying processes that may affect the pain experience has indeed become a topic of interest in the literature [37], and further consideration of these distinctive relationships between pain outcomes and psychological processes has the potential to optimize treatment recommendations.

A comparison of pre- and posttreatment scores demonstrates that the administered intensive and interdisciplinary treatment significantly lessened negative cognitions and emotions associated with chronic pain, as well as subjects' perceived disability level, but had less effect on self-reported pain intensity and opioid use. Regarding the lack of improvement in pain intensity, this suggests that decreases in disability were not necessarily a function of decreases in pain intensity and is consistent with the extant literature and with the VHA National Pain Strategy [8], which calls for improvements in both physical and psychosocial functioning. Although decreases in pain intensity following interdisciplinary rehabilitation often occur, such reductions may not be necessary for improvements in functioning [38, 39]. This directly supports the foundational theory of the Acceptance and Commitment Therapy (ACT) treatment model, which hypothesizes that one's orientation to a distressing experience can be altered without an alteration in the distressing experience itself [29, 40]. Also, in line with the ACT model, decreases of negative psychological states, for example, depression and pain catastrophizing, may facilitate increases in behavioral flexibility. Increases in behavioral flexibility allow patients to re-engage in life activities reflecting personal values and thus decrease disability. Although behavioral flexibility was not measured in this initial sample of Veterans undergoing IPRP, it is plausible that our integrative treatment that improved depression and pain catastrophizing may have decreased disability by giving patients the option to engage in more value-based behaviors which they may have been avoiding previously [41, 42]. The significant impact that depression and catastrophizing may have on decreasing disability further supports the idea that decreases in pain intensity may not be needed for functional improvement.

Likewise, we found that opioid medication use did not show significant decrease although reduction tendencies were noted. Given the current state of the opioid epidemic [43, 44] and its relevance to the veteran population in particular [45–47], this observation warrants particular attention. Given that opioid dose reduction was not an explicit treatment goal of IPRP, lack of significant decrease in opioid medication use is not surprising. While there is evidence that similar interdisciplinary programs may be effective in reducing opioid intake, these programs often focus on opioid use reduction as part of their treatment or mandate cessation of opioids altogether [48, 49]. However, our findings are consistent with the existing literature [50] suggesting that decreases in opioid use may not be related to decreases in pain-related disability and/or improvements in psychological outcomes. This finding is promising as many patients who refuse to reduce opioid intake for fear of worsening of their pain symptoms may still be able to make functional gains. If such functional gains are made, patients may be more willing to initiate changes in their opioid use with the help of their treatment providers. Importantly, future follow-up investigations should examine whether participants require more time after treatment has completed to solidify newly acquired functional gains that would support greater reductions in opioids use.

Finally, exploratory regression analyses indicated that only changes in depressive symptoms severity significantly predicted changes in pain-related disability in the current sample. While other studies also found that changes in catastrophizing may also be predictive of improvements in pain disability, which we did not observe, our results lend further support to the strong relationship between depression and pain-related disability which has been noted in the existing literature [21, 51–53]. In line with the present finding, investigations have repeatedly found that depressive symptoms in patients with chronic pain are associated with increased levels of disability [19, 54]. Additionally, a longitudinal investigation of a non-Veterans sample by Scott et al. [53] found that reductions in depression significantly predicted both decreases in disability days and decreased likelihood of severe disability. Contrary to our findings, Scott et al. [53] found that levels of pain catastrophizing also predicted decreased levels of high disability and disability days, although the effect size was moderate compared to the effects of depression in their study. Thus, focusing on lowering depressive symptoms through value-based actions, cognitive restructuring, and other psychological techniques may be critical in increasing functional improvements in veteran population. Yet another study showed that that catastrophizing had a larger role in predicting disability levels than depression [21]. Although the findings regarding whether depression or catastrophizing is more important for pain-related disability are mixed, the literature is consistent in indicating that both psychological factors play an important role. Thus, future investigations of catastrophizing in a larger sample of Veterans in interdisciplinary treatment may indeed predict changes in disability.

Several limitations of the present study should be noted. Firstly, the current sample was restricted to those patients who had minimal missing data (<10%), which limited the research and associated conclusions in the following ways: (a) possible introduction of selection bias, (b) limited sample size, and (c) lack of posttreatment follow-up data. Such limitations indeed impact the generalizability of our findings, and further research with a larger and more inclusive sample is needed. Thus, our initial findings should be interpreted with caution, particularly regarding the non-significant reduction in average reported pain intensity. We are currently collecting data in a larger sample of Veterans and at multiple assessment time points. Additionally, a future examination with a larger and less restrictive sample would also allow for a more fine-grained analysis of the outcome variables and identification of potential mechanisms of change. Furthermore, all data collected were self-reported, and results are subject to possible over- and underreporting. Future examinations should include additional objective measures of functioning, such as physical therapy outcomes. Despite these limitations, these initial results are promising and clearly demonstrate the need for further evaluations in our veteran population. Specifically, due to apparent lack of comparative efficacy trials for nonpharmacological pain treatment options available to our Veterans, the investigation of the efficacy of such a program via a randomized controlled trial is desperately needed.

## 5. Conclusion

Chronic pain is a major concern among Veterans, leading to immense suffering and disability. Interdisciplinary treatment of chronic pain has been recommended by the VHA, and appraisal of such a nonpharmacological treatment in this specific population is needed. Preliminary evaluation of such a treatment program shows intensive and interdisciplinary pain rehabilitation to be a promising treatment for Veterans with chronic pain. Patients overall exhibited positive gains in cognitions and emotions related to their pain experience, as well as improved functioning. These improvements among this sample are promising and are a call to action to conduct efficacy trials going forward.

## Disclosure

The views expressed in this article are those of the authors and do not necessarily represent the position or policy of the Department of Veterans Affairs.

## Acknowledgments

This work was supported in part by I01-CX-000816 (IAS) from the United States Department of Veterans Affairs Clinical Sciences Research and Development Service. The authors thank the University of California San Francisco Open Access Publishing Fund for the support.

## References

[1] R. D. Kerns, E. J. Philip, A. W. Lee, and P. H. Rosenberger, "Implementation of the veterans health administration national pain management strategy," *Translational Behavioral Medicine*, vol. 1, no. 4, pp. 635–643, 2011.

[2] J. L. Goulet, R. D. Kerns, M. Bair et al., "The musculoskeletal diagnosis cohort: examining pain and pain care among veterans," *Pain*, vol. 157, no. 8, pp. 1696–1703, 2016.

[3] R. L. Nahin, "Severe pain in veterans: the effect of age and sex, and comparisons with the general population," *Journal of Pain*, vol. 18, no. 3, pp. 247–254, 2017.

[4] S. H. Snook and B. S. Webster, "The cost of disability," *Clinical Orthopaedics and Related Research*, vol. 221, pp. 77–84, 1987.

[5] K. Seal, W. Becker, J. Tighe, Y. Li, and T. Rife, "Managing chronic pain in primary care: it really does take a village," *Journal of General Internal Medicine*, vol. 32, no. 8, pp. 931–934, 2017.

[6] H. Flor, T. Fydrich, and D. C. Turk, "Efficacy of multidisciplinary pain treatment centers: a meta-analytic review," *Pain*, vol. 49, no. 2, pp. 221–230, 1992.

[7] Interagency Pain Research Coordinating Committee, *National Pain Strategy: A Comprehensive Population Health-Level Strategy for Pain*, Department of Health and Human Services, Washington, DC, USA, 2015.

[8] Department of Veterans Affairs, *Pain Management (VHA Directive 2009-053)*, Veterans Health Administration, Department of Veterans Affairs, Washington, DC, USA, 2009.

[9] R. J. Gatchel, Y. B. Peng, M. L. Peters, P. N. Fuchs, and D. C. Turk, "The biopsychosocial approach to chronic pain: scientific advances and future directions," *Psychological Bulletin*, vol. 133, no. 4, p. 581, 2007.

[10] R. J. Gatchel, D. D. McGeary, C. A. McGeary, and B. Lippe, "Interdisciplinary chronic pain management: past, present, and future," *American Psychologist*, vol. 69, no. 2, p. 119, 2014.

[11] R. J. Gatchel and A. Okifuji, "Evidence-based scientific data documenting the treatment and cost-effectiveness of comprehensive pain programs for chronic nonmalignant pain," *Journal of Pain*, vol. 7, no. 11, pp. 779–793, 2006.

[12] S. H. Sanders, R. N. Harden, and P. J. Vicente, "Evidence-based clinical practice guidelines for interdisciplinary rehabilitation of chronic nonmalignant pain syndrome patients," *Pain Practice*, vol. 5, no. 4, pp. 303–315, 2005.

[13] I. A. Strigo, A. N. Simmons, and S. C. Matthews, "Increased affective bias revealed using experimental graded heat stimuli in young depressed adults: evidence of "emotional allodynia"," *Psychosomatic Medicine*, vol. 70, no. 3, p. 338, 2008.

[14] C. Villemure and C. M. Bushnell, "Cognitive modulation of pain: how do attention and emotion influence pain processing?," *Pain*, vol. 95, no. 3, pp. 195–199, 2002.

[15] M. J. Sullivan, *The Pain Catastrophizing Scale: User Manual*, McGill University, Montreal, Canada, 2009.

[16] M. J. Sullivan, M. E. Lynch, A. J. Clark, T. Mankovsky, and J. Sawynok, "Catastrophizing and treatment outcome: differential impact on response to placebo and active treatment outcome," *Contemporary Hypnosis*, vol. 25, no. 3-4, pp. 129–140, 2008.

[17] A. Ushinsky, L. E. Reinhardt, A. N. Simmons, and I. A. Strigo, "Further evidence of emotional allodynia in unmedicated young adults with major depressive disorder," *PLoS One*, vol. 8, no. 11, article e80507, 2013.

[18] K. J. Bär, S. Brehm, M. K. Boettger, S. Boettger, G. Wagner, and H. Sauer, "Pain perception in major depression depends on pain modality," *Pain*, vol. 117, no. 1-2, pp. 97–103, 2005.

[19] M. J. Bair, R. L. Robinson, W. Katon, and K. Kroenke, "Depression and pain comorbidity: a literature review," *Archives of Internal Medicine*, vol. 163, no. 20, pp. 2433–2445, 2003.

[20] M. L. Loggia, J. S. Mogil, and M. C. Bushnell, "Experimentally induced mood changes preferentially affect pain unpleasantness," *Journal of Pain*, vol. 9, no. 9, pp. 784–791, 2008.

[21] B. A. Arnow, C. M. Blasey, M. J. Constantino et al., "Catastrophizing, depression and pain-related disability," *General Hospital Psychiatry*, vol. 33, no. 2, pp. 150–156, 2011.

[22] R. R. Edwards, R. H. Dworkin, M. D. Sullivan, D. C. Turk, and A. D. Wasan, "The role of psychosocial processes in the development and maintenance of chronic pain," *Journal of Pain*, vol. 17, no. 9, pp. T70–T92, 2016.

[23] R. R. Edwards, C. Cahalan, G. Mensing, M. Smith, and J. A. Haythornthwaite, "Pain, catastrophizing, and depression in the rheumatic diseases," *Nature Reviews Rheumatology*, vol. 7, no. 4, pp. 216–224, 2011.

[24] S. J. Linton and W. S. Shaw, "Impact of psychological factors in the experience of pain," *Physical Therapy*, vol. 91, no. 5, pp. 700–711, 2011.

[25] C. J. Main, N. Foster, and R. Buchbinder, "How important are back pain beliefs and expectations for satisfactory recovery from back pain?," *Best Practice & Research Clinical Rheumatology*, vol. 24, no. 2, pp. 205–217, 2010.

[26] J. E. Bialosky, M. D. Bishop, and J. A. Cleland, "Individual expectation: an overlooked, but pertinent, factor in the treatment of individuals experiencing musculoskeletal pain," *Physical Therapy*, vol. 90, no. 9, pp. 1345–1355, 2016.

[27] S. Morley, C. Eccleston, and A. Williams, "Systematic review and meta-analysis of randomized controlled trials of cognitive behaviour therapy and behaviour therapy for chronic pain in adults, excluding headache," *Pain*, vol. 80, no. 1, pp. 1–3, 1999.

[28] B. M. Hoffman, R. K. Papas, D. K. Chatkoff, and R. D. Kerns, "Meta-analysis of psychological interventions for chronic low back pain," *Health Psychology*, vol. 26, no. 1, p. 1, 2007.

[29] L. Dindo, J. R. Van Liew, and J. J. Arch, "Acceptance and commitment therapy: a transdiagnostic behavioral intervention for mental health and medical conditions," *Neurotherapeutics*, vol. 14, no. 3, pp. 546–553, 2017.

[30] K. E. Vowles, L. M. McCracken, and J. Z. O'Brien, "Acceptance and values-based action in chronic pain: a three-year follow-up analysis of treatment effectiveness and process," *Behaviour Research and Therapy*, vol. 49, no. 11, pp. 748–755, 2011.

[31] C. Anagnostis, R. J. Gatchel, and T. G. Mayer, "The pain disability questionnaire: a new psychometrically sound measure for chronic musculoskeletal disorders," *Spine*, vol. 29, no. 20, pp. 2290–2302, 2004.

[32] R. J. Gatchel, T. G. Mayer, and B. R. Theodore, "The pain disability questionnaire: relationship to one-year functional and psychosocial rehabilitation outcomes," *Journal of Occupational Rehabilitation*, vol. 16, no. 1, pp. 72–91, 2006.

[33] A. Osman, F. X. Barrios, P. M. Gutierrez, B. A. Kopper, T. Merrifield, and L. Grittmann, "The pain catastrophizing scale: further psychometric evaluation with adult samples," *Journal of Behavioral Medicine*, vol. 23, no. 4, pp. 351–365, 2000.

[34] K. Kroenke, R. L. Spitzer, and J. B. Williams, "The PHQ-9: validity of a brief depression severity measure," *Journal of General Internal Medicine*, vol. 16, pp. 606–613, 2001.

[35] A. Martin, W. Rief, A. Klaiberg, and E. Braehler, "Validity of the brief patient health questionnaire mood scale (PHQ-9) in the general population," *General Hospital Psychiatry*, vol. 28, no. 1, pp. 71–77, 2006.

[36] M. E. Clark, R. J. Gironda, and R. W. Young, "Development and validation of the pain outcomes questionnaire-VA,"

[37] K. E. Weiss, A. Hahn, D. P. Wallace, B. Biggs, B. K. Bruce, and T. E. Harrison, "Acceptance of pain: associations with depression, catastrophizing, and functional disability among children and adolescents in an interdisciplinary chronic pain rehabilitation program," *Journal of Pediatric Psychology*, vol. 38, no. 7, pp. 756–765, 2013.

[38] K. E. Vowles, K. Witkiewitz, J. Levell, G. Sowden, and J. Ashworth, "Are reductions in pain intensity and pain-related distress necessary? An analysis of within-treatment change trajectories in relation to improved functioning following interdisciplinary acceptance and commitment therapy for adults with chronic pain," *Journal of Consulting and Clinical Psychology*, vol. 85, no. 2, p. 87, 2017.

[39] J. C. Ballantyne and M. D. Sullivan, "Intensity of chronic pain—the wrong metric?," *New England Journal of Medicine*, vol. 373, no. 22, pp. 2098-2099, 2015.

[40] J. D. Herbert, "Acceptance and Commitment Therapy: An Experiential Approach to Behavior Change," S. C. Hayes, K. D. Strosahl, and K. G. Wilson, Eds., Guilford Press, New York, NY, USA, 1999.

[41] R. K. Wicksell and K. E. Vowles, "The role and function of acceptance and commitment therapy and behavioral flexibility in pain management," *Pain Management*, vol. 5, no. 5, pp. 319–322, 2015.

[42] M. D. Sullivan and K. E. Vowles, "Patient action: as means and end for chronic pain care," *Pain*, vol. 158, no. 8, pp. 1405–1407, 2017.

[43] L. Laxmaiah, S. Helm, B. Fellows et al., "Opioid epidemic in the United States," *Pain Physician*, vol. 15, pp. 2150–1149, 2012.

[44] L. S. Nelson, D. N. Juurlink, and J. Perrone, "Addressing the opioid epidemic," *JAMA*, vol. 314, no. 14, pp. 1453-1454, 2015.

[45] J. L. Clarke, A. Skoufalos, and R. Scranton, "The American opioid epidemic: population health implications and potential solutions. Report from the National Stakeholder Panel," *Population Health Management*, vol. 19, no. S1, pp. S-1–S-10, 2016.

[46] A. S. Bohnert, M. A. Ilgen, J. A. Trafton et al., "Trends and regional variation in opioid overdose mortality among Veterans Health Administration patients, fiscal year 2001 to 2009," *Clinical Journal of Pain*, vol. 30, no. 7, pp. 605–612, 2014.

[47] K. H. Seal, Y. Shi, G. Cohen et al., "Association of mental health disorders with prescription opioids and high-risk opioid use in US veterans of Iraq and Afghanistan," *JAMA*, vol. 307, no. 9, pp. 940–947, 2012.

[48] J. W. Frank, T. I. Lovejoy, W. C. Becker et al., "Patient outcomes in dose reduction or discontinuation of long-term opioid therapy: a systematic review," *Annals of Internal Medicine*, vol. 167, no. 3, pp. 181–191, 2017.

[49] J. L. Murphy, K. M. Phillips, and S. Rafie, "Sex differences between Veterans participating in interdisciplinary chronic pain rehabilitation," *Journal of Rehabilitation Research & Development*, vol. 53, no. 1, pp. 83–94, 2016.

[50] J. E. MacLaren, R. T. Gross, J. A. Sperry, and J. T. Boggess, "Impact of opioid use on outcomes of functional restoration," *Clinical Journal of Pain*, vol. 22, no. 4, pp. 392–398, 2006.

[51] M. Ericsson, W. S. C. Poston, J. Linder, J. E. Taylor, C. K. Haddock, and J. P. Foreyt, "Depression predicts disability in long-term chronic pain patients," *Disability and Rehabilitation*, vol. 24, no. 6, pp. 334–340, 2002.

[52] M. N. Raftery, K. Sarma, A. W. Murphy, D. De la Harpe, C. Normand, and B. E. McGuire, "Chronic pain in the Republic of Ireland—community prevalence, psychosocial profile and predictors of pain-related disability: results from the Prevalence, Impact and Cost of Chronic Pain (PRIME) study, part 1," *Pain*, vol. 152, no. 5, pp. 1096–1103, 2011.

[53] E. L. Scott, K. Kroenke, J. Wu, and Z. Yu, "Beneficial effects of improvement in depression, pain catastrophizing, and anxiety on pain outcomes: a 12-month longitudinal analysis," *Journal of Pain*, vol. 17, no. 2, pp. 215–222, 2016.

[54] C. E. Dionne, T. D. Koepsell, M. Von Korff, R. A. Deyo, W. E. Barlow, and H. Checkoway, "Predicting long-term functional limitations among back pain patients in primary care settings," *Journal of Clinical Epidemiology*, vol. 50, no. 1, pp. 31–43, 1997.

# 3

# Patient and Physician Satisfaction with Analgesic Treatment: Findings from the Analgesic Treatment for Cancer Pain in Southeast Asia (ACE) Study

**Dang Huy Quoc Thinh,**[1] **Wimonrat Sriraj,**[2] **Marzida Mansor,**[3] **Kian Hian Tan,**[4]
**Cosphiadi Irawan,**[5] **Johan Kurnianda,**[6] **Yen Phi Nguyen,**[7] **Annielyn Ong-Cornel,**[8]
**Yacine Hadjiat ⓘ,**[9] **Hanlim Moon ⓘ,**[9] **and Francis O. Javier ⓘ**[10]

[1]*Department of Radiation Oncology, HCMC Oncology Hospital, Ho Chi Minh City, Vietnam*
[2]*Department of Anesthesiology, Faculty of Medicine, Srinagarind Hospital, Khon Kaen University, Khon Kaen, Thailand*
[3]*Department of Anesthesiology, Faculty of Medicine, University of Malaya, Kuala Lumpur, Malaysia*
[4]*Department of Anaesthesiology, Singapore General Hospital, Singapore*
[5]*Department of Internal Medicine, Cipto Mangunkusumo General Hospital (RSCM), University of Indonesia, Jakarta Pusat, Indonesia*
[6]*Department of Internal Medicine, Dr. Sardjito General Hospital, Gadjah Mada University, Yogyakarta, Indonesia*
[7]*Department of Palliative Care and Pain Management, K Hospital, Vietnam National Cancer Hospital, Hanoi, Vietnam*
[8]*Veterans Memorial Medical Centre, Quezon City, Philippines*
[9]*APAC LATAM MEA, Mundipharma, Singapore*
[10]*Pain Management Center, St. Luke's Medical Center, Quezon City, Philippines*

Correspondence should be addressed to Francis O. Javier; drfrancisjavier@yahoo.com

Academic Editor: José W. Geurts

*Aim.* The aim of this study was to examine patients' and physicians' satisfaction, and concordance of patient-physician satisfaction with patients' pain control status. *Methods.* This cross-sectional observational study involved 465 adults prescribed analgesics for cancer-related pain from 22 sites across Indonesia, Malaysia, Philippines, Singapore, Thailand, and Vietnam. Pain intensity, pain control satisfaction, and adequacy of analgesics for pain control were documented using questionnaires. *Results.* Most patients (84.4%) had stage III or IV cancer. On a scale of 0 (no pain) to 10 (worse pain), patients' mean worst pain intensity over 24 hours was 4.76 (SD 2.47). More physicians (19.0%) than patients (8.0%) reported dissatisfaction with patient's pain control. Concordance of patient-physician satisfaction was low (weighted kappa 0.36; 95% CI 0.03–0.24). Most physicians (71.2%) found analgesics to be adequate for pain control. Patients' and physicians' satisfaction with pain control and physician-assessed analgesic adequacy were significantly different across countries ($P < 0.001$ for all). *Conclusions.* Despite pain-related problems with sleep and quality of life, patients were generally satisfied with their pain control status. Interestingly, physicians were more likely to be dissatisfied with patients' pain control. Enhanced patient-physician communication, physicians' proactivity in managing opioid-induced adverse effects, and accessibility of analgesics have been identified to be crucial for successful cancer pain management. This study was registered at ClinicalTrials.gov (identifier NCT02664987).

## 1. Introduction

Pain associated with cancer is prevalent and negatively affects a patient's psychological and emotional states [1]. Approximately 70–80% of patients with advanced cancer experience moderate to severe pain [2]. The WHO "analgesic ladder" guidelines recommend treating pain in a stepwise approach, starting with nonopioids (step I), then, as necessary, weak opioids (step II), and finally strong opioids (step III) until the patient is free of pain [2, 3].

Patient satisfaction may be used as a key indicator of the effectiveness of cancer pain management in terms of analgesic treatment outcomes [4]. Previous studies have shown that higher patient satisfaction directly influences treatment adherence [5, 6]. Notably, patients' satisfaction levels with pain control vary considerably across different countries and regions. A study conducted across four Northern European countries (Denmark, Germany, Sweden, and United Kingdom) revealed that more than three-quarters (76%) of cancer patients were satisfied with opioid-induced pain relief despite 60% reporting severe pain [7]. In contrast, only 44% of Korean cancer patients with severe pain reported satisfaction with pain control [8].

Despite established cancer pain management guidelines and effective pain medications, a substantial number of patients with cancer pain in Southeast Asia (SEA) still remain inadequately treated for pain symptoms [2, 9]. Although many studies have evaluated patients' satisfaction with pain control status, very few studies have assessed physicians' satisfaction with patients' pain control status in parallel with that of their patients'. As patient-physician relationship also affects patient satisfaction with treatment [5], gaining insights into the alignment of patient-physician satisfaction will hopefully improve future treatment approaches. The objective of the Analgesic treatment for Cancer pain in SouthEast Asia (ACE) study was to provide real-world information on analgesic prescription patterns and patient-reported pain outcomes among cancer patients with pain in SEA. The aim of the current report was to examine patient and physician satisfaction with patient's pain control status in the ACE cohort, and concordance between the two. In addition, we sought to explore the variations in satisfaction with pain control as well as analgesic prescription doses between the 6 participating SEA countries.

## 2. Methods

*2.1. Study Design and Participants.* This was a multicenter, multinational, cross-sectional, observational study conducted between October 2015 and December 2015 at 22 sites in 6 SEA countries (Indonesia, Malaysia, the Philippines, Singapore, Thailand, and Vietnam). Eligible patients were recruited based on these criteria: at least 18 years old; diagnosed with cancer pathologically; outpatients with cancer pain due to cancer itself or its treatment; and treated with any analgesics for more than one month for the management of cancer pain. Patients were excluded from the study if they met any of the following criteria: had an operation for any reason within 3 months; had an oncologic emergency; had any interventional therapy (e.g., nerve block, and neurolytic procedures) related to cancer pain within the past 6 weeks; and current participation in any other interventional clinical trials for cancer treatment or supportive care. All patients provided written informed consent before study enrolment.

Study protocol, case report forms, and documents used for obtaining patients' informed consent were reviewed and approved by the local ethics committee at each study site. All study procedures were conducted in accordance with the Declaration of Helsinki and in compliance with local regulatory requirements.

*2.2. Study Assessments.* Patient demographics, cancer characteristics, treatment histories, and current analgesic prescriptions were obtained from medical records. Questionnaires were administered to patients for self-assessment of worst pain intensity over the past 24 hours (scored on a numeric rating scale (NRS), from 0 (no pain) to 10 (worst pain imaginable) [10, 11]), sleep disturbance due to cancer pain within the past 7 days, quality of life (assessed using the EuroQol Group 5-Dimension Self-Report Questionnaire 3 Level (EQ-5D-3L) system [12, 13]), and patients' satisfaction with pain control status (scored on a 5-point scale: very satisfied, satisfied, acceptable, dissatisfied, and very dissatisfied [14–16]). Attending physicians assessed their satisfaction with their patients' pain control status (scored on a 5-point scale: very satisfied, satisfied, acceptable, dissatisfied, and very dissatisfied) and adequacy of analgesics for pain control (adequate and not adequate).

*2.3. Statistical Analyses.* Of 465 patients recruited into the study, 462 patients met eligibility requirements and were included in the analyses. Patient demographics, cancer characteristics, treatment histories, pain intensities, EQ-5D-3L responses, satisfaction with pain control, and total daily dose of analgesics prescribed were summarized using descriptive statistics. Quantitative variables were summarized as mean (SD) whereas qualitative variables were expressed as number (percentage). Concordance of satisfaction with pain control between patient and physician was evaluated by weighted kappa statistics and McNemar test. $P$ values $< 0.05$ were considered statistically significant. All statistical analyses were performed using R version 3.1.3 (R Development Core Team, Vienna, Austria, 2015).

## 3. Results

*3.1. Patient Demographics and Characteristics.* A total of 465 patients from 6 SEA countries (81 from Indonesia, 100 from Malaysia, 105 from the Philippines, 8 from Singapore, 100 from Thailand, and 71 from Vietnam) were recruited into the study. Three patients did not fulfil eligibility criteria and were excluded from the analysis (two had an operation within three months and one was not treated with analgesics for more than one month), leaving 462 patients in the analysis population.

The analysis population consisted of 46.3% males and 53.7% females, and the mean age of patients was 55.14 (13.39) years. The majority of patients (84.4%) were diagnosed with stage III or IV cancer, and 93.1% had received surgery, radiotherapy, or chemotherapy (Table 1).

More than half of all patients (53.7%, $n = 248$) were prescribed a combination of nonopioid and opioid analgesics to manage their cancer pain. On the other hand, 37.0% ($n = 171$) received only opioid analgesics, while 9.3% ($n = 43$) received only nonopioid analgesics. Of those who received opioid analgesics ($n = 419$), more received at least

TABLE 1: Demographics and characteristics of the analysis population ($n = 462$).

| | |
|---|---|
| Age (years) | |
| Mean (SD) | 55.14 (13.39) |
| Age group, $n$ (%) | |
| 18–29 years | 17 (3.7) |
| 30–39 years | 54 (11.7) |
| 40–49 years | 74 (16.0) |
| 50–59 years | 139 (30.1) |
| 60–69 years | 113 (24.5) |
| 70–79 years | 53 (11.5) |
| 80+ years | 12 (2.6) |
| Gender, $n$ (%) | |
| Male | 214 (46.3) |
| Female | 248 (53.7) |
| Cancer stage, $n$ (%) | |
| 0 | 4 (0.9) |
| I | 11 (2.4) |
| II | 32 (6.9) |
| III | 79 (17.1) |
| IV | 311 (67.3) |
| Not available | 25 (5.4) |
| Metastasis, $n$ (%) | |
| Yes | 303 (65.6) |
| No | 144 (31.2) |
| Unknown | 15 (3.2) |
| Received surgery/radiotherapy/ chemotherapy, $n$ (%) | |
| Yes | 430 (93.1) |
| No | 32 (6.9) |
| Site of pain, $n$ (%)[†] | |
| Head | 48 (10.4) |
| Neck | 50 (10.8) |
| Chest | 103 (22.3) |
| Abdomen | 90 (19.5) |
| Upper back | 46 (10.0) |
| Lower back | 107 (23.2) |
| Joints | 56 (12.1) |
| Others | 125 (27.1) |
| Worst pain intensity over the past 24 hours | |
| Mean (SD) | 4.76 (2.47) |
| Median (min, max) | 5.00 (0.00, 10.00) |
| Sleep disturbance, $n$ (%) | |
| Yes | 253 (54.8) |
| No | 209 (45.2) |
| Quality of life assessed by EQ-5D-3L | |
| Mobility, $n$ (%) | |
| No problems | 193 (41.8) |
| Problems | 269 (58.2) |
| Self-care, $n$ (%) | |
| No problems | 281 (60.8) |
| Problems | 181 (39.2) |
| Usual activities, $n$ (%) | |
| No problems | 158 (34.2) |
| Problems | 304 (65.8) |
| Pain/discomfort, $n$ (%) | |
| No problems | 82 (17.7) |
| Problems | 380 (82.3) |
| Anxiety/depression, $n$ (%) | |
| No problems | 202 (43.7) |
| Problems | 260 (56.3) |

SD: standard deviation; [†]patients may experience more than one site of pain, percentages may not add up to 100%.

one strong opioid (57.8%) than weak opioids alone (42.2%). Morphine (42.0%, $n = 194$) and tramadol (40.9%, $n = 189$) were the most frequently prescribed strong and weak opioids, respectively.

*3.2. Pain Intensity, Quality of Life, and Sleep Disturbance.* Based on NRS scoring, mean worst pain intensity over the past 24 hours was 4.76 (2.47). Responses to the EQ-5D-3L questionnaire revealed that 82.3% of patients experienced problems with pain/discomfort, 65.8% with usual activities, 58.2% with mobility, 56.3% with anxiety/depression, and 39.2% with self-care (Table 1). More than half (54.8%) reported sleep disturbance due to pain in the past 7 days.

*3.3. Patient and Physician Satisfaction with Patients' Pain Control Status.* Patient and physician assessment of satisfaction with pain control are presented in Table 2. The majority of patients (60.2%) were either very satisfied (18.6%) or satisfied (41.6%) with their pain control status, while 30.3% found it to be acceptable. A small proportion, however, were dissatisfied (8.0%) or very dissatisfied (1.5%) with pain control. Patient satisfaction with pain control varied significantly across countries ($P < 0.001$); satisfaction was the highest in the Philippines and the lowest in Malaysia (Supplementary Table 1). More physicians (19.0%) than patients (8.0%) reported dissatisfaction with patients' pain control (Table 2). Physician satisfaction with pain control varied significantly across countries ($P < 0.001$); satisfaction was the highest in Singapore and the lowest in Indonesia (Supplementary Table 1).

Patients who were more satisfied with pain control appeared to have reported lower median pain intensity (very satisfied: median 3, interquartile range 2–5; satisfied: median 5, interquartile range 2–6) than those who were less satisfied with pain control (very dissatisfied: median 8, interquartile range 5.5–8.5; dissatisfied: median 7, interquartile range 6–8; Figure 1(a)). A similar trend was observed for physician satisfaction with patients' pain control (Figure 1(b)).

Overall, 71.2% of physicians described prescribed analgesics to be "adequate" while 28.8% described it to be "not adequate" for pain control. Physician assessment of analgesic adequacy for pain control varied significantly across countries ($P < 0.001$); adequacy was assessed to be the highest in Singapore and the lowest in Indonesia (Supplementary Table 2).

*3.4. Concordance of Patients' and Physicians' Satisfaction with Patients' Pain Control Status.* Concordance of patient-physician satisfaction with patients' pain control status is depicted in Figure 2. Satisfaction levels reported by patients and physicians were the same in 45.5% of cases; 19.2% of patients were less satisfied with their pain control compared with their physicians, whereas 35.2% of physicians were less satisfied with their patients' pain control than patients themselves (Figure 2). The disagreement between patients' and physicians' assessment of satisfaction with pain control was significant ($P < 0.001$, McNemar's test).

TABLE 2: Patient and physician assessment of satisfaction with pain control ($n = 462$). Data presented as $n$ (%).

|  | Patient | Physician |
| --- | --- | --- |
| Very satisfied | 86 (18.6%) | 56 (12.1%) |
| Satisfied | 192 (41.6%) | 194 (42.0%) |
| Acceptable | 140 (30.3%) | 117 (25.3%) |
| Dissatisfied | 37 (8.0%) | 88 (19.0%) |
| Very dissatisfied | 7 (1.5%) | 7 (1.5%) |

Evaluating overall concordance of satisfaction with pain control between physicians and patients, a weighted kappa of 0.36 (95% CI, 0.30 to 0.43) was obtained, suggesting low overall agreement on satisfaction with pain control. Concordance of patient-physician satisfaction based on weighted kappa appears to be highest in the Philippines and lowest in Indonesia (Supplementary Table 3).

*3.5. Doses of Analgesics Prescribed.* The median daily doses of prescribed strong and weak opioids, as well as nonopioids, are listed in Table 3. Median daily doses of prescribed opioids, fentanyl, morphine, and tramadol were 0.89 mg, 30.00 mg, and 150.00 mg, respectively. Prescribed median daily doses of opioids were highest in Vietnam and lowest in Indonesia (Supplementary Table 4). On the other hand, median daily doses of prescribed nonopioids, gabapentin, paracetamol, and pregabalin were 900.00 mg, 1300.00 mg, and 150.00 mg, respectively. Prescribed median doses of nonopioids were the highest in Singapore and the lowest in Indonesia (Supplementary Table 5).

## 4. Discussion

Levels of patient and physician satisfaction with analgesic treatment for pain management can be indicators of the effectiveness and appropriateness of current analgesic prescription practices. Using a cohort of SEA cancer patients undergoing analgesic treatment for cancer pain, the present analysis examined levels of patient and physician satisfaction with pain control and analysed the degree of patient-physician agreement with respect to pain control satisfaction. Our key findings were (i) most patients were satisfied with pain control despite unrelieved moderate pain, (ii) low concordance between patient- and physician-reported satisfaction with patients' pain control status, and (iii) physicians tended to be less satisfied with the level of pain control than their patients.

Interestingly, patient satisfaction with pain control was unexpectedly high (60.2%) in our cohort despite clear evidence of unrelieved moderate pain (mean worst pain intensity in the last 24 hours: 4.76 (SD 2.47)). This phenomenon was particularly perplexing given that the majority of patients also reported problems with pain/discomfort (82.3%) and sleep disturbance due to pain (54.8%). Notably, the coexistence of patient satisfaction with pain control and unrelieved moderate to high pain has been reported by others in the literature [16–18]. Some insight into the reasons for this high pain-high satisfaction paradox was provided through patient interviews

conducted by Beck et al.; patients conveyed that they expected some pain and believed that their pain cannot be completely relieved or that having unrelieved pain was a choice as they opted not to take their pain medication more frequently [18]. Importantly, cultural perceptions of cancer may also influence the individual's concept of cancer pain; compared to patients of other cultures, Asian patients were inclined to disregard pain [19] and to view their pain as retribution [20] or as an unavoidable consequence of cancer [21]. Others have suggested that the degree of satisfaction with analgesic treatment may be positively influenced by the patients' perception of having control over their pain [22], faster onset of pain relief following administration of pain medication [23], better communication with healthcare professionals [1, 5, 18, 24–26], and prompt management of side effects [18], even though pain continues to be unrelieved. An effective pain management plan coupled with proactive management of analgesic-induced adverse effects would thus be vital for patient satisfaction with analgesic treatment and pain control. Nevertheless, although patient satisfaction with analgesic treatment is a desired outcome, our findings taken together with several others [16–18] suggest that patient-reported satisfaction alone may not be indicative of the patient's pain control status. An all-round assessment of cancer pain and its associated effects (including patient-reported pain intensity, sleep disturbance due to pain, quality of life, and satisfaction with analgesic treatment) may perhaps provide more insight into the pain status of the cancer patient and contribute to better pain management.

A recent study found a discrepancy in reported cancer pain intensity between patients and physicians, suggesting that clinical assessments by patients and physicians may not always be aligned [27]. Indeed, we noted low concordance between patient- and physician-reported satisfaction with pain control in our cohort, with physicians more likely to be dissatisfied than their patients. The specific reasons for physician dissatisfaction with pain control in the present study were not explored. However, high patient loads and the resultant decline in individual patient-contact time may be a plausible source of physician dissatisfaction [28]. Especially in Asia, where shortage of pain management services is perceived to be a barrier to cancer pain management [16], medical consultations may often be too brief for pain specialists to provide quality patient care (e.g., detailed explanation of treatment options and adverse effects and attention to psychosocial aspects of patient complaints). In addition, a large-scale survey of physicians across Asia revealed that physicians generally agreed on the effectiveness of opioids, but excessive regulatory barriers to the use of opioids were identified as a problem by almost half of the physicians surveyed [16]. Based on physician's knowledge of unexplored analgesic options and their potential to effectively manage pain control, we speculate that regulatory barriers may be a contributory factor to physician dissatisfaction with pain control. Indeed, more than 1 in 4 physicians indicated that prescribed analgesics were inadequate for pain control in the present study. As physician satisfaction directly influences quality and delivery of care [29], more needs to be done to establish the sources of physician dissatisfaction with pain management and why they were

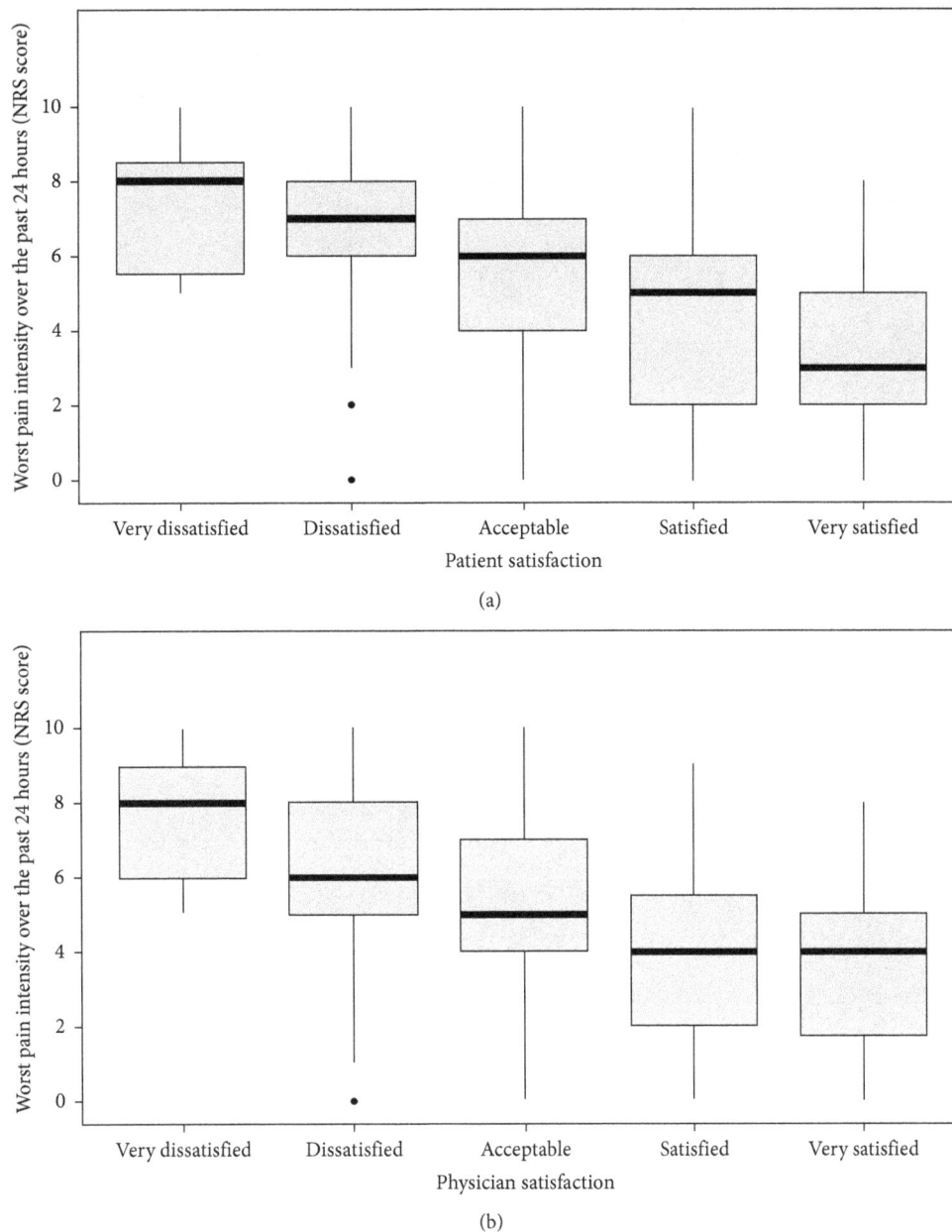

FIGURE 1: Box plots showing patients' worst pain intensity over the past 24 hours and (a) patients' and (b) physicians' satisfaction with patients' pain control. Horizontal line within the box plot indicates the median; boundaries of the box represent the 25th- and 75th-percentile; filled symbols denote outliers.

more likely to be dissatisfied with pain control than their patients.

The small proportion of patients who were less satisfied with their pain control compared to their physicians also contributed to the low patient-physician concordance in satisfaction observed in the present study. Patient-physician contact time is an underrated yet crucial determining factor for both patient satisfaction and physician satisfaction with cancer pain management [28]. Patients who spent less time with their physicians were likely to be less satisfied than their counterparts who had more contact time with the physician [28]. Lack of experience, awareness, and empathy towards cancer pain management on the physician's part could also

contribute to perceived poor pain control by patients [30, 31]. Patients may be educated on how to talk about pain with their physicians [32], or on their prescribed therapeutic interventions, such as course of treatment [33], dosage, and concerns about tolerance or addiction [34]. The goal of education would be to raise awareness about self-management of pain and to dispel misconceptions regarding analgesic treatment [35]. Ongoing education is also likely to keep physicians abreast of dynamic cancer pain management approaches [33, 36]. The low concordance between patient- and physician-reported satisfaction with pain control in our cohort highlights the need for improved patient-physician communication about analgesic treatment expectations, as

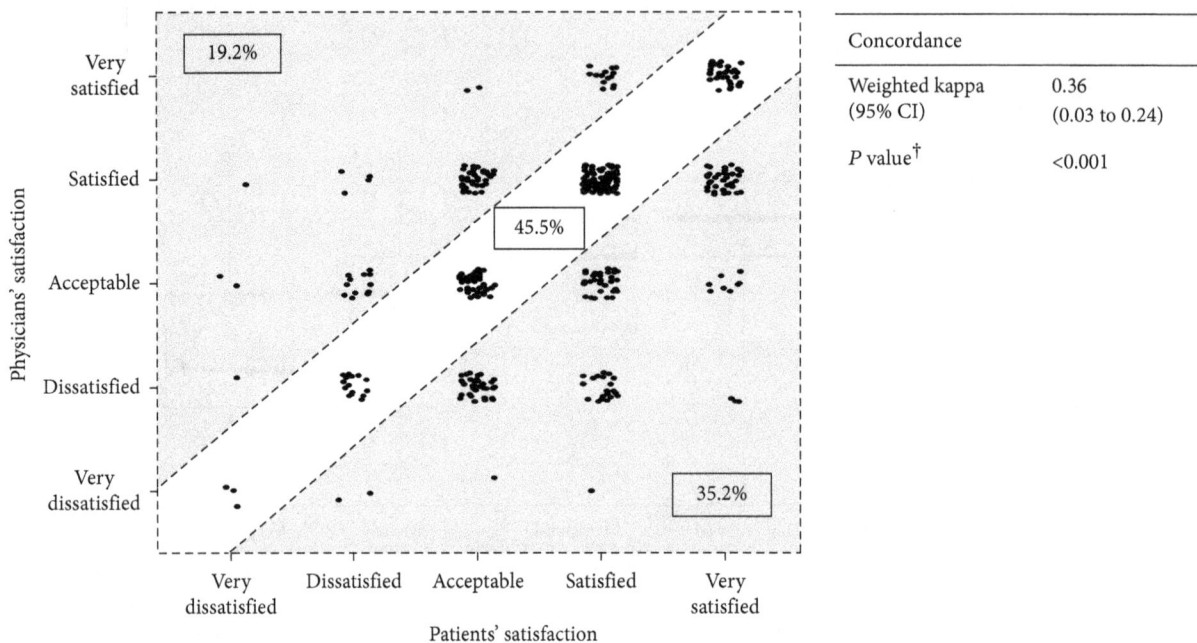

FIGURE 2: Concordance of patients' and physicians' satisfaction with patients' pain control status ($n = 462$). [†]McNemar's test. CI: confidence interval.

TABLE 3: Total daily dose of analgesics prescribed.

| | Median dose (mg) | Minimum, Maximum dose (mg) |
|---|---|---|
| Opioids | | |
| Fentanyl[†] | 0.89 | 0.29, 4.49 |
| Morphine | 30.00 | 2.00, 300.00 |
| Tramadol | 150.00 | 30.00, 420.00 |
| Nonopioids | | |
| Gabapentin | 900.00 | 100.00, 3600.00 |
| Paracetamol | 1300.00 | 325.00, 4000.00 |
| Pregabalin | 150.00 | 50.00, 750.00 |

Only analgesics with data across all six countries were included; all analgesics were orally administered unless otherwise stated; [†]transdermal.

well as pain management education for both patients and physicians in SEA [32, 33].

Amongst the 6 SEA countries included in the present study, Indonesia scored the lowest for physician satisfaction, patient-physician concordance in satisfaction with pain control, and adequacy of analgesics. In addition, median daily doses of the weak opioid, tramadol, and the strong opioids, fentanyl and morphine, were also the lowest in Indonesia amongst all studied countries. Notably, the median daily dose of prescribed morphine was only 20.00 mg in Indonesia—one third of the dose reported to be effective for opioid-tolerant patients with moderate pain [37]. These observations may be the consequence of heavy regulatory restrictions governing the prescription of opioids in Indonesia (e.g., duration of opioid prescription limited to a few days and burdensome procedures for reporting opioid prescription) [38]. Such burdensome regulatory procedures not only limit opioid prescription, but also occupy physician time and results in less time for patient care—a possible contributory factor towards the observed high levels of physician dissatisfaction in Indonesia. These findings highlight the broader picture of availability and/or accessibility

of analgesics, particularly those of opioids, which may influence prescription doses and satisfaction levels. National health policies and laws that impose strict regulations on opioid prescription may cause restrictions to opioid availability, inadvertently leading to under-management of pain [39, 40]. A shift towards less regulatory paperwork will allow physicians to focus more on patient care and possibly improve both patient and physician satisfaction with pain management. In less-developed countries whose healthcare infrastructure are under-developed, inaccessibility to opioids is often compounded by high costs and limited variety of opioids [41].

In the present study, study outcomes were primarily evaluated using self-reporting tools. Assessments depending solely on such tools are often one-dimensional and do not capture all aspects of the treatment experience (i.e., pain relief, quality of life, sleep disturbance, and satisfaction with pain control). In addition, owing to the cross-sectional study design, data on all variables were collected only once, and the associations identified between variables were difficult to interpret. The relationship between the variables measured and prescribed analgesics may be better reflected if the questionnaire had been administered before and after analgesic treatment. It is also important to note that variations across countries in patient education levels, types of hospitals (e.g., national, community, or local district hospitals), number of recruited patients (e.g., eight from Singapore compared with 70–100 from other countries), and physicians' education regarding cancer pain management were not taken into account in the comparison of data across countries. More importantly, our findings may not be representative of the whole range of clinical settings for pain management in SEA. Cancer pain management in less-developed regions of SEA is, therefore, likely to be more challenging in reality as issues with healthcare systems and analgesic accessibility and availability still persist.

## 5. Conclusions

The results of our study highlight the complexity of managing cancer pain in SEA. Despite relatively high patient-reported satisfaction with analgesic treatment for pain control, many patients still reported unrelieved pain, problems with quality of life, and sleep disturbance due to pain. In addition, there was low concordance between patients' and physicians' satisfaction with patients' pain control. Successful management of cancer pain will require action on a number of fronts—firstly, noting that patient-reported pain measures are often one-dimensional and do not capture all aspects of the patient's pain control status, an all-round assessment of patients' pain symptoms (including patient satisfaction, pain intensity, sleep disturbance due to pain, quality of life, and adverse effects) would be crucial in assessing the effectiveness of prescribed analgesics. Additionally, one important finding of this study is the evidence of a gap in satisfaction with pain control between patients and their physicians, which suggests a need for further improvements in patient-physician communication about analgesic treatment expectations and pain control. To improve patients' analgesic compliance and quality of life, physicians are also encouraged to proactively assess and manage opioid-induced adverse effects. Finally, national health policies that support and improve the accessibility of analgesics are welcomed so that patients can access the best possible analgesic treatment for their cancer pain.

## Acknowledgments

This study was funded by Mundipharma Pte. Ltd. Data management and statistical analyses were performed by Tech Observer Asia Pacific Pte. Ltd. (formerly known as Research2Trials Clinical Solutions Pte. Ltd.). Medical writing and editorial support was funded by Mundipharma Pte. Ltd. and provided by Wei Yi Kwok and Bao Hui Lee from Tech Observer Asia Pacific Pte. Ltd.

## References

[1] T. A. Baker, J. L. Krok-Schoen, and S. C. McMillan, "Identifying factors of psychological distress on the experience of pain and symptom management among cancer patients," *BMC Psychology*, vol. 4, no. 1, p. 52, 2016.

[2] A. Caraceni, G. Hanks, S. Kaasa et al., "Use of opioid analgesics in the treatment of cancer pain: evidence-based recommendations from the EAPC," *Lancet Oncology*, vol. 13, no. 2, pp. e58–e68, 2012.

[3] R. K. Portenoy and P. Lesage, "Management of cancer pain," *The Lancet*, vol. 353, no. 9165, pp. 1695–1700, 1999.

[4] T. A. Baker, J. L. Krok-Schoen, M. L. O'Connor, and A. K. Brooks, "The influence of pain severity and interference on satisfaction with pain management among middle-aged and older adults," *Pain Research and Management*, vol. 2016, Article ID 9561024, 7 pages, 2016.

[5] T. A. Baker, M. L. O'Connor, R. Roker, and J. L. Krok, "Satisfaction with pain treatment in older cancer patients: identifying variants of discrimination, trust, communication, and self-efficacy," *Journal of Hospice and Palliative Nursing*, vol. 15, no. 8, pp. 455–463, 2013.

[6] A. T. Hirsh, J. W. Atchison, J. J. Berger et al., "Patient satisfaction with treatment for chronic pain: predictors and relationship to compliance," *Clinical Journal of Pain*, vol. 21, no. 4, pp. 302–310, 2005.

[7] A. Davies, G. Zeppetella, S. Andersen et al., "Multi-centre European study of breakthrough cancer pain: pain characteristics and patient perceptions of current and potential management strategies," *European Journal of Pain*, vol. 15, no. 7, pp. 756–763, 2011.

[8] Y. H. Yun, D. S. Heo, I. G. Lee et al., "Multicenter study of pain and its management in patients with advanced cancer in Korea," *Journal of Pain and Symptom Management*, vol. 25, no. 5, pp. 430–437, 2003.

[9] S. L. Du Pen, A. R. Du Pen, N. Polissar et al., "Implementing guidelines for cancer pain management: results of a randomized controlled clinical trial," *Journal of Clinical Oncology*, vol. 17, no. 1, pp. 361–370, 1999.

[10] G. A. Hawker, S. Mian, T. Kendzerska, and M. French, "Measures of adult pain: Visual Analog Scale for Pain (VAS Pain), Numeric Rating Scale for Pain (NRS Pain), McGill Pain Questionnaire (MPQ), Short-Form McGill Pain Questionnaire (SF-MPQ), Chronic Pain Grade Scale (CPGS), Short Form-36 Bodily Pain Scale (SF-36 BPS), and Measure of Intermittent and Constant Osteoarthritis Pain (ICOAP)," *Arthritis Care & Research*, vol. 63, no. 11, pp. S240–S252, 2011.

[11] M. P. Jensen, "The validity and reliability of pain measures in adults with cancer," *Journal of Pain*, vol. 4, no. 1, pp. 2–21, 2003.

[12] N. J. Devlin and R. Brooks, "EQ-5D and the EuroQol Group: past, present and future," *Applied Health Economics and Health Policy*, vol. 15, no. 2, pp. 127–137, 2017.

[13] R. Rabin and F. de Charro, "EQ-5D: a measure of health status from the EuroQol Group," *Annals of Medicine*, vol. 33, no. 5, pp. 337–343, 2001.

[14] K. M. Rau, J. S. Chen, H. B. Wu et al., "Cancer-related pain: a nationwide survey of patients' treatment modification and satisfaction in Taiwan," *Japanese Journal of Clinical Oncology*, vol. 47, no. 11, pp. 1060–1065, 2017.

[15] Y. S. Choi, S. H. Kim, J. S. Kim et al., "Change in patients' satisfaction with pain control after using the Korean cancer pain assessment tool in Korea," *Journal of Pain and Symptom Management*, vol. 31, no. 6, pp. 553–562, 2006.

[16] ACHEON Working Group, Y. C. Kim, J. S. Ahn et al., "Current practices in cancer pain management in Asia: a survey of patients and physicians across 10 countries," *Cancer Medicine*, vol. 4, no. 8, pp. 1196–1204, 2015.

[17] R. Dawson, J. A. Spross, E. S. Jablonski, D. R. Hoyer, D. E. Sellers, and M. Z. Solomon, "Probing the paradox of patients' satisfaction with inadequate pain management," *Journal of Pain and Symptom Management*, vol. 23, no. 3, pp. 211–220, 2002.

[18] S. L. Beck, G. L. Towsley, P. H. Berry, K. Lindau, R. B. Field, and S. Jensen, "Core aspects of satisfaction with pain management: cancer patients' perspectives," *Journal of Pain and Symptom Management*, vol. 39, no. 1, pp. 100–115, 2010.

[19] W. Kwok and T. Bhuvanakrishna, "The relationship between ethnicity and the pain experience of cancer patients: a systematic review," *Indian Journal of Palliative Care*, vol. 20, no. 3, pp. 194–200, 2014.

[20] E. O. Im, S. H. Lee, Y. Liu, H. J. Lim, E. Guevara, and W. Chee, "A national online forum on ethnic differences in cancer pain experience," *Nursing Research*, vol. 58, no. 2, pp. 86–94, 2009.

[21] C. H. Chen, S. T. Tang, and C. H. Chen, "Meta-analysis of cultural differences in Western and Asian patient-perceived barriers to managing cancer pain," *Palliative Medicine*, vol. 26, no. 3, pp. 206–221, 2012.

[22] T. A. Pellino and S. E. Ward, "Perceived control mediates the relationship between pain severity and patient satisfaction," *Journal of Pain and Symptom Management*, vol. 15, no. 2, pp. 110–116, 1998.

[23] L. M. Torres, J. Revnic, A. D. Knight, and M. Perelman, "Relationship between onset of pain relief and patient satisfaction with fentanyl pectin nasal spray for breakthrough pain in cancer," *Journal of Palliative Medicine*, vol. 17, no. 10, pp. 1150–1157, 2014.

[24] T. F. Hack, L. F. Degner, P. A. Parker, and SCRN Communication Team, "The communication goals and needs of cancer patients: a review," *Psycho-Oncology*, vol. 14, no. 10, pp. 831–845, discussion 846–837, 2005.

[25] T. A. Baker, R. Roker, H. R. Collins et al., "Beyond race and gender: measuring behavioral and social indicators of pain treatment satisfaction in older black and white cancer patients," *Gerontology and Geriatric Medicine*, vol. 2, p. 2333721415625688, 2016.

[26] A. Anton, J. Montalar, J. Carulla et al., "Pain in clinical oncology: patient satisfaction with management of cancer pain," *European Journal of Pain*, vol. 16, no. 3, pp. 381–389, 2012.

[27] S. N. Lim, H. S. Han, K. H. Lee et al., "A satisfaction survey on cancer pain management using a self-reporting pain assessment tool," *Journal of Palliative Medicine*, vol. 18, no. 3, pp. 225–231, 2015.

[28] D. C. Dugdale, R. Epstein, and S. Z. Pantilat, "Time and the patient-physician relationship," *Journal of General Internal Medicine*, vol. 14, no. 1, pp. S34–40, 1999.

[29] R. Grol, H. Mokkink, A. Smits et al., "Work satisfaction of general practitioners and the quality of patient care," *Family Practice*, vol. 2, no. 3, pp. 128–135, 1985.

[30] M. Glajchen, "Chronic pain: treatment barriers and strategies for clinical practice," *Journal of the American Board of Family Practice*, vol. 14, no. 3, pp. 211–218, 2001.

[31] M. L. Levin, J. I. Berry, and J. Leiter, "Management of pain in terminally ill patients: physician reports of knowledge, attitudes, and behavior," *Journal of Pain and Symptom Management*, vol. 15, no. 1, pp. 27–40, 1998.

[32] C. R. Green, K. O. Anderson, T. A. Baker et al., "The unequal burden of pain: confronting racial and ethnic disparities in pain," *Pain Medicine*, vol. 4, no. 3, pp. 277–294, 2003.

[33] C. Prandi, L. Garrino, P. Mastromarino et al., "Barriers in the management of cancer-related pain and strategies to overcome them: findings of a qualitative research involving physicians and nurses in Italy," *Annali dell'Istituto Superiore di Sanità*, vol. 51, no. 1, pp. 71–78, 2015.

[34] B. Rimer, M. H. Levy, M. K. Keintz, L. Fox, P. F. Engstrom, and N. MacElwee, "Enhancing cancer pain control regimens through patient education," *Patient Education and Counseling*, vol. 10, no. 3, pp. 267–277, 1987.

[35] J. W. Oliver, R. L. Kravitz, S. H. Kaplan, and F. J. Meyers, "Individualized patient education and coaching to improve pain control among cancer outpatients," *Journal of Clinical Oncology*, vol. 19, no. 8, pp. 2206–2212, 2001.

[36] M. Z. Cohen, M. K. Easley, C. Ellis et al., "Cancer pain management and the JCAHO's pain standards: an institutional challenge," *Journal of Pain and Symptom Management*, vol. 25, no. 6, pp. 519–527, 2003.

[37] S. Mercadante, "Opioid titration in cancer pain: a critical review," *European Journal of Pain*, vol. 11, no. 8, pp. 823–830, 2007.

[38] F. O. Javier, C. Irawan, M. B. Mansor, W. Sriraj, K. H. Tan, and D. H. Q. Thinh, "Cancer pain management insights and reality in southeast asia: expert perspectives from six countries," *Journal of Global Oncology*, vol. 2, no. 4, pp. 235–243, 2016.

[39] F. Brennan, D. B. Carr, and M. Cousins, "Pain management: a fundamental human right," *Anesthesia and Analgesia*, vol. 105, no. 1, pp. 205–221, 2007.

[40] N. I. Cherny, J. Cleary, W. Scholten, L. Radbruch, and J. Torode, "The Global Opioid Policy Initiative (GOPI) project to evaluate the availability and accessibility of opioids for the management of cancer pain in Africa, Asia, Latin America and the Caribbean, and the Middle East: introduction and methodology," *Annals of Oncology*, vol. 24, no. 11, pp. xi7–xi13, 2013.

[41] L. De Lima, C. Sweeney, J. L. Palmer, and E. Bruera, "Potent analgesics are more expensive for patients in developing countries: a comparative study," *Journal of Pain & Palliative Care Pharmacotherapy*, vol. 18, no. 1, pp. 59–70, 2004.

# 4

# Dutch Translation and Validation of the Headache-Specific Locus of Control Scale (HSLC-DV)

**Marceline C. Willekens ⓘ,[1] Don Postel,[2] Martin D. M. Keesenberg,[2] and Robert Lindeboom[3]**

[1]*Health Center "het Wantveld", Noordwijk, Netherlands*
[2]*Corpus Mentis, Center for Physical Therapy & Science, Leiden, Netherlands*
[3]*Academic Medical Center, Department of Clinical Epidemiology and Biostatistics, University of Amsterdam, Amsterdam, Netherlands*

Correspondence should be addressed to Marceline C. Willekens; marceline.willekens@gmail.com

Academic Editor: Federica Galli

*Background and Objective*. The assessment of locus of control forms an important part of headache treatment, and there is need to adapting them to the Dutch population. *Methods*. Forward-backward translation was used to obtain the Headache-Specific Locus of Control Scale–Dutch Version (HSLC-DV). The response of 87 participants with migraine, tension-type headache, and cervicogenic headache, aged between 18 and 55 years (75% female), is used. Test-retest reliability was measured by intraclass correlations. Construct validity was assessed by correlations with corresponding domains of the Pain Coping and Cognition List (PCCL) and by confirmation of known groups hypotheses. Structural validity was evaluated by factor analysis (principal axis factoring). *Results*. The intraclass correlations for the External, Internal, and Chance domains were 0.79, 0.89, and 0.73, respectively. Internal consistencies for domains exceeded 0.73 and were similar to those observed in the original study. Convergent correlations were as expected and three of the seven known groups hypotheses were confirmed. Structural validity was supported by results of the factor analysis that matched the proposed structure of the original instrument. *Conclusions*. The HSLC-DV is a valid and reliable questionnaire for measuring the locus of control.

## 1. Introduction

Migraine and tension-type headaches are highly prevalent and have a strong impact on society [1, 2]. Locus of Control (LoC) is related to the impact of headaches and chronic pain [3]. The extent patients believe they can control events affecting their pain is influenced by the degree of LoC [4, 5]. Individuals with internal LoC believe that events in their life derive primarily from their own actions. Individuals with External LoC attribute outcomes of events to external circumstances, for example, "the intervention of powerful others such as health-care professionals." Chance LoC represents unordered forces such as fate and luck [6]. Cognitive-behavioral therapy (CBT) is a successful and most common psychological approach in treating pain and

is effective in reducing disability and catastrophic reaction [2]. Positive outcomes have been detected also in patients with chronic daily headaches [2]. CBT helps to reduce pain by learning how to manage the LoC in headaches [2].

Influencing the level of LoC of patients with headache leads to faster and more sustained recovery from headaches [7]. The patient empowerment proceeds from the perspective that optimal outcomes of an intervention are achieved when patients become active participants in their treatment process [3, 7].

The Headache-Specific Locus of Control Scale (HSLC) by Martin en Holroyd [4] was developed in the US using the framework from Rotter's social learning theory [8]. The original US English version [4] of the HSLC showed promising psychometric properties. Three-week test-retest reliabilities of the subscales ranged between 0.72 and 0.78. Internal consistency reliabilities ranged between 0.84 and 0.88 [6]. Danish [5] and Spanish [9] versions are available. The Danish version was reliable and valid in a multiethnic sample from a tertiary care headache center.

To assess LoC in Dutch patients with headache, the Pain Coping and Cognition List (PCCL) is used. However, the PCCL includes two domains measuring more global internal and external pain management and was not specifically developed for patients with headache. Headache-specific instruments can be useful to screen patients on their Internal or External LoC before the treatment as it may affect the outcome [7]. We argue that there is a need for a specific instrument to measure LoC in patients with headache in Dutch. We developed a Dutch version of the HSLC (HSLC-DV). The aim of the present study is to investigate the reliability and validity of the HSLC-DV.

## 2. Methods

### 2.1. Translation Procedure.
After obtaining permission from the developer (Professor Kenneth Holroyd, Ohio University), the original HSLC questionnaire was translated by a translation agency. Two translators independently translated the original US English version of the HSLC into Dutch. A third independent translator merged these two Dutch HSLC versions into the best suitable Dutch translation for each item. Subsequently, this Dutch version of the HSLC was backward translated into English by two other independent translators of the translation agency. These independent translators were unacquainted with the original US English version of the HSLC. Another independent translator translated again forward into Dutch.

A focus group consisting of four content experts with regard to the target group achieved consensus on comprehensibility and translation. Subsequently, 20 health-care professionals (10 psychologists and 10 general practitioners) evaluated the equivalence between the original and the translated version of the HSLC. After this assessment, the final Dutch version was composed, the HSLC-DV (Appendix).

### 2.2. Participants.
Eligible participants were patients with a history of headaches visiting two referral centers ("Corpus Mentis, Center for Physical Therapy & Science" or "het Wantveld") for treatment. Additionally, patients were recruited through the websites of the Dutch Association for Physical Therapy & Science (part of Corpus Mentis) and two patient support groups of the Dutch Migraine Association. The participants of the support groups were already diagnosed with migraine by visiting a physician in the past. Migraine patients were not recruited in the referral centers because they are not visiting a physiotherapist for their headache problems on a regular basis. Patients with migraine [4], cervicogenic headache [9], and tension-type headache [4], between the ages of 18 and 55 years old with headache complaints lasting longer than two months, were included. Thirty-five patients were allocated to the migraine group and 52 to the Tension-Type and Cervicogenic

Headache group. All participants were native Dutch speakers and signed informed consent after receiving information about the purpose and procedure of the research. Exclusion criteria were stroke, TIA, CVA, dementia, pregnancy/menopause, medication overuse or cluster headache, tumors, and use of alcohol or special medication.

### 2.3. Assessment Instruments and Procedure.
The participants included from Wantveld and Corpus Mentis were diagnosed by the physical therapist through history taking and physical examination, and after inclusion they filled out the survey. Patients completed the survey after inclusion (T0) and after three weeks (T1). The survey included the HSLC-DV (Appendix), the Pain Coping and Cognition List (PCCL [10]), and the numeric pain rating scale (NPRS [11]).

The HSLC [3] is a self-report questionnaire and contains 33 items with a Likert response scale ranging from 1 (strongly disagree) to 5 (strongly agree). The questionnaire has three subscales consisting of 11 items each: Internal LoC, External LoC, and Chance LoC. Each subscale score may range from 11 to 55 points. Lower scores reflect lower levels of the trait being measured by a subscale [12].

The PCCL [10] has 42 items and measures dealing with pain, LoC, and pain cognitions, within four subscales: Pain Coping (11 items), Catastrophizing (12 items), Internal Pain Management (11 items), and External Pain Management (8 items). It uses a 6-point Likert scale: 1 (totally disagree) to 6 (totally agree). The total scores and subscale scores may range from 1 to 6 points (total score divided by number of questions that were answered).

The NPRS [11] was used as a global measure of the experienced pain intensity and runs from 0 (no pain) to 10 (the worst pain you can imagine). The patient was instructed to circle the number that reflects the severity of the pain in the past week.

A Global Rating of Change (GRC) was included at T1 to inquire to what extent the headache complaints were changed at follow-up. A score of −5 indicates much worsened symptoms compared to the previous measurement, 0 indicates unchanged, and +5 indicates a maximum improvement compared to the previous measurement.

Patients were recruited from May 2014 to February 2015. Questions on demographic and clinical characteristics were included in the T0 survey. Patients provided self-reported information including headache intensity, headache episodes and headache duration, age and gender as well as work status, children, doctors' visits, sport, education level, civil status, and medication use (Table 1).

The survey was provided on paper and as an online version. Participants who did not respond to the request to fill out the questionnaires received a reminder by e-mail after 10 days. After two reminders, patients were excluded from the analysis.

### 2.4. Reliability.
Reproducibility of the HSLC-DV domain scores was assessed by comparing the scores on T0 and T1 using intraclass correlations (ICCs), (consistency model, single measures). The reproducibility of the item scores was

TABLE 1: Baseline characteristics.

| | Total sample ($N = 87$) | Lost to follow-up ($N = 16$) |
|---|---|---|
| Gender | | |
| Male | 21 (24%) | 3 (19%) |
| Mean (SD) age in years | 36 (9) | 35 (7) |
| Headache type | | |
| Migraine | 35 (40%) | 5 (31%) |
| Tension type and cervicogenic headache | 52 (60%) | 11 (69%) |
| Median (range) headache days per month | 8 (1–31) | 8 (4–30) |
| Median duration of headache in years | 13 (1–45) | 13 (3–30) |
| Median duration of headache period in days | 3 (0.5–31) | 2 (0.5–6) |
| Headache treatment | 34 (39%) | 4 (25%) |
| Work | | |
| Full-time | 40 (46%) | 7 (44%) |
| Part-time | 32 (37%) | 7 (44%) |
| No paid work | 11 (13%) | 1 (6%) |
| Freelance | 4 (4%) | 1 (6%) |
| Median (range) number of children | 0 (0–6) | 1 (0–3) |
| Sports or moderate physical activity for 30 min a day[1] | | |
| No sports or moderate physical activity | 26 (30%) | 9 (56%) |
| Moderate physical activity only | 32 (37%) | 4 (25%) |
| >2x a week sport | 29 (33%) | 3 (19%) |
| Education[2] | | |
| Low | 44 (51%) | 8 (50%) |
| High | 43 (49%) | 8 (50%) |
| Civil status | | |
| Single | 18 (21%) | 2 (13%) |
| Relation, living with partner, (re)married | 65 (75%) | 13 (81%) |
| Divorced | 4 (5%) | 1 (6%) |
| Medication | | |
| Pain medication | 63 (72%) | 13 (81%) |
| Beta-blocker | 2 (2%) | 0 (0%) |
| Blood pressure-lowering drugs | 3 (3%) | 0 (0%) |
| Doctors visit in median times a year | 2 (0–25) | 2 (0–6) |
| HSLC | | |
| External | 24.2 (6.9) | 23.4 (5.2) |
| Internal | 34.9 (9.3) | 37.8 (9.5) |
| Chance | 33.8 (7.0) | 35.0 (5.3) |

Numbers are frequencies (%), mean (SD), or median (range). [1]Dutch norm for healthy exercise. [2]High education = higher vocational education and science education.

investigated using weighted kappas. Weighted kappas were estimated by calculating ICCs [13]. Random and systematic measurement error of the HSLC-DV was evaluated through the method of Bland & Altman that examines the magnitude of the mean score differences between T0 and T1 and by calculating limits of agreement (LoA) [14]. LoA were calculated as the mean sumscore differences between T0 and T1 $\pm 1.96 \times$ the standard deviation of the differences. LoA were calculated for the total sample and for the subsample with GRC scores between −1 and +1 who were considered unchanged in their headache severity at follow-up. Internal consistency was evaluated by Cronbach's alpha and item-rest correlations. Cronbach's alpha values for the subscales were compared to those of the original US version [4] study and with the Danish version [5]. Item-rest correlations of >0.30 were considered as adequate [15].

2.5. *Construct Validity.* Validity of the Dutch HSLC was evaluated by the correlations of HSLC-DV domains with corresponding domains of the PCCL. We regarded correlations between 0.1 and 0.3 as low, between 0.3 and 0.5 as medium, and between 0.5 and 0.7 as high [16]. We expected a medium/high correlation ($r > 0.40$) between the domains Internal LoC and External LoC of the HSLC-DV and PCCL and between the HSLC-DV Chance LoC and PCCL Catastrophizing (convergent correlations) [4, 9]. We expected low correlations between dissimilar domains of both instruments (divergent correlations). In addition, we also tested mean score differences between subgroups based on the following hypotheses ("known groups" validation):

(1) We expected lower Internal LoC scores for the Tension-Type and Cervicogenic Headache group compared to the Migraine-Type group. Tension-type headache and cervicogenic headache are more often the results of stress and burnout complaints that are in turn associated with lower Internal LoC scores [17, 18].

(2) We expected higher Internal scores for higher educated people compared to lower educated people.

According to Pellino and Oberst, a higher educational level may indicate that the individual has more problem-solving ability or a higher level of self-efficacy in dealing with chronic pain [19].

(3) We expected higher Internal LoC scores for men compared to woman. Men were found to be more inclined to believe that headache problems and headache relief are determined by their own actions or behaviors [19–21].

(4) We expected higher Internal LoC scores for subjects who actively practiced sports or engaged daily in at least 30 minutes of moderate physical activity compared to those who did not. The positive influence of sports activity on the production of endorphins reduces the stress hormone cortisol [22]. Previous studies found that subjects who actively practice sports have higher scores on the Internal LoC than others [18].

(5) We expected higher External LoC scores for subjects under (medical) headache treatment compared to no-headache treatment. Higher levels of medication use and preference for medical treatment were associated with External LoC in the original US study and the Spanish validation [4, 9].

(6) We expected higher Chance LoC scores with more frequent headache days per month [4].

(7) We expected higher Chance LoC scores with longer duration in days of headache episodes [4].

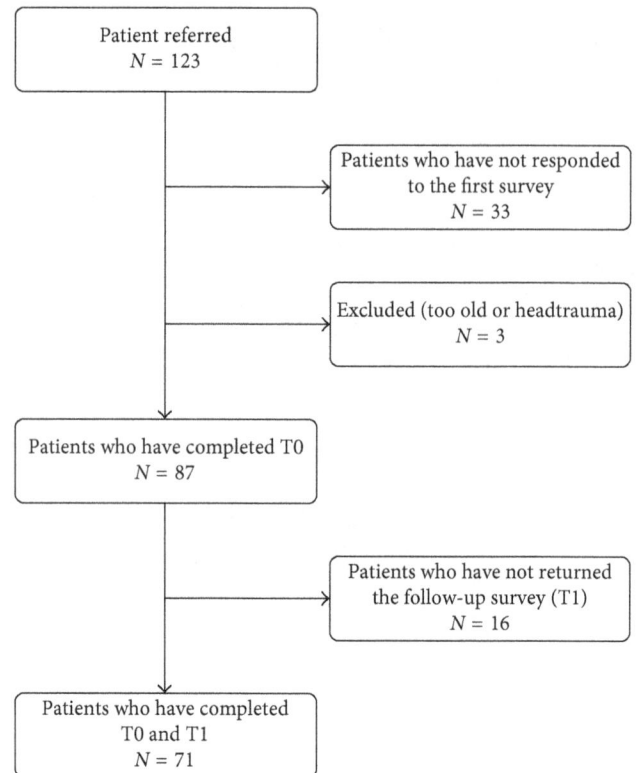

FIGURE 1: Flowchart.

### 2.6. Structural Validity.

Structural validity of the HSLC-DV was examined by a principal axis factoring analysis with orthogonal (Varimax) rotation in order to test the purported subscale structure of the HSLC-DV. A forced three-factor structure was used. Factor loadings > 0.40 for individual items were considered indicative of subscale domain membership. Kaiser–Meyer–Olkin test was used to examine whether the data are suited for factor analysis. KMO test values may range between 0 and 1. Values below 0.50 are deemed unacceptable. KMO measure of sampling adequacy was 0.69 indicating that the sample was large enough to conduct a principal component analysis.

### 2.7. Statistical Analysis.

Numerical data were presented as mean (SD) or median (range) as appropriate. Differences between clinical subgroups were assessed with independent $t$-test or a one-way ANOVA in case of >2 groups or a nonparametric variant when assumptions of equal variances and normality were not met. All hypotheses were tested two-sided. In our analyses, $P < 0.05$ signified statistical significance. Differences in baseline and follow-up scores of respondents were tested with paired $t$-tests. Convergent and divergent (Pearson's) correlations between the HSLC and subscales of the PCCL were obtained by bootstrapping based on 1000 bootstrap samples.

There were no missing values on individual HSLC-DV items on T0. For the respondents on T1, one patient had 3 missing items, two had two missing items, and seven patients had one missing item. Little's MCAR test was not significant, and missing item values were imputed by expectation-maximization.

## 3. Results

A total of 87 patients with headache completed the survey at T0, and 16 patients did not return or completed the survey after three weeks at T1 (Figure 1). The baseline characteristics of the 16 patients that were lost to follow-up were not notably different. Baseline LoC subscale scores of the total sample were approximately normally distributed and were comparable to those of the patients who did not complete the study (Table 1). The online version was completed by 81 patients and six completed the paper version at T0. At T1, 6 patients completed the paper version and 65 patients completed the online version. The participants were outpatients from the referral centers (52 patients) or patient the support groups (35 patients).

### 3.1. Reliability of the HSLC-DV.

The reproducibility and internal consistency results are summarized in Table 2. Cronbach's alpha ranged from 0.73 for Chance LoC to 0.89 for Internal LoC. These results are in line with the Danish study and the original US study. All item-rest correlations exceeded 0.30 except for two items of the External subscale and two items of the Chance subscale. Weighted kappas, as estimated using ICCs, for the items of the External LoC,

TABLE 2: Reproducibility and internal consistency of the HSLC-DV ($N$ = 87).

| | Weighted kappa | Item-rest correlation | Cronbach's alpha if item deleted | Cronbach's alpha |
|---|---|---|---|---|
| External LoC | | | | 0.79 (0.75*) (0.88**) |
| HSLC6 | 0.24 | 0.12 | 0.80 | |
| HSLC8 | 0.43 | 0.47 | 0.77 | |
| HSLC10 | 0.44 | 0.56 | 0.76 | |
| HSLC12 | 0.34 | 0.28 | 0.79 | |
| HSLC14 | 0.61 | 0.54 | 0.76 | |
| HSLC15 | 0.34 | 0.26 | 0.79 | |
| HSLC16 | 0.69 | 0.55 | 0.76 | |
| HSLC22 | 0.69 | 0.51 | 0.76 | |
| HSLC24 | 0.77 | 0.47 | 0.77 | |
| HSLC27 | 0.58 | 0.44 | 0.77 | |
| HSLC30 | 0.62 | 0.61 | 0.75 | |
| Internal LoC | | | | 0.89 (0.88*) (0.86**) |
| HSLC2 | 0.57 | 0.60 | 0.88 | |
| HSLC4 | 0.21 | 0.56 | 0.88 | |
| HSLC5 | 0.60 | 0.66 | 0.88 | |
| HSLC7 | 0.59 | 0.52 | 0.89 | |
| HSLC11 | 0.59 | 0.67 | 0.88 | |
| HSLC17 | 0.68 | 0.79 | 0.87 | |
| HSLC19 | 0.62 | 0.73 | 0.87 | |
| HSLC21 | 0.53 | 0.61 | 0.88 | |
| HSLC26 | 0.44 | 0.38 | 0.89 | |
| HSLC28 | 0.70 | 0.67 | 0.88 | |
| HSLC32 | 0.55 | 0.57 | 0.88 | |
| Chance LoC | | | | 0.73 (0.71*) (0.84**) |
| HSLC1 | 0.60 | 0.49 | 0.70 | |
| HSLC3 | 0.66 | 0.60 | 0.68 | |
| HSLC9 | 0.63 | 0.43 | 0.71 | |
| HSLC13 | 0.57 | 0.56 | 0.69 | |
| HSLC18 | 0.58 | −0.02 | 0.77 | |
| HSLC20 | 0.43 | 0.32 | 0.72 | |
| HSLC23 | 0.60 | 0.53 | 0.70 | |
| HSLC25 | 0.61 | 0.55 | 0.69 | |
| HSLC29 | 0.68 | 0.06 | 0.76 | |
| HSLC31 | 0.51 | 0.39 | 0.71 | |
| HSLC33 | 0.56 | 0.36 | 0.72 | |

LoC = Locus of Control subscale. Numbers correspond to the original HSLC scale. *Danish study. **Original US study.

Internal LoC, and Chance LoC ranged from 0.24 to 0.77 (median 0.58), 0.21 to 0.70 (median 0.59), and 0.43 to 0.68 (median 0.60), respectively.

The intraclass correlations (95%CI) for the External, Internal, and Chance domains were 0.77 (0.65–0.85), 0.81 (0.70–0.88), and 0.79 (0.67–0.86), respectively.

The mean difference between the External scores on the HSLC-DV between T0 and T1 was −0.42 points, and limits of agreement (LoA) were −11.2 to 10.4 points. The mean differences (LoA) for the Internal scores and the Chance scores were −0.94 (−12.1–10.2) and 0.85 (−8.7–10.4), respectively. For a subsample of the participants with GRC scores −1 to +1 ($N$ = 35), these were respectively 0.88 (−7.0–8.8), −0.96 (−11.7–9.8), and −0.97 (−9.0–7.1). Intraclass correlations in the subsample were practically equal to those calculated for the total sample: 0.83 (0.68–0.91), 0.82 (0.67–0.91), and 0.81 (0.66–0.90) for the External, Internal, and Chance scales, respectively.

TABLE 3: Pearson correlations between HSLC subscales and similar domains of the PCCL ($N$ = 87).

| | PCCL external | PCCL internal | PCCL catastrophizing |
|---|---|---|---|
| HSLC external | **0.64**\*\* | 0.12 | 0.20 |
| HSLC internal | −0.10 | **0.42**\*\* | −0.02 |
| HSLC chance | 0.27* | −0.35** | **0.36**\*\* |

Convergent correlations are given in bold. HSLC = Headache-Specific Locus of Control Scale; PCCL = Pain Coping and Cognition List. *$P < 0.05$. **$P < 0.01$.

### 3.2. Construct Validity of the HSLC-DV.

Table 3 shows the correlations between HSLC-DV subscale scores and PCCL subscale scores. All convergent and divergent correlations were as hypothesized except for those between the HSLC Chance and PCCL Catastrophizing that had a correlation of 0.36 ($P < 0.01$). Pearson correlations between HSLC-DV

TABLE 4: Known groups and hypotheses ($N = 87$).

|     |                                                              | External      | Internal       | Chance         |
| --- | ------------------------------------------------------------ | ------------- | -------------- | -------------- |
|     | Migraine ($N = 35$)                                          | 24.98 (7.20)  | 32.88 (9.78)   | 33.68 (6.68)   |
| (1) | Tension type + cervicogenic headache ($N = 52$)             | 23.61 (6.65)  | 36.24 (8.87)   | 33.93 (7.25)   |
|     |                                                              | $P = 0.34$    | **P= 0.15**    | $P = 0.76$     |
|     | Education, low ($N = 44$)                                    | 25.47 (6.87)  | 34.65 (9.52)   | 34.36 (6.90)   |
| (2) | Education, high ($N = 43$)                                   | 22.82 (6.67)  | 35.13 (9.26)   | 33.29 (7.12)   |
|     |                                                              | $P = 0.08$    | **P= 0.93**    | $P = 0.37$     |
|     | Male ($N = 21$)                                              | 23.97 (6.27)  | 37.70 (7.04)   | 32.34 (8.05)   |
| (3) | Female ($N = 66$)                                            | 24.22 (7.09)  | 33.99 (9.84)   | 34.30 (6.61)   |
|     |                                                              | $P = 0.89$    | **P= 0.40**    | $P = 0.30$     |
|     | No sport ($N = 26$)                                          | 23.30 (5.65)  | 38.71 (9.74)   | 32.68 (5.92)   |
| (4) | Moderate activity + 2x wk sports ($N = 61$)                 | 24.53 (7.34)  | 33.26 (8.75)   | 34.32 (7.39)   |
|     |                                                              | 0.47          | **P= 0.01***   | $P = 0.19$     |
|     | No treatment ($N = 53$)                                      | 22.99 (6.15)  | 35.39 (9.97)   | 33.54 (6.44)   |
| (5) | Treatment ($N = 34$)                                         | 25.99 (7.59)  | 34.11 (8.36)   | 34.27 (7.85)   |
|     |                                                              | **P= 0.04***  | $P = 0.45$     | $P = 0.43$     |
|     | 0–8 headache days per month ($N = 44$)                      | 23.73 (6.01)  | 35.76 (8.34)   | 31.22 (6.35)   |
| (6) | 9–31 headache days per month ($N = 43$)                     | 24.60 (7.69)  | 34.00 (10.29)  | 36.50 (6.65)   |
|     |                                                              | $P = 0.54$    | $P = 0.92$     | **P < 0.001*** |
|     | 0–3 days per headache period ($N = 58$)                     | 24.14 (6.1)   | 34.84 (8.89)   | 32.54 (6.46)   |
| (7) | 4–31 days per headache period ($N = 29$)                    | 24.20 (8.30)  | 36.75 (9.05)   | 36.40 (7.40)   |
|     |                                                              | $P = 0.99$    | $P = 0.56$     | **P= 0.01***   |

$P$ values for construct validity hypotheses are given in bold. HSLC = Headache-Specific Locus of Control Scale. Scores are mean (SD). Score differences are tested using the Mann–Whitney $U$ test. *$P < 0.05$.

subscales and PCCL pain or NPRS at T0 and T1 were generally small and not significant ($r < 0.20$, not shown in Table 3).

Table 4 shows the mean scores of clinical subgroups to test the construct validity hypotheses. From the seven HSLC hypotheses, three were confirmed (headache treatment, headache frequency, and headache duration) and four hypothesis were not confirmed (headache type, education, gender, and sports/moderate physical activity). For example, contrary to what was hypothesized, there was a higher mean score on Internal LoC for the Tension-Type and Cervicogenic Headache group compared with the Migraine group. Similarly, subjects who exercised at least 30 minutes of moderate physical activity or who actively engaged in sports had lower Internal LoC scores than those who did not (33.3 versus 38.7, $P = 0.01$). Higher educated subjects had, as hypothesized, higher Internal scores (35.13 versus 34.65), however not significant ($P = 0.93$).

*3.3. Structural Validity of the HSLC-DV.* The factor analysis (Table 5) largely confirmed the proposed three-factor structure of the HSLC-DV except for item 6 (Internal scale, low loading on all 3 factors) and items 18 (Chance item, loaded on External factor) and 29 (Chance item with low loading). The extracted factors explained 41% of the variance.

## 4. Discussion

We translated and validated the HSLC in a Dutch sample. The item reproducibility over a similar time interval as the original US study was generally good, except for item 4

(prevent headaches by not getting emotionally upset) and item 6 (prevent headaches by doctor). We found a comparable internal consistency as reported in the US and Danish validation studies. Most items contributed to the internal consistency although some items (items 6, 18, and 29) did not. The convergent correlations (>0.40) and divergent correlations (<0.30) between subscales of the HSLC-DV and related subscales of the PCCL were as expected. Only the HSLC Chance subscale correlated somewhat lower with the PCCL Catastrophizing scale (0.36). Catastrophizing in the US study was considered as a strategy for coping with headaches when chance or fate play a primary role in the onset of headache episodes. This is similar to what is measured by the HSLC Chance scale. Structural validity of the HSLC-DV was supported by the principal component analysis results. The vast majority of the items exclusively loaded on the intended subscales.

We expected a difference between men and woman. Men were found to be more inclined to believe that headache problems and headache relief are determined by their own actions or behaviors. This difference was not found in our results, comparable with Cano-García et al. [3].

From the seven HSLC known groups hypotheses, five were confirmed of which two reached no statistical significance. For example, contrary to what was expected, the mean Internal LoC score in the Tension-Type and Cervicogenic Headache group was higher than that in the Migraine-type group. We argue that the HSLC measures symptoms that may be present in all the three types of headaches. Hence, the hypotheses outcomes were not as expected for the different types.

TABLE 5: Structural validity: factor loadings on the purported subscales of the HSLC-DV scale.

|  |  | Internal LoC eigenvalue = 6.8 | External LoC eigenvalue = 4.3 | Chance LoC eigenvalue = 2.4 |
| --- | --- | --- | --- | --- |
| External LoC | HSLC6* | 0.168 | **0.100** | 0.228 |
|  | HSLC8 | 0.190 | **0.512** | 0.229 |
|  | HSLC10 | 0.230 | **0.687** | −0.080 |
|  | HSLC12 | 0.056 | **0.336** | 0.118 |
|  | HSLC14 | −0.108 | **0.643** | 0.153 |
|  | HSLC15* | −0.093 | **0.356** | 0.145 |
|  | HSLC16 | −0.112 | **0.720** | 0.028 |
|  | HSLC22 | 0.220 | **0.619** | −0.134 |
|  | HSLC24 | −0.052 | **0.639** | 0.188 |
|  | HSLC27 | 0.030 | **0.534** | 0.037 |
|  | HSLC30 | 0.062 | **0.702** | 0.057 |
| Internal LoC | HSLC2 | **0.660** | −0.013 | −0.123 |
|  | HSLC4 | **0.596** | 0.037 | −0.157 |
|  | HSLC5 | **0.699** | 0.000 | −0.195 |
|  | HSLC7 | **0.638** | 0.147 | 0.023 |
|  | HSLC11 | **0.729** | −0.012 | −0.076 |
|  | HSLC17 | **0.796** | 0.061 | −0.216 |
|  | HSLC19 | **0.845** | 0.054 | 0.037 |
|  | HSLC21 | **0.600** | 0.084 | −0.353 |
|  | HSLC26 | **0.429** | −0.067 | −0.281 |
|  | HSLC28 | **0.742** | −0.041 | −0.083 |
|  | HSLC32 | **0.618** | 0.019 | −0.201 |
| Chance LoC | HSLC1 | −0.224 | −0.148 | **0.650** |
|  | HSLC3 | −0.205 | −0.217 | **0.707** |
|  | HSLC9 | −0.249 | 0.019 | **0.568** |
|  | HSLC13 | −0.142 | 0.122 | **0.650** |
|  | HSLC18* | 0.479 | 0.114 | **0.096** |
|  | HSLC20 | 0.041 | 0.162 | **0.423** |
|  | HSLC23 | −0.020 | 0.186 | **0.694** |
|  | HSLC25 | −0.129 | 0.271 | **0.674** |
|  | HSLC29* | −0.032 | −0.223 | **0.088** |
|  | HSLC31 | −0.130 | 0.163 | **0.484** |
|  | HSLC33 | −0.276 | −0.181 | **0.415** |

Three factors explained 41% of the total variance in HSLC-DV scores. *Cross-loadings or items that do not load (<0.40) on the purported subscale.

Migraine patients are usually comorbid to depression [2]. The comorbidity with major affective disorders is more prevalent in subjects suffering from the chronic type of migraine, hence these patients report more frequently high levels of hopelessness and suicidal risk [2]. In our study, differences between chronic migraine and migraine were not investigated. Because we focused on the validation of the questionnaire, the factor depression was not processed in the analyses nor comorbidity factors in patients with headache.

No difference was observed for "sports or moderate physical activity for 30 min a day" with lower Internal LoC scores for physically active subjects.

*4.1. Study Limitations.* In our study, the relatively small sample size for the Principal Component Analysis is the first limitation. Further research in larger sample sizes should be completed to reach more definite conclusions regarding the structural validity of the HSLC-DV. A second limitation of this study is possible selection bias. A part of the sample may not be representative of the regular headache subjects

visiting the referral centers for treatment because we also recruited patients from patient-support groups. This could have led to inclusion of patients with chronic headache with longer disease duration. We argue that patients with longer sustained headaches were more willing to participate in this study, as we can see in the high median duration of headaches in years at baseline of this group. In our study, more women (75%) were included than men. We argue that this could be a representative reflection of the headache population because women are affected 2 to 4 times more often by headaches than men [23]. A third limitation is the classification of headache types based on self-report. Patients of the support groups were not verified or seen by a physician and had to classify their type of headaches according to the given symptoms and definitions in the survey. The patient-support groups were associated with the Dutch Migraine Association and were approached for the inclusion of migraine patients, the most prevalent headache type. These participants were assumed confirmed migraine cases. We did not rule out possible secondary headaches in the migraine group. Despite this limitation, we argue that for the validation of this questionnaire, the importance is more on headache characteristics (localization, intensity, and duration) than on the underlying mechanism. The accuracy of the diagnosis is fundamental, and we want to promote more researches that could provide reliable results.

Finally, Nilsson and Bove have classified TTH and CH together as "musculoskeletal headache" [24]. We argue that the myogene headache group and migraine group represented a good heterogeneity for validation of the LoC questionnaire. For the validation of the HSLC, inclusion of these headache types better reflects the characteristics of the general population of patients with headache.

# 5. Conclusions

We conclude that the HSLC-DV is a reliable and valid instrument to measure LoC in a Dutch sample of patients with headache. Therefore, we strongly recommend the use of the HSLC-DV in the treatment counseling of patients with headache. Future research is necessary to determine cutoff points for the different scales of the HSLC-DV to identify patients with poor outcome on the headache treatment.

# Appendix

## Hoofdpijn-Specifiek Locus of Control (HSLC-DV)

*Instructies*: Deze vragenlijst geeft inzicht in de klachten die u ervaart door de hoofdpijn. Hieronder staan 33 stellingen waarmee u het eens of oneens bent. Naast iedere stelling staan de getallen 1 tot en met 5. Hiermee geeft u aan in welke mate u het eens of oneens bent met de stelling. De 1 staat voor "Volkomen oneens" en de 5 staat voor "Volkomen eens." Omcirkel het getal dat correspondeert met de mate waarin u het eens of oneens bent met de stelling. Zorg ervoor dat u achter *alle 33 stellingen* een getal heeft omcirkeld. *Slechts één getal* per stelling kan worden omcirkeld. De antwoorden die u geeft zijn uw persoonlijk mening. Er zijn dan ook geen goede of foute antwoorden mogelijk.

  1 = Volkomen oneens

  2 = Gematigd oneens

  3 = Neutraal

  4 = Gematigd eens

  5 = Volkomen eens

TABLE 6: Hoofdpijn-Specifiek Locus of Control (HSLC-DV) scale

| | | |
|---|---|---|
| 1. | Als ik hoofdpijn heb is er niets wat ik kan doen om het beloop te veranderen | 1 2 3 4 5 |
| 2. | Ik ben in staat een deel van mijn hoofdpijn te voorkomen door het vermijden van bepaalde stressvolle situaties | 1 2 3 4 5 |
| 3. | Ik ben compleet machteloos met betrekking tot mijn hoofdpijn | 1 2 3 4 5 |
| 4. | Ik kan hoofdpijn soms voorkomen door niet overstuur te raken | 1 2 3 4 5 |
| 5. | Wanneer ik zorg voor voldoende rust heb ik minder vaak hoofdpijn | 1 2 3 4 5 |
| 6. | Alleen mijn arts kan mij aanwijzingen geven om mijn hoofdpijn te voorkomen | 1 2 3 4 5 |
| 7. | Mijn hoofdpijn is soms erger omdat ik overactief ben | 1 2 3 4 5 |
| 8. | Mijn hoofdpijn kan minder erg zijn wanneer medische professionals mij goede zorg verlenen. (Artsen, zusters, etc.) | 1 2 3 4 5 |
| 9. | Ik heb geen enkele invloed op mijn hoofdpijn | 1 2 3 4 5 |
| 10. | De behandeling van mijn arts kan mij helpen tegen hoofdpijn | 1 2 3 4 5 |
| 11. | Wanneer ik mij zorgen maak of pieker over iets heb ik een grotere kans op hoofdpijn | 1 2 3 4 5 |
| 12. | Alleen al een bezoek aan mijn arts helpt tegen mijn hoofdpijn | 1 2 3 4 5 |
| 13. | Ongeacht wat ik doe: als ik hoofdpijn zal krijgen, dan krijg ik het ook | 1 2 3 4 5 |
| 14. | Regelmatig contact met mijn arts is de beste manier voor mij om controle te krijgen over mijn hoofdpijn | 1 2 3 4 5 |
| 15. | Wanneer ik hoofdpijn heb dien ik een medische deskundige te raadplegen | 1 2 3 4 5 |
| 16. | Het zorgvuldig volgen van de door mijn arts uitgeschreven medicijnenkuur is de beste manier om hoofdpijn te voorkomen | 1 2 3 4 5 |
| 17. | Wanneer ik teveel van mijzelf vraag krijg ik hoofdpijn | 1 2 3 4 5 |
| 18. | Geluk speelt een grote rol bij het bepalen hoe snel ik zal herstellen van hoofdpijn | 1 2 3 4 5 |
| 19. | Door er voor te zorgen dat ik niet overactief of geïrriteerd raak voorkom ik veel hoofdpijn | 1 2 3 4 5 |
| 20. | Het niet krijgen van hoofdpijn is voornamelijk een kwestie van geluk | 1 2 3 4 5 |
| 21. | De dingen die ik doe beïnvloeden de kans op hoofdpijn | 1 2 3 4 5 |
| 22. | Gewoonlijk herstel ik van een hoofdpijn na het ontvangen van goede medische zorg | 1 2 3 4 5 |
| 23. | Ik heb een grote kans op hoofdpijn, ongeacht wat ik doe | 1 2 3 4 5 |
| 24. | Wanneer ik niet de juiste medicatie heb, heb ik last van hoofdpijn | 1 2 3 4 5 |
| 25. | Vaak heb ik het gevoel dat wat ik ook doe ik toch hoofdpijn zal krijgen | 1 2 3 4 5 |
| 26. | Ik ben zelf verantwoordelijk voor het krijgen van hoofdpijn | 1 2 3 4 5 |
| 27. | Wanneer mijn arts een vergissing maakt, ben ik degene die daaronder lijdt door hoofdpijn | 1 2 3 4 5 |
| 28. | Mijn hoofdpijn wordt erger wanneer ik met stress te maken heb | 1 2 3 4 5 |
| 29. | Wanneer ik hoofdpijn krijg moet ik de natuur gewoon zijn gang laten gaan | 1 2 3 4 5 |
| 30. | Professionele medische deskundigen zorgen dat ik geen hoofdpijn krijg | 1 2 3 4 5 |
| 31. | Ik heb simpelweg geluk wanneer ik een maand geen hoofdpijn heb | 1 2 3 4 5 |
| 32. | Wanneer ik niet goed voor mezelf zorg heb ik een grote kans op hoofdpijn | 1 2 3 4 5 |
| 33. | Het is een kwestie van toeval of ik hoofdpijn krijg | 1 2 3 4 5 |

Explanation domains:

(i) External subscale: 6, 8, 10, 12, 14, 15, 16, 22, 24, 27, 30.

(ii) Internal subscale: 2, 4, 5, 7, 11, 17, 19, 21, 26, 28, 32.

(iii) Chance subscale: 1, 3, 9, 13, 18, 20, 23, 25, 29, 31, 33.

## Acknowledgments

The authors want to thank Kenneth Holroyd for providing copies of the original versions of HSLC and useful advice on the process to accomplish this study. Additionally, the authors want to express their gratitude to the Dutch Association for Physical Therapy & Science for providing an online survey and all the support in recruiting the patients for this study. Furthermore, the authors thank the focus group for assessing equivalence between the original and the translated version of the HSLC. The authors thank the psychologists from Primary Care Psychology (PEP) "Wantveld" and general practitioners from Health Center "Wantveld" for assistance in recruiting patients with headache symptoms.

## References

[1] L. J. Stovner, K. Hagen, R. Jensen et al., "The global burden of headache: a documentation of headache prevalence and disability worldwide," *Cephalalgia*, vol. 27, no. 3, pp. 193–210, 2007.

[2] C. Tassorelli, M. Tramontano, M. Berlangieri et al., "Assessing and treating primary headaches and cranio-facial pain in patients undergoing rehabilitation for neurological diseases," *Journal of Headache and Pain*, vol. 18, no. 1, p. 99, 2017.

[3] F. J. Cano-García, L. Rodríguez-Franco, and A. M. López-Jiménez, "Locus of control patterns in headaches and chronic pain," *Pain Research & Management*, vol. 18, pp. 48–54, 2013.

[4] N. J. Martin, K. A. Holroyd, and D. B. Penzien, "The headache-specific locus of control scale: adaptation to recurrent headaches," *Headache: The Journal of Head and Face Pain*, vol. 30, no. 11, pp. 729–734, 1990.

[5] J. S. Hansen, L. Bendtsen, and R. Jensen, "Psychometric properties of the Danish version of headache-specific locus of controls scale and headache management self-efficacy scale," *Journal of Headache and Pain*, vol. 10, no. 5, pp. 341–347, 2009.

[6] M. E. Lachman, "Locus of control in aging research: a case for multidimensional and domain-specific assessment," *Psychology and Aging*, vol. 1, no. 1, pp. 34–40, 1986.

[7] W. R. Stanton and G. A. Jull, "Cervicogenic headache: locus of control and success of treatment," *Headache: The Journal of Head and Face Pain*, vol. 43, no. 9, pp. 956–961, 2003.

[8] J. B. Rotter, "Generalised expectancies for internal and external control of reinforcement," *Psychological Monographs: General and Applied*, vol. 80, no. 1, pp. 1–28, 1966.

[9] J. Francisco, F. J. Cano-García, L. Rodríguez-Franco, and A. M. López-Jiménez, "A shortened version of the headache-specific locus of control scale in Spanish population," *Headache*, vol. 50, no. 8, pp. 1335–1345, 2010.

[10] S. G. M. Stom-van den Berg, J. W. S. Vlaeyen, M. M. ter Kuile et al., *Measures of Chronic Pain: Part 3. Pain Coping and Cognition List, Validation and Norms*, Pijn en Kennis Centrum, Maastricht, Netherlands, in Dutch, 2003.

[11] J. A. Cleland, J. D. Childs, and J. M. Whitman, "Psychometric properties of the neck disability index and numeric pain rating scale in patients with mechanical neck pain," *Archives of Physical Medicine and Rehabilitation*, vol. 89, no. 1, pp. 69–74, 2008.

[12] H. M. Lefcourt, *Research with the Locus of Control Construct: Assessment Methods*, Vol. 1, Academic Press, New York, NY, USA, 1981.

[13] J. L. Fleiss and J. Cohen, "The equivalence of weighted kappa and the intraclass correlation coefficient as measures of reliability," *Educational and Psychological Measurement*, vol. 33, pp. 613–619, 1973.

[14] J. M. Bland and D. G. Altman, "Agreed statistics: measurement method comparison," *Anesthesiology*, vol. 116, no. 1, pp. 182–185, 2012.

[15] A. Field, *Discovering Statistics Using SPSS*, SAGE, London, UK, 3rd edition, 2009.

[16] J. Cohen, *Statistical Power Analysis for the Behavioral Sciences*, Chapter 3, Lawrence Erlbaum Associates, New Jersey, NY, USA, 2nd edition, 1988.

[17] H. Ettekoven van and C. Lucas, "Efficacy of physiotherapy including a craniocervical training programme for tension-type headache, a randomized clinical trial," *Cephalalgia*, vol. 26, no. 8, pp. 983–991, 2006.

[18] N. Schitz, W. Neumann, and R. Oppermann, "Stress, burnout and locus of control in German nurses," *International Journal of Nursing Studies*, vol. 37, no. 2, pp. 95–99, 2000.

[19] T. A. Pellino and M. T. Oberst, "Perception of control and appraisal of illness in chronic low back pain," *Orthopedic Nursing*, vol. 11, no. 1, pp. 22–26, 1992.

[20] F. H. Walkey, "Internal control, powerful others, and chance: a confirmation of Levenson's factor structure," *Journal of Personality Assessment*, vol. 43, no. 5, pp. 532–535, 1979.

[21] M. A. Morowatisharifabad, S. S. Mahmoodabad, M. H. Baghianimoghadam, and N. R. Tonekboni, "Relationship between locus of control and adherence to diabetes regimen in a sample of Iranians," *International Journal Of Diabetes in Developing Countries*, vol. 30, no. 1, pp. 27–32, 2010.

[22] E. Heyman, F. X. Gamelin, M. Goekint et al., "Intense exercise increases circulating endocannabinoid and BDNF levels in humans–possible implications for reward and depression," *Psychoneuroendocrinology*, vol. 37, no. 6, pp. 844–851, 2012.

[23] G. Bronfort, W. J. J. Assendelft, R. Evans, M. Haas, and L. Bouter, "Efficacy of spinal manipulation for chronic headache: a systematic review," *Journal of Manipulative and Physiological Therapeutics*, vol. 24, no. 7, pp. 457–466, 2001.

[24] N. Nilsson and G. Bove, "Evidence that tension-type headache and cervicogenic headache are distinct disorders," *Journal of Manipulative and Physiological Therapeutics*, vol. 23, no. 4, pp. 288-289, 2000.

# 5

# The Patient-Reported Outcomes Thermometer –5-Item Scale (5T-PROs): Validation of a New Tool for the Quick Assessment of Overall Health Status in Painful Rheumatic Diseases

**Fausto Salaffi** ⓘ,[1] **Marco Di Carlo** ⓘ,[1] **Marina Carotti** ⓘ,[2] and **Sonia Farah** ⓘ[1]

[1]*Rheumatological Clinic, Università Politecnica delle Marche, Jesi, Ancona, Italy*
[2]*Department of Radiology, Università Politecnica delle Marche, Ancona, Italy*

Correspondence should be addressed to Marco Di Carlo; dica.marco@yahoo.it

Academic Editor: Parisa Gazerani

*Objective.* To investigate the construct validity, reliability (internal consistency and retest reliability), and feasibility of the patient-reported outcomes thermometer–5-item scale (5T-PROs), a new tool to measure overall health status in patients with painful chronic rheumatic diseases such as rheumatoid arthritis (RA), psoriatic arthritis (PsA), axial spondyloarthritis (axialSpA), and fibromyalgia (FM). *Methods.* Consecutive patients have been involved in this study. The following analyses were performed to establish the validity of the 5T-PROs: (1) principal component factor analysis was used to identify the presence of a relatively small number of underlying latent factors than can be used to represent relations among sets of many variables; (2) Cronbach's alpha was calculated as an indicator of internal consistency; and (3) Pearson product-moment correlations were conducted to assess the convergent validity. The 5T-PROs was also administered a second time (two weeks after the initial administration) to a subset of sample ($n = 426$) to allow for calculation of test-retest reliability. We used the intraclass correlation coefficient (ICC) as an estimate of test-retest reliability. Additionally, discriminant validity was tested using analysis of variance (ANOVA) with Bonferroni post hoc multiple comparisons, in different disease conditions. Feasibility was analyzed by the time taken in completing the 5T-PROs and the proportion of patients able to complete the 5 item. *Results.* 1,199 patients (572 with RA, 251 with axialSpA, 150 with PsA, and 226 with FM) were examined. The mean age was 55.7 (standard deviation: 13.1; range: 20 to 80) years. Factor analysis yielded two factors which accounted for 62.54% of the variance of the 5T-PROs. The first factor "Symptom Summary Score" (35.57% of the variance) revealed a good internal consistency (alpha = 0.88); the internal consistency of the second factor "Psychological Summary Score" (26.97% of the variance) was moderate (alpha = 0.69). The reliability of the whole instrument was good (alpha = 0.82). A very high correlation was obtained between Symptom Summary Score and SF-36 PCS and between pain thermometer intensity and SF-36 bodily pain. For all five items and summary scale scores of the SF-36, there was strong evidence that the mean rank of the scores differs significantly between the groups (Kruskal–Wallis tests, $p < 0.001$). Discriminant validity, assessed by comparing the 5T-PRO dimensions in patients with different states of disease activity, showed that the 5T-PROs show moderate association with the presence of comorbidities. It was also noted that it was inversely correlated ($p = 0.01$) to years of formal education. *Conclusion.* The 5T-PROs is easily administered, reliable and a valid instrument for evaluating the extensive multidimensional impact associated with chronic painful rheumatic conditions.

## 1. Introduction

Rheumatoid arthritis (RA), axial spondyloarthritis (axial-SpA), and psoriatic arthritis (PsA) are common chronic painful rheumatic diseases characterized by systemic inflammation, joint destruction, and impairment in physical function and health-related quality of life (HRQoL).

Fibromyalgia (FM) is a chronic disease characterized by muscle pain and other multisymptoms such as fatigue, morning stiffness, memory, and mood issues. RA is the most frequent inflammatory rheumatic disease, with a prevalence of 0.5% in the general adult population [1]. Patients with active RA showed to suffer deficits in HRQoL, along with a number of limitations in physical functioning and mental health dimensions: pain, fatigue, and disability are common challenges that may subsequently lead to psychological distress [2]. Furthermore, patients with RA who have significant functional disability have a 3-fold increased risk of mortality compared with that of the general population, and this risk is comparable with that of individuals of the general population in the highest quintile for systolic and diastolic blood pressure, cholesterol level, or pack-years of smoking [3]. AxialSpA has a heterogeneous clinical presentation and does not have a single pathognomonic feature that distinguishes the disease from other conditions with similar symptoms. In daily rheumatological practice, a diagnosis of axialSpA is generally made in patients with chronic back pain on the basis of a combination of symptoms from medical history, physical examination, laboratory investigations, and findings on imaging. Similar to other chronic diseases, axialSpA can affect quality of life, morbidity, mortality, participation in paid and unpaid work, and healthcare costs [4]. PsA is an inflammatory peripheral and/or axial arthritis associated with psoriasis, usually seronegative for rheumatoid factor. In Italy, it has been estimated to be 36% in psoriatic subjects and 0.42% in general population [1]. In addition to the peripheral joint disease, patients with PsA have a debilitating skin disease, and up to 50% may also have spinal disease [5]. Compared to RA and ankylosing spondylitis (AS), there is less information about the burden of illness in PsA [6, 7]. Although considered a benign disease in the majority of cases given in previous reports or in population-based samples [8], clinical cohort studies described PsA as a progressive, disabling disease, particularly when polyarticular peripheral arthritis is present [9]. FM affects approximately 2-3% of the general population (more than 90% of the patients are female), and usually pain is the most important symptom [1, 10]. FM has a deep impact on global well-being [8] and has been found to be associated with high rates of use of healthcare resource and an increased risk of being unable to work [11]. Traditional methods of evaluation, focused on the musculoskeletal system and measures of impairment, may fail to describe the extensive multidimensional issues associated with chronic painful rheumatic conditions. Consideration of HRQoL has become increasingly important on decisions regarding resource allocation, intervention design, and pharmacological treatment with biologic agents of individuals with chronic inflammatory disabling conditions [12, 13]. Improvements in pain, fatigue, physical function, emotional well-being, and patient global ratings of health are often more important and meaningful in disease assessment than improvements in composite disease activity measures [14–16]. The relevance of patients preference is highlighted by the Outcome Measures in Rheumatology (OMERACT) [17, 18], by the American College of Rheumatology (ACR) (http://www.rheumatology.org/Practice/Clinical/Clinical_Support/2015), by the European League Against Rheumatism recommendations (EULAR), by the Group for Research and Assessment of Psoriasis and Psoriatic Arthritis (GRAPPA) [19, 20], by the Assessment in Spondyloarthritis International Society (ASAS) [21], and in the US Food and Drug Administration guidance

[22]. All the scientific societies underline the importance of including clinically relevant patient-reported outcomes (PROs) when designing clinical trials in rheumatic diseases [23–26].

The increasing focus on PROs in rheumatology has had the positive effect of giving prominence to the views and experiences of patients [14].

PROs have been implemented globally and have correlated significantly with objective values in rheumatologic diseases and other chronic pathologies (i.e., cancer, asthma, hypertension, heart disease, stroke, psychiatric illness, migraines, and diabetes) [27–29]. Despite the proliferation of tools and the burgeoning theoretical literature devoted to these measurements, no unified approach has been devised for PROs application in clinical practice, and little agreement has been attained about mean this lack of standardization of outcome measures, limiting the usefulness of clinical trial evidence to inform healthcare decisions; moreover, PROs can be difficult to be administered, scored, and interpreted in clinical practice.

Of utmost importance is the graphic presentation that influences the psychometric properties of each instrument. Usually numerical rating scales (NRS) and verbal descriptor scales (VDS) are preferred for older adults, which may be find more difficulties with other types of scales [30]. The thermometer scales, a modified vertical VDS alongside a graphic thermometer, have also been validated as a measure for pain in older adults and are recommended and commonly used in clinical practice in inflammatory arthritis [31].

Time constrains usually hinder the evaluation of HRQoL through long and difficult to compute instruments. Thus, we developed the Patient-Reported Outcomes Thermometer–5-item scale (5T-PROs), a simple tool made of 5 "thermometers" combining NRS and VDS (Figure 1), exploring the main domains of HRQoL, namely, pain, fatigue, physical function, depression, and general health status.

The aims of this study were to investigate the construct validity, reliability (internal consistency and retest reliability), and feasibility of this new tool in patients suffering from chronic inflammatory joint diseases and FM.

## 2. Materials and Methods

*2.1. Study Population.* Participants at this study were part of an ongoing longitudinal project measuring rheumatic disease outcomes, started in 2005. This longitudinal project involves consecutive adult patients coming from the Rheumatological Clinic of the Università Politecnica delle Marche, Jesi (Ancona). The study population was represented by patients suffering from RA, PsA, axialSpA, and FM. All the diagnoses were made according to the international criteria for each disease [32–36].

All procedures performed were approved by the institutional review board (Comitato Etico Unico Regionale), and written informed consent for anonymous analysis of data was obtained from all individual participants.

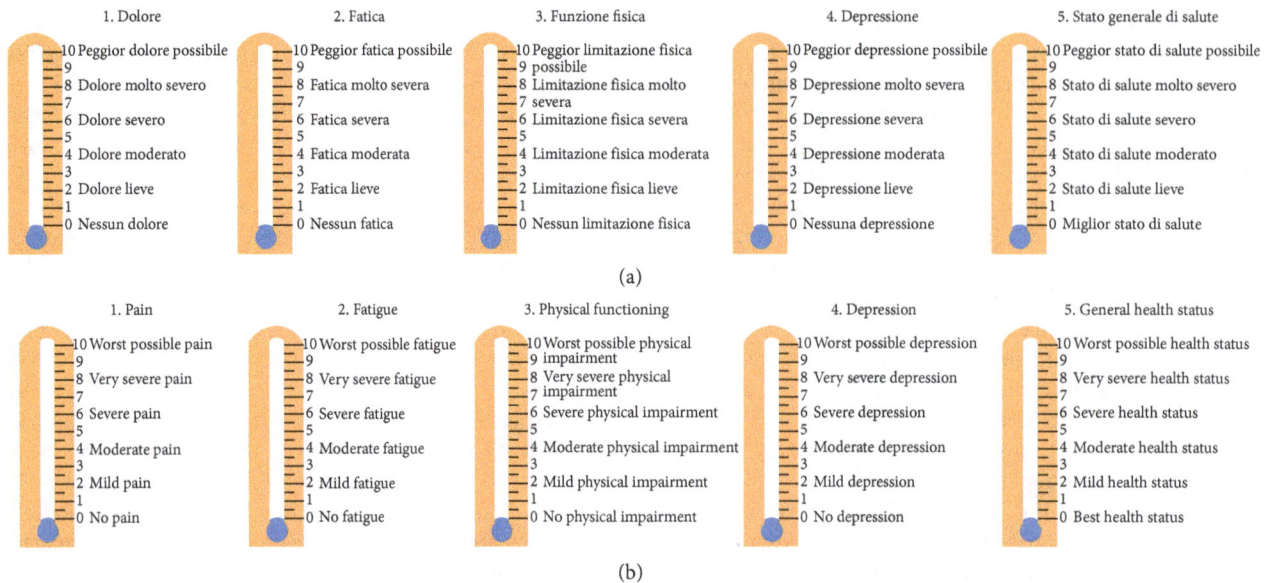

FIGURE 1: The Italian (a) and English (b) versions of the Patient-Reported Outcomes Thermometer–5-item scale (5T-PROs).

*2.2. Measurements and Instruments.* A comprehensive questionnaire package (including sociodemographic data, disease duration—years since fulfilment of the classification criteria of the disease, quality of life measuring tools, and disease-related variables) was administered to the patients. The sociodemographic variables assessed were age, sex, and level of education (primary; secondary; and high school/university). Furthermore, the presence of comorbidities were assessed using additional questions asking for the presence of nine specific comorbid conditions (hypertension, myocardial infarction, lower extremity arterial disease, major neurological problem, diabetes, gastrointestinal disease, chronic respiratory disease, kidney disease, and poor vision). The algebraic sum of positive responses was calculated for each subject, giving a comorbidity factor with a possible range from 0 to 9.

*2.3. Disease-Related Characteristics.* Disease-related characteristics included the measures for disease activity. The Clinical Disease Activity Index (CDAI) was used to evaluate disease activity in patients with RA [37], the Disease Activity index for PSoriatic Arthritis (DAPSA) was employed for peripheral PsA [38], while the Ankylosing Spondylitis Disease Activity Score C-reactive protein (ASDAS-CRP) was used to assess disease activity in patients with axialSpA [39]. FM was evaluated trough the Fibromyalgia Impact Questionnaire—revised version (FIQ-R) [40].

The CDAI is based on the simple sum of the swollen/tender joint counts-28 joints, along with patient and physician global assessment (PaGA and PhGA, respectively) of disease activity (on a 0–10 VAS scale) [37]. The CDAI result can range from 0 to 76. High disease activity is defined as a CDAI > 22, moderate disease activity with 10 < CDAI ≤ 22, low disease activity 2.8 < CDAI ≤ 10, and remission as a CDAI ≤ 2.8 [41].

DAPSA was adapted from the Disease Activity Index for Reactive Arthritis (DAREA), a score developed and validated to assess reactive arthritis. Developed from a clinical cohort [38] and validated using clinical trial data [42], DAPSA comprises 68 tender and 66 swollen joints count, PaGA, pain (0–10 NRS), and CRP in mg/dl. The final score is the sum of these variables. Recently, DAPSA cutoffs for disease activity states and treatment response have been derived using patient level data from three PsA randomized controlled trials [43]; therefore, this index is now usable and interpretable.

The ASDAS is the first validated disease activity index that considers together self-reported items and objective measures including back pain, duration of morning stiffness, peripheral joint pain and/or swelling, PaGA, and a serologic marker of inflammation (ESR or CPR) [39]. The cutoffs defining the disease activity ranks are as follows: <1.3 inactive disease, ≥1.3 and <2.1 moderate disease activity, ≥2.1 and <3.5 high disease activity, and ≥3.5 for very high disease activity.

The FIQ-R is an updated version of the FIQ [44]. The new version, validated in Italy for its use in patients with FM [45], has 21 items (all based on an 11-point NRS, with 10 being the "worst") and covers the three domains of function (9 items), overall impact (2 items), and symptoms (10 items). The questions are framed in the context of the previous seven days, and the total maximum score is 100 (higher scores indicating greater disease impact). The FIQ-R score is the sum of the three domain scores: the summed score for the 9-item function domain (range 0–90) is divided by three; the summed score for the 2-item overall impact domain (range 0–20) remains as it is; and the summed score for the 10-item symptom domain (range 0–100) is divided by two.

*2.4. Health-Related Quality of Life (HRQoL) Assessment.* HRQoL was assessed using well-validated generic instruments such as the self-administered SF-36 questionnaire [46] and EuroQoL-5 dimensions (EQ-5D) [47]. The

Short-Form 6-dimensions (SF-6D) was estimated from the SF-36 [48].

The 36 items are comprised in the eight scales cover the following health domains: physical functioning (PF), role limitations due to physical function (RP), bodily pain (BP), general health (GH), mental health (MH), role limitations due to emotional health (RE), social functioning (SF), and vitality (VT). One additional item pertains to health transition. The raw scores were encoded and reweighted (items summed and transformed to the eight 0–100 scales, with a final value ranging from 0 = worst health to 100 = best health) [46]. The SF-36 has been validated for use in Italy [49] and can be completed within 15 minutes by the majority of the subjects. Two psychometrical summary measures can be derived from SF-36: the physical and the mental component summary score (PCS and MCS) [46].

EQ-5D is directed to the domains of mobility, self-care, usual activities, pain/discomfort, and anxiety/depression. Each domain has one question, and each question has three levels: one denoting no problems and three denoting severe problems [47]. The Italian population-based values were used to convert patient responses to the health status classifier into a single index which produces scores from 1 to −0.38 [50, 51]. In addition, patients were asked to rate their current health status on a vertical, graduated 20 cm VAS (EQ-5D VAS), ranging from 0 (worst possible health state) to 100 (best possible health status).

Finally, the SF-6D was collected. Derived from the SF-36 [49], SF-6D is focused on six of the eight health domains: PF, role participation (combining RP and RE), SF, BP, MH, and VT. The SF-6D is calculated using a definite scoring function [48] in order to create a weighted index score ranging from 1.0, no difficulty in any dimensions (or perfect health), to 0.296 (severely impaired levels in all dimensions). Table 1 provides an overview of the HRQoL instruments.

*2.5. The Patient-Reported Outcomes Thermometer–5-Item-Scale (5T-PROs).* The 5T-PROs is a five-item measure which consists of thermometers with numerals displayed vertically from 0 to 10. It has a broader perspective and better coverage of the domains in the International Classification of Functioning, Disability and Health (ICF), and identified as important by people with rheumatic disorders [52, 53].

Patients rate the five thermometers with a recall of one week: 0 indicates no pain, fatigue, physical impairment, depression and best health status, and 10 indicates worst possible pain, fatigue, physical impairment, depression, and general health status. These five measures afford a simple and rapid administration and increased comprehension and completion rates. The 5T-PROs is a tool that can help both the person and staff to begin a conversation with each other about the wider range of difficulties, together with the services and resources that may be helpful in addressing them. The advantages of this tool are the brevity of the questionnaire, the ease of assessing the results, and its less-stigmatizing format. In this study, we administered the 5T-PROs using a single sheet of paper (Figure 1).

*2.6. Statistical Analysis.* The Kolmogorov–Smirnov test was used to assess distribution of the 5T-PROs, SF-36, EQ-5D, and EQ-6D scores. The interval measurements were normally distributed, and therefore several parametric tests were employed to analyze data. The critical values for significance were set at $p < 0.05$. Following standard guidelines for the evaluation of measurement properties of quality of life instruments [54–56], we tested validity, reliability, and feasibility of 5T-PROs. Construct validity was assessed by performing principal components factor analysis on individual 5T-PROs scales. An eigenvalue criterion of 1.0 was used to select factors, and the results are given in terms of the percentage of variance in the scale score explained by the principal factor. Convergent validity was tested by correlating (Pearson's $r$) the scores of the 5T-PRO subscales with the other measures applied in the study. One-way ANOVA was performed to test for differences. A particular subscale is expected to converge with the scores of those instruments targeting the same construct and to deviate from the scores given by instruments or scales assessing a different one (divergent validity). To investigate a possible influence of patient characteristics, such as age, gender, educational level, and the number of comorbid conditions on the 5T-PROs, the associations between the total score and these features were also analyzed. The internal structure and reliability of the 5T-PROs scales were evaluated by means of internal consistency (Chronbach's alpha coefficient) and test-retest reliability [55]. Chronbach's alpha statistic measures the overall correlation between items within a scale. It ranges from zero to 1, and values equal or greater than 0.80 indicate adequate internal consistency for a scale [57]. Inter-item correlations compares scores on individual items with the total score of the scale. Items with item-total correlations less than 0.4 should be considered as rejects. To evaluate reproducibility, 434 randomly selected patients (189 with RA, 67 with PsA, 45 with axialSpa and 133 with FM) completed the 5T-PROs twice with a time interval of 7 days. The opinions regarding the appropriate interval vary from an hour to a year depending on the task, but a test-retest interval of two to 14 days is common for this type of questionnaire [54]. Reproducibility concerns the degree to which repeated measurements in stable persons provide similar results. Test-retest reliability (reproducibility) was evaluated using intraclass correlation coefficient (ICC) [55], that assesses the correlation of scales at two different measure points. The values of ICC vary from 1 (perfectly reliable) to 0 (totally unreliable), and values above 0.80 were considered as evidence of excellent reliability [56]. The Bland and Altman method was used to quantify agreement, by calculating the mean difference (Mean Δ) between the two measurements and the standard deviation (SD) of this difference [58]. Finally, to assess the patient's acceptance and feasibility of 5T-PROs, the participants filled out an additional questionnaire. The patient's acceptance was established by asking the following questions: (a) is the 5T-PROs easy to use? (b) Is the 5T-PROs format user-friendly? (c) Is the 5T-PROs easy to understand? (d) The 5T-PROs works well (is reliable)? (e) In general, are

TABLE 1: Overview of the health-related quality of life assessment instruments.

| Instrument | Description | Scale |
|---|---|---|
| EQ-5D domains* | (i) Subject report, addressing 5 questions:<br>(a) Mobility<br>(b) Self-care<br>(c) Usual activities<br>(d) Pain/discomfort<br>(e) Anxiety/depression | 0-1 points<br><br>(Worst to best) |
| EQ-5D VAS | (i) Vertical 20 cm used to score the patient's health perception | 100 representing the best and 0 the worst health |
| SF-36 domains* | (i) Patient report, 36 items<br>(a) Physical functioning<br>(b) Role-Physical<br>(c) Bodily Pain<br>(d) General health<br>(e) Vitality<br>(f) Role-emotional<br>(g) Social functioning<br>(h) Mental health | 0–100 mm<br><br><br>(Worst to best) |
| SF-36 PCS and MCS scores | (i) calculated based upon domain scores | Normative value: mean = 50, SD = 10 |
| SF-6D* | (i) Patient report, 11 items<br>(a) Physical functioning<br>(b) Role participation (RP and RE)<br>(c) Bodily pain<br>(d) Vitality<br>(e) Mental health | 0-1 points |

*Based on transformed scale scores. Abbreviations: HRQoL = health-related quality of life; MCS = mental component summary; PCS = physical component summary; SF-36 = 36-Item Short-Form Health Survey version 2; EQ-5D = EuroQol-five dimensions; SF-6D = Short-Form-six dimensions.

you satisfied with using the 5T-PROs? Further, feasibility was evaluated by the time taken to complete the 5T-PROs, which was recorded by a research assistant using a stopwatch and the time taken to complete the questionnaire. Finally, we assessed the presence of floor and ceiling effects, by examining the frequency of the highest and lowest possible scores at baseline. Floor effects were considered to be present if more than 15% of the patients had a minimal score at the baseline, and the ceiling effects were considered to be present if 15% of the patients had a maximum baseline score [59]. Data were stored in a FileMaker 7.0 relational database and has been processed with the SPSS 11.0 and MedCalc 17.8 for statistical software packages for Windows XP.

## 3. Results

*3.1. Demographic and Clinical Data.* Of the 1,298 patients enrolled, 1,199 (92.4%) subjects (572 with RA, 251 with axialSpa, 150 with PsA, and 226 with FM) completed the clinical assessment and the questionnaires, ninety-nine (7.6%) were excluded because of incomplete data and nonrespondents were significantly older ($p < 0.001$). The majority of the sample were women with primary or secondary educational level. The respondents' age ranged from 19 to 80 years, with a mean of 55.5 years (SD = 12.2 years). The age and sex distributions of the patients with RA, PsA, axialSpA, and FM were significantly different

($p < 0.001$). The mean (±SD) age was 57.6 ± 14.5 years for RA, 60.4 ± 12.1 years for PsA, 53.1 ± 10.4 years for axialSpA, and 50.7 ± 10.1 years for FM. Slightly more than one quarter of the patients with RA, more than two thirds of the patients with axialSpA, and slightly less than an half of the patients with PsA were male. In FM patients, only 16.4% were male. Mean (±SD) disease duration was similar in PsA and axialSpA (4.6 ± 3.3 and 4.5 ± 3.2 years, respectively), while it was higher ($p = 0.02$) in RA (6.7 ± 4.4 years) and in FM (5.9 ± 4.1 years). The educational level among patients with RA was lower than among patients with PsA and axialSpA ($p < 0.02$). Of the 1,199 subjects enrolled, 867 (72.3%) reported one or more medical comorbidities. The frequency of multimorbidity was higher in those subjects classified with PsA followed by that of those classified as RA, axialSpA, and with FM. The most prevalent combinations were with arterial hypertension (10.8%), hypercholesterolemia (7.9%), digestive diseases (6.3%), cardiologic diseases (5.4%), and diabetes mellitus (3.5%). The demographic and disease characteristics of patients enrolled in the study are shown in Table 2.

*3.2. Disease Activity and Health-Related Quality of Life.* Table 3 provides statistics summaries: the mean and SD for each of the aspects of health status covered by the SF-36, EQ-5D, SF-6D, and 5T-PROs and by the disease activity indices for the different diagnostic groups.

TABLE 2: Characteristics of patients with rheumatoid arthritis (RA), psoriatic arthritis (PsA), axial spondyloarthritis (AxialSpA), and fibromyalgia (FM).

| | RA (n = 572) | PsA (n = 150) | AxialSpA (n = 251) | FM (n = 226) |
|---|---|---|---|---|
| Women (n, %) | 412 (72.0) | 102 (68.0) | 99 (39,8) | 189 (83.6) |
| Age, years (mean (±SD)) | 57.6 (14.5) | 60.4 (12.1) | 53.1 (10.4) | 50.7 (10.1) |
| Disease duration, years (mean (±SD)) | 6.7 (4.4) | 4.6 (3.3) | 4.5 (3.2) | 5.9 (4.1) |
| Educational level, years (mean (±SD)) | 11.3 (3.6) | 8.5 (3.5) | 8.6 (3.7) | 9.2 (3.8) |
| Comorbid conditions, n (%) | | | | |
| (i) None | 161 (28.1) | 25 (16.6) | 75 (29.8) | 71 (31.4) |
| (ii) 1 | 98 (17.1) | 39 (26.0) | 108 (43.0) | 99 (43.8) |
| (iii) 2 | 255 (44.6) | 45 (30.0) | 48 (19.2) | 38 (16.8) |
| (iv) 3 or more | 58 (10.1) | 41 (27.3) | 20 (7.9) | 18 (8.0) |

TABLE 3: Distribution analysis of the Patient-Reported Outcomes Thermometer–5-item scale (5T-PROs) total score.

| 5T-PROs total score | |
|---|---|
| Lowest value | 16.38 |
| Highest value | 40.99 |
| Arithmetic mean | 26.46 |
| 95% CI for the mean | 26.27 to 26.66 |
| Median | 26.50 |
| 95% CI for the median | 26.21 to 26.60 |
| Variance | 11.91 |
| Standard deviation | 3.45 |
| Relative standard deviation | 0.13 (13.04%) |
| Standard error of the mean | 0.099 |
| Coefficient of Skewness | 0.23 ($P = 0.0010$) |
| Coefficient of Kurtosis | 0.57 ($P = 0.0010$) |
| Kolmogorov–Smirnov test for normal distribution | Accept normality ($P = 0.097$) |

*3.3. Score Distribution.* The number of patients receiving floor or ceiling effects was low for the 5T-PROs subscales, with one exception. The 5T-PROs total score distribution is described in Table 3. Figure 2 presents the estimates of central tendency and distributions for 5T-PROs total score and domains. The bar on the left of each graph represents the number of subjects with a score of 0 (floor effect), and the bar on the right represents the number of subjects with a maximum possible score (ceiling effect).

All the eight health concepts of the SF-36 and those of utility scores (EQ-5D, EQ-VAS and SF-6D) were impaired in the four categories of rheumatic disorders (Table 4). Figure 3 compares the scores in each domain of the 5T-PROs in the different diseases. Overall, the dimensions typically affected were depression and general global health; the disease with the worst HRQoL for those dimensions was FM. The mean depression score of FM patients was 6.87 (SD = 0.77). The mean 5T-PROs global health status of FM patients was 6.00 (SD = 0.98). Regarding the HRQoL dimensions involving physical function, patients with RA score generally higher than the FM patients (Figure 3).

*3.4. Construct Validity.* Factor analysis was carried out to examine the factorial structure of the Italian version of the 5T-PROs. Items were accepted on the final factors if they had a loading of more than 0.50 on the corresponding factor. The analysis revealed a two-factor solution (eigenvalues 1.819 and 1.308) (Table 5). The first factor, namely, the 5T-PRO physical summary score, accounted for the 35.57% of the explained variance and represents the patients rating of the grade of pain, disability, and global health perception in different areas of daily life he or she is suffering from. The second factor, the 5T-PROs psychological summary score, accounted for the 26.97% of the explained variance, representing the patients rating of his medium emotional complaints.

Table 5 shows the loading of each question after varimax rotation with Kaiser normalization on the two factors. Each factor loading represents the correlation between that item and the underlying factor. Both the two dimensions of 5T-PROs (physical and psychological summary scores) correlated significantly with each other ($r = 0.548$; $p < 0.001$).

*3.5. Internal Reliability.* Cronbach's alpha was 0.81 for the 5T-PROs. Both subscales of the 5T-PROs showed satisfying to good internal consistency. Cronbach's alpha was 0.81 for the first factor (physical summary score) and 0.85 for the second factor (psychological summary score). Item-total correlations, which are another measure of internal consistency, compare scores on individual items with the total score of the scale. Items with item-total correlations less than 0.4 should be considered for rejection. In our analysis, item-total correlations for the subscales were moderate up to high (Table 6).

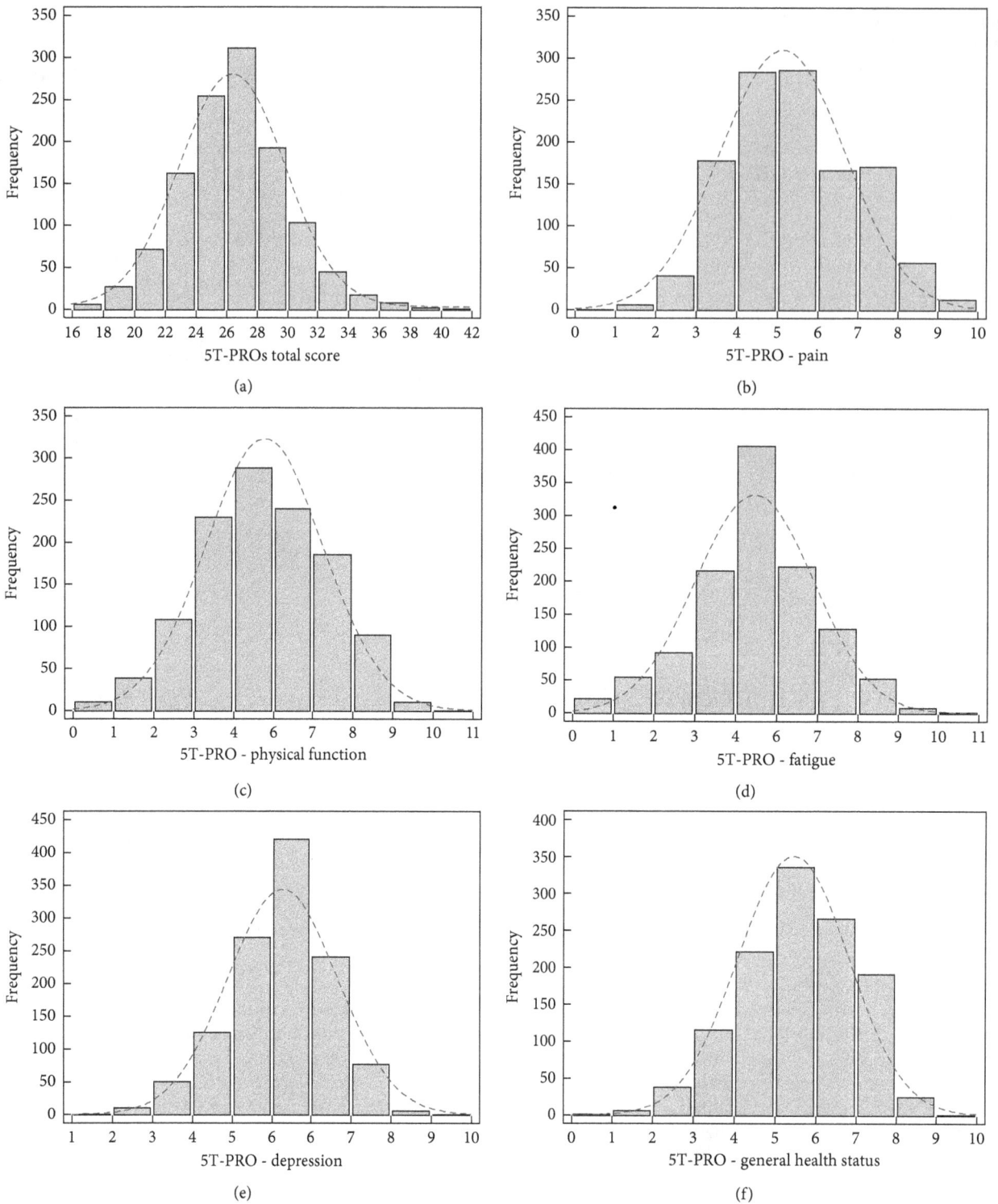

Figure 2: Distribution of the Patient-Reported Outcomes Thermometer–5-item scale (5T-PROs): Total score (a) and the five domains (b)–(f) in 1,199 patients with chronic rheumatic diseases. Floor effect is noted by the percentage of values at 0 for each item. Ceiling effect is indicated by the percentage of values at 100. For descriptive purposes, normal distribution, displayed as vertical lines, has been superimposed on the histogram.

*3.6. Reproducibility.* Equivalence between the two administrations of the 5T-PROs was measured by calculating single-measurement ICCs between corresponding scales.

The ICCs ranged from 0.822 ("fatigue" domain) to 0.913 ("general health status" domain) for all the domains in the 5T-PRO, indicating excellent agreement between two

TABLE 4: Summary statistics table of the 36-Item Short-Form Health Survey (SF-36) subscales, of the utility questionnaires, of the Patient-Reported Outcomes Thermometer–5-item scale (5T-PROs) subscales, and of the disease activity indices.

| | RA (n = 572) | | PsA (n = 150) | | AxialSpA (n = 251) | | FM (n = 226) | |
|---|---|---|---|---|---|---|---|---|
| | Mean | SD | Mean | SD | Mean | SD | Mean | SD |
| SF-36 subscales | | | | | | | | |
| BP | 28.63 | 16.33 | 38.19 | 19.04 | 44.29 | 17.47 | 35.56 | 9.69 |
| RP | 29.19 | 14.86 | 32.58 | 23.26 | 38.42 | 28.17 | 38.81 | 17.24 |
| GH | 43.60 | 19.46 | 45.69 | 18.18 | 47.31 | 20.96 | 34.41 | 11.09 |
| PF | 39.14 | 19.83 | 46.69 | 21.31 | 52.13 | 20.24 | 49.96 | 17.35 |
| MH | 49.05 | 22.79 | 49.46 | 20.36 | 53.55 | 20.95 | 36.91 | 13.32 |
| RE | 36.25 | 40.83 | 33.30 | 36.02 | 43.09 | 30.54 | 36.86 | 23.99 |
| SF | 46.16 | 20.81 | 48.80 | 22.21 | 52.02 | 19.49 | 39.64 | 13.82 |
| VT | 43.63 | 17.30 | 47.86 | 17.29 | 48.10 | 17.68 | 38.51 | 11.81 |
| SF-36 MCS | 44.74 | 12.23 | 41.23 | 11.33 | 40.75 | 10.18 | 32.12 | 7.50 |
| SF-36 PCS | 30.64 | 6.20 | 34.18 | 6.71 | 36.88 | 8.12 | 38.85 | 4.78 |
| Utility questionnaires | | | | | | | | |
| SF-6D | 0.56 | 0.07 | 0.60 | 0.07 | 0.62 | 0.07 | 0.56 | 0.05 |
| EQ-5D | 0.43 | 0.14 | 0.51 | 0.14 | 0.54 | 0.13 | 0.45 | 0.11 |
| 5T-PROs | | | | | | | | |
| 5T-PROs pain | 5.03 | 1.57 | 5.17 | 1.46 | 5.09 | 1.58 | 5.34 | 1.448 |
| 5T-PROs fatigue | 4.77 | 1.60 | 4.78 | 1.72 | 4.82 | 1.77 | 5.37 | 1.06 |
| 5T-PROs physical function | 5.57 | 1.62 | 4.87 | 1.56 | 5.23 | 1.56 | 4.70 | 1.55 |
| 5T-PROs depression | 5.18 | 1.17 | 6.12 | 1.09 | 5.76 | 1.07 | 6.87 | 0.77 |
| 5T-PROs general health status | 5.65 | 1.39 | 5.13 | 1.29 | 4.65 | 1.26 | 6.00 | 0.92 |
| 5T-PROs total score | 26.23 | 3.51 | 26.08 | 3.24 | 25.57 | 3.08 | 28.31 | 3.16 |
| Disease activity indices | | | | | | | | |
| CDAI | 23.81 | 7.84 | | | | | | |
| DAPSA | | | 28.04 | 10.36 | | | | |
| ASDAS-CRP | | | | | 2.50 | 1.13 | | |
| FIQ-R | | | | | | | 50.01 | 16.0 |

Abbreviations: RA = rheumatoid arthritis; PsA = psoriatic arthritis; AxialSpA = axial spondyloarthritis; FM = fibromyalgia; SF-36 = 36-Item Short-Form Health Survey; BP = bodily pain; RP = role limitations due to physical function; GH = general health; PF = physical functioning; MH = mental health; RE = role limitations due to emotional health; SF = social functioning; VT = vitality; MCS = mental component summary score; PCS = physical component summary score; SF-6D = Short-Form 6-dimensions; EQ-5D = EuroQoL-5 dimensions; CDAI = Clinical Disease Activity Index; DAPSA = Disease Activity index for PSoriatic Arthritis; ASDAS-CRP = Ankylosing Spondylitis Disease Activity Score C-reactive protein; FIQ-R = Fibromyalgia Impact Questionnaire Revised Version.

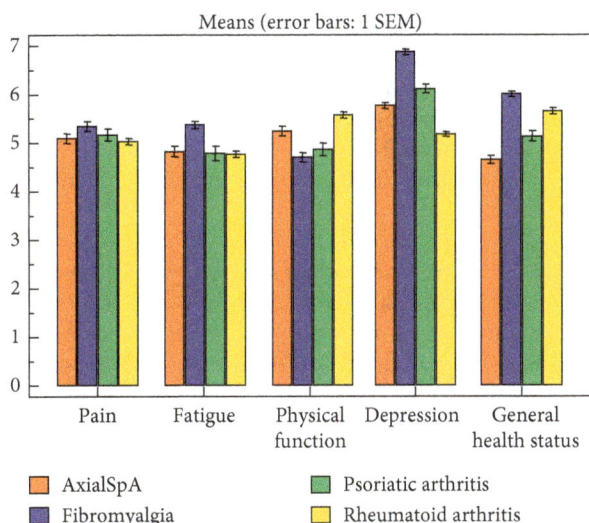

FIGURE 3: The Patient-Reported Outcomes Thermometer–5-item scale (5T-PROs) domains in the four rheumatic disorders. Bars to show mean and SEM of pain, physical function, fatigue, depression, and global health status in patients with axial spondyloarthritis, psoriatic arthritis, fibromyalgia, and rheumatoid arthritis.

administrations (Table 7). All scales met Cicchetti's criterion of 0.75 [60].

Agreement between scores was also illustrated by Bland and Altman plots, in which the difference between scores was plotted on the $y$-axis against the average of scores on the $x$-axis. According to Bland and Altman analysis, there was no systematic error in scores of 5T-PROs (Figure 4).

3.7. Convergent Validity. In testing for convergent validity between instruments, we found that correlation coefficients for the comparable dimension of the 5T-PROs and the SF-36 questionnaires ranged from 0.049 to 0.626. Generally, higher significant correlations were seen when comparing 5T-PROs scales to SF-36 scales with a high ability to measure similar health concept (convergent construct validity) (Table 8).

Of special interest are the correlations between the 5T-PROs total score and disease activity indices such as CDAI for RA ($r = -0.709$; $p < 0.001$), DAPSA for PsA ($r = 0.479$; $p < 0.001$), and ASDAS-CRP for axialSpA ($r = 0.549$; $p < 0.001$), and between 5T-PROs total score and FIQ-R for FM ($r = 0.722$; $p < 0.0001$). Positive correlations between the

TABLE 5: Principal component analysis—total variance explained.

| Component | Initial eigenvalues | | | Extraction sums of squared loadings | | | Rotation sums of squared loadings | | |
|---|---|---|---|---|---|---|---|---|---|
| | Total | % of variance | Cumulative % | Total | % of variance | Cumulative % | Total | % of variance | Cumulative % |
| 1 | 1.819 | 36.373 | 36.373 | 1.819 | 36.373 | 36.373 | 1.778 | 35.569 | 35.569 |
| 2 | 1.308 | 26.169 | 62.542 | 1.308 | 26.169 | 62.542 | 1.349 | 26.973 | 62.542 |
| 3 | 0.903 | 18.068 | 80.610 | | | | | | |
| 4 | 0.568 | 11.359 | 91.969 | | | | | | |
| 5 | 0.402 | 8.031 | 100.000 | | | | | | |

Extraction method: principal component analysis.

TABLE 6: Principal component analysis—rotated component matrix.

| Rotated component matrix[a] | | |
|---|---|---|
| 5T-PROs | Component | |
| | Factor 1 physical component | Factor 2 psychological component |
| 5T-PROs pain | 0.865 | 0.112 |
| 5T-PROs fatigue | 0.158 | 0.755 |
| 5T-PROs function | 0.823 | −0.155 |
| 5T-PROs depression | −0.053 | 0.845 |
| 5T-PROs general health status | 0.571 | 0.165 |

Extraction method: principal component analysis. Rotation method: varimax with Kaiser normalization. Abbreviation: 5T-PROs = Patient-Reported Outcomes Thermometer–5-item scale.

TABLE 7: Agreement between the Patient-Reported Outcomes Thermometer–5-item-scale (5T-PROs) scores assessed by intraclass correlation coefficient (ICC).

| 5T-PROs | Intraclass correlation coefficient | 95% Confidence Interval |
|---|---|---|
| 5T-PROs pain | 0.871 | 0.857 to 0.885 |
| 5T-PROs fatigue | 0.822 | 0.799 to 0.842 |
| 5T-PROs function | 0.871 | 0.856 to 0.885 |
| 5T-PROs depression | 0.844 | 0.826 to 0.861 |
| 5T-PROs general health status | 0.913 | 0.896 to 0.927 |

total 5T-PROs score were also found with the number of comorbidities ($r = 0.93$; $p = 0.001$) and educational level ($r = 101$; $p = 0.001$).

*3.8. Acceptance and Feasibility of 5T-PROs.* The mean time to complete the 5T-PROs was 3.1 ± 1.3 minutes (range 2.2–9.3 minutes). Overall, the 5T-PROs was correctly completed by most respondents. Less than 3% of each of the 5T-PROs questions had missing values. In subjects who expressed a preference, the majority rated that the tool was easy to fulfill. Patients' preference was not related to sex or age.

## 4. Discussion

There is growing recognition of the importance of placing patients at the center of healthcare by developing patient-centered care models and integrating patient-valued outcomes into shared decision-making [61]. PROs contribute fundamental information from the point of view of people that live with a chronic painful disease, and its treatments about the status of or a change in their physical, emotional, and social health outcomes [62] have become increasingly popular as measurement instruments in epidemiological studies.

In RA and SpA, three PROs have been included within the American College of Rheumatology core set of outcome measures recommended for use in randomized clinical trials [63] as a part of the OMERACT PsA Core Domain Set [64] and the International Classification of Functioning, Disability and Health Core Set for AS [65] and clinical care including global ratings of disease activity or health, pain, and physical function; more recently, fatigue and emotional distress also has been recommended for inclusion [25, 63, 66, 67].

Pain is the most prominent symptom in the majority of the subjects with chronic musculoskeletal conditions, and is the most important determinant of disability. Accurate assessment of pain intensity, which is a necessary prerequisite to rational choice of medical and rehabilitation interventions, represents a clinically challenging proposition. In recent years, several studies began to address the psychometric properties of a variety of pain intensity assessment scales. Among them, the pain thermometer, a modified vertical VDS alongside a graphic thermometer, has also been validated as a measure for pain in older adults [68]. A growing number of studies showed that pain is the strongest factor driving the patient global assessment in inflammatory rheumatic diseases [68, 69].

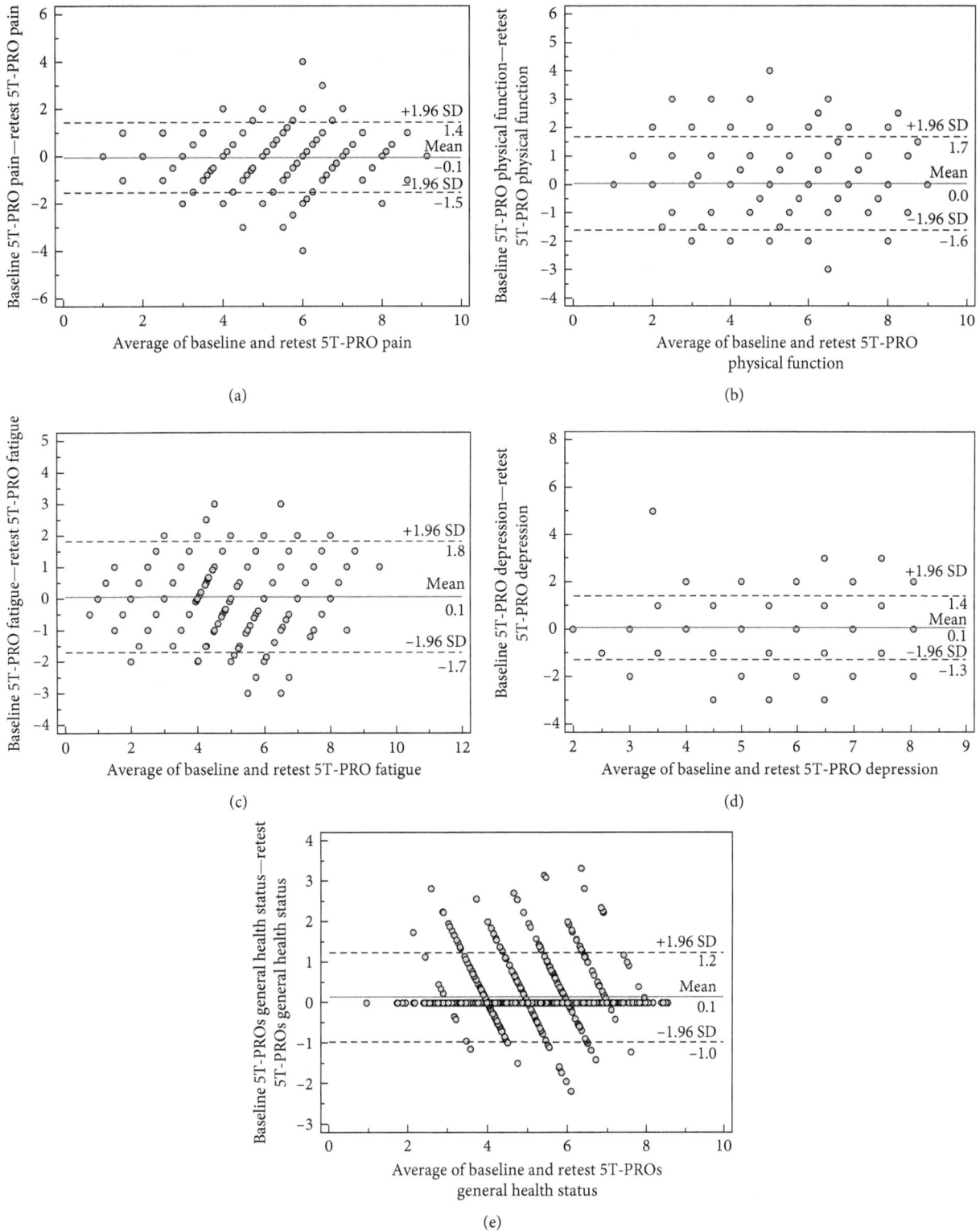

FIGURE 4: Bland and Altman plot of repeatability with the differences in the Patient-Reported Outcomes Thermometer–5-item scale (5T-PROs). Subscales values ((a) pain; (b) physical function; (c) fatigue; (d) depression; (e) general health status) plotted against average values for the 434 randomly selected patients (189 with rheumatoid arthritis, 67 with psoriatic arthritis, 45 with axial spondyloarthritis, and 133 with fibromyalgia) who completed the 5T-PROs twice with a time interval of 7 days. Ninety-five percent of the differences against the means were less than two standard deviations (SD; dotted lines).

TABLE 8: Convergent construct validity analysis: correlation matrix of the Patient-Reported Outcomes Thermometer–5-item scale (5T-PROs) component scores and their components versus the eight SF-36 subscales.

| | BP | GH | PF | RP | RE | MH | SF | VT | 5T-PROs depression | 5T-PROs fatigue | 5T-PROs physical function | 5T-PROs global health |
|---|---|---|---|---|---|---|---|---|---|---|---|---|
| GH | 0.164 | | | | | | | | | | | |
| | <0.001 | | | | | | | | | | | |
| PF | 0.392 | 0.289 | | | | | | | | | | |
| | <0.001 | <0.001 | | | | | | | | | | |
| RP | 0.251 | 0.163 | 0.425 | | | | | | | | | |
| | <0.001 | <0.001 | <0.001 | | | | | | | | | |
| RE | 0.240 | 0.308 | 0.313 | 0.311 | | | | | | | | |
| | <0.001 | <0.001 | <0.001 | <0.001 | | | | | | | | |
| | 1199 | 1199 | 1199 | | | | | | | | | |
| MH | 0.184 | 0.479 | 0.309 | 0.124 | 0.411 | | | | | | | |
| | <0.001 | <0.001 | <0.001 | <0.001 | <0.001 | | | | | | | |
| SF | 0.218 | 0.254 | 0.295 | 0.101 | 0.252 | 0.460 | | | | | | |
| | <0.001 | <0.001 | <0.001 | <0.001 | <0.001 | <0.001 | | | | | | |
| VT | 0.206 | 0.395 | 0.346 | 0.178 | 0.373 | 0.636 | 0.357 | | | | | |
| | <0.001 | <0.001 | <0.001 | <0.001 | <0.001 | <0.001 | <0.001 | | | | | |
| 5T-PROs depression | 0.049 | −0.352 | −0.054 | 0.058 | −0.322 | −0.626 | −0.377 | −0.507 | | | | |
| | 0.088 | <0.001 | 0.061 | 0.045 | <0.001 | <0.001 | <0.001 | <0.001 | | | | |
| 5T-PROs fatigue | 0.148 | 0.258 | 0.310 | 0.211 | 0.275 | 0.385 | 0.152 | 0.679 | −0.272 | | | |
| | <0.001 | <0.001 | <0.001 | <0.001 | <0.001 | <0.001 | <0.001 | <0.001 | <0.001 | | | |
| 5T-PROs physical function | −0.039 | 0.124 | −0.072 | 0.028 | 0.099 | 0.134 | 0.071 | 0.141 | −0.204 | 0.132 | | |
| | 0.174 | <0.001 | 0.012 | 0.333 | 0.001 | <0.001 | 0.013 | <0.001 | <0.001 | <0.001 | | |
| 5T- PROs global health | −0.480 | −0.432 | −0.632 | −0.260 | −0.377 | −0.568 | −0.443 | −0.462 | 0.342 | −0.268 | −0.109 | |
| | <0.001 | <0.001 | <0.001 | <0.001 | <0.001 | <0.001 | <0.001 | <0.001 | <0.001 | <0.001 | <0.001 | |
| 5T-PROs pain | 0.101 | 0.134 | 0.202 | 0.147 | 0.154 | 0.151 | 0.067 | 0.150 | −0.085 | 0.242 | 0.531 | −0.195 |
| | <0.001 | <0.001 | <0.001 | <0.001 | <0.001 | <0.001 | 0.020 | <0.001 | 0.003 | <0.001 | <0.001 | <0.001 |

The pain, and the consequent physical disability, affects social functioning and mental health, further diminishing the patient's quality of life [70].

The second factor considered is the fatigue, a frequent symptom in several inflammatory diseases. Overman et al. evaluating 30 rheumatic diseases showed that severe fatigue is a widespread and highly prevalent problem across rheumatic diseases [71] exacerbating pain and depressive symptoms that have a devastating effect on daily functioning and overall well-being [72]. Therefore, addressing the management of fatigue may also improve a larger cluster of symptoms, like decreased strength accompanied by a feeling of weariness, sleepiness, and irritability [73, 74]. In rheumatic diseases, the association between fatigue and pain has been well established [75, 76]. In RA, it is an important outcome to evaluate according to OMERACT [77], and it has been associated with the Disease Activity Score-28 joints (DAS28) and the CDAI. In SpA, fatigue is part of the Bath Ankylosing Spondylitis Disease Activity Index (BASDAI), and it is more strongly related to the disease process than patient-related variables [78]. Furthermore, fatigue is common in various rheumatic conditions, although most publications concerned fatigue in RA or SpA [79]. In these pathologies, the frequency of fatigue ranges from 42% to 80% depending on the definition and methods of assessment [76, 80, 81]. For 75% of patients with AS and 50% of those with RA, fatigue was considered severe [76, 82]. The fatigue experienced by people with AS is reported to be related to

disease activity, poorer functional ability, pain, stiffness, depression, lower global well-being, impaired working, and enthesitis [83–90]. Severe fatigue, more than just being tired, is a typical feature also of FM, affecting up to 4 out of 5 subjects. For patients with FM, fatigue is a complicated, multifactorial, and persistent, as evidenced by longitudinal studies over 5 years [71, 91]. Patients with FM may experience fatigue physically (lack of energy and physical exhaustion), emotionally (lack of motivation), cognitively (inability to think or concentrate), or via the symptom's impact on virtually any aspect of living, such as the ability to work, meet family needs, or engage in social activities [92].

Depression is more common in RA than in the general population and has been associated with increased pain, fatigue, reduced HRQoL, increased levels of physical disability, affected patient global assessment, and increased healthcare costs [93–102]. Depressed RA patients have poorer long-term outcomes and more comorbidities [103] and increased mortality levels [104]. However, prevalence estimates for depression in RA range between 9.5% [105] and 41.5% [106], making it difficult to establish the likely impact of depression in this patient group. Recently, psychological disorders such as depression have been frequently reported in patients with axialSpA [107]. Depression was associated with clinically significantly worse physical functioning, measured with both the Health Assessment Questionnaire and the SF-36 in RA [108]. Moussavi et al. found that the combination of depression and arthritis was cross-sectionally correlated with lower health status, more than depression alone, arthritis alone, or 2 somatic conditions [109]. Morris et al. showed that depression and even intermittent depression over time was associated with low self-reported health status and disability after 18 years [110]. Anxiety and depression are major factors affecting a HRQoL of patients with FM, and the associated symptoms (inability to concentrate, loss of motivation, disturbed sleep, fatigue, and pessimistic mood) may affect their response to treatment and rehabilitation programs [12–111]. Furthermore, negative mood seems to contribute to the persistence of chronic widespread pain [112].

A major use of health measurement scales is to detect health status changes over time, and a priority may be efficiency, i.e., responses achieved using the shortest possible questionnaire [113, 114]. A shorter version would further enhance its applicability in epidemiologic studies, clinical trials, and daily clinical practice [115] since short questionnaires result in improved patient compliance and response rates and are thought to improve the quality of the response [116–118].

Developing an instrument is an ongoing consuming process; effort, costs, and testing validity arise not from a single powerful experiment, but from a series of converging experiments [54]. The current study was conducted to examine and to validate the psychometric properties of the 5T-PROs, a five-item measure which consists of "thermometers" with numerals displayed vertically from 0 to 10, within a population of patients with RA, PsA, axialSpA, and FM. There were three main findings, the first regarding construct validity, specifically, factorial analysis in patients with rheumatic diseases generally supports the factorial validity of the 5T-PROs and suggests the use of separate scores for physical and psychological aspects. Altogether, they explain 69.2% of the variance of the entire questionnaire and indicate high construct validity. The second finding was that the final version of the 5T-PROs showed very good internal consistency; the Cronbach's alpha ranged from 0.74 to 0.91, and this indicates that the items measure the same general construct; and that the tool is stable. In addition, the 5T-PROs showed excellent test-retest reliability, with ICC ranging from 0.83 to 0.96. Our third finding concerned the convergent validity, in particular, the 5T-PROs total score was significantly associated with the physical and mental component scores of the SF-36 and clinical measures, and in fact satisfactory significant correlations were found between the PCS score and most of the 5T-PROs domains, especially mobility level, walking and bending, and pain.

This study has a number of strengths, including the use of a large sample of treatment-seeking individuals with rheumatic diseases. However, the study also has limitations; the main concern is that this study did not provide evidence for responsiveness to change or other psychometric tests. Secondly, criterion validity cannot be assessed because there is no previously accepted "gold standard" instrument for measuring the extensive multidimensional impact associated with chronic rheumatic conditions. Nevertheless, this study represents a structured and carefully conducted approach to validate the 5T-PROs in a large number of sample patients with RD. Finally, patients were recruited from tertiary center, and the results might not be generalizable to patients with chronic painful rheumatic disorders treated by a general practitioner or in small practices.

## 5. Conclusion

The present study is an initial step in evaluating psychometric properties of a new instrument to measure the multidimensional impact on patients with chronic rheumatic conditions. The 5T-PROs demonstrated to be feasible and easy to be administered, with reasonably good scale internal validity, reliability, and external validity in the primary setting. It covers most important areas of HRQoL, rarely assessed as primary end-point in studies and in the everyday clinical practice; the 5T-PROs might help clinicians with substantial advantages to assess fundamental health features in patients suffering from chronic painful diseases. However, its sensitivity to change needs still to be studied.

## References

[1] F. Salaffi, R. De Angelis, and W. Grassi, "Prevalence of musculoskeletal conditions in an Italian population sample: results of a regional community-based study. The MAPPING study," *Clinical and Experimental Rheumatology*, vol. 23, no. 6, pp. 819–828, 2005.

[2] L. Gettings, "Psychological well-being in rheumatoid arthritis: a review of the literature," *Musculoskeletal Care*, vol. 8, no. 2, pp. 99–106, 2010.

[3] M. Cross, E. Smith, D. Hoy et al., "The global burden of rheumatoid arthritis: estimates from the global burden of disease 2010 study," *Annals of the Rheumatic Diseases*, vol. 73, no. 7, pp. 1316–1322, 2014.

[4] R. Ramonda, A. Marchesoni, A. Carletto et al., "Patient-reported impact of spondyloarthritis on work disability and working life: the ATLANTIS survey," *Arthritis Research & Therapy*, vol. 1, no. 18, p. 78, 2016.

[5] A. Kerschbaumer, D. Baskar, J. S. Smolen, and D. Aletaha, "The effects of structural damage on functional disability in psoriatic arthritis," *Annals of the Rheumatic Diseases*, vol. 76, no. 12, pp. 2038–2045, 2017.

[6] W.-H. Boehncke WH and A. Menter, "Burden of disease: psoriasis and psoriatic arthritis," *American Journal of Clinical Dermatology*, vol. 14, no. 5, pp. 377–388, 2013.

[7] M. Di Carlo, A. Becciolini, V. Lato, C. Crotti, E. G. Favalli, and F. Salaffi, "The 12-item psoriatic arthritis impact of disease questionnaire: construct validity, reliability, and interpretability in a clinical setting," *Journal of Rheumatology*, vol. 44, no. 3, pp. 279–285, 2017.

[8] F. Salaffi, R. De Angelis, A. Stancati, W. Grassi, MArche Pain, and Prevalence INvestigation Group (MAPPING) study, "Health-related quality of life in multiple musculoskeletal conditions: a cross-sectional population based epidemiological study. II. The MAPPING study," *Clinical and Experimental Rheumatology*, vol. 23, no. 6, pp. 829–839, 2005.

[9] F. Salaffi, M. Carotti, S. Gasparini, M. Intorcia, and W. Grassi, "The health-related quality of life in rheumatoid arthritis, ankylosing spondylitis, and psoriatic arthritis: a comparison with a selected sample of healthy people," *Health and Quality of Life Outcomes*, vol. 7, no. 1, p. 25, 2009.

[10] A. J. Masi, L. M. Carmona, M. Valverde, B. Ribas, and the EPISER Study Group, "Prevalence and impact of fibromyalgia on function and quality of life in individuals from the general population: results from a nationwide study in Spain," *Clinical and Experimental Rheumatology*, vol. 26, no. 4, pp. 519–526, 2008.

[11] M. Kivimäki, P. Leino-Arjas, L. Kaila-Kangas et al., "Increased sickness absence among employees with fibromyalgia," *Annals of the Rheumatic Diseases*, vol. 66, no. 1, pp. 65–69, 2007.

[12] F. Salaffi, P. Sarzi-Puttini, A. Ciapetti, and F. Atzeni, "Assessment instruments for patients with fibromyalgia: properties, applications and interpretation," *Clinical and Experimental Rheumatology*, vol. 27, no. 56, pp. S92–S105, 2009.

[13] F. Salaffi, P. Sarzi-Puttini, A. Ciapetti, and F. Atzeni, "Clinimetric evaluations of patients with chronic widespread pain," *Best Practice & Research: Clinical Rheumatology*, vol. 25, no. 2, pp. 249–270, 2011.

[14] L. H. van Tuyl and M. Boers, "Patient-reported outcomes in core domain sets for rheumatic diseases," *Nature Reviews Rheumatology*, vol. 11, no. 12, pp. 705–712, 2015.

[15] L. Idzerda, T. Rader, P. Tugwell, and M. Boers, "Can we decide which outcomes should be measured in every clinical trial? A scoping review of the existing conceptual frameworks and processes to develop core outcome sets," *Journal of Rheumatology*, vol. 41, no. 5, pp. 986–993, 2014.

[16] P. S. Tugwell, I. F. Petersson, M. Boers et al., "Domains selection for patient-reported outcomes: current activities and options for future methods," *Journal of Rheumatology*, vol. 38, no. 8, pp. 1702–1710, 2011.

[17] K. Toupin-April, J. Barton, L. Fraenkel et al., "Toward the development of a core set of outcome domains to assess shared decision-making interventions in rheumatology: results from an OMERACT Delphi survey and consensus meeting," *Journal of Rheumatology*, vol. 44, no. 10, pp. 1544–1550, 2017.

[18] L. Trenaman, A. Boonen, F. Guillemin et al., "OMERACT quality-adjusted life-years (QALY) working group: do current QALY measures capture what matters to patients?," *Journal of Rheumatology*, vol. 44, no. 12, pp. 1899–1903, 2017.

[19] P. J. Mease, C. E. Antoni, D. D. Gladman, and W. J. Taylor, "Psoriatic arthritis assessment tools in clinical trials," *Annals of the Rheumatic Diseases*, vol. 64, no. 2, pp. ii49–ii54, 2005.

[20] A. Ogdie, M. de Wit, K. Callis Duffin et al., "Defining outcome measures for psoriatic arthritis: a report from the GRAPPA-OMERACT working group," *Journal of Rheumatology*, vol. 44, no. 5, pp. 697–700, 2017.

[21] U. Kiltz, D. van der Heijde, A. Boonen et al., "Measuring impairments of functioning and health in patients with axial spondyloarthritis by using the ASAS Health Index and the Environmental Item Set: translation and cross-cultural adaptation into 15 languages," *RMD Open*, vol. 4, no. 2, article e000311, 2016.

[22] C. F. Snyder, M. E. Watson, J. D. Jackson, D. Cella, and M. Y. Halyard, Mayo/FDA Patient-Reported Outcomes Consensus Meeting Group, "Patient-reported outcome instrument selection: designing a measurement strategy," *Value Health*, vol. 10, no. 2, pp. S76–S85, 2007.

[23] J. R. Kirwan, S. E. Hewlett, T. Heiberg et al., "Incorporating the patient perspective into outcome assessment in rheumatoid arthritis–progress at OMERACT 7," *Journal of Rheumatology*, vol. 32, pp. 2250–2256, 2005.

[24] N. Bellamy, M. Boers, D. Felson et al., "Health status instruments/utilities," *Journal of Rheumatology*, vol. 22, pp. 1203–1207, 1995.

[25] J. R. Kirwan, P. Minnock, A. Adebajo et al., "Patient perspective: fatigue as a recommended patient centered outcome measure in rheumatoid arthritis," *Journal of Rheumatology*, vol. 34, no. 5, pp. 1174–1177, 2007.

[26] V. Strand, M. Boers, L. Idzerda et al., "It's good to feel better but it's better to feel good and even better to feel good as soon as possible for as long as possible. Response criteria and the importance of change at OMERACT 10," *Journal of Rheumatology*, vol. 38, no. 8, pp. 1720–1727, 2011.

[27] D. L. Patrick, L. B. Burke, J. H Power et al., "Patient-reported outcomes to support medical product labeling claims: FDA perspective," *Value in Health*, vol. 10, no. 2, pp. S125–S137, 2017.

[28] K. Fiscella, S. Ransom, P. Jean-Pierre et al., "Patient-reported outcome measures suitable to assessment of patient navigation," *Cancer*, vol. 117, no. S15, pp. 3603–3617, 2011.

[29] N. E. Rothrock, R. D. Hays, K. Spritzer, S. E. Yount, W. Riley, and D. Cella, "Relative to the general US population, chronic diseases are associated with poorer health-related quality of life as measured by the Patient-Reported Outcomes Measurement Information System (PROMIS)," *Journal of Clinical Epidemiology*, vol. 63, no. 11, pp. 1195–1204, 2010.

[30] F. Salaffi, P. Sarzi-Puttini, and F. Atzeni, "How to measure chronic pain: new concepts," *Best Practice & Research: Clinical Rheumatology*, vol. 29, no. 1, pp. 164–186, 2015.

[31] L. R. Benesh, E. Szigeti, F. R. Ferraro, and J. N. Gullicks, "Tools for assessing chronic pain in rural elderly women," *Home Healthcare Nurse*, vol. 15, no. 3, pp. 207–211, 1997.

[32] D. Aletaha, T. Neogi, A. J. Silman et al., "2010 Rheumatoid arthritis classification criteria: an American College of Rheumatology/European League against Rheumatism collaborative initiative," *Annals of the Rheumatic Diseases*, vol. 69, no. 9, pp. 1580–1588, 2010.

[33] M. Rudwaleit, R. Landewé, D. van der Heijde et al., "The developement of Assessment of SpondyloArthritis international Society classification criteria for axial spondyloarthritis (part I): classification of paper patients by expert opinion including uncertainty appraisal," *Annals of the Rheumatic Diseases*, vol. 68, no. 6, pp. 770–776, 2009.

[34] M. Rudwaleit, D. van der Heijde, R. Landewé et al., "The developement of Assessment of Spondyloarthritis international Society classification criteria for axial spondyloarthritis (part II): validation and final selection," *Annals of the Rheumatic Diseases*, vol. 68, no. 6, pp. 777–783, 2009.

[35] W. Taylor, D. Gladman, P. Helliwell et al., "Classification criteria for psoriatic arthritis: development of new criteria from a large international study," *Arthritis & Rheumatism*, vol. 54, no. 8, pp. 2665–2673, 2006.

[36] F. Wolfe, D. J. Clauw, M. A. Fitzcharles et al., "The American College of Rheumatology preliminary diagnostic criteria for fibromyalgia and measurement of symptom severity," *Arthritis Care & Research*, vol. 62, no. 5, pp. 600–610, 2010.

[37] D. Aletaha, V. P. Nell, T. Stamm et al., "Acute phase reactants add little to composite disease activity indices for rheumatoid arthritis: validation of a clinical activity score," *Arthritis Research & Therapy*, vol. 7, no. 4, pp. R796–R806, 2005.

[38] G. Eberl, A. Studnicka-Benke, H. Hitzelhammer et al., "Development of a disease activity index for the assessment of reactive arthritis (DAREA)," *Rheumatology*, vol. 39, no. 2, pp. 148–155, 2000.

[39] C. Lukas, R. Landewé, J. Sieper et al., "Development of an ASAS-endorsed disease activity score (ASDAS) in patients with ankylosing spondylitis," *Annals of the Rheumatic Diseases*, vol. 68, no. 1, pp. 18–24, 2009.

[40] R. M. Bennett, R. Friend, K. D. Jones, R. Ward, B. K. Han, and R. L. Ross, "The revised fibromyalgia impact questionnaire (FIQR): validation and psychometric properties," *Arthritis Research & Therapy*, vol. 11, no. 4, p. R120, 2009.

[41] M. Mierau, M. Schoels, G. Gonda, J. Fuchs, D. Aletaha, and J. S. Smolen, "Assessing remission in clinical practice," *Rheumatology*, vol. 46, no. 6, pp. 975–979, 2007.

[42] V. P. Nell-Duxneuner, T. A. Stamm, K. P. Machold, S. flugbeil, D. Aletaha, and J. S. Smolen, "Evaluation of the appropriateness of composite disease activity measures for assessment of psoriatic arthritis," *Annals of the Rheumatic Diseases*, vol. 69, no. 3, pp. 546–549, 2010.

[43] M. M. Schoels, D. Aletaha, F. Alasti, and J. S. Smolen, "Disease activity in psoriatic arthritis (PsA): defining remission and treatment success using the DAPSA score," *Annals of the Rheumatic Diseases*, vol. 75, no. 5, pp. 811–818, 2016.

[44] C. S. Burckhardt, S. R. Clark, and R. M. Bennett, "The fibromyalgia impact questionnaire: development and validation," *Journal of Rheumatology*, vol. 18, no. 5, pp. 728–733, 1991.

[45] F. Salaffi, F. Franchignoni, A. Giordano, A. Ciapetti, P. Sarzi-Puttini, and M. Ottonello, "Psychometric characteristics of the Italian version of the revised Fibromyalgia Impact Questionnaire using classical test theory and Rasch analysis," *Clinical and Experimental Rheumatology*, vol. 31, no. 79, pp. S41–S49, 2013.

[46] J. E. Ware and C. D. Sherbourne, "The MOS 36-item short form health survey (SF-36). I. Conceptual framework and item selection," *Medical Care*, vol. 30, no. 6, pp. 473–483, 1992.

[47] P. Kind, "The EuroQol instrument: an index of health-related quality of life," in *Quality of Life and Pharmaeconomics in Clinical Trials*, B. Spiler, Ed., Lippincott-Raven, Philadelphia, PA, USA, 1996.

[48] R. Ara and J. Brazier, "Predicting the short form-6D preference based index using the eight mean short form-36 health dimension scores: estimating preference-based health-related utilities when patient level data are not available," *Value Health*, vol. 12, no. 2, pp. 346–353, 2009.

[49] G. Apolone and P. Mosconi, "The Italian SF-36 Health Survey: translation, validation and norming," *Journal of Clinical Epidemiology*, vol. 51, no. 11, pp. 1025–1036, 1998.

[50] L. Scalone, P. A. Cortesi, R. Ciampichini et al., "Italian population-based values of EQ-5D health states," *Value Health*, vol. 16, no. 5, pp. 814–822, 2013.

[51] A. E. Savoia, M. P. Fantini, P. P. Pandolfi, O. L. Dallolio, and N. Collina, "Assessing the construct validity of the Italian version of the EQ-5D: preliminary results from a cross-sectional study in North Italy," *Health and Quality of Life Outcomes*, vol. 4, no. 1, p. 47, 2006.

[52] T. Pincus and T. Sokka, "Quantitative measures for assessing rheumatoid arthritis in clinical trials and clinical care," *Best Practice & Research: Clinical Rheumatology*, vol. 17, no. 5, pp. 753–781, 2003.

[53] S. Lillegraven and T. K. Kvien, "Measuring disability and quality of life in established rheumatoid arthritis," *Best Practice & Research: Clinical Rheumatology*, vol. 21, no. 5, pp. 827–840, 2007.

[54] G. L. Steiner and D. R. Norman, *Health Measurement Scales: a Practical Guide to Their Development and Use*, Oxford University Press, Oxford, UK, 2nd edition, 1996.

[55] G. Bravo and L. Potvin, "Estimating the reliability of continuous measures with Cronbach's alpha or the intraclass correlation coefficient: toward the integration of two traditions," *Journal of Clinical Epidemiology*, vol. 44, no. 4-5, pp. 381–390, 1991.

[56] J. C. Nunnally and I. R. Bernstein, *Psychometric Theory*, McGraw-Hill, New York, NY, USA, 1994.

[57] N. Bellamy, *Musculosceletal Clinical Metrology*, Kluwer Academic Publishers Group, Dordrecht, Netherlands, 1993.

[58] J. M. Bland and D. G. Altman, "Statistical methods for assessing agreement between two methods of clinical measurement," *The Lancet*, vol. 1, no. 8476, pp. 307–310, 1986.

[59] C. A. McHorney and A. R. Tarlov, "Individual-patient monitoring in clinical practice: are available health status surveys adequate?," *Quality of Life Research*, vol. 4, no. 4, pp. 293–307, 1995.

[60] D. V. Cicchetti, "Guidelines, criteria, and rules of thumb for evaluating normed and standardized assessment instruments in psychology," *Psychological Assessment*, vol. 6, no. 4, pp. 284–290, 1994.

[61] J. V. Selby, A. C. Beal, and L. Frank, "The Patient-Centered Outcomes Research Institute (PCORI) national priorities for research and initial research agenda," *JAMA*, vol. 307, no. 15, pp. 1583-1584, 2012.

[62] Food and Drug Administration, "Guidance for industry on patient-reported outcome measures: use in medical product development to support labeling claims," *Federal Register*, vol. 74, no. 235, pp. 65132-65133, 2009.

[63] D. T. Felson, J. J. Anderson, M. Boers et al., "The American College of Rheumatology preliminary core set of disease activity measures for rheumatoid arthritis clinical trials. The Committee on Outcome Measures in Rheumatoid Arthritis Clinical Trials," *Arthritis & Rheumatism*, vol. 36, no. 6, pp. 729–740, 1993.

[64] D. D. Gladman, P. J. Mease, V. Strand et al., "Consensus on a core set of domains for psoriatic arthritis," *Journal of Rheumatology*, vol. 34, no. 5, pp. 1167–1170, 2007.

[65] U. Kiltz, D. van der Heijde, A. Boonen, and J. Braun, "The ASAS Health Index (ASAS HI)—a new tool to assess the health status of patients with spondyloarthritis," *Clinical and Experimental Rheumatology*, vol. 32, no. 85, pp. S105–S108, 2014.

[66] C. O. Bingham 3rd, R. Alten, S. J. Bartlett et al., "Identifying preliminary domains to detect and measure rheumatoid arthritis flares: report of the OMERACT 10 RA Flare Workshop," *Journal of Rheumatology*, vol. 38, no. 8, pp. 1751–1758, 2011.

[67] T. Sanderson, M. Morris, M. Calnan, P. Richards, and S. Hewlett, "What outcomes from pharmacologic treatments are important to people with rheumatoid arthritis? Creating the basis of a patient core set," *Arthritis Care & Research*, vol. 62, no. 5, pp. 640–646, 2010.

[68] N. A. Khan, H. J. Spencer, E. A. Abda et al., "Patient's global assessment of disease activity and patient's assessment of general health for rheumatoid arthritis activity assessment: are they equivalent?," *Annals of the Rheumatic Diseases*, vol. 71, no. 12, pp. 1942–1949, 2012.

[69] P. Studenic, H. Radner, J. S. Smolen, and D. Aletaha, "Discrepancies between patients and physicians in their perceptions of rheumatoid arthritis disease activity," *Arthritis & Rheumatism*, vol. 64, no. 9, pp. 2814–2823, 2012.

[70] M. Hakala, P. Nieminen, and O. Koivisto, "More evidence from a community based series of better outcome in rheumatoid arthritis. Data on the effect of multidisciplinary care on the retention of functional ability," *Journal of Rheumatology*, vol. 21, no. 8, pp. 1432–1437, 1994.

[71] C. L. Overman, M. B. Kool, J. A. Da Silva, and R. Geenen, "The prevalence of severe fatigue in rheumatic diseases: an international study," *Clinical Rheumatology*, vol. 35, no. 2, pp. 409–415, 2016.

[72] F. Wolfe, D. J. Hawley, and K. Wilson, "The prevalence and meaning of fatigue in rheumatic disease," *Journal of Rheumatology*, vol. 23, no. 8, pp. 1407–1417, 1996.

[73] R. P. Riemsma, J. J. Rasker, E. Taal, E. N. Griep, J. M. Wouters, and O. Wiegman, "Fatigue in rheumatoid arthritis: the role of self-efficacy and problematic social support," *British Journal of Rheumatology*, vol. 37, no. 10, pp. 1042–1046, 1998.

[74] S. Stebbings and G. J. Treharne, "Fatigue in rheumatic disease: an overview," *International Journal of Clinical Rheumatology*, vol. 5, no. 4, pp. 487–502, 2010.

[75] M. J. Bergman, S. H. Shahouri, T. S. Shaver et al., "Is fatigue an inflammatory variable in rheumatoid arthritis (RA)? Analyses of fatigue in RA, osteoarthritis, and fibromyalgia," *Journal of Rheumatology*, vol. 36, no. 12, pp. 2788–2794, 2009.

[76] L. C. Pollard, E. H. Choy, J. Gonzalez, B. Khoshaba, and D. L. Scott, "Fatigue in rheumatoid arthritis reflects pain, not disease activity," *Rheumatology*, vol. 45, no. 7, pp. 885–889, 2006.

[77] J. Kirwan, T. Heiberg, S. Hewlett et al., "Outcomes from the patient perspective workshop at OMERACT 6," *Journal of Rheumatology*, vol. 30, no. 4, pp. 868–872, 2003.

[78] K. Chauffier, S. Paternotte, V. Burki et al., "Fatigue in spondyloarthritis: a marker of disease activity. A cross-sectional study of 266 patients," *Clinical and Experimental Rheumatology*, vol. 31, no. 6, pp. 864–870, 2013.

[79] K. B. Norheim, G. Jonsson, and R. Omdal, "Biological mechanisms of chronic fatigue," *Rheumatology*, vol. 50, no. 6, pp. 1009–1018, 2011.

[80] H. Repping-Wuts, J. Fransen, T. van Achterberg, G. Bleijenberg, and P. van Riel, "Persistent severe fatigue in patients with rheumatoid arthritis," *Journal of Clinical Nursing*, vol. 16, no. 11, pp. 377–378, 2007.

[81] L. Gossec, M. Dougados, M.-A. D'Agostino, and B. Fautrel, "Fatigue in early axial spondyloarthritis. Results from the French DESIR cohort," *Joint Bone Spine*, vol. 83, no. 4, pp. 427–431, 2016.

[82] K. L. Haywood, J. C. Packham, and K. P. Jordan, "Assessing fatigue in ankylosing spondylitis: the importance of frequency and severity," *Rheumatology*, vol. 53, no. 3, pp. 552–556, 2013.

[83] H. Dagfinrud, N. K. Vollestad, J. H. Loge, T. K. Kvien, and A. M. Mengshoel, "Fatigue in patients with ankylosing spondylitis: a comparison with the general population and associations with clinical and self-reported measures," *Arthritis & Rheumatism*, vol. 53, no. 1, pp. 5–11, 2005.

[84] R. Gunaydin, A. Goksel Karatepe, N. Cesmeli, and T. Kaya, "Fatigue in patients with ankylosing spondylitis: relationships with disease-specific variables, depression, and sleep disturbance," *Clinical Rheumatology*, vol. 28, no. 9, pp. 1045–1051, 2009.

[85] Y. Turan, M. T. Duruoz, S. Bal, A. Guvenc, L. Cerrahoglu, and A. Gurgan, "Assessment of fatigue in patients with ankylosing spondylitis," *Rheumatology International*, vol. 27, no. 9, pp. 847–852, 2007.

[86] van Tubergen, J. Coenen, R. Landewe, A. Spoorenberg, A. Chorus, and A. Boonen, "Assessment of fatigue in patients with ankylosing spondylitis: a psychometric analysis," *Arthritis & Rheumatism*, vol. 47, no. 1, pp. 8–16, 2002.

[87] S. Hultgren, J. E. Broman, B. Gudbjornsson, J. Hetta, and U. Lindqvist, "Sleep disturbances in outpatients with ankylosing spondylitis a questionnaire study with gender implications," *Scandinavian Journal of Rheumatology*, vol. 29, no. 6, pp. 365–369, 2000.

[88] S. A. Fernandez, X. Juanola Roura, A. Alonso Ruiz et al., "Clinical utility of the ASDAS index in comparison with BASDAI in patients with ankylosing spondylitis (Axis Study)," *Rheumatology International*, vol. 37, no. 11, pp. 1817–1823, 2017.

[89] W. H. Koh, I. Pande, A. Samuels, S. D. Jones, and A. Calin, "Low dose amitriptyline in ankylosing spondylitis: a short term, double blind, placebo controlled study," *Journal of Rheumatology*, vol. 24, no. 11, pp. 2158–2161, 1997.

[90] Y. Yacoub, B. Amine, A. Laatiris, R. Abouqal, and N. Hajjaj-Hassouni, "Assessment of fatigue in Moroccan patients with ankylosing spondylitis," *Clinical Rheumatology*, vol. 29, no. 11, pp. 1295–1299, 2010.

[91] F. Wolfe, J. Anderson, D. Harkness et al., "Health status and disease severity in fibromyalgia: results of a six-center longitudinal study," *Arthritis & Rheumatism*, vol. 40, no. 9, pp. 1571–1579, 1997.

[92] L. Humphrey, R. Arbuckle, P. Mease, D. A. Williams, B. D. Samsoe, and C. Gilbert, "Fatigue in fibromyalgia: a conceptual model informed by patient interviews," *BMC Musculoskeletal Disorders*, vol. 20, no. 11, p. 216, 2010.

[93] P. Waraich, E. M. Goldner, J. M. Somers, and L. Hsu, "Prevalence and incidence studies of mood disorders: a systematic review of the literature," *Canadian Journal of Psychiatry*, vol. 49, no. 2, pp. 124–138, 2004.

[94] S. A. Atal, E. Ceceli, M. Okumu et al., "The evaluation of pain in patients with rheumatoid arthritis," *Pain Practice*, vol. 9, p. 31, 2009.

[95] D. van Hoogmoed, J. Fransen, G. Bleijenberg, and P. van Riel, "Physical and psychosocial correlates of severe fatigue in rheumatoid arthritis," *Rheumatology*, vol. 49, no. 7, pp. 1294–1302, 2010.

[96] T. Mikuls, K. Saag, L. Criswell, L. Merlino, and J. R. Cerhan, "Health related quality of life in women with elderly onset rheumatoid arthritis," *Journal of Rheumatology*, vol. 30, no. 5, pp. 952–957, 2003.

[97] Y. M. Miedany and A. H. El Rasheed, "Is anxiety a more common disorder than depression in rheumatoid arthritis?," *Joint Bone Spine*, vol. 69, pp. 300–306, 2002.

[98] D. N. Challa, C. S. Crowson, and J. M. Davis 3rd, "The patient global assessment of disease activity in rheumatoid arthritis: identification of underlying latent factors," *Rheumatology and Therapy*, vol. 4, no. 1, pp. 201–208, 2017.

[99] D. N. Challa, Z. Kvrgic, A. L. Cheville et al., "Patient-provider discordance between global assessments of disease activity in rheumatoid arthritis: a comprehensive clinical evaluation," *Arthritis Research & Therapy*, vol. 19, no. 1, p. 212, 2017.

[100] N. Inanc, S. Yilmaz-Oner, M. Can, T. Sokka, and H. Direskeneli, "The role of depression, anxiety, fatigue, and

fibromyalgia on the evaluation of the remission status in patients with rheumatoid arthritis," *Journal of Rheumatology*, vol. 41, no. 9, pp. 1755–1760, 2014.

[101] M. M. Ward, "Are patient self-report measures of arthritis activity confounded by mood? A longitudinal study of patients with rheumatoid arthritis," *Journal of Rheumatology*, vol. 21, no. 6, pp. 1046–1050, 1994.

[102] A. T. Joyce, P. Smith, R. Khandker et al., "Hidden cost of rheumatoid arthritis (RA): estimating cost of comorbid cardiovascular disease and depression among patients with RA," *Journal of Rheumatology*, vol. 36, no. 4, pp. 743–752, 2009.

[103] P. P. Katz and E. H. Yelin, "Prevalence and correlates of depressive symptoms among persons with rheumatoid arthritis," *Journal of Rheumatology*, vol. 20, no. 5, pp. 790–796, 1993.

[104] D. C. Ang, H. Choi, K. Kroenke, and F. Wolfe, "Comorbid depression is an independent risk factor for mortality in patients with rheumatoid arthritis," *Journal of Rheumatology*, vol. 32, no. 6, pp. 1013–1019, 2005.

[105] E. Y. Lok, C. C. Mok, C. W. Cheng, and E. F. Cheung, "Prevalence and determinants of psychiatric disorders in patients with rheumatoid arthritis," *Psychosomatics*, vol. 51, no. 4, p. 338, 2010.

[106] A. Isik, S. S. Koca, A. Ozturk, and O. Mermi, "Anxiety and depression in patients with rheumatoid arthritis," *Clinical Rheumatology*, vol. 26, no. 6, pp. 872–878, 2007.

[107] J. Hakkou, S. Rostom, M. Mengat, N. Aissaoui, R. Bahiri, and N. Hajjaj-Hassouni, "Sleep disturbance in Moroccan patients with ankylosing spondylitis: prevalence and relationships with disease-specific variables, psychological status and quality of life," *Rheumatology International*, vol. 33, no. 2, pp. 285–290, 2013.

[108] J. van den Hoek, L. D. Roorda, H. C. Boshuizen, G. J. Tijhuis, G. A. van den Bos, and J. Dekker, "Physical and mental functioning in patients with established rheumatoid arthritis over an 11-year followup period: the role of specific comorbidities," *Journal of Rheumatology*, vol. 43, no. 2, pp. 307–314, 2016.

[109] S. Moussavi, S. Chatterji, E. Verdes, A. Tandon, V. Patel, and B. Ustun, "Depression, chronic diseases, and decrements in health: results from the World Health Surveys," *The Lancet*, vol. 370, no. 9590, pp. 851–858, 2007.

[110] A. Morris, E. H. Yelin, P. Panopalis, L. Julian, and P. P. Katz, "Long-term patterns of depression and associations with health and function in a panel study of rheumatoid arthritis," *Journal of Health Psychology*, vol. 16, no. 4, pp. 667–677, 2011.

[111] F. Salaffi, P. Sarzi-Puttini, R. Girolimetti, F. Atzeni, S. Gasparini, and W. Grassi, "Health-related quality of life in fibromyalgia patients: a comparison with rheumatoid arthritis patients and the general population using the SF-36 health survey," *Clinical and Experimental Rheumatology*, vol. 27, no. 56, pp. S67–S74, 2009.

[112] P. M. Nicassio, E. G. Moxham, C. E. Schuman et al., "The contribution of pain, reported sleep quality, and depressive symptoms to fatigue in fibromyalgia," *Pain*, vol. 100, no. 3, pp. 271–279, 2002.

[113] F. Tubach, G. Baron, B. Falissard et al., "Using patients' and rheumatologists' opinions to specify a short form of the WOMAC function subscale," *Annals of the Rheumatic Diseases*, vol. 64, no. 1, pp. 75–79, 2005.

[114] L. A. Moran, G. H. Guyatt, and G. R. Norman, "Establishing the minimal number of items for a responsive, valid, health-related quality of life instrument," *Journal of Clinical Epidemiology*, vol. 54, no. 6, pp. 571–579, 2001.

[115] J. Coste, F. Guillemin, J. Pouchot, and J. Fermanian, "Methodological approaches to shortening composite measurement scales," *Journal of Clinical Epidemiology*, vol. 50, no. 3, pp. 247–252, 1997.

[116] K. G. Auw Yang, N. J. H. Raijmakers, A. J. Verbout, W. J. Dhert, and D. B. Saris, "Validation of the short-form WOMAC function scale for the evaluation of osteoarthritis of the knee," *Journal of Bone and Joint Surgery*, vol. 89, no. 1, pp. 50–56, 2007.

[117] J. S. Kalantar and N. J. Tally, "The effects of lottery incentive and length of questionnaire on health survey response rates: a randomised study," *Journal of Clinical Epidemiology*, vol. 52, no. 11, pp. 1117–1122, 1999.

[118] A. J. Mitchell, "Pooled results from 38 analyses of the accuracy of distress thermometer and other ultra-short methods of detecting cancer-related mood disorders," *Journal of Clinical Oncology*, vol. 25, no. 29, pp. 4670–4680, 2007.

# 6

# Pleasant Pain Relief and Inhibitory Conditioned Pain Modulation: A Psychophysical Study

Nathalie Bitar,[1,2] Serge Marchand ⓘ,[3,4] and Stéphane Potvin ⓘ[1,2]

[1]*Centre de recherche de l'Institut Universitaire en Santé Mentale de Montréal, Montreal, QC, Canada*
[2]*Department of Psychiatry, Faculty of Medicine, Université de Montréal, Montréal, QC, Canada*
[3]*Centre de recherche du Centre Hospitalier de l'Université de Sherbrooke, Sherbrooke, QC, Canada*
[4]*Department of Surgery, Faculty of Medicine and Health Sciences, Université de Sherbrooke, Sherbrooke, QC, Canada*

Correspondence should be addressed to Stéphane Potvin; stephane.potvin@umontreal.ca

Academic Editor: Manfred Harth

*Background.* Inhibitory conditioned pain modulation (ICPM) is one of the principal endogenous pain inhibition mechanisms and is triggered by strong nociceptive stimuli. Recently, it has been shown that feelings of pleasantness are experienced after the interruption of noxious stimuli. Given that pleasant stimuli have analgesic effects, it is therefore possible that the ICPM effect is explained by the confounding effect of pleasant pain relief. The current study sought to verify this assumption. *Methods.* Twenty-seven healthy volunteers were recruited. Thermal pain thresholds were measured using a Peltier thermode. ICPM was then measured by administering a tonic thermal stimulus before and after a cold-pressor test (CPT). Following the readministration of the CPT, pleasant pain relief was measured for 4 minutes. According to the opponent process theory, pleasant relief should be elicited following the interruption of a noxious stimulus. *Results.* The interruption of the CPT induced a *mean* and *peak* pleasant pain relief of almost 40% and 70%, respectively. Pleasant pain relief did not correlate with ICPM amplitude but was positively correlated with pain level during the CPT. Finally, a negative correlation was observed between pleasant pain relief and anxiety. *Discussion.* Results show that the cessation of a strong nociceptive stimulus elicits potent pleasant pain relief. The lack of correlation between ICPM and pleasant pain relief suggests that the ICPM effect, as measured by sequential paradigms, is unlikely to be fully explained by a pleasant pain relief phenomenon.

## 1. Introduction

Chronic pain affects approximately 22% of the adult population [1] and is a complex phenomenon resulting from biological, psychological, and social factors. Among these factors, the importance of central mechanisms, such as the activity of endogenous pain excitatory and inhibitory systems, is increasingly acknowledged [2–4]. Indeed, growing evidence suggests that endogenous pain modulation mechanisms are impaired in nearly every type of chronic pain disorders, and that alterations are particularly significant in neuropathic and functional pain syndromes [5–7].

*Inhibitory conditioned pain modulation* (ICPM) is one of the principal endogenous pain inhibition mechanisms [8–10]. The ICPM theory postulates that a nociceptive stimulation will reduce another nociceptive stimulation if it occurs on a body surface distant from the pain surface [11, 12]. Preclinical studies have shown that the ICPM effect is mediated by brain stem and bulbospinal mechanisms [13–16]. When triggered, ICPM causes a diffuse diminution of pain throughout the body.

From an experimental point of view, two types of paradigms are used to measure ICPM: in the *parallel* ICPM paradigm, a noxious stimulus (test stimulus) is applied before and at the same time as a heterotopic conditioning painful stimulus, while in the *sequential* paradigm, the test stimulus is applied before and after a heterotopic conditioning painful stimulus [17]. Considering that it is unclear if the *parallel* ICPM paradigm truly measures the ICPM effect or a distracting effect, some investigators prefer the *sequential* paradigm which removes the potential effect of distraction [18–20]. It is indeed well known that pain experience is reduced when individuals are engaged in cognitive tasks (e.g., arithmetic and working memory) [10]. This raises the possibility that the conditioning stimulus actually distracts participants from their pain when it is concomitantly administered at the same time as the test stimulus. Conversely, some laboratories have made mention of their preference of the *parallel* ICPM paradigm over the *sequential* one, considering that ICPM effect gradually fades over time and that the precise duration of this effect remains uncertain [21].

Another potential limitation of *sequential* ICPM paradigms that has gone unnoticed is that the pain reduction observed using these paradigms may be confounded by the pleasant pain relief phenomenon. According to the opponent process theory, when a stimulus causing deviation from homeostasis is terminated, the opposite sensation will be felt [22]. Consistently with this theory, recent research has shown that the interruption of a noxious stimulus causes a feeling of pleasantness [23], similar to the feeling often observed in reaction to analgesic drugs [23]. Given that pleasant stimuli (e.g., music, odors, and attractive faces) are well known for producing analgesic effects [24–26], it is therefore possible that the interruption of the conditioning stimulus elicits a pleasant feeling, which in turn decreases pain perception when the second test stimulus is reapplied. If so, the reduction in pain perception observed during the second test stimulus would not reflect a pure ICPM effect but rather a pleasure-induced analgesic effect, at least partially.

In the past, our research team has pursued several studies on ICPM using a sequential paradigm, consisting in the application of a tonic noxious heat stimulation to the left forearm of participants eliciting moderate pain, administered before and after the immersion of their right arm in a bath of cold water. This paradigm has allowed us, among others, to show that pain perception is reduced during the second application of the test stimulus, relative to the first one, indicating that endogenous pain inhibition mechanisms have been recruited [27, 28]. In the current study, we sought to examine a hypothetical association between ICPM and pleasant pain relief, using our validated ICPM procedure [3]. Thus far, most studies on pleasant pain relief have used heating thermodes to elicit the phenomenon [23, 29]. The current study differed from the latter, and we measured pleasant pain relief after the interruption of the cold-pressor test, given that it is the conditioning stimulus used in our *sequential* paradigm to trigger the ICPM effect. The secondary objective of the current study was to examine the potential associations between pleasant pain relief and anxiodepressive subclinical symptoms. Although several experimental studies have shown that anxiety and depression influence pain perception in experimental settings [30–32], the influence of these variables on pleasant pain relief is unknown.

## 2. Method

### 2.1. Participants.
We recruited a total of 27 (14 women) healthy participants, aged between 18 and 35 years old (mean age 25.1 years ± 4.27, mean ± standard error of the mean (SEM)) (Table 1). Exclusion criteria were the following: (1) any DSM-V axis psychiatric disorder (including substance use disorders); (2) centrally acting medications; (3) neurologic disorders; and (4) any unstable medical condition. In

TABLE 1: Characteristics of the participants.

| Characteristics | M (%) |
|---|---|
| Age (M ± SEM) | 25.1 ± 0.82 |
| Sex (%) | |
| Male | 40.6 |
| Female | 43.8 |
| Ethnicity (%) | |
| Caucasian | 50 |
| Afro-American | 6.3 |
| Latin American | 3.1 |
| Asian | 6.3 |
| Other | 18.8 |
| Level of education (%) | |
| College degree | 15.6 |
| Bachelor's degree | 40.6 |
| Graduate studies | 28.1 |
| Employment status (%) | |
| Employed | 46.9 |
| Unemployed | 6.3 |
| Loan or bursary | 15.6 |
| Others (i.e., independent worker and welfare) | 15.6 |
| Psychological symptoms (M ± SEM) | |
| BDI-II | 5.11 ± 1.07 |
| STAI-S | 46.68 ± 0.83 |
| SHPS | 48.81 ± 0.65 |

BDI-II = Beck Depression Inventory; SHPS = Snaith–Hamilton Pleasure Scale; STAI = State and Trait Inventory; SEM = standard error of the mean; M = mean.

particular, none of the participants suffered from chronic pain and none had significant acute painful symptoms as determined with the *Brief Pain Inventory* (mean pain = 0.9 ± 0.4) [33, 34]. Subclinical psychological symptoms (e.g., depression, anxiety, anhedonia, and pain) were evaluated, respectively, with the French versions of the *Beck Depression Inventory-II* (BDI-II) [35], the *State and Trait Anxiety Inventory*-state subscale (STAI-S) [36, 37], and the *Snaith–Hamilton Pleasure Scale* (SHPS) [38, 39]. Recruitment was made via word of mouth and through online advertisement (Kijiji). Each participant signed a detailed consent form, and the local ethics committee approved the research.

### 2.2. Inhibitory Conditioned Pain Modulation (ICPM) Paradigm

#### 2.2.1. Heat Pain Threshold and Tolerance.
Thermal pain threshold and tolerance were measured by applying a 3 cm² Peltier thermode (TSA II, Medoc, Advanced Medical Systems, Ramat Yishai, Israel) on the left forearm of participants [28]. This heating plate was connected to a computer and allowed a precise control of temperatures. Experimental temperatures were initially set at 32°C and gradually increased at a rate of 0.3°C per second. To ensure that there would be no peripheral sensitization, the thermode was moved to a different area of the forearm for every test. Participants were asked to report the moment at which sensation changed from heat to pain (thermal pain threshold, VAS = 1) [23, 28] and the moment the sensation of pain was at its highest (most intense pain tolerable) (thermal pain tolerance, VAS = 100). For each

participant, the temperature inducing moderate pain (T50) was also measured. Upon the first application, these measures were taken verbally to ensure the participant's comprehension of the procedure. During the second and third applications, these measures were reported by the participants using a computerized visual analog scale (VAS). This scale ranged from 0 (no pain) to 100 (most intense pain tolerable) [28].

*2.2.2. Tonic Heat Pain Perception.* The *test stimulus* consisted of a continuous heat stimulation that induced moderate pain (T50) for 2 minutes [28]. This heat stimulation was administered with a thermode on the left forearm of the participants. The temperature of the thermode quickly reached T50, an individually predetermined temperature (baseline at 32°C and increase rate of 0.3°C per second), and then remained constant for the remaining time. However, participants were not told that the temperature was kept constant [40]. During the administration of the test stimulus, individuals were instructed to measure pain intensity using the same COVAS as previously mentioned. The test stimulus was administered twice, separated by the administration of the cold-pressor test (CPT) (e.g., the conditioning stimulus).

*2.2.3. Conditioning Stimulus.* The CPT consisted the immersion of the opposite arm (right arm) into a bath of ice water that was kept constant at 10°C, for a maximum of 2 minutes, by continuously recirculating the water (Julabo F33-HL heating/refrigerated circulator). The temperature was chosen to be painful enough to elicit the endogenous analgesic effect yet tolerable for 2 minutes [28]. During the administration of the conditioning stimulus, participants were instructed to verbally report pain intensity and pain unpleasantness on a scale of 0 to 100. In order to differentiate between pain intensity and pain unpleasantness, two scenarios were presented to the participants. For pain intensity, they were asked to imagine themselves at their favourite concert; the music is extremely loud and it damages their eardrums. In this scenario, the intensity is very high; however, it is not unpleasant because they enjoy the music. On the contrary, for pain unpleasantness, they were asked to imagine themselves studying the day before a final exam with loud construction noise outside their house. In the second scenario, the intensity of the noise is not high; however, it is extremely unpleasant. The measures for pain intensity and pain unpleasantness were taken at the moment the arm was immersed into the bath of cold water and afterwards every 30 seconds, until 120 seconds. With these measures, the mean pain intensity and mean pain unpleasantness were calculated for each participant. By measuring pain perception (using the test stimulus) before and after the conditioning stimulus, it was possible to measure ICPM. In other words, ICPM is defined as the reduction in pain perception observed between both administrations of the test stimulus (before and after the conditioning stimulus) [20].

*2.2.4. Pleasant Pain Relief.* Pleasant pain relief was measured immediately after the conditioning stimulus. In order

to explain to participants the pleasant pain relief phenomenon, we provided an example similar to the one used by Leknes et al. [23]. Participants were asked to imagine themselves walking in a −30°C snowstorm for 20 minutes and finally arriving home to feel the warmth of the air inside the house. This warmth would induce the feeling of both pain relief and of pleasure [23]. Considering that the ICPM effect lasts for a short time span (approximately 10 minutes), it was important that the administration of the second test stimulus quickly follows the conditioning stimulus [5]. Consequently, following the conditioning stimulus, the measure of pleasant pain relief was taken only once in order to avoid delaying the administration of the second test stimulus. The second test stimulus was then administered immediately after the score of pleasant pain relief was taken. To fully capture the dynamics of pleasant pain relief, thirty minutes after the full administration of the sequential ICPM paradigm, we readministered the conditioning stimulus for 2 minutes. During the second administration of the conditioning stimulus, participants were again instructed to verbally report pain intensity and pain unpleasantness using the same scale as mentioned earlier (Section 2.2.3). Pleasant pain relief was measured immediately after the end of the immersion and every 30 seconds afterwards for 4 minutes. To assess the pleasant pain relief, participants were asked to rate their level of pleasant pain relief on a scale of 0 ("I feel relief, but no pleasure") to 100 ("I feel relief and the most intense pleasure possible"). These ratings were used to calculate the mean and peak (the highest score) pleasant pain relief of each participant.

# 3. Statistical Analyses

Two paired-sample *t*-tests were conducted. Firstly, we compared pain ratings of the test stimulus before and after the conditioning stimulus, as an index of ICPM efficacy. Secondly, we compared two pleasant pain relief scores, measured after the separate administrations of the conditioning stimulus. To determine the relationship between the conditioning stimulus, ICPM, pleasant pain relief, and subclinical symptoms, Pearson's correlation analyses were performed. We examined potential correlations (i) between pain intensity and pain unpleasantness during the conditioning stimulus and pleasant pain relief (mean and peak), (ii) between ICPM efficacy and pleasant pain relief (mean and peak), (iii) between pain intensity and unpleasantness during the conditioning stimulus and ICPM efficacy, (iv) between psychological symptoms (STAI-S, BDI-II, and SHPS) and pleasant pain relief (mean and peak), and finally (v) between psychological symptoms (STAI-S, BDI-II, and SHPS) and pain (intensity and unpleasantness). The interclass correlation coefficient (ICC) estimate along with the 95% confidence intervals (CI) was calculated for mean pain intensity scores taken during each conditioning stimulus, mean pain unpleasantness scores taken during each conditioning stimulus, and for pleasant pain relief (first pleasant pain relief score taken immediately after each conditioning stimulus). The ICC was calculated using a one-way random effect model, and single measures were reported [41]. This

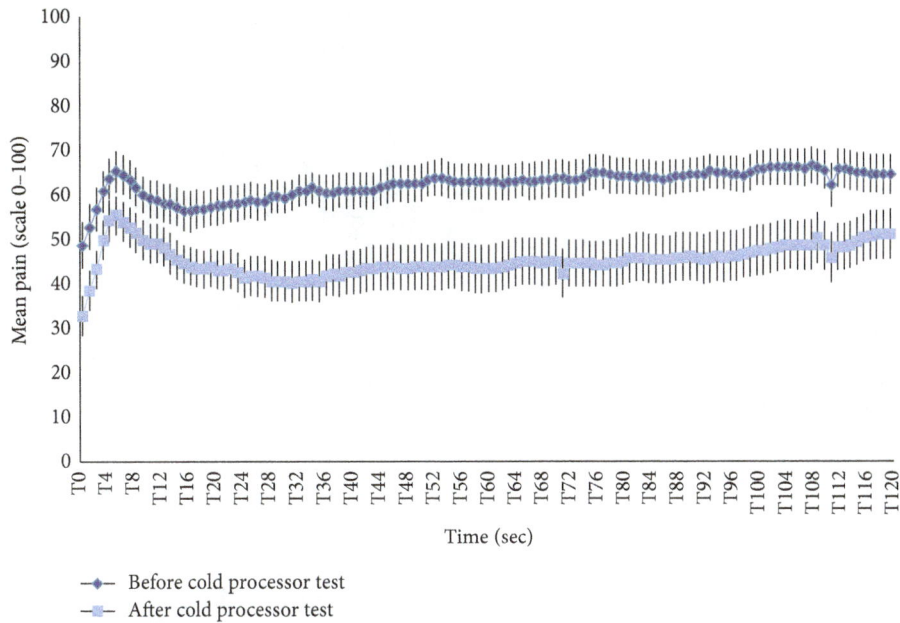

FIGURE 1: Inhibitory conditioned pain modulation. This figure shows the pain perception of participants during both administrations of the test stimulus for 2 minutes (120 seconds). Pain perception during the test stimulus was evaluated twice, once before (in dark blue) and once after (in pale blue) the administration of the conditioning stimulus. Each time point shows the mean and SEM.

allowed us to determine the test-retest reliability of pain intensity and unpleasantness during both administrations of the conditioning stimulus and of both measures of pleasant pain relief. Values of the ICC that are less than 0.5 are indicative of poor reliability, values between 0.5 and 0.75 are indicative of moderate reliability, and finally, values between 0.75 and 0.90 are indicative of excellent reliability [41]. All variables had a normal distribution, as determined with the Shapiro–Wilk test for normality. All results are presented as mean ± standard error of the mean (SEM) and are considered significant at $p < 0.05$. All analyses were performed using SPSS, version 24.

## 4. Results

### 4.1. Inhibitory Conditioned Pain Modulation Paradigm

*4.1.1. Heat Pain Threshold and Tolerance.* During the pretest, the thermal pain threshold of participants was 42.3°C ± 0.7, the thermal pain tolerance was 47.2°C ± 0.5, and the T50 was 45.9°C ± 0.4.

*4.1.2. Tonic Pain Perception.* The mean pain ratings for the test stimulus administered before the conditioning stimulus were 67.4 ± 3.3 and were reduced to 51.2 ± 4.7 after the conditioning stimulus (mean difference = 16.1 ± 3.0) (Figure 1). The difference between these pain ratings was significant ($t(26) = 5.4$; $p < 0.001$). During the conditioning stimulus, the mean pain intensity and mean pain unpleasantness were, respectively, 50.9 ± 3.0 and 51.1 ± 4.0.

*4.1.3. Pleasant Pain Relief.* During the second administration of the conditioning stimulus (30 minutes later), the mean pain

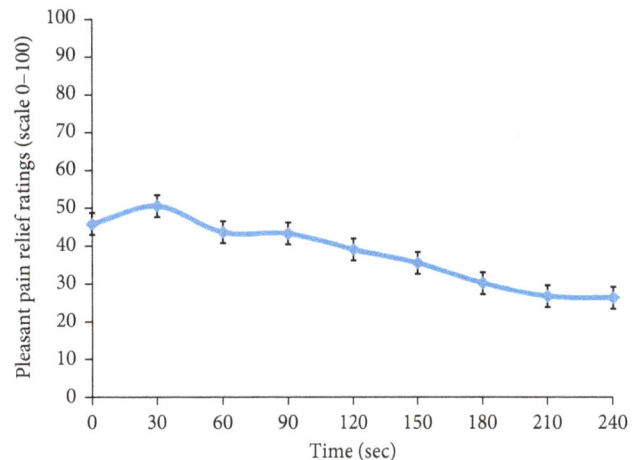

FIGURE 2: Perception of pleasant pain relief during 240 seconds. This figure illustrates the pleasant pain relief reported by participants for 4 minutes following the second administration of the conditioning stimulus. The mean and SEM are displayed for each time point.

intensity and mean pain unpleasantness were, respectively, 47.8 ± 3.4 and 47.9 ± 4.0. After this conditioning stimulus, pleasant pain relief measures were taken every 30 seconds for 4 minutes. The mean pleasant pain relief was 40.0 ± 3.8 (Figure 2), and the *peak* pleasant pain relief was 69.3 ± 4.4. It is noteworthy that pleasant pain relief was also measured after the first administration of the conditioning stimulus. No significant difference was found between the two measures ($t(26) = 0.81$; $p = 0.936$).

*4.2. Correlations of Pleasant Pain Relief with Other Psychophysical Measures.* A significant correlation was observed between *mean* pleasant pain relief and pain intensity during

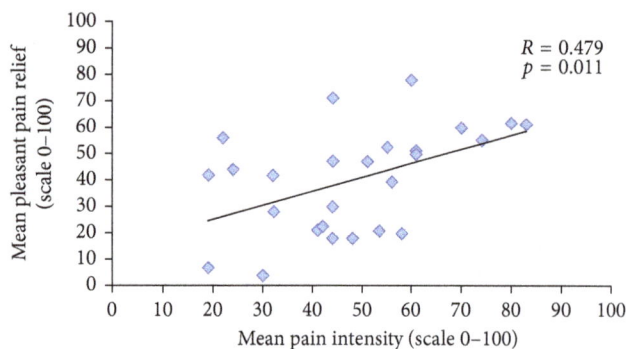

FIGURE 3: Correlation between pain intensity during the cold-pressor test and mean pleasant pain relief. This figure illustrates the correlation between the mean pain intensity, during the second application of the conditioning stimulus, and the mean pleasant pain relief, measured following the second conditioning stimulus.

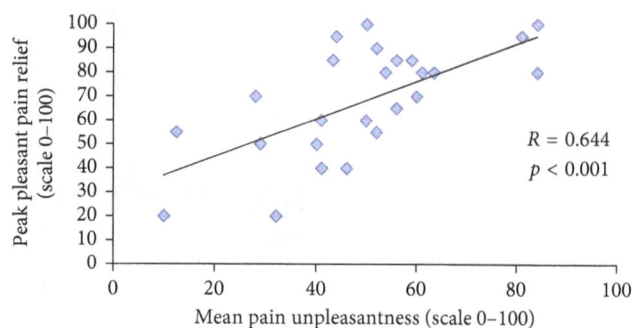

FIGURE 4: Correlation between pain unpleasantness during the cold-pressor test and peak pleasant pain relief. This figure illustrates the correlation between the mean pain unpleasantness, during the second application of the conditioning stimulus, and peak pleasant pain relief, measured following the second conditioning stimulus.

the conditioning stimulus ($r = 0.479$; $p = 0.011$) (Figure 3). Likewise, a significant correlation was also found between *peak* pleasant pain relief and pain unpleasantness during the conditioning stimulus ($r = 0.644$; $p < 0.001$) (Figure 4). Conversely, no significant correlations were found between pleasant pain relief (measured after the first conditioning stimulus) and ICPM efficacy ($r = 0.113$; $p = 0.576$), as well as between *mean* and *peak* pleasant pain relief (measured after the second conditioning stimulus) and ICPM efficacy (resp., $r = 0.144$, $p = 0.47$; $r = 0.090$, $p = 0.656$). Finally, no significant correlations were found between pain intensity during the conditioning stimulus and ICPM efficacy ($r = 0.107$; $p = 0.601$), as well as between pain unpleasantness during the conditioning stimulus and ICPM efficacy ($r = 0.126$; $p = 0.532$).

*4.3. Correlations of Pleasant Pain Relief and Subclinical Psychological Symptoms.* Significant correlations were found between mean pleasant pain relief and STAI-S ($r = -0.402$; $p = 0.038$). No significant correlations were found between mean pleasant pain relief and BDI-II ($r = 0.814$; $p = 0.359$) and mean pleasant pain relief and SHPS ($r = -0.136$; $p = 0.498$). Finally, no significant correlations were found between BDI-II, STAI-S, and SHPS and pain unpleasantness or pain intensity during the conditioning stimulus ($p > 0.4$).

*4.4. Test-Retest Reliability.* Reliability was evaluated for mean pain intensity and mean pain unpleasantness, taken during two separate administrations of the conditioning stimulus, as well as between each value of pleasant pain relief, taken 10 s after each conditioning stimulus. The ICC correlations along with their 95% CI for mean pain intensity, mean pain unpleasantness, and pleasant pain relief were, respectively, ICC (1,1) = 0.692, 95% CI = 0.434–0.846; ICC (1,1) = 0.870, 95% CI = 0.738–0.939; and ICC (1,1) = 0.638, 95% CI = 0.35–0.816.

## 5. Discussion

The main objective of this study was to examine if there is a relationship between the ICPM efficacy and the pleasant

pain relief experienced after the administration of the same conditioning stimulus used to trigger endogenous pain inhibition mechanisms. Associations between pleasant pain relief and other psychophysical measures and subclinical psychological symptoms were also examined. As shown by several previous investigations [5, 7, 42], the conditioning stimulus (e.g., cold-pressor test) produces significant analgesia, as illustrated by a significant reduction in pain perception during the second test stimulus, compared to the first one. Our study showed that significant pleasure was experienced after the interruption of the conditioning stimulus. Greater pain intensity and unpleasantness during the conditioning stimulus was associated with greater pleasant pain relief. However, there was no correlation between ICPM efficacy and the magnitude of pleasant pain relief. Finally, we found that anxiety was negatively correlated with pleasant pain relief.

Prior to analyzing any potential association between ICPM efficacy and the magnitude of pleasant pain relief, it was important to first establish that the interruption of the conditioning stimulus produces significant pleasant pain relief. This was the case. Indeed, in addition to having the mean pleasant pain relief close to 40% and the peak pleasant pain relief close to 70%, the effect also lasted at least 4 minutes in most participants (at endpoint, the pleasant pain relief was 26.3%). By comparison, Leknes et al. [23] measured pleasant pain relief after the interruption of a $15 \times 20$ mm thermode on the left forehead of the participants during 3 seconds and found that the peak pleasant pain relief was about 35% and lasted about 8 seconds. As in the study from Leknes et al. [23], we found that both pain intensity and unpleasantness during the conditioning stimulus were positively correlated with the magnitude of pleasant pain relief after cessation of the conditioning stimulus. Taken together, these results strengthen the validity of using the cold-pressor test as a conditioning stimulus to elicit pleasant pain relief.

Although the conditioning stimulus elicited strong pleasant pain relief and significant ICPM, pleasant pain relief and ICPM were not significantly correlated. From a methodological point of view, this is an important observation, considering that several teams of investigators use *sequential*

ICPM paradigms [28, 43, 44]. A significant positive correlation between the two phenomena would have suggested that the analgesic effects triggered by the conditioning stimulus could be confounded by pleasant pain relief triggered at the end of the conditioning stimulus. The lack of correlation observed here suggests that ICPM assessment is not significantly confounded by the pleasant pain relief effect, although both phenomena co-occur in time.

Another implication of the current study lies in the fact that it provides a new potential explanation for the strong link between pain and anxiety. Although we found no significant relationship in the current study, several previous experimental studies have shown that noxious stimuli cause anxiety, and that anxiety increases pain perception in healthy volunteers [8, 45, 46]. At the moment, however, the reasons for the association between pain and anxiety remain elusive. Despite inconsistent results, some studies have found a negative association between anxiety and the ability to experience pleasure [47, 48]. Comparatively, the link between anxiety and pleasure has been less investigated in experimental settings. Therefore, the finding of a negative correlation between pleasant pain relief and anxiety, as observed in the current study, suggests that anxiety acutely disrupts the homeostatic balance between pleasure and pain. Conversely, a lower ability to experience pleasant pain relief may have caused participants to feel more anxious.

The current study has a few limitations. Firstly, the most prolonged measure of pleasant pain relief (e.g., 240 seconds) was not assessed at the same time as endogenous pain inhibition. However, we found no correlation between pleasant pain relief and ICPM efficacy even when we used the first assessment of pleasant pain relief (e.g., after the first of the conditioning stimulus). This makes it unlikely that the lack of correlation between ICPM efficacy and pleasant pain relief would be confounded by the passage of time. Another limitation of the current study is that the sample size could have been larger, meaning that the lack of correlation between ICPM and pain relief pleasantness could be explained by a lack of statistical power. However, this does not seem very likely given that the correlation between ICPM and pleasant pain relief was very weak. Another limitation has to do with the fact that participants were explicitly introduced to the concept of pleasant pain relief before the experimental session, and this may have influenced participants' expectations of experiencing ICPM. Previous research has shown that the magnitude of ICPM is influenced by expectations [49]. Finally, it is important to remember that the current study used a correlational design, which means that it cannot be concluded from the present results that pleasant pain relief and ICPM are independent phenomena. The experimental manipulation of variables would be required in order to reach a firm conclusion.

## 6. Conclusion

The current study showed, for the first time, that strong feelings of pleasantness are elicited after the cessation of the conditioning stimulus and that ICPM and pleasant pain relief both co-occur but are not significantly correlated.

These results provide support for the use of the cold-pressor test as a conditioning stimulus to study pleasant pain relief and suggest that the results of *sequential* ICPM paradigms are not strongly confounded by co-occurring pleasant pain relief. The current results also provide novel insights on the complex link between anxiety and pain perception. Future studies will need to examine the influence of psychophysical properties of nociceptive stimuli (e.g., spatial and temporal summation) on the magnitude of pleasant pain relief and to investigate the neural pathways that are specifically and/or commonly involved in ICPM and pleasant pain relief. Finally, the precise influence of anxiety on pleasant pain relief will need to be determined.

## Abbreviation

ICPM: Inhibitory conditioned pain modulation.

## Acknowledgments

Stéphane Potvin is a holder of the Eli Lilly Canada Chair on schizophrenia research and a supported member from the Fondation de l'Institut Universitaire en Santé Mentale de Montréal.This study was funded by a discovery grant to Stéphane Potvin from the Natural Sciences and Engineering Research Council of Canada.

## References

[1] S. Tamburin, S. Paolucci, N. Smania, and G. Sandrini, "The burden of chronic pain and the role of neurorehabilitation: consensus matters where evidence is lacking," *Journal of Pain Research*, vol. 10, pp. 101–103, 2017.

[2] J. DeSantana and K. Sluka, "Central mechanisms in the maintenance of chronic widespread noninflammatory muscle pain," *Current Pain and Headache Reports*, vol. 29, no. 5, pp. 338–343, 2012.

[3] Y. Tousignant-Laflamme, S. Pagé, P. Goffaux, and S. Marchand, "An experimental model to measure excitatory and inhibitory pain mechanisms in humans," *Brain Research*, vol. 1230, pp. 73–79, 2008.

[4] M. Kwon, M. Altin, H. Duenas, and L. Alev, "The role of descending inhibitory pathways on chronic pain modulation and clinical implications," *Pain Practice*, vol. 14, no. 7, pp. 656–667, 2014.

[5] G. N. Lewis, L. Heales, D. A. Rice, K. Rome, and P. J. McNair, "Reliability of the conditioned pain modulation paradigm to assess endogenous inhibitory pain pathways," *Pain Research and Management*, vol. 17, no. 2, pp. 98–102, 2012.

[6] C. J. Woolf, "Central sensitization: implications for the diagnosis and treatment of pain," *Pain*, vol. 152, no. 3, pp. S2–S15, 2011.

[7] D. Yarnitsky, "Role of endogenous pain modulation in chronic pain mechanisms and treatment," *Pain*, vol. 156, no. 2, pp. S24–S31, 2015.

[8] H. Nahman-Averbuch, Y. Granovsky, R. C. Coghill, D. Yarnitsky, E. Sprecher, and I. Weissman-Fogel, "Waning of 'conditioned pain modulation': a novel expression of subtle pronociception in migraine," *Headache: The Journal of Head and Face Pain*, vol. 53, no. 7, pp. 1104–1115, 2013.

[9] G. N. Lewis, D. A. Rice, and P. J. McNair, "Conditioned pain modulation in populations with chronic pain: a systematic review and meta-analysis," *Journal of Pain*, vol. 13, no. 10, pp. 936–944, 2012.

[10] R. Moont, Y. Crispel, R. Lev, D. Pud, and D. Yarnitsky, "Temporal changes in cortical activation during distraction from pain: a comparative LORETA study with conditioned pain modulation," *Brain Research*, vol. 1435, pp. 105–117, 2011.

[11] D. Le Bars, A. H. Dickenson, and J.-M. Besson, "Diffuse noxious inhibitory controls (DNIC). I. Effects on dorsal horn convergent neurones in the rat," *Pain*, vol. 6, no. 3, pp. 283–304, 1979.

[12] D. Le Bars, A. H. Dickenson, and J. Besson, "Diffuse noxious inhibitory controls (DNIC). II. Lack of effect on non-convergent neurones, supraspinal involvement and theoretical implications," *Pain*, vol. 6, no. 3, pp. 305–327, 1979.

[13] A. I. Basbaum and H. L. Fields, "Endogenous pain control mechanisms: review and hypothesis," *Annals of Neurology*, vol. 4, no. 5, pp. 451–462, 1978.

[14] J. C. Willer, D. Bouhassira, and D. Le Bars, "Bases neurophysiologiques du phénomène de contre-irritation: les contrôles inhibiteurs diffus induits par stimulations nociceptives," *Neurophysiologie Clinique/Clinical Neurophysiology*, vol. 29, no. 5, pp. 379–400, 1999.

[15] S. Marchand, "The physiology of pain mechanisms: from the periphery to the brain," *Rheumatic Disease Clinics of North America*, vol. 34, no. 2, pp. 285–309, 2008.

[16] M. J. Millan, "Descending control of pain," *Progress in Neurobiology*, vol. 66, no. 6, pp. 355–474, 2002.

[17] D. L. Kennedy, H. I. Kemp, D. Ridout, D. Yarnitsky, and A. S. C. Rice, "Reliability of conditioned pain modulation," *Pain*, vol. 157, no. 11, pp. 2410–2419, 2016.

[18] S. S. Olesen, H. Van Goor, S. A. W. Bouwense, O. H. G. Wilder-Smith, and A. M. Drewes, "Reliability of static and dynamic quantitative sensory testing in patients with painful chronic pancreatitis," *Regional Anesthesia and Pain Medicine*, vol. 37, no. 5, pp. 530–536, 2012.

[19] C. Valencia, L. L. Kindler, R. B. Fillingim, and S. Z. George, "Investigation of central pain processing in shoulder pain: converging results from two musculoskeletal pain models," *Journal of Pain*, vol. 13, no. 1, pp. 81–89, 2012.

[20] C. Valencia, R. B. Fillingim, M. Bishop et al., "Investigation of central pain processing in post-operative shoulder pain and disability," *Clinical Journal of Pain*, vol. 30, no. 9, pp. 775–786, 2014.

[21] D. Pud, Y. Granovsky, and D. Yarnitsky, "The methodology of experimentally induced diffuse noxious inhibitory control (DNIC)-like effect in humans," *Pain*, vol. 144, no. 1, pp. 16–19, 2009.

[22] M. Andreatta, A. Mühlberger, and P. Pauli, "When does pleasure start after the end of pain? The time course of relief," *Journal of Comparative Neurology*, vol. 524, no. 8, pp. 1653–1667, 2016.

[23] S. Leknes, J. C. W. Brooks, K. Wiech, and I. Tracey, "Pain relief as an opponent process: a psychophysical investigation," *European Journal of Neuroscience*, vol. 28, no. 4, pp. 794–801, 2008.

[24] C. E. Dobek, M. E. Beynon, R. L. Bosma, and P. W. Stroman, "Music modulation of pain perception and pain-related activity in the brain, brain stem, and spinal cord: a functional magnetic resonance imaging study," *Journal of Pain*, vol. 15, no. 10, pp. 1057–1068, 2014.

[25] J. Prescott and J. Wilkie, "Pain tolerance selectively increased by a sweet-smelling odor," *Psychological Science*, vol. 18, no. 4, pp. 308–311, 2007.

[26] J. Younger, A. Aron, S. Parke, N. Chatterjee, and S. Mackey, "Viewing pictures of a romantic partner reduces experimental pain: involvement of neural reward systems," *PLoS One*, vol. 5, no. 10, Article ID e13309, 2010.

[27] E. Normand, S. Potvin, I. Gaumond, G. Cloutier, J.-F. Corbin, and S. Marchand, "Pain inhibition is deficient in chronic widespread pain but normal in major depressive disorder," *Journal of Clinical Psychiatry*, vol. 72, no. 2, pp. 219–224, 2011.

[28] S. Potvin and S. Marchand, "Pain facilitation and pain inhibition during conditioned pain modulation in fibromyalgia and in healthy controls," *Pain*, vol. 157, no. 8, pp. 1704–1710, 2016.

[29] C. Mohr, S. Leyendecker, I. Mangels et al., "Central representation of cold-evoked pain relief in capsaicin induced pain: an event-related fMRI study," *Pain*, vol. 139, no. 2, pp. 416–430, 2008.

[30] E. W. De Heer, M. M. J. G. Gerrits, A. T. F. Beekman et al., "The association of depression and anxiety with pain: a study from NESDA," *PLoS One*, vol. 9, no. 10, Article ID e106907, 2014.

[31] R. Defrin, S. Schreiber, and K. Ginzburg, "Paradoxical pain perception in posttraumatic stress disorder: the unique role of anxiety and dissociation," *Journal of Pain*, vol. 16, no. 10, pp. 961–970, 2015.

[32] S. Zambito Marsala, M. Pistacchi, P. Tocco et al., "Pain perception in major depressive disorder: a neurophysiological case-control study," *Journal of the Neurological Sciences*, vol. 357, no. 1-2, pp. 19–21, 2015.

[33] T. M. Atkinson, T. R. Mendoza, L. Sit et al., "The brief pain inventory and its "pain at its worst in the last 24 hours" item: clinical trial endpoint considerations," *Pain Medicine*, vol. 11, no. 3, pp. 337–346, 2010.

[34] J. Poundja, D. Fikretoglu, S. Guay, and A. Brunet, "Validation of the French version of the brief pain inventory in Canadian veterans suffering from traumatic stress," *Journal of Pain and Symptom Management*, vol. 33, no. 6, pp. 720–726, 2007.

[35] K. Lahlou-Laforêt, F. Ledru, R. Niarra, and S. M. Consoli, "Validity of Beck Depression Inventory for the assessment of depressive mood in chronic heart failure patients," *Journal of Affective Disorders*, vol. 184, pp. 256–260, 2015.

[36] L. L. B. Barnes, D. Harp, and W. S. Jung, "Reliability generalization of scores on the Spielberger state-trait anxiety inventory," *Educational and Psychological Measurement*, vol. 62, no. 4, pp. 603–618, 2002.

[37] J. Gauthier and S. Bouchard, "Adapatation canadienne-française de la forme revisée du State-Trait Anxiety Inventory de Spielberger," *Canadian Journal of Behavioural Science*, vol. 25, no. 4, pp. 559–578, 1993.

[38] R. Ameli, D. A. Luckenbaugh, N. F. Gould et al., "SHAPS-C: the Snaith-Hamilton pleasure scale modified for clinician administration," *PeerJ*, vol. 2, p. e429, 2014.

[39] G. Loas, S. Dubal, P. Perot, F. Tirel, P. Nowaczkowski, and A. Pierson, "Validation of the French version of the Snaith-Hamilton Pleasure Scale (SHAPS, Snaith et al. 1995).

Determination of the statistical parameters in 208 normal subjects and 103 hospitalized patients presenting with depression or schizophrenia," *L'Encéphale*, vol. 23, no. 6, pp. 454–458, 1997.

[40] S. Potvin, E. Stip, A. Tempier et al., "Pain perception in schizophrenia: no changes in diffuse noxious inhibitory controls (DNIC) but a lack of pain sensitization," *Journal of Psychiatric Research*, vol. 42, no. 12, pp. 1010–1016, 2008.

[41] T. K. Koo and M. Y. Li, "A guideline of selecting and reporting intraclass correlation coefficients for reliability research," *Journal of Chiropractic Medicine*, vol. 15, no. 2, pp. 155–163, 2016.

[42] S. Mlekusch, A. Y. Neziri, A. Limacher, P. Jüni, L. Arendt-Nielsen, and M. Curatolo, "Conditioned pain modulation in patients with acute and chronic low back pain," *Clinical Journal of Pain*, vol. 32, no. 2, pp. 116–121, 2016.

[43] P. D. Drummond and L. Knudsen, "Central pain modulation and scalp tenderness in frequent episodic tension-type headache," *Headache*, vol. 51, no. 3, pp. 375–383, 2011.

[44] G. Leonard, P. Goffaux, D. Mathieu, J. Blanchard, B. Kenny, and S. Marchand, "Evidence of descending inhibition deficits in atypical but not classical trigeminal neuralgia," *Pain*, vol. 147, no. 1, pp. 217–223, 2009.

[45] J. L. Rhudy and M. W. Meagher, "Fear and anxiety: divergent effects on human pain thresholds," *Pain*, vol. 84, no. 1, pp. 65–75, 2000.

[46] K. C. Prabhat, S. Maheshwari, S. K. Verma et al., "Dental anxiety and pain perception associated with the use of miniscrew implants for orthodontic anchorage," *Journal of Indian Orthodontic Society*, vol. 48, pp. 163–167, 2014.

[47] D. G. Dillon, A. J. Holmes, A. L. Jahn, R. Bogdan, L. L. Wald, and D. A. Pizzagalli, "Dissociation of neural regions associated with anticipatory versus consummatory phases of incentive processing," *Psychophysiology*, vol. 45, no. 1, pp. 36–49, 2008.

[48] H. R. Cremers, I. M. Veer, P. Spinhoven, S. A. R. B. Rombouts, and K. Roelofs, "Neural sensitivity to social reward and punishment anticipation in social anxiety disorder," *Frontiers in Behavioral Neuroscience*, vol. 8, pp. 1–9, 2015.

[49] P. Goffaux, W. J. Redmond, P. Rainville, and S. Marchand, "Descending analgesia–when the spine echoes what the brain expects," *Pain*, vol. 130, no. 1-2, pp. 137–143, 2007.

# 7

# Electromyographic Analysis of Masticatory Muscles in Cleft Lip and Palate Children with Pain-Related Temporomandibular Disorders

Liliana Szyszka-Sommerfeld ⓘ,[1] Teresa Matthews-Brzozowska,[2] Beata Kawala ⓘ,[3] Marcin Mikulewicz ⓘ,[4] Monika Machoy ⓘ,[1] Włodzimierz Więckiewicz ⓘ,[5] and Krzysztof Woźniak[1]

[1]Department of Orthodontics, Pomeranian Medical University of Szczecin, Al. Powstańców Wlkp. 72, Szczecin 70111, Poland
[2]Department and Clinic of Maxillofacial Orthopaedics and Orthodontics, Poznan University of Medical Sciences, 70 Bukowska Street, Poznań 60812, Poland
[3]Department of Maxillofacial Orthopaedics and Orthodontics, Wroclaw Medical University, 26 Krakowska Street, Wrocław 50425, Poland
[4]Department of Maxillofacial Orthopaedics and Orthodontics, Division of Facial Abnormalities, Wroclaw Medical University, 26 Krakowska Street, Wrocław 50425, Poland
[5]Department of Prosthetic Dentistry, Wroclaw Medical University, 26 Krakowska Street, Wrocław 50425, Poland

Correspondence should be addressed to Liliana Szyszka-Sommerfeld; liliana.szyszka@gmail.com

Academic Editor: Shiau Yuh-Yuan

*Aim.* The aim of this study was to assess the electrical activity of temporalis and masseter muscles in children with cleft lip and palate (CLP) and pain-related temporomandibular disorders (TMD-P). *Methods.* The sample consisted of 31 CLP patients with a TMD-P (mean age 9.5 ± 1.8 years) and 32 CLP subjects with no TMD (mean age 9.2 ± 1.7 years). The children were assessed for the presence of temporomandibular disorders (TMD) using Axis I of the Research Diagnostic Criteria for TMD (RDC/TMD). Electromyographical (EMG) recordings were performed using a DAB-Bluetooth Instrument (Zebris Medical GmbH, Germany) in the mandibular rest position and during maximum voluntary contraction (MVC). *Results.* The rest activity of the temporalis and masseter muscles was significantly higher in TMD-P group compared with non-TMD children. A significant decrease in temporalis muscle activity during MVC was observed in TMD-P patients. There was a significant increase in the Asymmetry Index for temporalis and masseter muscle rest activity in the TMD-P group. *Conclusion.* Cleft children diagnosed with TMD-P have altered masticatory muscle activity, and this can affect their muscle function.

## 1. Introduction

Cleft lip and palate (CLP) is one of the most common congenital deformities of the craniofacial area requiring long-term functional and aesthetic rehabilitation [1]. Complete clefts of the lip and/or palate are immediately recognizable disruptions of normal facial structure [2]. In addition to dysfunctional facial expressions, patients with CLP may have serious functional problems with sucking, swallowing, breathing, chewing, speaking, hearing, and social integration [3, 4].

The prevalence of malocclusions in CLP patients is relatively high [5]. The most common occlusal disorders in patients with clefts are crossbites and class III malocclusions [6, 7]. Malocclusions, particularly of the transverse type where disrupted symmetry of the dental arches can be clinically observed, are a potential cause of functional disorders of the stomatognathic system [8]. Hence, patients with CLPs are potentially at risk of developing temporomandibular disorders (TMD), due to psychosocial burdens and malocclusions predisposing them to this condition [6, 9]. This is consistent with previous reports [10–12]. The importance of a patient's lower socioeconomic status as a likely important factor in the development of TMD in CLP patients has also been noted [13].

Temporomandibular disorders (TMD) are a collective term embracing a number of clinical problems affecting the masticatory muscles, the temporomandibular joint (TMJ), and associated structures [14]. Pain-related temporomandibular disorders (TMD-P) are the most prevalent conditions among TMD [15]. They comprise myalgia, arthralgia, and headaches attributed to TMD [16]. The primary manifestations of TMD-P are pain of a persistent, recurring, or chronic nature in the masticatory muscles, TMJ, or in adjacent structures [17, 18]. The other major symptoms include limitation in the range of mandibular motion and joint noises [14, 17]. The pain may radiate to different regions, such as the dental arches, ears, temples, forehead, occiput, and the cervical region of spine or shoulder girdle [18]. The aetiology of pain-related TMD is considered to be multifactorial and to result from a complex interaction between biological, psychological, social, and environmental variables [19, 20].

The prevalence of TMD signs and symptoms in children and adolescents in the general population ranges from 1 to 50%, and TMD-P from 1% to 22% [21–26]. The prevalence of objective and subjective symptoms of TMD in children with CLP is relatively higher [13].

Surface electromyography (sEMG) is the study of muscle function based on an analysis of the electrical signals produced during muscular contraction. The sEMG method is painless and innocuous, and these are important factors when conducting studies involving children [27, 28]. It has been widely used in research settings for the assessment and follow-up of patients with TMD [29, 30], and numerous studies have demonstrated altered electromyographical (EMG) values in the masticatory muscles of patients with TMDs [31–34]. Subjects diagnosed with TMD-P alter the recruitment of their jaw muscles [35]. Free nerve endings act as nociceptors activated by noxious stimulation such as temporomandibular joint (TMJ) overloads and/or masticatory muscle ischemia, if it is prolonged and associates with muscle contractions [36, 37]. A correlation has been observed between a decrease in the motor unit firing rate and muscle pain intensity, although the central mechanisms involved remain unclear [38]. Maximum EMG activity is greater in pain-free subjects than in patients with pain-related TMD [33, 39]. Nevertheless, to the authors' knowledge, until now there have been no EMG studies on masticatory muscle activity in cleft lip and palate subjects with a TMD-pain diagnosis. The identification of the electromyographic pattern of the mastication muscles is necessary in order to achieve functional improvement in the stomatognathic system, particularly in cleft children. For these reasons, it is essential to determine temporalis and masseter muscle activity in cleft lip and palate children with pain-related TMD by means of electromyography (EMG).

The aim of this study was to determine whether the electrical activity of temporalis and masseter muscles in children with complete CLP and pain-related TMD differs from that observed in CLP individuals with no TMD. The null hypothesis was that there are no differences between CLP individuals with TMD-P and non-TMD with regard to the electrical activity of the temporalis and masseter muscles in the mandibular rest position and during maximum voluntary teeth clenching.

## 2. Material and Methods

The clinical research was registered as a case-control study in the ClinicalTrials.gov database and assigned the number NCT03308266.

*2.1. Study Sample.* The sample comprised 63 children with cleft lip and palate and mixed dentition. In accordance with the outcomes of Axis I of the Research Diagnostic Criteria for Temporomandibular Disorders (RDC/TMD) [17], the children were divided into two groups: a TMD-pain group and a non-TMD group. The groups were matched for age and gender. The TMD-pain group included 31 children (15 girls and 16 boys) aged between 6.4 and 13.9 (mean $9.5 \pm 1.8$) with complete cleft lip and palate and a pain-related TMD diagnosis. The control group consisted of 32 subjects (14 girls and 18 boys) aged between 6.7 and 11.7 years (mean $9.2 \pm 1.7$) with CLP and no TMD diagnosis. The subjects were selected from a total of 90 patients who had been referred to three Cleft Care Centres in Szczecin, Poznań, and Wrocław, Poland, between November and December 2015. All had undergone lip and palate surgery at one of four different Plastic Surgery Clinics in Poland according to the following protocols: A. a two-stage lip and palate repair procedure, that is, a lip operation at the age of 3–6 months, followed by palate closure (hard and soft palate in one-step procedure) at the age of approximately 12 months; B. single-stage lip and palate repair in children at the age of about 6 months, that is, the lip and hard and soft palate were closed in a single operation. The application of the adopted inclusion and exclusion criteria resulted in 27 of the subjects being excluded from the study and 63 of the participants qualifying for further examination. The inclusion criteria for the TMD-pain group were as follows: meeting Axis I of the RDC/TMD diagnosis criteria with pain (arthrogenous or myogenous TMD), children of both sexes with mixed dentition, undergoing lip and palate surgery, the presence of a cleft lip and palate without a syndrome, a sequence or karyotype abnormalities, and consent to participate voluntarily in the study. The inclusion criteria for control group were as follows: children without any TMD diagnosis according to the RDC/TMD protocol, children of both sexes with mixed dentition, undergoing lip and palate surgery, the presence of a cleft lip and palate without a syndrome, a sequence, or karyotype abnormalities, and consent to participate voluntarily in the study. The exclusion criteria for both groups included: meeting Axis I of the RDC/TMD diagnosis criteria without pain, the presence of systemic or rheumatologic diseases, a history of cervical spine or temporomandibular joint (TMJ) surgery, trauma or malformations, and completed orthodontic or masticatory motor system dysfunction treatment.

Masticatory motor system function was assessed on the basis of a clinical examination and electromyographic procedures.

*2.2. Clinical Examination.* Anamnestic interviews were conducted, which covered the patients' general medical history and provided detailed information on the patients' masticatory motor systems, including subjective TMD symptoms, such as jaw pain during function, frequent headaches, jaw stiffness/fatigue, difficulty in opening the mouth wide, teeth grinding, and TMJ sounds. The children were assessed for the presence of temporomandibular disorders using Axis I of the Research Diagnostic Criteria for TMD (RDC/TMD) by a single trained examiner. This helped ensure standardized procedures for epidemiological studies, unified TMD diagnostic and exploratory criteria, and a comparison with the results of other similar studies [17, 40]. The clinical signs were assessed using the RDC/TMD criteria, including pain on palpation, mandibular range of motion (mm), associated pain (jaw opening pattern, unassisted opening, maximum assisted opening, mandibular excursive, and protrusive movements), sounds coming from the TMJ, and tenderness induced by muscle and joint palpation. Generally, the RDC/TMD criteria classify forms of TMD into three diagnostic categories:

(i) Group I: muscle disorders (Group Ia with myofascial pain and Group Ib with myofascial pain with limited opening);

(ii) Group II: disc displacement (Group IIa with reduction, Group IIb without reduction with limited opening, and Group IIc without reduction but without limited opening);

(iii) Group III: arthralgia (Group IIIa) or arthritis (Group IIIb/IIIc).

RDC/TMD specifies distinct operational criteria for each TMD subtype; for example, a myalgia diagnosis is made if a person reports pain in the face or mastication muscles at rest or during function, as well as the presence of pain upon palpation at 3 or more sites. An arthralgia diagnosis includes pain upon palpation of the TMJ and joint-related pain during movements of the opening mouth, mandibular excursive, and protrusive movements; a diagnosis of arthritis includes pain in addition to reported clicking sounds upon palpation. Thus, every TMD subject could have both a masticatory muscle pain diagnosis and/or a TMJ pain diagnosis.

Replicate measurements of clinical signs of TMD were recorded for twenty randomly selected children in order to assess intraexaminer reliability. For this purpose, intraclass correlation coefficients (ICCs) were calculated for both continuous and dichotomous variables of the RDC/TMD examination. The considered ICC values were as follows: ICC < 0.4 which corresponds to poor reliability;

$0.4 \leq ICC \leq 0.75$—fair to good reliability; ICC > 0.75—excellent reliability [41, 42].

The intraoral examination included an analysis of the dental arch shape on three planes together with a reciprocal analysis of both dental arches. The following occlusal characteristics were evaluated: sagittal relationship of the permanent first molar according to Angle's classification, posterior crossbite, overbite, overjet, and lateral open bite.

*2.3. Electromyographical Examination.* We followed the methods by Szyszka-Sommerfeld et al. [43]. The EMG recordings were taken with a DAB-Bluetooth Instrument (Zebris Medical GmbH, Germany) by a single experienced researcher. During the recordings, each patient sat in a comfortable chair without a head support and was instructed to assume a natural head position [44]. This position allows us to eliminate or limit any unintentional movements from other parts of the body.

Surface EMG signals were detected with four silver/silver chloride (Ag/AgCl), disposable, self-adhesive, bipolar electrodes (Naroxon Dual Electrode, Naroxon, USA) with a fixed interelectrode distance of 20 mm. The electrodes were precisely positioned on the anterior temporalis muscle and the superficial masseter on both the left and the right sides parallel to the muscular fibres. The placement of the electrodes was exactly the same as previously described by Ferrario et al. [45] The temporalis anterior muscle: vertically along the anterior margin of the muscle; the masseter muscle: parallel to the muscular fibres with the upper pole of the electrode located at the intersection between the tragus-labial commissura and exocanthion-gonion lines. A reference electrode was applied inferior and posterior to the right ear.

The surface of the patient's skin was cleaned of impurities and degreased with a 70% ethyl alcohol solution by wiping it several times with disposable cotton wool. Slight reddening of the skin after cleaning is a clinical indicator that the site has been properly prepared. To confirm that the tested area had been properly prepared, an impedance test was performed with Metex P-10 a measuring device (Metex Instruments Corporation, Korea) with an accuracy of 2%. This device measures the resistance between a pair of electrodes for a period of 5 minutes from the placing of the electrodes. Further examinations would be conducted if the test produced a positive result (low skin tissue impedance).

The EMG recordings were taken 5 minutes later. The electrical activity of the temporalis and masseter muscles was then measured during the course of three different tests:

(1) Rest activity of the masticatory muscles in the clinical rest position;

(2) Maximum voluntary clench (MVC) in the intercuspal position where the patient was asked to clench as hard as possible for 5 seconds;

(3) Maximum voluntary clench (MVC) with two 10-mm thick cotton rolls placed on the mandibular second premolars and molars or on the mandibular second milk molars and the first permanent molars and the

patient was asked to clench as hard as possible for 5 seconds.

To avoid any effects of fatigue, a rest period of at least 5 minutes was allowed between each of these recordings. The EMG recordings were repeated at least three times to ascertain stability. The first recordings were eliminated as a "learning" sequence since they were frequently observed to be dissimilar to the other two repetitions. In a single subject, all EMG data were the arithmetic means of these last two surface EMG recordings. The patients were allowed to relax for 1 minute between each activity.

The DAB-Bluetooth Instrument was interfaced with a computer, which presented the data graphically and recorded it for further analysis. The EMG signals were amplified, digitized, and digitally filtered. The basic component of the data analysis was the normalization process. Normalization involved referring the raw results (the mean values of the EMG potentials) to the data obtained from each patient after clenching on two cotton rolls (reference values) according to the following formula: mean values ($\mu$V) during rest position or MVC/mean values ($\mu$V) during MVC with two 10 mm cotton rolls $\times$ 100%. For each muscle, the EMG potentials were expressed as a percentage of the MVC value using cotton rolls (unit $\mu$V/$\mu$V%). This procedure was essential for the preliminary processing of raw data to ensure intercomparisons and further analysis. In order to compare EMG recordings among different subjects, it was necessary to relate all measurements to the electrical muscle activity detected during certain standardization recordings, such as MVC. The EMG potentials collected in MVC are reported to have the highest repeatability. Among the various protocols, MVC on cotton rolls is reported to have the lowest interindividual variability, and a method based on this standardization is now commonly used [45–48]. According to this protocol, normalized EMG data will provide information on the impact of occlusion (teeth contact) on neuromuscular activity, while avoiding individual variability (anatomical variations, physiological and psychological status, etc.) and technical variations (muscle cross-talk, electrode position, skin and electrode impedance, etc.).

Finally, the Asymmetry Index (As, unit %) was recorded to assess asymmetry between the activity of the left and right jaw muscles according to a formula ranging from 0% (total symmetry) to 100% (total asymmetry) [49].

$$\text{As} = \frac{\sum_{i=1}^{N} |R_i - L_i|}{\sum_{i=1}^{N} (R_i + L_i)} \cdot 100 \qquad (1)$$

To investigate the repeatability of the recording protocol, duplicate EMG evaluations were performed on the 20 subjects by the same operator, after a gap of 15 minutes between the two recordings. We asked the subjects to remain relaxed during this 15-minute break once the electrodes had been removed from their muscles and to walk around the laboratory if they needed to. The results of the first and second set of experiments demonstrated the repeatability of the EMG measurements. The data were presented as the mean values of the electrical activity of the temporalis and

masseter muscles in rest position and during MVC. The repeatability of electrode positioning was maintained by using a standard procedure for positioning the electrodes. To assure standard results during the EMG examination, the electrodes were placed accurately at the area of muscle belly contraction [50].

*2.4. Statistical Analysis.* The homogeneity of variance was evaluated using the Levene test. The normality test applied was the Kolmogorov–Smirnov test. The results of the EMG recordings and the repeatability of the EMG measurements were analysed using Student's $t$-test and the Mann–Whitney $U$ test to determine differences between the mean values of the independent variables. The chi-square test was used to determine differences in the prevalence of malocclusions between the groups of participants. The level of significance was set at $P = 0.05$.

# 3. Results

The reliability value for the RDC/TMD clinical examination ranged from good to excellent (from 0.62 to 1.0). Table 1 presents the distribution of TMD-P subjects according to their RDC/TMD diagnosis. Myofascial pain with no limited mouth opening (Group Ia) and arthralgia (Group IIIa) were diagnosed in 38.7% of the TMD-P patients, while 9.7% of the children were diagnosed with myofascial pain with limited mouth opening (Group Ib) and 12.9% of the subjects received a mixed TMD-pain diagnosis (Groups Ia and IIIa or Ib and IIIa).

The occlusal characteristics for both groups of children are presented in Table 2. There were no significant differences between TMD-pain group and control subjects in terms of the prevalence of malocclusions ($P > 0.05$).

Table 3 shows the results of the repeatability of the recording protocol. The differences between first and second evaluations of the electrical potentials of the masticatory muscles were not statistically significant in the case of any of the aforementioned activities ($P > 0.05$).

Analysis of the EMG recordings showed that the rest activity of both the temporalis and the masseter muscles was higher in subjects with CLP and TMD-P compared with non-TMD subjects (for temporalis muscles, $P = 0.0102$; for masseter muscles, $P = 0.0188$) (Table 4).

A significant increase was observed in the Asymmetry Index in relation to the rest activity of the temporalis ($P = 0.0218$) and masseter muscles ($P = 0.0010$) in patients with TMD-P compared with non-TMD children (Table 4).

Temporalis muscle activity during MVC was significantly lower in children from the TMD-pain group compared with children with no TMD ($P = 0.0477$). There were no significant differences in masseter muscle activity during MVC between the TMD-pain group and control subjects ($P = 0.3163$) (Table 5).

There were no differences between TMD-P and non-TMD subjects in terms of the Asymmetry Index for the temporalis and masseter muscles during MVC (temporalis muscle $P = 0.0858$, masseter muscle $P = 0.0773$) (Table 5).

TABLE 1: The distribution of TMD-pain subjects according to RDC/TMD diagnosis.

| Diagnosis | TMD-pain group ($n = 31$) | |
|---|---|---|
| | n | % |
| Myofascial pain without limited mouth opening (Group Ia) | 12 | 38.7 |
| Myofascial pain with limited mouth opening (Group Ib) | 3 | 9.7 |
| Arthralgia (Group IIIa) | 12 | 38.7 |
| Group Ia and IIIa | 3 | 9.7 |
| Group Ib and IIIa | 1 | 3.2 |

TABLE 2: The occlusal characteristics in the children studied.

| Variable | | TMD-pain group | | Non-TMD group | |
|---|---|---|---|---|---|
| | | n | % | n | % |
| Vertical overlap | Normal[1] | 12 | 38.7 | 19 | 59.4 |
| | Increased[2] | 7 | 22.6 | 7 | 21.9 |
| | Absence[3] | 12 | 38.7 | 6 | 18.7 |
| Overjet | Normal[4] | 8 | 25.8 | 13 | 40.6 |
| | Increased[5] | 7 | 22.6 | 7 | 21.9 |
| | Anterior crossbite | 17 | 54.8 | 13 | 40.6 |
| Posterior crossbite | No | 7 | 22.6 | 12 | 37.5 |
| | Yes | 24 | 77.4 | 20 | 62.5 |
| Angle class | I | 10 | 32.3 | 17 | 53.1 |
| | II | 7 | 22.6 | 5 | 15.6 |
| | III | 14 | 45.2 | 10 | 31.2 |
| Lateral open bite | No | 22 | 71.0 | 24 | 75.0 |
| | Yes | 9 | 29.0 | 8 | 25.0 |

[1]Upper incisors is one-third of the clinical crown of lower incisors; [2]categorized as ≥3 mm; [3]the overlap absence (anterior open bite); [4]upper central incisors did not exceed 3 mm; [5]categorized as ≥3 mm.

TABLE 3: The results of the repeatability of the recording protocol.

| Region | Activity | 1 examination | | 2 examination | | P value |
|---|---|---|---|---|---|---|
| | | Mean | SD | Mean | SD | |
| Temporalis muscles | Rest | 6.06 | 2.12 | 6.21 | 2.07 | 0.916 |
| | MVC | 109.63 | 41.01 | 109.98 | 41.09 | 0.994 |
| Masseter muscles | Rest | 5.25 | 2.10 | 5.41 | 2.14 | 0.948 |
| | MVC | 107.41 | 34.29 | 107.82 | 34.22 | 0.993 |

In the rest position, differences between girls and boys in the TMD-pain and control groups with regard to the Asymmetry Index of the masseter muscles were statistically significant (for girls-$P = 0.0080$ and for boys-$P = 0.0478$) (Table 4). During MVC, a significant difference was observed in the Asymmetry Index of the masseter muscles between girls from the TMD-pain and the non-TMD group ($P = 0.0330$) (Table 5).

## 4. Discussion

The present clinical study was designed to evaluate the electrical potentials of the masticatory muscles in cleft lip and palate children with pain-related temporomandibular disorders. Muscle activity was analysed in the mandibular rest position and during maximum isometric contraction (MVC). The EMG recordings showed that children diagnosed with CLP and pain-related TMD have greater temporalis and masseter muscle activity at rest, reduced temporalis muscle activity during maximum voluntary contraction, and a higher Asymmetry Index for the temporalis and masseter muscles in the rest position.

We used surface electrodes in this examination. They have the advantage of being noninvasive and for this reason are better tolerated by patients [51]. The repetition of the main experiment confirmed the repeatability of electrode positioning, as well as the entire protocol. No study on method error was performed with regard to the positioning of subjects in the "natural head position". On the other hand, we employed a method that is considered one of the most repeatable, especially in adults (data about children are not so clear).

The study revealed hyperfunction of both temporalis and masseter muscles at rest position in patients with CLP and TMD-pain diagnoses. This means that, at rest, the EMG activity of the masticatory muscles was higher in CLP children with pain-related TMD than in subjects with no TMD. This behaviour may be explained by the need for greater muscle recruitment in individuals with TMD and pain when the mandible is at rest [52, 53]. This is probably due to sensorial-motor interactions, of which pain can modify the generation of action potentials and, eventually, myoelectric activity [54]. Riise [55] found that the activity of the temporalis muscle in the rest position was higher when occlusal interferences existed. In the long term, hyperactivity may be followed by structural adaptations, such as tooth movement, muscular reactions, and remodelling of the temporomandibular joints or it could lead to pathologic changes in the masticatory system.

Reduced temporalis activity in the cleft group diagnosed with TMD-pain during MVC suggests that there is an alteration in masticatory muscle recruitment compared to children without TMD. These alterations may be employed as an effective protective mechanism for damaged TMJs [56]. The specific recruitment of the temporalis muscle appears to be the result of descending central modulation subsequent to nociceptive stimuli of the affected TMJ and/or myofascial and/or periodontal nociceptors [36].

A higher Asymmetry Index for the temporalis and masseter muscles at rest in the TMD-P group indicates differential left-right muscle activity. Moreover, the increased Asymmetry Index in TMD-P patients may confirm a higher frequency of unilateral TMD in this group.

The results of the study indicate that in comparison to non-TMD cleft patients children diagnosed with CLP and TMD-P have altered masticatory muscle activity. As mentioned earlier, CLPs are strongly associated with the presence of malocclusions [5], which in turn could be a potential cause of TMD and can affect electrical muscle activity [8, 11, 12, 57]. Nevertheless, the prevalence of malocclusions in this study was similar in both children with TMD-P and in non-TMD children. However, other malocclusion-related

TABLE 4: Electrical activity of the masticatory muscles at clinical mandibular rest position in the children studied.

| Region | Variable | Gender | TMD-pain group | | | Non-TMD group | | | P value |
|---|---|---|---|---|---|---|---|---|---|
| | | | n | Mean | SD | n | Mean | SD | |
| Temporalis muscles | Electrical activity (μV/μV%) | Females | 15 | 6.79 | 1.43 | 14 | 5.80 | 1.24 | 0.0554 |
| | | Males | 16 | 7.53 | 2.43 | 18 | 6.06 | 1.95 | 0.0596 |
| | | Total | 31 | 7.17 | 2.01 | 32 | 5.94 | 1.66 | 0.0102* |
| | Asymmetry index (%) | Females | 15 | 15.81 | 7.66 | 14 | 10.19 | 4.97 | 0.1557 |
| | | Males | 16 | 16.13 | 7.62 | 18 | 9.94 | 4.68 | 0.0807 |
| | | Total | 31 | 15.99 | 7.02 | 32 | 10.06 | 4.33 | 0.0218* |
| Masseter muscles | Electrical activity (μV/μV%) | Females | 15 | 5.18 | 2.37 | 14 | 3.98 | 1.97 | 0.1516 |
| | | Males | 16 | 6.08 | 2.11 | 18 | 4.64 | 2.01 | 0.0509 |
| | | Total | 31 | 5.64 | 2.25 | 32 | 4.35 | 1.98 | 0.0188* |
| | Asymmetry index (%) | Females | 15 | 14.35 | 7.01 | 14 | 5.53 | 2.44 | 0.0080* |
| | | Males | 16 | 12.04 | 6.67 | 18 | 6.08 | 3.42 | 0.0478* |
| | | Total | 31 | 13.25 | 6.69 | 32 | 5.81 | 2.46 | 0.0010* |

*Statistically significant difference.

TABLE 5: Electrical activity of the masticatory muscles at maximal voluntary contraction (MVC) in the children studied.

| Region | Variable | Gender | TMD-pain group | | | Non-TMD group | | | P value |
|---|---|---|---|---|---|---|---|---|---|
| | | | n | Mean | SD | n | Mean | SD | |
| Temporalis muscles | Electrical activity (μV/μV%) | Females | 15 | 99.83 | 37.05 | 14 | 110.55 | 40.04 | 0.4607 |
| | | Males | 16 | 102.98 | 26.68 | 18 | 129.78 | 48.20 | 0.0576 |
| | | Total | 31 | 101.46 | 31.61 | 32 | 121.37 | 45.17 | 0.0477* |
| | Asymmetry index (%) | Females | 15 | 15.93 | 7.30 | 14 | 7.53 | 3.03 | 0.0607 |
| | | Males | 16 | 5.81 | 2.48 | 18 | 5.91 | 2.87 | 0.9563 |
| | | Total | 31 | 10.71 | 5.21 | 32 | 6.62 | 2.93 | 0.0858 |
| Masseter muscles | Electrical activity (μV/μV%) | Females | 15 | 98.24 | 31.53 | 14 | 102.56 | 31.33 | 0.7144 |
| | | Males | 16 | 103.01 | 35.33 | 18 | 115.29 | 41.76 | 0.3649 |
| | | Total | 31 | 100.70 | 33.08 | 32 | 109.72 | 37.54 | 0.3163 |
| | Asymmetry index (%) | Females | 15 | 15.31 | 7.32 | 14 | 8.09 | 4.85 | 0.0330* |
| | | Males | 16 | 6.75 | 3.34 | 18 | 6.59 | 3.38 | 0.9418 |
| | | Total | 31 | 10.89 | 5.59 | 32 | 7.24 | 3.50 | 0.0773 |

*Statistically significant difference.

factors, for example, the severity of malocclusion, were not determined. Further research would be needed to explore the association between TMD and muscle EMG activity in CLP subjects including factors that may contribute to TMD problems and changes in EMG pattern (e.g., malocclusion).

It is important to note that the children who participated in the study were still in the developmental stage. The alterations in masticatory muscle electrical activity showed by EMG recordings in children with TMD-P affect their muscle function. The altered muscle function in a growing stomatognathic system can result in malocclusion, or in the exacerbation of an already existing malocclusion, and this will be a significant risk factor promoting the development or progression of TMD problems in the future. Early investigation of the electromyographic characteristics of children could facilitate the development of treatment strategies aimed at normalizing muscle activity so as to achieve functional improvement in these patients. Of course, further studies that could be repeated for the same group of children in the future would provide evidence for a validity of EMG on the progression of their TMD.

This is the first report concerning masticatory muscle activity in children diagnosed with CLP and TMD-P based on the RDC/TMD criteria. As there have been no similar studies, it is difficult to compare our results with others. Nevertheless, the data obtained in our study could be referred to Li et al. [12], who evaluated masticatory muscle activity in patients with unilateral cleft lip and palate and anterior crossbite. The examined group included 29 individuals with CLP ranging in age from 11 to 21 years. Among them, 22 cleft patients had one or more symptoms of TMD on clinical examination. The control group consisted of 28 volunteers with no cleft abnormalities and normal occlusion. They found that compared to noncleft controls, patients with unilateral CLP had the following parameters for temporalis and masseter muscles: higher activation levels in the rest position, lower activity recorded during maximum clenching in the intercuspid position, and a higher Asymmetry Index.

An analysis of masticatory muscle EMG activity in children with TMD was the subject conducted by Chaves et al. [58]. They assessed the EMG activity of the masseter, temporalis, and suprahyoid muscles in 34 children aged 8–12 years: 17 children with TMD and 17 without TMD. The results of this study demonstrated a lower mean electromyographic ratio for masseter muscles and anterior temporalis muscles (sEMG-M/AT ratio) during maximum voluntary clenching in the TMD group. These results can be explained by three factors acting together: the lower mean raw activity of the masseter muscle compared to the anterior temporalis muscle in the TMD children, the lower mean raw activity of the masseter muscle in the TMD group compared to the control group, and the higher mean raw activity of the anterior temporalis muscle in the TMD group compared to the non-TMD group.

The relationship between TMD and TMD-P and the electrical activity of the masticatory muscles in adult females has been described by Rodrigues et al. [54] and Berni et al. [33]. They analysed the EMG potentials of the anterior temporalis, masseter, and suprahyoid muscles at rest position and during MVC on parafilm. They both found that EMG activity of the masticatory muscles at rest was higher in a TMD group than in a control group with no TMD. Rodrigues et al. [54] observed no differences with regard to MVC between such groups. However, Berni et al. [33] reported significantly lower activity in the masseter muscle. Similarly, Tartaglia et al. [34] and Liu et al. [59] found that temporalis and masseter muscle activity was significantly lower in TMD subjects than in non-TMD patients during MVC. Moreover, Liu et al. [59] observed greater EMG activity at rest position in the anterior temporalis muscle.

Khawaja et al. [15] assessed associations between masticatory muscle activity levels both when awake and during sleep among pain-related TMD diagnostic groups. Twenty-six adult subjects were classified into those diagnosed with TMD-P (myalgia and arthralgia) and those who were diagnosed with no pain. The data suggest a tendency towards increased masseter muscle activity in the TMD-pain group both when awake and during sleep. However, the same tendency was not noted in the temporalis muscle. They observed that temporalis muscle activity was only found to be higher in the pain-related TMD diagnoses group at extreme activity levels (<25% and ≥80% ranges).

The importance of such a parameter as muscular symmetry was noted by Liu et al. [59] and Tartaglia et al. [34]. Tartaglia et al. [34] found that symmetry in the temporalis muscles was greater in the control group than in TMD patients. Liu et al. [59] reported that asymmetry of the masseter muscle during MVC was significantly pronounced in TMD patients compared to normal subjects. The asymmetry of the anterior temporalis muscle was more pronounced in TMD patients during 70% MVC and was estimated at 28.6%, compared with 19.6% in normal subjects.

The results of the aforementioned studies suggest that an association exists between TMD and pain-related TMD and masticatory muscle EMG activity. Our study also revealed the influence of TMD-P on masticatory muscle EMG potentials in children with cleft lip and palate. Cleft children diagnosed with TMD-P have altered temporalis and masseter muscle activity compared with non-TMD subjects. From a clinical point of view, what is important is the fact that alteration of the pattern of muscle electrical activity in TMD-P patients can affect muscle fatigue, and can, as a consequence, have an impact on every function they perform in the stomatognathic system [60]. Such knowledge is essential when it comes to developing treatment protocols to normalize muscle activity and improve muscle function in these patients. However, we ought to be aware of the study's limitations, such as the relatively small number of subjects involved. In addition, the groups studied cover a comparatively wide age range. Hence, some differences between patients may result from variations in neuromuscular system development. Another possible limitation of the study might be the fact that the TMD-pain group included both joint- and muscle-related pain disorders, since EMG activity may vary in these subgroups of patients. In this context, further studies involving a larger number of patients are needed to confirm the study results.

## 5. Conclusions

The EMG recordings showed that in comparison to non-TMD cleft patients, children diagnosed with CLP and pain-related TMD have greater temporalis and masseter muscle activity at rest, reduced temporalis muscle activity during maximum voluntary contraction, and a higher Asymmetry Index for the temporalis and masseter muscles in the rest position. The altered masticatory muscle activity in TMD-P children can affect their muscle function.

## Ethical Approval

The present study was previously approved by the Local Bioethics Committee of the Medical University and assigned number KB-0012/08/15. All the children's parents were informed about the examination procedures and gave their consent to all the procedures performed.

## References

[1] P. A. Mossey, J. Little, R. G. Munger, M. J. Dixon, and W. C. Shaw, "Cleft lip and palate," *The Lancet*, vol. 374, no. 9703, pp. 1773–1785, 2009.

[2] D. J. Desmedt, T. J. Maal, M. A. Kuijpers, E. M. Bronkhorst, A. M. Kuijpers-Jagtman, and P. S. Fudalej, "Nasolabial symmetry and esthetics in cleft lip and palate: analysis of 3D facial images," *Clinical Oral Investigations*, vol. 19, no. 8, pp. 1833–1842, 2015.

[3] R. H. Lithovius, V. Lehtonen, T. J. Autio et al., "The association of cleft severity and cleft palate repair technique on hearing outcomes in children in northern Finland," *Journal of Craniomaxillofacial Surgery*, vol. 43, no. 9, pp. 1863–1867, 2015.

[4] L. Szyszka-Sommerfeld, K. Woźniak, T. Matthews-Brzozowska, B. Kawala, and M. Mikulewicz, "Electromyographic analysis of superior orbicularis oris muscle function in children surgically treated for unilateral complete cleft lip and palate," *Journal of Craniomaxillofacial Surgery*, vol. 45, no. 9, pp. 1547–1151, 2017.

[5] M. V. Vettore and A. E. Sousa Campos, "Malocclusion characteristics of patients with cleft lip and/or palate,"

*European Journal of Orthodontics*, vol. 33, no. 3, pp. 311–317, 2011.

[6] A. Paradowska-Stolarz and B. Kawala, "Occlusal disorders among patients with total clefts of lip, alveolar bone, and palate," *Biomed Research International*, vol. 2014, Article ID 583416, 5 pages, 2014.

[7] P. R. Shetye and C. A. Evans, "Midfacial morphology in adult unoperated complete unilateral cleft lip and palate patients," *Angle Orthodontist*, vol. 76, no. 5, pp. 810–816, 2006.

[8] K. Woźniak, L. Szyszka-Sommerfeld, and D. Lichota, "The electrical activity of the temporal and masseter muscles in patients with TMD and unilateral posterior crossbite," *Biomed Research International*, vol. 2015, Article ID 259372, 7 pages, 2015.

[9] A. Marcusson, T. List, G. Paulin, and S. Dworkin, "Temporomandibular disorders in adults with repaired cleft lip and palate: a comparison with controls," *European Journal of Orthodontics*, vol. 23, no. 2, pp. 193–204, 2001.

[10] A. P. Vanderas, "Craniomandibular dysfunction in children with clefts and noncleft children with and without unpleasant life events: a comparative study," *ASDC Journal of Dentistry for Children*, vol. 63, no. 5, pp. 333–337, 1996.

[11] A. P. Vanderas, "The relationship between craniomandibular dysfunction and malocclusion in white children with unilateral cleft lip and cleft lip and palate," *Cranio*, vol. 7, no. 3, pp. 200–204, 1989.

[12] W. Li, J. Lin, and M. Fu, "Electromyographic investigation of masticatory muscles in unilateral cleft lip and palate patients with anterior crossbite," *Cleft Palate Craniofacial Journal*, vol. 35, no. 5, pp. 415–418, 1998.

[13] A. P. Vanderas and D. N. Ranalli, "Evaluation of craniomandibular dysfunction in children 6 to 10 years of age with unilateral cleft lip or cleft lip and palate: a clinical diagnostic adjunct," *Cleft Palate Journal*, vol. 26, no. 4, pp. 332–337, 1989.

[14] S. J. Scrivani, D. A. Keith, and L. B. Kaban, "Temporomandibular disorders," *New England Journal of Medicine*, vol. 359, no. 25, pp. 2693–2705, 2008.

[15] S. N. Khawaja, W. McCall Jr., R. Dunford et al., "Infield masticatory muscle activity in subjects with pain-related temporomandibular disorders diagnoses," *Orthodontics and Craniofacial Research*, vol. 18, no. 1, pp. 137–145, 2015.

[16] E. Schiffman, R. Ohrbach, E. Truelove et al., "Diagnostic criteria for temporomandibular disorders (DC/TMD) for clinical and research applications: recommendations of the international RDC/TMD consortium network∗ and orofacial pain special interest groupdagger," *Journal of Oral and Facial Pain and Headache*, vol. 28, no. 1, pp. 6–27, 2014.

[17] S. F. Dworkin and L. LeResche, "Research diagnostic criteria for temporomandibular disorders: review, criteria, examinations and specifications, critique," *Journal of Craniomandibular Disorders*, vol. 6, no. 4, pp. 301–355, 1992.

[18] M. Wieckiewicz, K. Boening, P. Wiland, Y. Y. Shiau, and A. Paradowska-Stolarz, "Reported concepts for the treatment modalities and pain management of temporomandibular disorders," *Journal of Headache and Pain*, vol. 16, p. 106, 2015.

[19] C. S. Greene, "Diagnosis and treatment of temporomandibular disorders: emergence of a new care guidelines statement," *Oral Surgery, Oral Medicine, Oral Pathology, Oral Radiology, and Endodontics*, vol. 110, no. 2, pp. 137–139, 2010.

[20] M. Wieckiewicz, A. Paradowska-Stolarz, and W. Wieckiewicz, "Psychosocial aspects of bruxism: the paramount factor influencing teeth grinding," *Biomed Research International*, vol. 2014, Article ID 469187, 7 pages, 2014.

[21] I. Egermark, G. E. Carlsson, and T. Magnusson, "A 20-year longitudinal study of subjective symptoms of temporomandibular disorders from childhood to adulthood," *Acta Odontologica Scandinavica*, vol. 59, no. 1, pp. 40–48, 2001.

[22] R. M. Feteih, "Signs and symptoms of temporomandibular disorders and oral parafunctions in urban Saudi Arabian adolescents: a research report," *Head and Face Medicine*, vol. 16, no. 2, pp. 25, 2006.

[23] A. A. Köhler, A. N. Helkimo, T. Magnusson, and A. Hugoson, "Prevalence of symptoms and signs indicative of temporomandibular disorders in children and adolescents. A cross-sectional epidemiological investigation covering two decades," *European Archives of Paediatric Dentistry*, vol. 10, no. 1, pp. 16–25, 2009.

[24] A. Moyaho-Bernal, C. Lara-Muñoz Mdel, I. Espinosa-De Santillana, and G. Etchegoyen, "Prevalence of signs and symptoms of temporomandibular disorders in children in the State of Puebla, Mexico, evaluated with the research diagnostic criteria for temporomandibular disorders (RDC/TMD)," *Acta Odontologica Latinoamericana*, vol. 23, no. 3, pp. 228–233, 2010.

[25] M. Muhtaroğullari, F. Demirel, and G. Saygili, "Temporomandibular disorders in Turkish children with mixed and primary dentition: prevalence of signs and symptoms," *Turkish Journal of Pediatrics*, vol. 46, no. 2, pp. 159–163, 2004.

[26] I. M. Nilsson, T. List, and M. Drangsholt, "Prevalence of temporomandibular pain and subsequent dental treatment in Swedish adolescents," *Journal of Orofacial Pain*, vol. 19, no. 2, pp. 144–150, 2005.

[27] S. Hugger, H. J. Schindler, B. Kordass, and A. Hugger, "Clinical relevance of surface EMG of the masticatory muscles. (Part 1): resting activity, maximal and submaximal voluntary contraction, symmetry of EMG activity," *International Journal of Computerized Dentistry*, vol. 15, no. 4, pp. 297–314, 2012.

[28] K. Woźniak, D. Piątkowska, M. Lipski, and K. Mehr, "Surface electromyography in orthodontics—a literature review," *Medical Science Monitor*, vol. 19, pp. 416–423, 2013.

[29] D. Manfredini, F. Cocilovo, L. Favero, G. Ferronato, S. Tonello, and L. Guarda-Nardini, "Surface electromyography of jaw muscles and kinesiographic recordings: diagnostic accuracy for myofascial pain," *Journal of Oral Rehabilitation*, vol. 38, no. 11, pp. 791–799, 2011.

[30] M. A. Al-Saleh, S. Armijo-Olivo, C. Flores-Mir, and N. M. Thie, "Electromyography in diagnosing temporomandibular disorders," *Journal of American Dental Association*, vol. 143, no. 4, pp. 351–362, 2012.

[31] U. Santana-Mora, M. López-Ratón, M. J. Mora, C. Cadarso-Suárez, J. López-Cedrún, and U. Santana-Penín, "Surface raw electromyography has a moderate discriminatory capacity for differentiating between healthy individuals and those with TMD: a diagnostic study," *Journal of Electromyography and Kinesiology*, vol. 24, no. 3, pp. 332–340, 2014.

[32] C. A. Rodrigues, M. O. Melchior, L. V. Magri, W. Mestriner Jr., and M. O. Mazzetto, "Is the masticatory function changed in patients with temporomandibular disorders?," *Brazilian Dental Journal*, vol. 26, no. 2, pp. 181–185, 2015.

[33] K. C. Berni, A. V. Dibai-Filho, P. F. Pires, and D. Rodrigues-Bigaton, "Accuracy of the surface electromyography RMS processing for the diagnosis of myogenous temporomandibular disorder," *Journal of Electromyography and Kinesiology*, vol. 25, no. 4, pp. 596–602, 2015.

[34] G. M. Tartaglia, M. A. Moreira Rodrigues da Silva, S. Bottini, C. Sforza, and V. F. Ferrario, "Masticatory muscle activity

during maximum voluntary clench in different research diagnostic criteria for temporomandibular disorders (RDC/TMD) groups," *Manual Theraphy*, vol. 13, no. 5, pp. 434–440, 2008.

[35] I. L. Nielsen, C. McNeill, W. Danzig, S. Goldman, J. Levy, and A. J. Miller, "Adaptation of craniofacial muscles in subjects with craniomandibular disorders," *American Journal of Orthodontics and Dentofacial Orthopedics*, vol. 97, no. 1, pp. 20–34, 1990.

[36] B. J. Sessle, "Acute and chronic craniofacial pain: brainstem mechanisms of nociceptive transmission and neuroplasticity, and their clinical correlates," *Critical Reviews in Oral Biology and Medicine*, vol. 11, no. 1, pp. 57–91, 2000.

[37] E. Tanaka, M. S. Detamore, and L. G. Mercuri, "Degenerative disorders of the temporomandibular joint: etiology, diagnosis, and treatment," *Journal of Dental Research*, vol. 87, no. 4, pp. 296–307, 2008.

[38] D. Farina, L. Arendt-Nielsen, R. Merletti, and T. Graven-Nielsen, "Effect of experimental muscle pain on motor unit firing rate and conduction velocity," *Journal of Neurophysiology*, vol. 91, no. 3, pp. 1250–1259, 2004.

[39] A. G. Glaros, E. G. Glass, and D. Brockman, "Electromyographic data from TMD patients with myofascial pain and from matched control subjects: evidence for statistical, not clinical, significance," *Journal of Orofacial Pain*, vol. 11, no. 2, pp. 125–129, 1997.

[40] M. Wieckiewicz, N. Grychowska, K. Wojciechowski et al., "Prevalence and correlation between TMD based on RDC/TMD diagnoses, oral parafunctions and psychoemotional stress in Polish university students," *Biomed Research International*, vol. 2014, Article ID 472346, 7 pages, 2014.

[41] J. L. Fleiss, *Statistical Methods for Rates and Proportions*, Wiley, New York, NY, USA, 1981.

[42] D. V. Cicchetti and S. S. Sparrow, "Developing criteria for establishing interrater reliability of specific items: applications to assessment of adaptive behaviour," *American Journal of Mental Deficiency*, vol. 87, pp. 127–137, 1981.

[43] L. Szyszka-Sommerfeld, K. Woźniak, T. Matthews-Brzozowska, B. Kawala, M. Mikulewicz, and M. Machoy, "The electrical activity of the masticatory muscles in children with cleft lip and palate," *International Journal of Paediatric Dentistry*, vol. 28, no. 2, pp. 257–265, 2018.

[44] K. Woźniak, D. Piątkowska, and M. Lipski, "The influence of natural head position on the assessment of facial morphology," *Advances in Clinical and Experimental Medicine*, vol. 21, no. 6, pp. 743–749, 2012.

[45] V. F. Ferrario, C. Sforza, A. Colombo, and V. Ciusa, "An electromyographic investigation of masticatory muscles symmetry in normo-occlusion subjects," *Journal of Oral Rehabilitation*, vol. 27, no. 1, pp. 33–40, 2000.

[46] C. M. De Felício, F. V. Sidequersky, G. M. Tartaglia, and C. Sforza, "Electromyographic standardized indices in healthy Brazilian young adults and data reproducibility," *Journal of Oral Rehabilitation*, vol. 36, no. 8, pp. 577–583, 2009.

[47] S. E. Forrester, S. J. Allen, R. G. Presswood, A. C. Toy, and M. T. Pain, "Neuromuscular function in healthy occlusion," *Journal of Oral Rehabilitation*, vol. 37, no. 9, pp. 663–669, 2010.

[48] G. M. Targalia, G. Lodetti, G. Paiva, C. M. De Felício, and C. Sforza, "Surface electromyographic assessment of patients with long lasting temporomandibular joint disorder pain," *Journal of Electromyography and Kinesiology*, vol. 21, no. 4, pp. 659–664, 2011.

[49] M. Naeije, R. S. McCarroll, and W. A. Weijs, "Electromyographic activity of the human masticatory muscles during submaximal clenching in the inter-cuspal position," *Journal of Oral Rehabilitation*, vol. 16, no. 1, pp. 63–70, 1989.

[50] S. Tecco, E. Epifania, and F. Festa, "An electromyographic evaluation of bilateral symmetry of masticatory, neck and trunk muscles activity in patients wearing a positioner," *Journal of Oral Rehabilitation*, vol. 35, no. 6, pp. 433–439, 2008.

[51] K. Woźniak, D. Piątkowska, L. Szyszka-Sommerfeld, and J. Buczkowska-Radlińska, "The impact of functional appliances on muscle activity: a surface electromyography study in children," *Medical Science Monitor*, vol. 21, pp. 246–253, 2015.

[52] J. Finsterer, "EMG-interference pattern analysis," *Journal of Electromyography and Kinesiology*, vol. 11, no. 4, pp. 231–246, 2001.

[53] G. C. Venezian, M. A. da Silva, R. G. Mazzetto et al., "Low level laser effects on pain to palpation and electromyographic activity in TMD patients: a double-blind, randomized, placebo-controlled study," *Cranio*, vol. 28, no. 2, pp. 84–91, 2010.

[54] D. Rodrigues, A. O. Siriani, and F. Berzin, "Effect of conventional TENS on pain and electromyographic activity of masticatory muscles in TMD patients," *Brazilian Oral Research*, vol. 18, no. 4, pp. 290–295, 2004.

[55] C. Riise and A. Sheikholeslam, "The influence of experimental interfering occlusal contacts on the postural activity of the anterior temporal and masseter muscles in young adults," *Journal of Oral Rehabilitation*, vol. 9, no. 5, pp. 419–425, 1982.

[56] J. C. Nickel, L. R. Iwasaki, R. D. Walker, K. R. McLachlan, and W. D. McCall Jr., "Human masticatory muscle forces during static biting," *Journal of Dental Research*, vol. 82, no. 3, pp. 212–217, 2003.

[57] J. A. Alarcon, C. Martin, and J. C. Palma, "Effect of unilateral posterior crossbite on the electromyographic activity of human masticatory muscles," *American Journal of Orthodontics and Dentofacial Orthopedics*, vol. 118, no. 3, pp. 328–334, 2000.

[58] T. C. Chaves, A. dos Santos Aguiar, L. R. Felicio, S. M. Greghi, S. C. Hallak Regalo, and D. Bevilaqua-Grossi, "Electromyographic ratio of masseter and anterior temporalis muscles in children with and without temporomandibular disorders," *International Journal of Pediatric Otorhinolaryngology*, vol. 97, pp. 35–41, 2017.

[59] Z. J. Liu, K. Yamagata, Y. Kasahara, and G. Ito, "Electromyographic examination of jaw muscles in relation to symptoms and occlusion of patients with temporomandibular joint disorders," *Journal of Oral Rehabilitation*, vol. 26, no. 1, pp. 33–47, 1999.

[60] L. G. K. Ries, M. D. Graciosa, L. P. Soares et al., "Effect of time of contraction and rest on the masseter and anterior temporal muscles activity in subjects with temporomandibular disorder," *Codas*, vol. 28, no. 2, pp. 155–162, 2016.

# 8

# Reliability and Validity of the Korean Version of the Multidimensional Fatigue Inventory (MFI-20): A Multicenter, Cross-Sectional Study

Sang-Wook Song ⓘ,[1] Sung-Goo Kang ⓘ,[1] Kyung-Soo Kim,[2] Moon-Jong Kim,[3] Kwang-Min Kim,[4] Doo-Yeoun Cho,[3] Young-Sang Kim ⓘ,[3] Nam-Seok Joo,[4] and Kyu-Nam Kim ⓘ[4]

[1]Department of Family Medicine, St. Vincent's Hospital, College of Medicine, The Catholic University of Korea, Suwon, Republic of Korea
[2]Department of Family Medicine, CMC Clinical Research Coordinating Center, Seoul St. Mary's Hospital, College of Medicine, The Catholic University of Korea, Seoul, Republic of Korea
[3]Department of Family Medicine, CHA Bundang Medical Center, CHA Medical University, Seongnam, Republic of Korea
[4]Department of Family Practice and Community Health, Ajou University School of Medicine, Suwon, Republic of Korea

Correspondence should be addressed to Sung-Goo Kang; hippo94@naver.com

Academic Editor: Bruno Gagnon

*Introduction.* A nonspecific symptom, fatigue accompanies a variety of diseases, including cancer, and can have a grave impact on patients' quality of life. As for multidimensional instruments, one of the most widely used is the Multidimensional Fatigue Inventory (MFI). This study aims to verify the reliability and validity of the MFI Korean (MFI-K) version. *Materials and Method.* This study was performed at four university hospitals in the Republic of Korea. Among outpatients visiting the Department of Family Medicine, those complaining of fatigue or visiting a chronic care clinic were enrolled in this study. A total of 595 participants were included, and the mean age was 42.2 years. *Results.* The Cronbach's alpha coefficient of the MFI-K was 0.88. The MFI-K had good convergent validity. Most subscales of the MFI-K were significantly correlated with the Visual Analogue Scale (VAS) and Fatigue Severity Scale (FSS). In particular, general and physical fatigue had the greatest correlation with the VAS and FSS. Although the English version of MFI had five subscales, the factor analysis led to four subscales in the Korean version. *Conclusion.* This study demonstrated the clinical usefulness of MFI-K instrument, particularly in assessing the degree of fatigue and performing a multidimensional assessment of fatigue.

## 1. Introduction

Fatigue is a largely subjective symptom and is one of the most common symptoms encountered in primary care. A nonspecific symptom, fatigue accompanies a variety of diseases, including cancer, and can have a grave impact on patients' quality of life [1–8]. The medical cause of fatigue remains undiscovered in about 59–64% of adults who claim to have it [1]. Because of this nonspecificity, differential diagnosis and management of fatigue is often difficult. Nevertheless, both patients and physicians alike tend to underestimate fatigue symptoms solely due to their high prevalence.

One study showed that the prevalence of fatigue varies widely in primary practice, from 7 to 45%. One reason for such wide variation might be its ambiguous definition and differences in measurement instruments used [1].

Instruments useful for assessing fatigue can be categorized as unidimensional and multidimensional. The most widely used unidimensional fatigue assessment instruments are the Visual Analogue Scale (VAS) and Fatigue Severity Scale (FSS) developed by Dr. Krupp [9, 10]. The FSS has already been translated into Korean and validated [11]. As for multidimensional instruments, one of the most widely used is the Multidimensional Fatigue Inventory (MFI) [12]. The MFI was developed by E. M. A. Smets, a Dutch doctor. The validities of the English [12], French, and Swedish versions [13, 14] of the scale have been verified. The MFI has five subscales: general fatigue, physical fatigue, reduced activity, reduced motivation, and mental fatigue. Gentile et al. [13] conducted factor analysis at the same time as they conducted a validation study of the French version of MFI. The subscale of the French version of MFI was different from that of the MFI of the original version. The structure of Korean sentences is very different from the structure of English sentences. Korean sentences have the structure of subject + object + verb. Even the meaning of positive and negative is placed at the end of the sentence. Therefore, the subscales of MFI Korean version are very likely to be different from the MFI original version.

Because of cultural differences, translated scales must be appropriately validated to be suitable to the corresponding culture. Although many studies on fatigue in various patient populations, including patients with cancer and COPD, are underway in South Korea, there is practically no multidimensional instrument with verified reliability and validity in Korean. While researchers have translated the MFI into Korean and used it in practice, the reliability and validity of the translated version have not been established. Therefore, this study aims to verify the reliability and validity of the MFI Korean (MFI-K) version and to establish a new factor structure for the Korean outpatient population.

## 2. Materials and Methods

*2.1. Study Population.* The study population comprised adults aged 19 years or older. This study was performed at four university hospitals based in Seoul ($n = 1$) and two cities in Gyeonggi Province: Suwon ($n = 2$) and Seongnam ($n = 1$). Since Seoul is a metropolitan city with a population of more than 10 million, and Seongnam and Suwon are also cities with populations of more than 1 million, the subjects of this study were all urban people. Among outpatients visiting the Department of Family Medicine, those complaining of fatigue or who were visiting a chronic care clinic were enrolled in this study. Individuals without fatigue symptoms who have visited the health improvement center for a routine health examination were established as the control group. On the first page of the questionnaire, participants were asked to choose one of the following responses regarding their level of fatigue over the past week, before continuing with the rest of the questionnaire: (1) rarely, (2) moderate, and (3) very severe.

*2.2. Translation of MFI-K.* The translation was performed after obtaining approval from Dr. Smets, the developer of the MFI. The translation process suggested by Guillemin et al. [15] and Beaton et al. [16] was followed. First, two Korean native translators proficient in English independently translated the English version into Korean. One of these translators was the first author of this study, and the other translator was

blinded to the purpose of the questionnaire to enhance the quality of the translation. Next, four specialists discussed and analyzed the differences between the two translations to merge them into a single complete translation. During the back-translation stage, two new back-translators independently translated the completed translation into the source language (English). The back-translators were native English speakers also proficient in Korean. In addition, they were not medical professionals and were blinded to the purpose of the questionnaire. Finally, four specialists discussed and analyzed the back-translated version to complete the final MFI-K. Dr. Smets reviewed the final version and approved the study using MFI-K.

*2.3. Visual Analogue Scale (VAS).* The VAS is 100 mm long, with the left end indicating "no exhaustion at all" and the right end indicating "complete exhaustion." We showed participants the VAS and instructed them to put a mark on the VAS line to indicate their level of fatigue. Then we measured the length (mm) from the left end of the line to the mark to indicate their score. A higher score indicated more severe fatigue.

*2.4. Fatigue Severity Scale (FSS).* To assess fatigue severity, we additionally used the FSS developed by Krupp et al. [10]. The FSS is a 9-item self-report questionnaire. Each item is rated on a seven-point scale, where respondents choose a score between 1 (no impairment at all) and 7 (severe impairment) corresponding to their perceived impairment. The total score is then divided by the total number of items to generate the mean score. This scale was translated into Korean previously and has been found to be clinically useful [11].

*2.5. Statistical Analysis.* All statistical analyses were performed using the PASW Statistics (i.e., SPSS) 18.0 for Windows. Items within the original five factors of the MFI-K were assessed for their internal consistency by using Cronbach's alpha. Principal component analysis was performed to examine the MFI-K's factor structure; factors with eigenvalues of >1 were extracted. The convergent validity of the total cognition score was tested using the Spearman rank-order correlation and Pearson correlation coefficients with the VAS and FSS. Differences between the fatigue groups were tested using the chi-square test and ANOVA.

*2.6. Ethics Statement.* This study was implemented in accordance with ethical and safety guidelines upon the approval of the Institutional Review Board in The Catholic University of Korea, St. Vincent's Hospital (IRB approval number: VC15QIMI0193). We provided adequate explanation of the aim, structure, content, and precautions of the study to all participants, and participants were given sufficient time to make decisions. The participants were then instructed to answer all questionnaire items after reading the instructions of each instrument. They were told to ask any questions they might have during the course of completing

TABLE 1: Baseline characteristics of the study population.

| | No or mild fatigue ($N$ = 76) | Moderate fatigue ($N$ = 342) | Severe fatigue ($N$ = 174) | $P$ value |
|---|---|---|---|---|
| Age (years) | $45.39 \pm 13.68$ | $42.39 \pm 12.20$ | $40.49 \pm 11.82$ | 0.014 |
| Sex | | | | 0.071 |
|   Male | 36 (16.8) | 122 (57.0) | 56 (26.2) | |
|   Female | 40 (10.6) | 222 (28.6) | 117 (30.9) | |
| BMI (kg/m$^2$) | $24.04 \pm 5.36$ | $23.39 \pm 10.01$ | $22.79 \pm 3.61$ | 0.506 |
| Sleep duration | $6.78 \pm 1.09$ | $6.43 \pm 1.08$ | $6.23 \pm 1.31$ | 0.002 |
| Smoking | | | | 0.161 |
|   Smoker | 9 (14.1) | 31 (48.4) | 25 (37.5) | |
|   Ex-smoker | 16 (19.8) | 44 (54.3) | 21 (25.9) | |
|   Nonsmoker | 50 (11.4) | 260 (59.5) | 127 (29.1) | |
| Marital condition | | | | 0.542 |
|   Single | 18 (10.7) | 98 (58.0) | 53 (31.4) | |
|   Married | 56 (13.9) | 231 (57.3) | 116 (28.8) | |
|   Others | 4 (19.0) | 13 (61.9) | 4 (19.0) | |
| Education | | | | 0.362 |
|   Under middle school | 6 (17.6) | 19 (55.9) | 9 (26.5) | |
|   High school or college | 37 (17.3) | 119 (55.6) | 58 (27.1) | |
|   Over university | 35 (10.1) | 205 (59.2) | 106 (30.6) | |

Others: separation, divorce, or bereavement, data are mean $\pm$ SD or $N$ (%); $P$ values were obtained by the one-way ANOVA or chi-square test.

TABLE 2: Principal component analysis after varimax rotation of MFI Korean version.

| Factors | Eigenvalue | % total of variance | Items | Interpretation of Korean dimensions |
|---|---|---|---|---|
| Factor 1 | 6.37 | 31.85 | 1, 5, 12, 14, 16, 20 | General and physical fatigue |
| Factor 2 | 2.48 | 12.41 | 7, 9, 11, 13, 18, 19 | Mental fatigue |
| Factor 3 | 1.38 | 6.92 | 2, 6, 10, 17 | Reduced activity |
| Factor 4 | 1.23 | 6.15 | 3, 4, 8, 15 | Motivation |

the questionnaire to ensure that they accurately understand the instrument items.

# 3. Results

*3.1. General Characteristics.* A total of 595 participants were included, and the mean age was $42.22 \pm 12.36$ years. A total of 380 (63.99%) participants were women and 215 (36.01%) were men. The study groups did not significantly differ in terms of body mass index, marital status, highest education level, and smoking status. Although statistically non-significant, women tended to experience more severe fatigue than did men. Participants who reported severe fatigue were younger and slept significantly less (Table 1).

Fifty-one (8.5%) participants said that the content of the questionnaire was slightly difficult to understand, while 8 participants (1.3%) said that the content of the questionnaire was very difficult to understand. The remaining 538 (90.2%) participants said that the content of the questionnaire was neither difficult nor easy to understand or was easy to understand.

Overall, the MFI-K was well received by the participants. About 99.5% of the participants completed the MFI-K without omissions. Extremely few questionnaires were submitted with missing items (less than 0.5%).

The time taken to complete the MFI-K did not significantly differ among the fatigue groups ($4.14 \pm 2.95$ versus $4.05 \pm 3.25$ versus $4.36 \pm 3.06$, $P$ = 0.557).

*3.2. Internal Consistency.* The Cronbach's alpha coefficient of the MFI-K was 0.88. The internal consistency of each of the five original subscales was as follows: general fatigue (0.84), physical fatigue (0.78), mental fatigue (0.67), reduced activity (0.66), and reduced motivation (0.52).

*3.3. Structure Validity.* The results of the principal component analysis (with a varimax rotation) are shown in Tables 2 and 3. Four factors explained 57.33% of the total variance. Factor 1 explains 31.9% of the total variance and included all of the "general fatigue" items and some "physical fatigue" items. Factor 2 explains 12.4% of the total variance and includes all "mental fatigue" items and "I don't feel like doing anything" items. Factor 3 mostly includes the "reduced activities" items, and most of the items are phrased negatively. Factor 4 included positively worded phrases about motivation. Although the English version had five subscales, the factor analysis led to four subscales in the Korean version.

*3.4. Convergent Validity.* The MFI-K had good convergent validity. Most subscales of the MFI-K were significantly correlated with the VAS. In particular, general fatigue had the greatest correlation with the VAS ($r$ = 0.533). Reduced activity had the lowest significant correlation with the VAS ($r$ = 0.084).

Similarly, the general fatigue subscale of the MFI-K had the strongest correlation with the FSS ($r$ = 0.725).

TABLE 3: Items of the new dimension of the MFI Korean version.

| New dimension Korean version | Items contribution |
| --- | --- |
| General and physical fatigue | 1. 나는 몸 상태가 좋다. (I feel fit.)<br>5. 나는 피곤함을 느낀다. (I feel tired.)<br>12. 나는 가뿐하다. (I am rested.)<br>14. 육체적으로 나는 몸 상태가 나쁘다고 생각한다. (Physically I feel I am in a bad condition.)<br>16. 나는 쉽게 피곤해진다. (I tire easily.)<br>20. 육체적으로 나는 몸 상태가 아주 좋다고 생각한다. (Physically I feel I am in an excellent condition.) |
| Mental fatigue | 7. 나는 어떤 일을 하는 동안 그 일에 대한 생각을 계속 유지할 수 있다. (When I am doing something, I can keep my thoughts on it.)<br>9. 나는 어떤 일을 하는 것이 염려스럽다. (I dread having to do things.)<br>11. 나는 집중을 잘 할 수 있다. (I can concentrate well.)<br>13. 어떤 일에 집중하기 위해서 많은 노력이 필요하다. (It takes a lot of effort to concentrate on things.)<br>18. 나는 어떠한 일도 하고 싶지 않다. (I don't feel like doing anything.)<br>19. 생각이 쉽게 산만해진다. (My thoughts easily wander.) |
| Reduced activities | 2. 육체적으로 나는 아주 가벼운 일 밖에 할 수 없다. (Physically I feel only able to do a little.)<br>6. 나는 하루 동안에 아주 많은 일을 해낸다고 생각한다. (I think I do a lot in a day.)<br>10. 나는 하루 동안에 아주 적은 일을 한다고 생각한다. (I think I do very little in a day.)<br>17. 나는 처리한 일이 거의 없다. (I get little done.) |
| Motivation | 3. 나는 매우 활동적이라고 생각한다. (I feel very active.)<br>4. 나는 온갖 흥미로운 일들에 빠져들기를 좋아한다. (I feel like doing all sorts of nice things.)<br>8. 육체적으로 나는 많은 일을 해낼 수 있다. (Physically I can take on a lot.)<br>15. 나는 계획하고 있는 일들이 많다. (I have a lot of plans.) |

The reduced activity subscale had the lowest correlation with the FSS ($r = 0.162$) but the correlation was statistically significant (Table 4). These results were also found for the new factor structure of the MFI-K (Tables 5 and 6).

*3.5. Differences in MFI-K Scores across Fatigue Groups.* The mean MFI-K score significantly varied across the fatigue groups. With the exception of reduced activities, all subgroup scores significantly differed across the groups. The VAS and FSS scores also significantly differed across groups. In all cases, the mean MFI-K score increased with increasing fatigue severity (Table 6).

TABLE 4: Correlation between MFI-K and VAS score and FSS score in English factor structure.

| Dimensions: English structure | VAS score | FSS score |
| --- | --- | --- |
| General fatigue | 0.533** | 0.725** |
| Physical fatigue | 0.378** | 0.578** |
| Mental fatigue | 0.241** | 0.403** |
| Reduced activity | 0.084* | 0.162** |
| Reduced motivation | 0.276** | 0.391** |
| MFI-K total score | 0.419** | 0.635** |

**$P < 0.01$, *$P < 0.05$; correlation coefficients were obtained by Spearman correlation analysis.

TABLE 5: Correlation between MFI-K and VAS score and FSS score in Korean factor structure.

| Dimensions: Korean structure | VAS score | FSS score |
| --- | --- | --- |
| General and physical fatigue | 0.519** | 0.718** |
| Mental fatigue | 0.333** | 0.506** |
| Reduced activity | 0.087* | 0.200** |
| Motivation | 0.159** | 0.248** |
| MFI-K total score | 0.419** | 0.635** |

**$P < 0.01$, *$P < 0.05$; correlation coefficients were obtained by Spearman correlation analysis.

## 4. Discussion

This study aimed to verify the reliability and validity of the Korean version of the MFI, one of the most widely used multidimensional fatigue scales. It was also the first study to examine a Korean version of the Multidimensional Fatigue Scale.

We tested the reliability of the MFI-K using Cronbach's alpha coefficients. Scales with Cronbach's alpha values of greater than 0.7 are considered reliable [17], and the Cronbach's alpha coefficient of the MFI-K was 0.88, suggesting high reliability. The subscales also showed reasonable internal consistency (>0.65), with the exception of reduced motivation. This was similar to the results presented by Dr. Smets, the developer of the MFI [12]. However, the internal consistency was generally lower than that of the French version of the MFI [13]. Although additional studies are needed to shed light on the causes of the difference between our findings and findings from other countries, it is nevertheless possible that differences in sentence structures are involved. For instance, unlike English and French, the verb is placed at the end of the sentence in Korean, which means that words suggesting a negative or positive tone are placed at the end of the sentence, requiring readers to focus on the end of each sentence in order to accurately understand the whole sentence. As proof of this, factor 3 mostly includes negatively worded phrases (except one item, 6, "I think I do a lot in a day") and factor 4 included positively worded phrases.

To know this more clearly, further research in Japan and China is needed to confirm whether this is a geographical, cultural, or sentence structural problem. Although Korea, China, and Japan have very close geographical and historical relations, the language structure of Chinese is similar to English, but the language structure of Japanese is similar to

TABLE 6: Univariate $F$-test for group differences on subclass of the MFI Korean structure.

| | No or mild fatigue | Moderate fatigue | Severe fatigue | $P$ value |
|---|---|---|---|---|
| MFI Korean structure | | | | |
| General and physical fatigue | $14.37 \pm 4.73$ | $20.67 \pm 4.30$ | $26.83 \pm 3.94$ | <0.001 |
| Mental fatigue | $9.66 \pm 2.62$ | $12.17 \pm 3.13$ | $14.07 \pm 3.78$ | <0.001 |
| Reduced activities | $8.46 \pm 3.33$ | $9.12 \pm 2.54$ | $9.22 \pm 3.23$ | 0.131 |
| Motivation | $8.94 \pm 3.14$ | $10.87 \pm 2.76$ | $11.11 \pm 3.64$ | <0.001 |
| MFI-K total score | $41.36 \pm 10.52$ | $52.85 \pm 9.63$ | $61.23 \pm 10.54$ | <0.001 |
| VAS score | $16.85 \pm 18.19$ | $33.02 \pm 26.53$ | $55.74 \pm 32.28$ | <0.001 |
| FSS score | $20.59 \pm 9.09$ | $31.26 \pm 10.25$ | $43.81 \pm 10.25$ | <0.001 |

Korean. Therefore, if MFI is translated into Chinese and Japanese, and factor analysis is performed, it is possible to know more exactly whether MFI-K differs from MFI of English version because of geographical and cultural differences or differences in language structure.

As anticipated, the general and physical fatigue subscale of the MFI-K had the strongest correlations with the VAS and FSS. This is in line with the findings of Dr. Smets [18] that the general fatigue subscale of the MFI-20 is compatible with the VAS for assessing fatigue in cancer patients, and with the findings of Rupp et al. [4] that the general fatigue and physical fatigue subscales of the MFI-20 had the highest correlations with the VAS in patients with rheumatoid arthritis. The subjects of this study were people who visited family medicine departments for (generally physical) fatigue or visited health promotion centers for routine health checkups. The correlation between general and physical fatigue subscale of the MFI-K and FSS was higher than 0.7 and showed a low correlation with other subscales. These results demonstrate the ability of the MFI-K to differentiate between the degree and the type of fatigue.

As for the structural validity, the MFI-K has only four subscales (Tables 2 and 3), whereas the English version has five. The English version of the MFI includes general fatigue (items 1, 5, 12, and 16), physical fatigue (items 2, 8, 14, and 20), reduced activity (items 3, 6, 10, and 17), reduced motivation (item 4, 9, 15, and 18), and mental fatigue (item 7, 11, 13, and 19) subscales (Table 3). In our study, it was difficult to distinguish general fatigue from physical fatigue, which is similar to the study by Dr. Smets and the study on the Swedish version of the MFI [19]. With the exception of item 2 and item 8, items corresponding to general fatigue and physical fatigue in the English version of MFI consisted of one factor (general and physical fatigue) in MFI-K. In the English version of MFI, item 2 and item 8 are included in the physical fatigue subscale. However, in MFI-K, item 2 ("Physically I feel only able to do a little") was more relevant to the reduced activities subscale, and item 8 ("Physically I can take on a lot") was more relevant to the motivation subscale. In the English version of MFI, item 9 and item 18 are included in the reduced motivation subscale. In MFI-K, item 9 ("I dread having to do things") and item 18 ("I don't feel like doing anything") were more relevant to the mental fatigue subscale. As mentioned earlier, in MFI-K, factor 3 (reduced activity) mostly included negatively worded phrases (except one item, 6, "I think I do a lot in a day") and factor 4 (motivation) included positively worded phrases. It is

a sentence of the same meaning, but depending on the English or Korean language, it can be conveyed to the person reading the item with a different feeling. In the end, the structure of the MFI-K was generally inconsistent with the English version of the MFI and was closer to the French version.

This study has a few limitations. First, the subjects of this study were all urban people. Rural people were not included in the study. However, as of 2016, 91.8% of the total population of Korea lives in cities [20]. Second, in this study, the employment status of the subjects was not investigated.

This study demonstrated the clinical usefulness of this instrument, particularly in assessing the degree of fatigue and performing a multidimensional assessment of fatigue. The general and physical fatigue subscale was strongly associated with the global fatigue measures (VAS and FSS), and the other subscales had fair relationships with the FSS. These results show that fatigue is a multidimensional concept and various aspects must be considered when dealing with patients with fatigue. Follow-up studies should be conducted on a more diverse study population for whom fatigue assessment using the MFI-K is important, such as cancer patients or families of cancer patients, as well as patients with chronic fatigue syndrome, fibromyalgia, or chronic obstructive pulmonary disease.

## 5. Conclusion

This study demonstrated the clinical usefulness of MFI-K instrument, particularly in assessing the degree of fatigue and performing a multidimensional assessment of fatigue. The MFI-K is the first validated tool to assess various aspects of fatigue in Koreans.

## Funding

This study was supported by the Daewoong Pharmaceutical company.

## Acknowledgments

The authors sincerely thank Dr. E. M. A. Smets for allowing the Korean version of MFI to be studied.

## References

[1] G. Lewis and S. Wessely, "The epidemiology of fatigue: more questions than answers," *Journal of Epidemiology and Community Health*, vol. 46, no. 2, pp. 92–97, 1992.

[2] J. E. Bower, K. Bak, A. Berger et al., "Screening, assessment, and management of fatigue in adult survivors of cancer: an American Society of Clinical oncology clinical practice guideline adaptation," *Journal of Clinical Oncology*, vol. 32, no. 17, pp. 1840–1850, 2014.

[3] J. P. Solano, B. Gomes, and I. J. Higginson, "A comparison of symptom prevalence in far advanced cancer, AIDS, heart disease, chronic obstructive pulmonary disease and renal disease," *Journal of Pain and Symptom Management*, vol. 31, no. 1, pp. 58–69, 2006.

[4] I. Rupp, H. C. Boshuizen, C. E. Jacobi, H. J. Dinant, and G. A. van den Bos, "Impact of fatigue on health-related quality of life in rheumatoid arthritis," *Arthritis and Rheumatology*, vol. 51, no. 4, pp. 578–585, 2004.

[5] S. O. Breukink, J. H. Strijbos, M. Koorn, G. H. Koeter, E. H. Breslin, and C. P. van der Schans, "Relationship between subjective fatigue and physiological variables in patients with chronic obstructive pulmonary disease," *Respiratory Medicine*, vol. 92, no. 4, pp. 676–682, 1998.

[6] M. J. Hjermstad, P. M. Fayers, K. Bjordal, and S. Kaasa, "Health-related quality of life in the general Norwegian population assessed by the European Organization for Research and Treatment of Cancer Core Quality-of-Life Questionnaire: The QLQ=C30 (+3)," *Journal of Clinical Oncology*, vol. 16, no. 3, pp. 1188–1196, 1998.

[7] H. Michelson, C. Bolund, B. Nilsson, and Y. Brandberg, "Healthrelated quality of life measured by the EORTC QLQ-C30 reference values from a large sample of Swedish population," *Acta Oncologica*, vol. 39, no. 4, pp. 477–484, 2000.

[8] M. Lavidor, A. Weller, and H. Babkoff, "Multidimensional fatigue, somatic symptoms and depression," *British Journal of Health Psychology*, vol. 7, no. 1, pp. 67–75, 2002.

[9] L. B. Krupp, L. A. Alvarez, N. G. LaRocca, and L. C. Scheinberg, "Fatigue in multiple sclerosis," *Archives of Neurology*, vol. 45, no. 4, pp. 435–437, 1988.

[10] L. B. Krupp, N. G. LaRocca, J. Muir-Nash, and A. D. Steinberg, "The fatigue severity scale application to patients with multiple sclerosis and systemic lupus erythematosus," *Archives of Neurology*, vol. 46, no. 10, pp. 1121–1123, 1989.

[11] K. I. Chung and C. H. Song, "Clinical usefulness of fatigue severity scale for patients with fatigue, and anxiety or depression," *Korean Journal of Psychosomatic Medicine*, vol. 9, no. 2, pp. 164–173, 2001.

[12] E. M. A. Smets, B. Garssen, B. Bonke, and J. C. J. M. De Haes, "The Multidimensional Fatigue Inventory (MFI) psychometric qualities of an instrument to assess fatigue," *Journal of Psychosomatic Research*, vol. 39, no. 3, pp. 315–325, 1995.

[13] S. Gentile, J. C. Delarozière, F. Favre, R. Sambuc, and J. L. San Marco, "Validation of the French 'multidimensional fatigue inventory' (MFI 20)," *European Journal of Cancer Care*, vol. 12, no. 1, pp. 58–64, 2003.

[14] A. Ericsson and K. Mannerkorpi, "Assessment of fatigue in patients with fibromyalgia and chronic widespread pain. Reliability and validity of the Swedish version of the MFI-20," *Disability and Rehabilitation*, vol. 29, no. 22, pp. 1665–1670, 2007.

[15] F. Guillemin, C. Bombardier, and D. Beaton, "Cross-cultural adaptation of health related quality of life measure: literature review and proposed guidelines," *Journal of Clinical Epidemiology*, vol. 46, pp. 1417–1432, 1993.

[16] D. E. Beaton, C. Bombardier, F. Guillemin, and M. B. Ferraz, "Guidelines for the process of cross cultural adaptation of self report measures," *Spine*, vol. 25, no. 24, pp. 3186–3191, 2000.

[17] L. J. Cronbach, "Coefficient alpha and the internal structure of tests," *Psychometrika*, vol. 16, no. 3, pp. 297–334, 1951.

[18] C. L. Hagelin, Y. Wengström, S. Runesdotter, and C. J. Fürst, "The psychometric properties of the Swedish Multidimensional Fatigue Inventory MFI-20 in four different populations," *Acta Oncologica*, vol. 46, no. 1, pp. 97–104, 2007.

[19] E. M. Smets, B. Garssen, A. Cull, and J. C. de Haes, "Application of the multidimensional fatigue inventory (MFI-20) in cancer patients receiving radiotherapy," *British Journal of Cancer*, vol. 73, no. 2, pp. 241–245, 1996.

[20] *Ministry of Land, Infrastructure and Transport (Republic of Korea)*, http://www.index.go.kr/potal/main/EachDtlPageDetail.do?idx_cd=1200.

# 9

# Efficacy of Pectoral Nerve Block Type II for Breast-Conserving Surgery and Sentinel Lymph Node Biopsy: A Prospective Randomized Controlled Study

Doo-Hwan Kim [ID],[1] Sooyoung Kim,[1] Chan Sik Kim [ID],[1] Sukyung Lee [ID],[1] In-Gyu Lee [ID],[1] Hee Jeong Kim [ID],[2] Jong-Hyuk Lee [ID],[1] Sung-Moon Jeong [ID],[1] and Kyu Taek Choi[1]

[1]Department of Anesthesiology and Pain Medicine, Asan Medical Center, University of Ulsan College of Medicine, Seoul, Republic of Korea
[2]Division of Breast and Endocrine Surgery, Department of Surgery, Asan Medical Center, University of Ulsan College of Medicine, Seoul, Republic of Korea

Correspondence should be addressed to Jong-Hyuk Lee; leejhpain@amc.seoul.kr

Academic Editor: Jacob Ablin

*Objectives.* The pectoral nerve block type II (PECS II block) is widely used for postoperative analgesia after breast surgery. This study evaluated the analgesic efficacy of PECS II block in patients undergoing breast-conserving surgery (BCS) and sentinel lymph node biopsy (SNB). *Methods.* Patients were randomized to the control group ($n = 40$) and the PECS II group ($n = 40$). An ultrasound-guided PECS II block was performed after induction of anesthesia. The primary outcome measure was opioid consumption, and the secondary outcome was pain at the breast and axillary measured using the Numerical Rating Scale (NRS) 24 hours after surgery. Opioid requirement was assessed according to tumor location. *Results.* Opioid requirement was lower in the PECS II than in the control group ($43.8 \pm 28.5$ g versus $77.0 \pm 41.9$ g, $p < 0.001$). However, the frequency of rescue analgesics did not differ between these groups. Opioid consumption in the PECS II group was significantly lower in patients with tumors in the outer area than that in patients with tumors in the inner area ($32.5 \pm 23.0$ g versus $58.0 \pm 29.3$ g, $p = 0.007$). The axillary NRS was consistently lower through 24 hr in the PECS II group. *Conclusion.* Although the PECS II block seemed to reduce pain intensity and opioid requirements for 24 h after BCS and SNB, these reductions may not be clinically significant. This trial is registered with Clinical Research Information Service KCT0002509.

## 1. Introduction

Breast-conserving surgery (BCS) and sentinel lymph node biopsy (SNB) are surgical methods designed to minimize intraoperative tissue injury, removing the cancer while leaving intact as much of the breast as possible. Moreover, because long-term survival rates are similar in patients undergoing BCS and radical mastectomy [1], the combination of BCS and SNB has become the standard treatment for patients with early-stage breast cancer [2].

Although BCS is minimally invasive surgery, it can lead to significant postoperative pain [3]. Because acute postoperative pain and BCS may be risk factors for persistent pain after breast cancer surgery, it is important to manage postoperative pain in patients undergoing BCS and SNB [4]. A thoracic epidural block used to be regarded as the gold-standard method for managing postoperative pain after breast surgery [5]. However, this technique is associated with serious complications, including intrathecal spread, nerve damage, epidural hematoma, and inadvertent intravascular injection [6]. A recently introduced pectoral nerve block type II (PECS II block) has been found to provide great pain relief and safety in patients undergoing radical mastectomy [7, 8]. Therefore, we hypothesized that the PECS II block may effectively alleviate acute postoperative pain in patients undergoing BCS and SNB. The present study evaluated the analgesic efficacy of PECS II block in patients undergoing BCS and SNB. In addition, this study assessed the efficacy of PECS II block according to breast cancer location and its comparative effects on breast and axillary pain.

## 2. Methods

*2.1. Patients.* This study enrolled patients with early breast cancer scheduled to undergo BCS and SNB between July 2016 and May 2017. The trial was approved by the Institutional Review Board (2016-0738) of Asan Medical Center and was registered at the Clinical Research Information Service (KCT 0002509). All patients provided written informed consent.

Patients were included if they were aged 20–70 years and had American Society of Anesthesiologists (ASA) physical status I and II. Patients were excluded if they had used an anticoagulant, did not cooperate with the study protocol, were allergic to local anesthetics, had serious neurological or psychiatric disorders, or were pregnant or breastfeeding. Patients with one and three incision sites were also excluded. Patients were randomized to two groups according to a computer-generated randomization schedule. Patients in the PECS II group received a PECS II block following the induction of general anesthesia, whereas patients in the control group did not receive any regional analgesia during the perioperative period.

*2.2. Process of Anesthesia and Analgesia.* Anesthesia was induced by administration of propofol (2 mg/kg). After the patient lost consciousness, rocuronium (0.6 mg/kg) was injected for smooth tracheal intubation. Desflurane and remifentanil were also used for induction. Remifentanil was administrated via target-controlled infusion using Orchestra (Fresenius Vial, Brezins, France). Anesthesia was maintained with desflurane 5-6% in 50% oxygen and 2–2.5 ng/ml of effect-site remifentanil concentration. After surgery, the patients were moved to the postanesthetic care unit (PACU) and administered fentanyl (0.4 μg/kg) when in need of analgesics or when analgesia was insufficient (Numerical Rating Scale (NRS) ≥ 4). Injection of fentanyl in the PACU was repeated until the patient was satisfied with analgesia. Upon being moved to the general ward, patients were administered 30 mg of the nonsteroidal anti-inflammatory drug (NSAID) ketorolac to reduce postoperative pain. Patients with sustained inadequate analgesia were administered meperidine 25 mg or tramadol 50 mg until 24 hours after surgery.

*2.3. Ultrasound-Guided PECS II Block.* Ultrasound-guided PECS II block was performed following general anesthesia to obviate any pain and anxiety associated with a regional block in conscious patients. This procedure was conducted according to the techniques described by Blanco et al. and therefore also included a PECS I block [9]. Patients were placed in the supine position on an operating table with their arm abducted. After sterile preparation for the procedure, a 12 MHz linear ultrasound probe (NextGen LOGIQ

e Ultrasound, GE Healthcare, USA) was positioned below the lateral third of the clavicle. The positions of the axillary artery and vein were confirmed, and the ultrasound probe was moved inferolaterally until the pectoralis major and minor and the serratus anterior muscles were identified in one plane at the level between the third and fourth ribs. A 23-gauge Quincke type spinal needle (TaeChang Industrial Co., Korea) was advanced in plane view of the ultrasound probe from the medial to lateral direction until it reached the interfascial plane between the pectoralis major and minor muscles. After the position of the needle tip was confirmed, 10 ml of 0.25% ropivacaine was administered. The needle was subsequently advanced further until its tip was located in the interfascial plane between the pectoralis minor and serratus anterior muscles, and an additional 20 ml of 0.25% ropivacaine was administered above the serratus anterior muscles (Figure 1). All of these nerve block procedures were performed by two anesthesiologists who were proficient and experienced in ultrasound-guided PECS II block.

*2.4. Outcome Measures and Data Collection.* All baseline and postoperative measurements were evaluated by an independent physician who was blinded to treatment allocation. Postoperative pain intensity was assessed using a single 11-point NRS (in which 0 = no pain and 10 = worst pain imaginable). The NRS was measured separately on the breast and axilla. To obtain a valid NRS value after the operation, all participants were instructed before the procedure about how to check the NRS correctly. Doses of all opioids administered to patients were converted to intravenous fentanyl equianalgesic doses according to published conversion factors (intravenous fentanyl 100 μg = meperidine 100 mg = tramadol 100 mg) [10]. Analgesic consumption and the NRS were measured 0, 0.5, 1, 2, 6, 9, 18, and 24 hours after the end of surgery. Opioid requirements were analyzed as a function of breast cancer location (quadrants, outer and inner areas, and upper and lower area; Figure 2). Complications associated with the PECS II block and with analgesics, such as pneumothorax, hematoma, nausea, vomiting, and urinary retention, were recorded. Vital signs (e.g., oxygen saturation, blood pressure, heart rate, and electrocardiography) were measured during the first 24 hours postoperatively. Differences in mean blood pressure and heart rate from before to after the incision were calculated. The sensory level of the block was evaluated using the cold test, performed by an independent physician after the operation.

A medical bandage was applied to the site of needle insertion in the PECS II group after the operation. To ensure patients were unaware whether the PECS II block had been performed, a bandage was also applied to a similar site in the control group.

The primary study outcome was the difference in 24-hour postoperative opioid consumption between the PECS II and control groups. Secondary outcomes included the NRS for each breast and axilla, changes in vital signs at incision, opioid requirements according to breast cancer location, side effects of analgesics (nausea, vomiting, dizziness, pruritus, sleeping

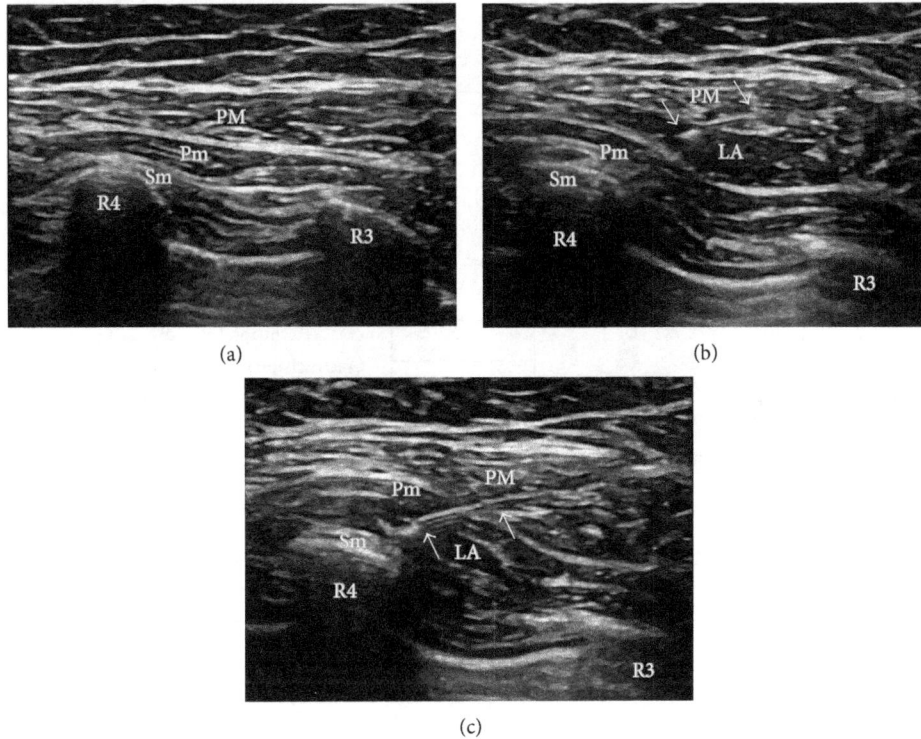

FIGURE 1: Ultrasound images of the introduction of a PECS II block. (a) Target areas of the PECS II block. (b) First injection of the PECS II block, showing spreading of local anesthetic in the interfascial plane between the pectoralis major and pectoralis minor muscles. (c) Second injection of the PECS II block, showing spreading of local anesthetic in the interfascial plane between the pectoralis minor and serratus anterior muscles. PM, pectoralis major muscle; Pm, pectoralis minor muscle; SA, serratus anterior muscle; LA, local anesthetic; R3, third rib; R4, fourth rib. The arrow indicates the 23-gauge Quincke needle.

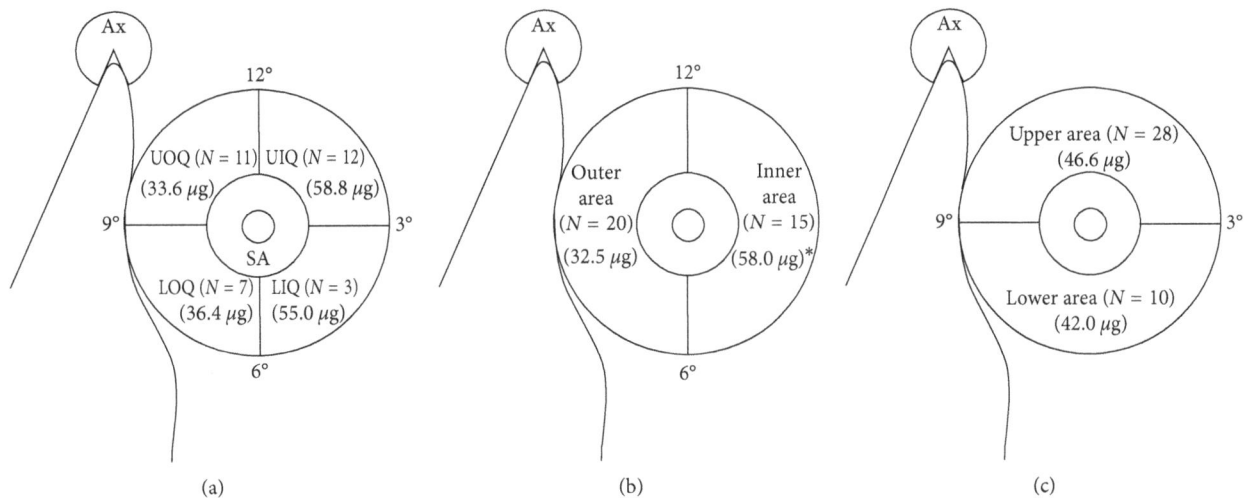

FIGURE 2: Opioid consumption as a function of breast cancer location. (a) Opioid consumption according to the quadrants of the breast. Patients with cancers located at 12, 3, 6, and 9 o'clock were not excluded because of the ambiguity of location. UOQ, upper outer quadrant; UIQ, upper inner quadrant; LOQ, lower outer quadrant; LIQ, lower inner quadrant; SA, subareolar; Ax, axilla; N, number of patients; values within parentheses denote mean fentanyl consumption. (b) Opioid consumption according to tumor location in the outer and inner areas of the breast, as determined by a line connecting the 12 o'clock and 6 o'clock positions. Patients with cancers located at 12 o'clock and 6 o'clock were not excluded, *p value < 0.05. (c) Opioid consumption according to tumor location in the upper and lower areas of the breast, as determined by a line connecting the 3 o'clock and 9 o'clock positions. Patients with cancers located at 3 o'clock and 9 o'clock were not excluded.

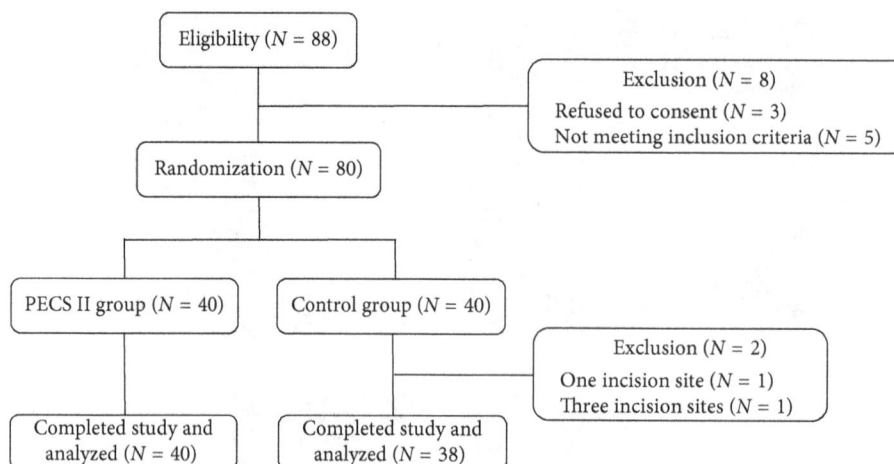

FIGURE 3: Study flow chart.

TABLE 1: Baseline demographic and clinical characteristics of study subjects.

| | PECS II group ($n = 40$) | Control group ($n = 38$) |
|---|---|---|
| Age (years) | 45.4 ± 9.9 | 45.2 ± 11.9 |
| BMI (kg/m$^2$) | 22.8 ± 2.8 | 23.9 ± 3.1 |
| ASA class (I/II) | 36 (90.0%)/4 (10.0%) | 29 (76.3%)/9 (23.7%) |
| Neoadjuvant CTx | 6 (15.0%) | 6 (15.8%) |
| Surgical time (min) | 93.5 ± 19.9 | 89.7 ± 24.9 |
| Intraoperative remifentanil dosage (μg) | 491.0 (440.0; 571.0) | 477.0 (420.0; 600.0) |
| Tumor location (left/right) | 14 (35.0%)/26 (65.0%) | 21 (55.3%)/17 (44.7%) |
| Tumor location (quadrant) | | |
| UOQ/LOQ | 11 (27.5%)/7 (17.5%) | 15 (39.5%)/7 (18.4%) |
| UIQ/LIQ | 12 (30.0%)/3 (7.5%) | 7 (18.4%)/3 (7.9%) |
| 12 o'clock/6 o'clock | 5 (12.5%)/0 (0.0%) | 1 (2.6%)/1 (2.6%) |
| 3 o'clock/9 o'clock | 0 (0.0%)/2 (5.0%) | 2 (5.2%)/1 (2.6%) |
| Subareolar | 0 (0.0%) | 1 (2.6%) |

Data are expressed as mean ± SD (standard deviation), number (%), or median (interquartile range). BMI, body mass index; ASA, American Society of Anesthesiologists Physical Status Classification; CTx, chemotherapy; UOQ, upper outer quadrant; LOQ, lower outer quadrant; UIQ, upper inner quadrant; LIQ, lower inner quadrant.

tendency, urinary retention, and respiratory depression), and complications of the PECS II block.

*2.5. Statistical Analysis.* The sample size was calculated based on our pilot study. If the mean ± standard deviation (SD) difference in opioid consumption between the PECS II and control groups was 48 ± 64 μg of fentanyl, with a significance level of 0.05 and a power of 0.9, and assuming a dropout rate of 5%, then 80 patients (40 per group) should be sufficient. Data were analyzed using the Statistical Package for the Social Sciences (SPSS version 21.0, SPSS Inc., Chicago, IL). Normal distribution of data was tested using the Kolmogorov–Smirnov test. Normally distributed continuous data were reported as mean ± SD and compared using Student's t-tests. Nonparametric continuous data were presented as median and interquartile range and compared using Mann–Whitney U tests. Categorical data were presented as numbers and percentages and compared using the chi-square test or Fisher's exact test. Opioid consumption as a function of breast cancer location was determined using the Kruskal–Wallis test. A $p$ value below 0.05 was considered statistically significant.

## 3. Results

Eighty patients were enrolled in this study, 40 in the PECS II group and 40 in the control group. Two patients in the control group, one with a single incision site and one with three incision sites, were excluded (Figure 3). The baseline demographic and clinical characteristics of the two groups are shown in Table 1. As expected, the changes in mean blood pressure and heart rate (from before to after the incision) were greater in the control than in the PECS II group. The side effect rates of analgesics were similar in the two groups (Table 2).

Opioid consumption during the first 24 hours after surgery was significantly lower in the PECS II group than in the control group (43.8 ± 28.5 μg versus 77.0 ± 41.9 μg, $p < 0.001$), but the frequency of rescue NSAIDs did not differ between these groups. The rates of side effects of analgesics were also similar in the two groups (Table 2). Analysis of patients in the PECS II group showed that opioid consumption was unrelated to the quadrant in which the breast cancer was located, that is, whether the tumor was located in the upper or lower area of the breast. However, opioid consumption was

TABLE 2: Opioid requirements, frequency of rescue NSAIDs, and incidence of side effects of analgesics in the PECS II and control groups during the 24 hours after the operation.

| | PECS II group ($n = 40$) | Control group ($n = 38$) | $p$ value |
|---|---|---|---|
| Total opioid requirements ($\mu$g) | $43.8 \pm 28.5$ | $77.0 \pm 41.9$ | $<0.001$ |
| Frequency of rescue NSAIDs | 1.0 (0.0; 1.0) | 1.0 (1.0; 1.0) | 0.213 |
| MBP after incision – MPB before incision (mmHg) | 5.0 (1.0; 10.5) | 16.0 (9.0; 24.0) | $<0.001$ |
| HR after incision – HR before incision (beats per minute) | 0.0 (−2.0; 2.5) | 3.0 (1.0; 5.0) | 0.002 |
| Side effects of analgesics (%) | 7 (17.5%) | 10 (26.3%) | 0.504 |

Data are expressed as mean ± SD (standard deviation), median (interquartile range), or number (%). NRS, Numerical Rating Scale; NSAID, nonsteroidal anti-inflammatory drug; MBP, mean blood pressure; HR, heart rate.

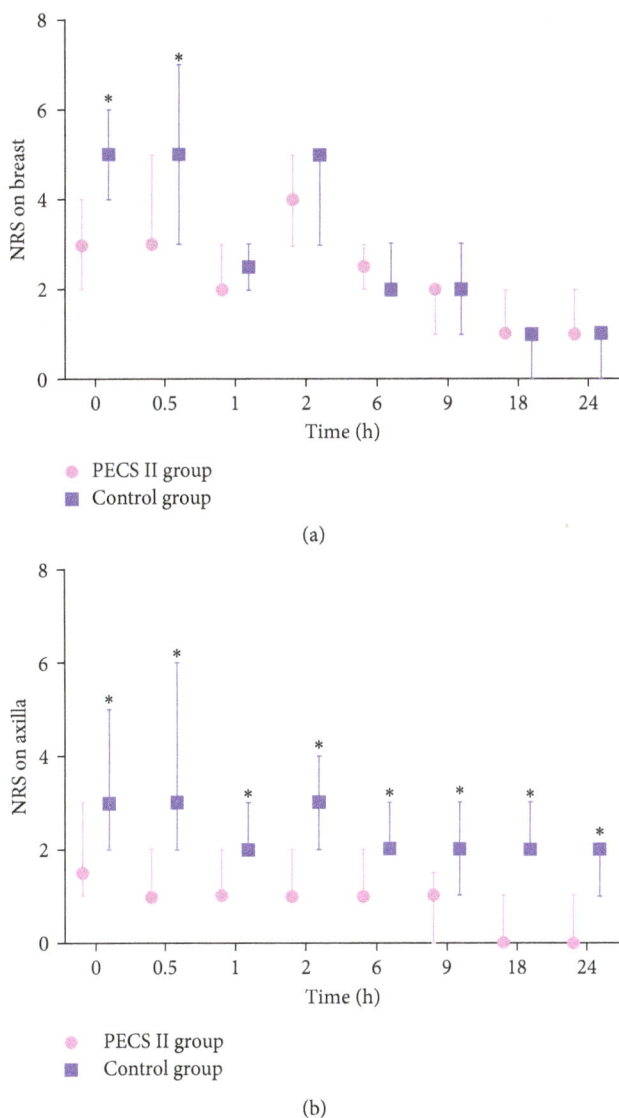

PECS II group
Control group

(a)

PECS II group
Control group

(b)

FIGURE 4: NRS of the breast (a) and axilla (b) in the PECS II and control groups. Data are expressed as the median (interquartile range). $^*$ $p$ value $< 0.05$.

significantly greater in PECS II patients with tumors in the inner area than in the outer area of the breast ($58.0 \pm 29.3\,\mu$g versus $32.5 \pm 23.0\,\mu$g, $p = 0.007$; Figure 2).

Mean NRS value of the breast was significantly lower in the PECS II than in the control group at 0 ($3.0 \pm 1.5$ versus $4.9 \pm 1.6$, $p < 0.001$) and 0.5 ($3.6 \pm 1.5$ versus $5.1 \pm 1.8$, $p < 0.001$) hours after the procedure. Median NRS value of the breast was not statistically lower in the PECS II than in the control group starting 1 hour after surgery. Median NRS value of the axilla, however, was significantly lower in the PECS II than in the control group throughout the first 24 hours after surgery (Figure 4). None of these patients reported complications associated with the PECS II block.

## 4. Discussion

This study had two main findings. First, although the PECS II block seemed to reduce pain severity and opioid consumption in patients undergoing BCS and SNB, it may not have clear clinical efficacy. Second, the PECS II block had a significantly greater effect in reducing axillary pain.

Since the introduction of PECS II block, several randomized controlled trials have shown that the PECS II block is effective in reducing pain in patients undergoing mastectomy [7–9, 11, 12]. To our knowledge, the present study is the first to test the efficacy of PECS II block only in patients undergoing BCS and SNB. The mean difference in opioid requirement between the two groups was only $33.2\,\mu$g of fentanyl. In other studies of interfascial plane block, the minimum difference in opioid consumption between the nerve block and control groups was 13 mg of morphine or $100\,\mu$g of fentanyl [13, 14]. The $33\,\mu$g difference in fentanyl consumption over 24 hours in the present study was less than $2\,\mu$g per hour, a quantitative difference lower than in other studies of regional analgesia. Similar to our results, two previous studies also found that the mean differences in 24-hour postoperative morphine consumption between the PECS II and control groups were 5.81 mg and 3.67 mg [12, 15]. Moreover, the frequency of rescue NSAIDs and the side effects of analgesics in the present study did not differ in the PECS II and control groups. These findings indicate that, although the PECS II block seemed to statistically significantly reduce rescue analgesic use, the difference may not have clinical significance. The present study also showed that the breast pain score was lower in the PECS II group than in the control group only for the first 30 min postoperatively. Moreover, the median difference in the NRS score between these groups was less than 1 at all other time points. This difference did not meet the threshold for a minimal clinically important difference in acute postoperative pain (i.e., a difference ≥10 on the 100 mm pain visual analogue scale)

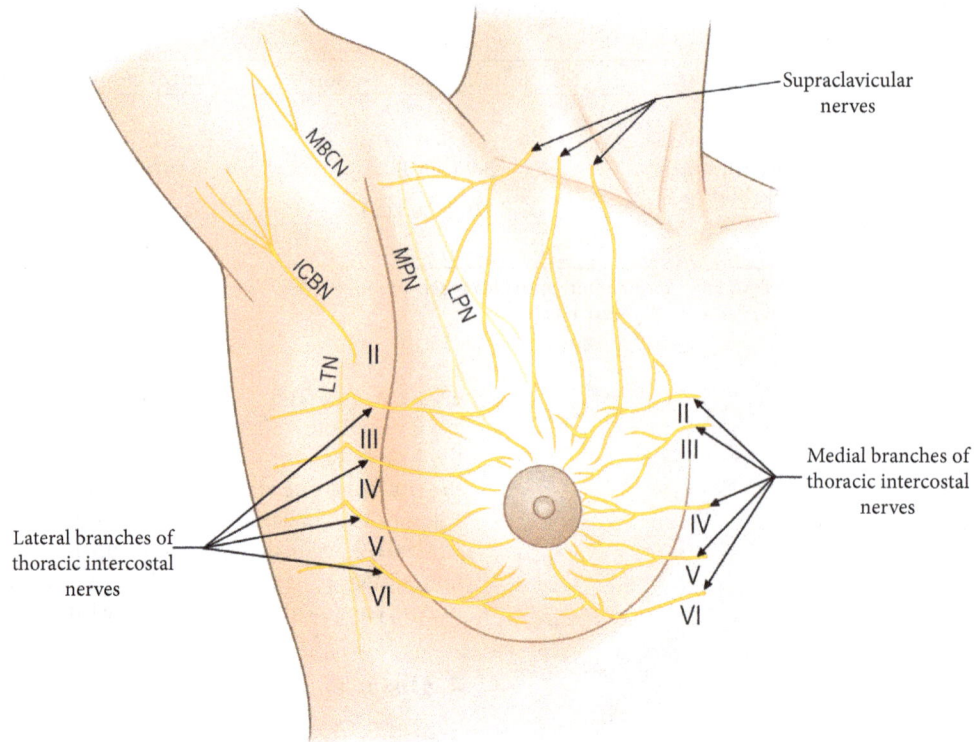

FIGURE 5: Diagrammatic representation of the nerves innervating the female breast and axilla. MPN, medial pectoral nerve; LPN, lateral pectoral nerve; MBCN, medial brachial cutaneous nerve; ICBN, intercostobrachial nerve; LTN, long thoracic nerve.

[16]. Therefore, the PECS II block appeared not to be clinically useful.

The lack of clinical significance of the PECS II block may have been due to its inability to block all the nerves innervating the breast. The breast is innervated by multiple nerve branches, including the lateral and anterior cutaneous branches of the second to sixth thoracic intercostal nerves (TICNs) and several branches of the supraclavicular nerves (Figure 5) [17, 18]. Thus, it is doubtful whether a single blocking method can provide adequate analgesia throughout the entire breast area. The targets of PECS II block include the medial and lateral pectoral nerves, including the lateral cutaneous branches of the TICNs (Figure 6). Local anesthetics cannot reach the anterior cutaneous branches of the TICNs by piercing the external and internal intercostal muscles. Therefore, they cannot block anterior cutaneous branches of the second to sixth TICNs and branches of the supraclavicular nerves. Although several recent studies have also mentioned these limitations of the PECS II block [15, 19, 20], those studies, in contrast to ours, did not demonstrate these limitations.

Additionally, we evaluated opioid requirements associated with tumor location in the breast (quadrant, outer/inner, and upper/lower areas). Opioid consumption did not differ significantly by breast tumor quadrant or in patients with tumors in the upper and lower areas. However, opioid requirements were greater in patients with tumors in the inner area than in the outer area of the breast. The inner area is primarily innervated by the anterior cutaneous branches of the TICN, whereas the outer area is primarily innervated by the lateral cutaneous branches of the TICN. Therefore, our finding suggests that the PECS II block could block the lateral, but not the anterior, cutaneous branches of the TICN.

Interestingly, axillary pain scores were significantly lower in the PECS II group than in the control group for up to 24 hours after surgery. The median difference in NRS between these groups was >1.5 at most evaluation times. These findings indicated that the PECS II block could be useful as regional analgesia for patients undergoing SNB. Local anesthetic administered into the interfascial plane likely reached the axilla via an axillary port, easily blocking the intercostobrachial and medial brachial cutaneous nerves, which innervate the axillary area. The spread of local anesthetic into the axilla has been demonstrated by dissection of cadavers and contrast distribution [9, 21]. The pectoral nerve block was also found to be beneficial for axillary surgery [22]. Consequently, the PECS II block may be effective at alleviating axillary pain.

In agreement with previous studies, no complications were associated with the PECS II block procedure. A PECS II block is conducted while patients are in the supine position, and the needle is manipulated relatively easily. Moreover, the target areas of a PECS II block are distant from the pleura and epidural space, but relatively close to the skin surface (Figure 6). Although the thoracoacromial artery may be present at the interfascial plane, it is easily visualized by ultrasonography. Direct intravascular injection of local anesthetics is performed very rarely due to a lack of vasculature at the interfascial plane [23, 24]. Therefore, a PECS II block seems to be a safe procedure.

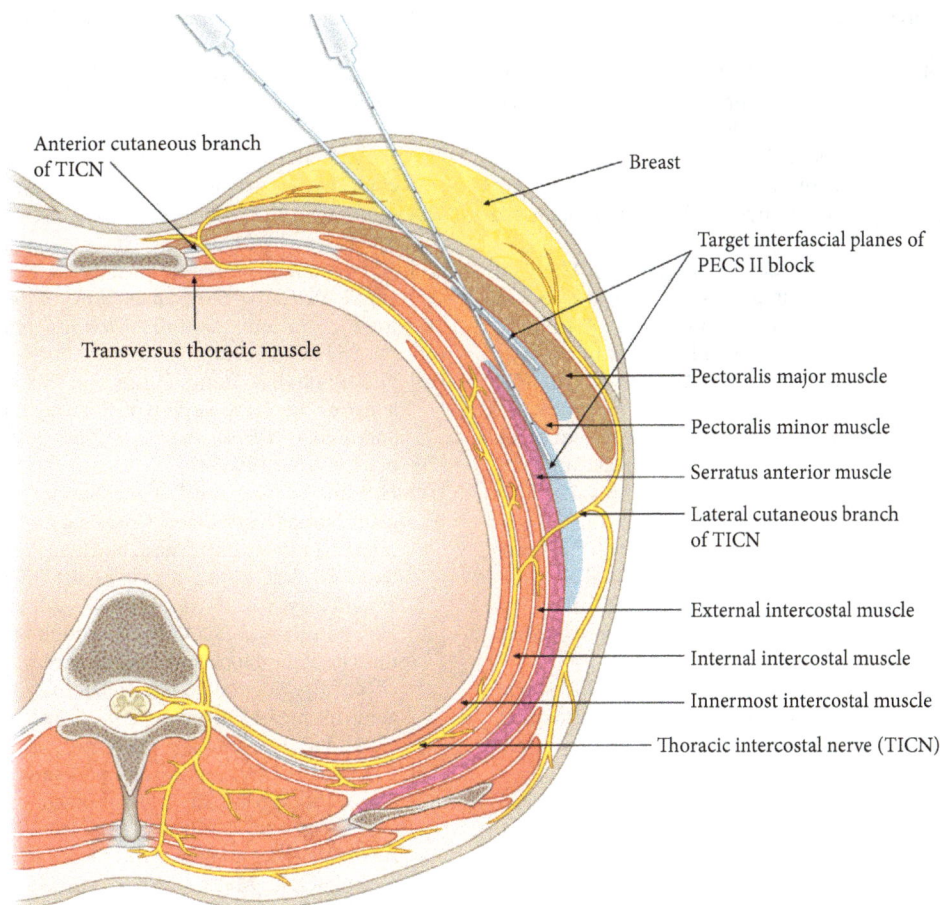

FIGURE 6: Illustration of target areas of the PECS II block. This agent can block the lateral cutaneous branches of the TICN in the interfascial plane between the pectoralis minor and serratus anterior muscles but cannot block the anterior cutaneous branch of the TICN.

This study had several limitations. First, the PECS II block was performed following the induction of general anesthesia to reduce procedural pain and anxiety, which may have affected postoperative pain [25]. Sensory level tests were performed in the PACU after the operation, with all patients in the PECS II group showing positive reactions on the cold test. However, in contrast to findings in a previous study, our patients did not express exact dermatome against cold tests [20], suggesting that wound dressing and a surgical brassiere may have interfered with these sensory examinations. Other reasons for inaccurate responses to sensory level tests include postoperative pain, the sedative effect of opioids, and anesthetic hangover. However, we speculated that the PECS II block was successfully performed based on the changes in mean blood pressure and heart rate during the incision and the positive reactions in the cold test. Consequently, this study did not present sensory test data. A second limitation of this study was our inability to perform a double-blind, placebo-controlled study. However, the patients and investigators were blinded to group assignment, suggesting that the lack of ability to perform a placebo-controlled study had little influence on the study outcomes.

In conclusion, although the PECS II block reduced pain intensity and opioid requirements for 24 hours in patients who underwent BCS and SNB, PECS II block may not be clinically useful. Because PECS II block could not completely block all the nerves innervating the breast, including the anterior cutaneous branch of the TICN, it could not provide complete postoperative analgesia after BCS and SNB. The PECS II block seemed to be more efficient at reducing axillary pain than breast pain. Therefore, PECS II block may lack the ability to provide sufficient postoperative analgesia after breast surgery.

## Acknowledgments

The authors thank the e-medical contents and e-learning teams at the Asan Medical Center for helping to draw Figures 5 and 6.

## References

[1] U. Veronesi, N. Cascinelli, L. Mariani et al., "Twenty-year follow-up of a randomized study comparing breast-conserving surgery with radical mastectomy for early breast cancer," *New England Journal of Medicine*, vol. 347, no. 16, pp. 1227–1232, 2002.

[2] S. Kashiwagi, N. Onoda, T. Takashima et al., "Breast conserving surgery and sentinel lymph node biopsy under local

anesthesia for breast cancer," *Journal of Cancer Therapy*, vol. 3, no. 5, pp. 810–813, 2012.

[3] H. Kehlet, T. S. Jensen, and C. J. Woolf, "Persistent post-surgical pain: risk factors and prevention," *The Lancet*, vol. 367, no. 9522, pp. 1618–1625, 2006.

[4] K. G. Andersen, H. M. Duriaud, H. E. Jensen, N. Kroman, and H. Kehlet, "Predictive factors for the development of persistent pain after breast cancer surgery," *Pain*, vol. 156, no. 12, pp. 2413–2422, 2015.

[5] E. P. Lynch, K. J. Welch, J. M. Carabuena, and T. J. Eberlein, "Thoracic epidural anesthesia improves outcome after breast surgery," *Annals of Surgery*, vol. 222, no. 5, p. 663, 1995.

[6] H. Freise and H. Van Aken, "Risks and benefits of thoracic epidural anaesthesia," *British Journal of Anaesthesia*, vol. 107, no. 6, pp. 859–868, 2011.

[7] S. S. Wahba and S. M. Kamal, "Thoracic paravertebral block versus pectoral nerve block for analgesia after breast surgery," *Egyptian Journal of Anaesthesia*, vol. 30, no. 2, pp. 129–135, 2014.

[8] S. Kulhari, N. Bharti, I. Bala, S. Arora, and G. Singh, "Efficacy of pectoral nerve block versus thoracic paravertebral block for postoperative analgesia after radical mastectomy: a randomized controlled trial," *British Journal of Anaesthesia (BJA)*, vol. 117, no. 3, pp. 382–386, 2016.

[9] R. Blanco, M. Fajardo, and T. P. Maldonado, "Ultrasound description of Pecs II (modified Pecs I): a novel approach to breast surgery," *Revista Espanola de Anestesiologia y Reanimacion*, vol. 59, no. 9, pp. 470–475, 2012.

[10] M. L. McPherson, *Demystifying Opioid Conversion Calculations: A Guide for Effective Dosing*, ASHP, Bethesda, MD, USA, 2009.

[11] G. M. N. Bashandy and D. N. Abbas, "Pectoral nerves I and II blocks in multimodal analgesia for breast cancer surgery: a randomized clinical trial," *Regional Anesthesia and Pain Medicine*, vol. 40, no. 1, pp. 68–74, 2015.

[12] K. Wang, X. Zhang, T. Zhang et al., "The efficacy of ultrasound-guided type ii pectoral nerve blocks in perioperative pain management for immediate reconstruction after modified radical mastectomy: a prospective, randomized study," *Clinical Journal of Pain*, vol. 34, pp. 231–236, 2018.

[13] N. Ma, J. K. Duncan, A. J. Scarfe, S. Schuhmann, and A. L. Cameron, "Clinical safety and effectiveness of transversus abdominis plane (TAP) block in post-operative analgesia: a systematic review and meta-analysis," *Journal of Anesthesia*, vol. 31, no. 3, pp. 432–452, 2017.

[14] J. F. Moller, L. Nikolajsen, S. A. Rodt, H. Ronning, and P. S. Carlsson, "Thoracic paravertebral block for breast cancer surgery: a randomized double-blind study," *Anesthesia and Analgesia*, vol. 105, no. 6, pp. 1848–1851, 2007.

[15] B. Versyck, G.-J. van Geffen, and P. Van Houwe, "Prospective double blind randomized placebo-controlled clinical trial of the pectoral nerves (Pecs) block type II," *Journal of Clinical Anesthesia*, vol. 40, pp. 46–50, 2017.

[16] P. Myles, D. Myles, W. Galagher et al., "Measuring acute postoperative pain using the visual analog scale: the minimal clinically important difference and patient acceptable symptom state," *British Journal of Anaesthesia (BJA)*, vol. 118, no. 3, pp. 424–429, 2017.

[17] A. Porzionato, V. Macchi, C. Stecco, M. Loukas, R. S. Tubbs, and R. De Caro, "Surgical anatomy of the pectoral nerves and the pectoral musculature," *Clinical Anatomy*, vol. 25, no. 5, pp. 559–575, 2012.

[18] N. Sarhadi, J. S. Dunn, F. Lee, and D. Soutar, "An anatomical study of the nerve supply of the breast, including the nipple and areola," *British Journal of Plastic Surgery*, vol. 49, no. 3, pp. 156–164, 1996.

[19] H. Kim, J. Shim, and I. Kim, "Surgical excision of the breast giant fibroadenoma under regional anesthesia by Pecs II and internal intercostal plane block: a case report and brief technical description: a case report," *Korean Journal of Anesthesiology*, vol. 70, no. 1, pp. 77–80, 2017.

[20] H. Ueshima and H. Otake, "Addition of transversus thoracic muscle plane block to pectoral nerves block provides more effective perioperative pain relief than pectoral nerves block alone for breast cancer surgery," *British Journal of Anaesthesia (BJA)*, vol. 118, no. 3, pp. 439–443, 2017.

[21] P. A. Torre, J. W. Jones Jr., S. L. Alvarez et al., "Axillary local anesthetic spread after the thoracic interfacial ultrasound block-a cadaveric and radiological evaluation," *Revista Brasileira De Anestesiologia*, vol. 67, no. 6, pp. 555–564, 2017.

[22] K. Yokota, T. Matsumoto, Y. Murakami, and M. Akiyama, "Pectoral nerve blocks are useful for axillary sentinel lymph node biopsy in malignant tumors on the upper extremities," *International Journal of Dermatology*, vol. 56, no. 3, pp. e64–e65, 2017.

[23] M. J. Young, A. W. Gorlin, V. E. Modest, and S. A. Quraishi, "Clinical implications of the transversus abdominis plane block in adults," *Anesthesiology Research and Practice*, vol. 2012, Article ID 731645, 11 pages, 2012.

[24] K. Okmen, B. M. Okmen, and S. Uysal, "Serratus anterior plane (SAP) block used for thoracotomy analgesia: a case report," *Korean Journal of Pain*, vol. 29, no. 3, pp. 189–192, 2016.

[25] R. Paolella, F. Guarnaccia, M. G. Baglieri, G. La Camera, and L. Maiolino, "Anxiety and postoperative pain," *Acta Medica*, vol. 29, p. 37, 2013.

# 10

# Pregabalin Prescription for Neuropathic Pain and Fibromyalgia: A Descriptive Study Using Administrative Database in Japan

Mikito Hirakata,[1,2] Satomi Yoshida,[1] Sachiko Tanaka-Mizuno,[1,3] Aki Kuwauchi,[1] and Koji Kawakami ⓘ[1]

[1]Department of Pharmacoepidemiology, Graduate School of Medicine and Public Health, Kyoto University, Yoshidakonoe-cho, Sakyo-ku, Kyoto 606-8501, Japan
[2]Toxicology and Pharmacokinetics Laboratories, Pharmaceutical Research Laboratories, Toray Industries, Inc., 10-1, Tebiro 6-chome, Kamakura, Kanagawa 248-8555, Japan
[3]Department of Medical Statistics, Shiga University of Medical Science, Seta Tsukinowa-cho, Otsu, Shiga 520-2192, Japan

Correspondence should be addressed to Koji Kawakami; kawakami.koji.4e@kyoto-u.ac.jp

Academic Editor: Jacob Ablin

*Objective*. To assess dose, characteristics, and coprescribed analgesics in patients newly prescribed pregabalin for neuropathic pain and fibromyalgia in Japan. *Methods*. Based on the medical and prescription information present in the Medical Data Vision database, we analyzed the initial and maximum daily doses, prescription period, coprescribed analgesics, and neuropathic pain-related disorders of patients newly prescribed pregabalin between 01 July 2010 and 31 December 2013. *Results*. A total of 45,331 patients (mean age 66.8 years, 48.7% men) were newly prescribed pregabalin during this period. The mean initial and maximum daily doses were 97.3 mg and 127.8 mg, respectively, and decreased yearly. The duration of the prescription period was 111.9 (mean) and 53 (median) days, and the frequently coprescribed analgesics included NSAIDs, opioids, and Neurotropin®. About one half of the patients had spinal disorders. *Conclusion*. In Japan during the period examined, the number of newly prescribed pregabalin users increased, but the initial and maximum daily doses decreased yearly after pregabalin went on the market. The maximum daily dose in Japan was lower than those reported in the USA and Europe. These differences might be associated with patient age and physical status and with anxiety about possible adverse events.

## 1. Introduction

Neuropathic pain and fibromyalgia are intractable chronic pains. Neuropathic pain is defined as "pain caused by a lesion or disease of the somatosensory system" and is classified as peripheral or central neuropathic pain according to the site of the lesion or disease [1, 2]. The prevalence of neuropathic pain was estimated at 6.9% to 10% in some countries [3]. Fibromyalgia is a disorder characterized by systemic pain accompanied by neuropsychiatric symptoms such as insomnia and depression and autonomic symptoms such as irritable bowel syndrome, gastroesophageal reflux disease, and over active bladder [4–6]. In Japan, the prevalence was estimated to be 1.7%–2.1% and about 60%–80% of sufferers were women [7, 8].

Pregabalin is a ligand for the $\alpha_2\delta$ subunit of the calcium channel and is used world wide to treat seizure, generalized anxiety disorder, neuropathic pain, and fibromyalgia. Pregabalin is a first- and/or second-line recommendation for neuropathic pain in many guidelines [9–12] and was approved for fibromyalgia in the USA but not in Europe. In Japan, pregabalin was approved for postherpetic neuralgia in April, 2010, and current indications have been expanded to neuropathic pain and first-line recommendation in the guideline for pharmacologic treatment of neuropathic pain [13]. Pregabalin was also approved for fibromyalgia in June, 2012, in Japan.

Pregabalin is approved to be started at 150 mg daily and titrated up to a maintenance daily dose range. In Japan and the USA, this dose range is 300–600 mg for neuropathic pain and 300–450 mg for fibromyalgia, and in Europe, 150–600 mg for neuropathic pain. However, the efficacy of 150 mg daily was inconsistent [14–16]. In the USA or European observation studies, the mean maximum (or average) daily dose was less than 300 mg (lower limit of approved maintenance dose range in the USA and Japan) or many patients were prescribed <300 mg for neuropathic pain [17–22] and fibromyalgia [23–25].

An interim report of postmarketing surveillance for peripheral neuropathic pain in Japan [26] showed that the mean initial and maximum daily doses of pregabalin were less than the approved initial and maintenance doses. However, the patient population of this study was small (2010 patients), and the observation period was short (13 weeks). Thus, in the present study, the real-world pregabalin prescription for neuropathic pain and fibromyalgia in Japan was examined using the Medical Data Vision database, a large medical and prescription database.

## 2. Methods

*2.1. Data Sources.* This descriptive study was conducted using the data collected and aggregated by the Medical Data Vision (MDV) Co. Ltd. from the hospitals using a novel medical reimbursement system for hospitalization, the Diagnosis Procedure Combination/Per-Diem Payment System (DPC/PDPS) in Japan [27, 28]. In April 2016, 1667 hospitals had introduced the DPC/PDPS, encompassing a total of about 495,227 beds. These constituted about 20% of all hospitals and 55% of the total hospital beds in Japan [29]. In May 2016, this database contained the anonymized data of 14,390,000 patients from 247 hospitals. These data contain medical and prescription data from both inpatients and outpatients. Prescription data consisted of individual records each containing one set of information comprising drug name, content, prescription date, daily volume or number of drug formulation, and the number of days prescribed. The study protocol was approved by Kyoto University Graduate School and Faculty of Medicine, Ethics Committee (Kyoto, Japan, Application number E2507).

*2.2. Patients.* We selected patients newly prescribed pregabalin between 01 July 2010 and 31 December 2013. *Newly prescribed* was defined as a first prescription in the database with no prescribed pregabalin in the previous 90 days. The date of newly prescribed pregabalin was designated as the *first prescription date*. Patients were excluded when the hospital's data collection had started within 90 days before the first prescription date. Records of prescribed pregabalin "as-needed" were excluded and patients whose first prescription was only "as-needed" were excluded.

*2.3. Daily Dose and Prescription Period.* The *daily dose of pregabalin* was calculated from the content and the daily number of capsules. When there were several records on the same prescription date, daily dose and the number of the days prescribed were estimated based on the number of days until the next pregabalin prescription date. The *last prescription date*

was defined as the last date of pregabalin prescription in the database or as the first date with no pregabalin prescription after 30 days plus the number of days of the last prescription. The *prescription period* was set to be the time between the first prescription date and the end of the time prescribed by the last prescription. When the duration of the prescription period was over 365 days, this duration was set at 365 days.

*2.4. Coprescribed Drugs. Coprescriptions* were defined as drugs that were coprescribed at the first prescription date of pregabalin, or before this first date but overlapping it and represcribed within 90 days after it. The number of kinds of coprescribed oral drugs was based on substance names. Coprescribed analgesic drugs were categorized as (1) first- and second-line drugs of the Japanese guideline (1-2-line drugs; oral formulation), including tricyclic antidepressants (TCAs; amitriptyline hydrochloride, imipramine hydrochloride, and nortriptyline hydrochloride), gabapentin, extract of cutaneous tissue of rabbit inoculated with vaccinia virus (Neurotropin), duloxetine hydrochloride, and mexiletine hydrochloride; (2) opioids, including fentanyl (transdermal patch), oxycodone (oral formulation), morphine (oral and injection formulations), buprenorphine (transdermal patch and oral mucosa patch), tramadol (oral and injection formulations), and acetaminophen/tramadol combination (oral formula); and (3) nonsteroidal anti-inflammatory drugs (NSAIDs; ATCcode M01A and N02B0, excluding pentazocine and acetaminophen/tramadol combination; oral formulation). Opioids were subcategorized by strength (weak (tramadol and acetaminophen/tramadol combination) and strong (the others)) and route (oral and nonoral).

*2.5. Neuropathic Pain-Related Disorders. Neuropathic pain-related disorders* were classified as follows: (1) spinal disorders (ICD-10 code: M47, M48, M50, M51, or M53), (2) postherpetic neuropathy (ICD-10 code: B02.2), (3) diabetic neuropathy (ICD-10 code: E10.4, E11.4, or E14.4), (4) cancer-related pain (disease name: cancer pain, or ICD-10 code: C00-C97 in combination with ICD-10 code: R52.1, R52.2, or R52.9), (5) trigeminal neuralgia (ICD-10 code: G50.0), (6) entrapment peripheral neuropathy of the upper limb (disease name: carpal-tunnel syndrome, Gion tunnel syndrome, cubital tunnel syndrome, or thoracic outlet syndrome), (7) other neuropathic pain (ICD-10 code: G62.9, G64, G96.9, or G98, not classified in the above categories), (8) fibromyalgia (disease name: fibromyalgia), and (9) others (not classified in the above categories).

*2.6. Analgesic Drugs Prescribed after Pregabalin Discontinuation Period.* Patients were analyzed whose pregabalin prescription period duration was less than 365 days. The *after pregabalin discontinuation period* was defined as the time between the day after the last prescription date and 90 days after the end of the pregabalin prescription period. The prescriptions of the analgesic drugs described above in this period were then summarized. The prescriptions after the pregabalin discontinuation period were compared with those during the pregabalin prescription period and

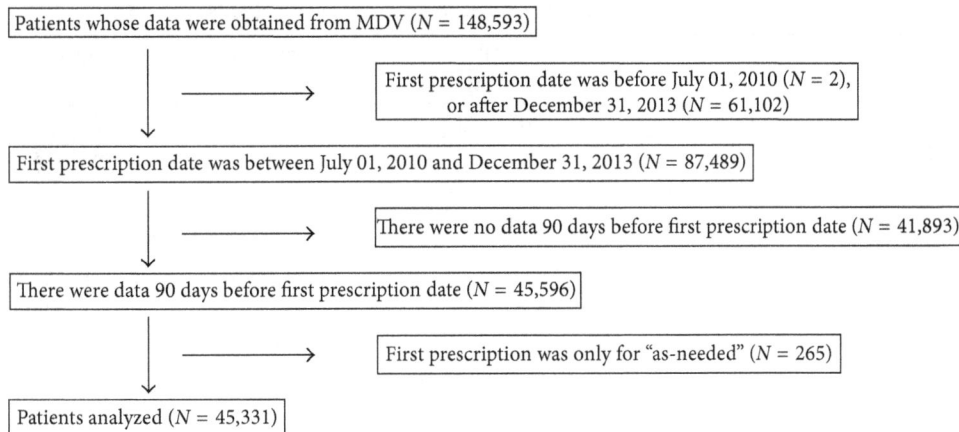

FIGURE 1: Patient selection flowchart.

categorized as follows: (1) *continued use*: when the same drug had been prescribed during the pregabalin prescription period without prescriptions of other drugs of the same category, (2) *new use*: when a drug or other drugs of the same category had not been prescribed during the pregabalin prescription period, (3) *changed/added drugs*: the drugs prescribed after the pregabalin discontinuation period were different from or added to other drugs of the same category prescribed during the pregabalin prescription period, (4) *changed/additions of the route*: the routes of the drugs coprescribed during the pregabalin prescription period were changed or new administration routes for the same drugs were added after the pregabalin discontinuation period, and (5) *changed/additions of the strength*: different strengths of opioids were prescribed after the pregabalin discontinuation period to change from or add to opioids prescribed during the pregabalin prescription period.

*2.7. Statistical Analysis.* Numerical data are presented as means ± their standard deviation, or as medians and their 25th and 75th percentiles, and categorical data are presented as numbers and percentages. Statistical comparisons were made using the $t$-test for numerical data and the chi-square test for categorical data and were conducted using the SAS version 9.4 (SAS Institute Inc.) statistical package.

# 3. Results

*3.1. Newly Prescribed Pregabalin Patients.* We obtained the data of 148,593 patients from the MDV database who had been prescribed pregabalin; 45,331 of those patients met the necessary criteria, and their data were analyzed further (Figure 1). The number of patients newly prescribed pregabalin increased dramatically in the first year after the launch of pregabalin in the second half of 2010. After that period, the number of these patients increased gradually (Figure 2).

*3.2. Characteristics of Pregabalin-Prescribed Patients.* Table 1 shows the characteristics of pregabalin-prescribed patients. At their first prescription date, 37,045 of the patients (81.7%) were prescribed pregabalin in an outpatient setting. The male ratio was 48.7%, and the mean age was

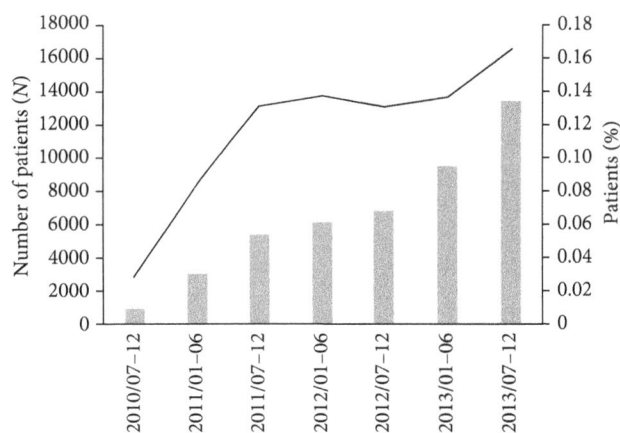

FIGURE 2: The number of patients newly prescribed pregabalin. Solid columns represent the number of patients newly prescribed pregabalin in each half year. Solid line represents the number of patients newly prescribed pregabalin in each half year divided by the total number of monthly patients in each half year in this database.

66.8 ± 13.9 years. The male ratio of inpatients was over 50%, and the mean age of inpatients was a little higher than that of outpatients. The mean initial daily dose and maximum daily dose were 97.3 ± 56.7 mg and 127.8 ± 87.0 mg, respectively, but these tended to decrease as time proceeded after the initial launch (Figure 3).

The mean and median durations of the prescription period were 111.9 ± 124.2 and 53 days, respectively. The duration of the prescription period was longer for outpatients than that for inpatients. The fraction of patients who changed from the initial daily dose to at least one another dose during the prescription period (change in dose) was only 26.9%, and these changes were higher for inpatients than they were for outpatients. The mean number of coprescribed oral drugs was 4.2 ± 3.7, and the number for inpatients was higher than that for outpatients.

The most frequently coprescribed analgesics for outpatients at the first pregabalin prescription date were NSAIDs (36.9%); the second most frequent was Neurotropin. Opioids were coprescribed for 5.7% of the outpatients, and most of these were oral formulas. For

TABLE 1: Characteristics of pregabalin-prescribed patients.

| | All | Outpatient | Inpatient | P value |
|---|---|---|---|---|
| N | 45331 | 37045 | 8286 | |
| Sex (male), N (%) | 22085 (48.7) | 17692 (47.8) | 4393 (53.0) | <0.001 |
| Age, mean (SD) | 66.8 (13.9) | 66.4 (14.0) | 69.0 (13.3) | <0.001 |
| Initial daily dose, mg | | | | |
| Mean (SD) | 97.3 (56.7) | 95.5 (55.7) | 105.4 (60.5) | <0.001 |
| N (%) | | | | |
| <50 mg | 5737 (12.7) | 4733 (12.8) | 1004 (12.1) | — |
| ≥50 mg, <75 mg | 8691 (19.2) | 7596 (20.5) | 1095 (13.2) | — |
| ≥75 mg, <150 mg | 13139 (29.0) | 10687 (28.8) | 2452 (29.6) | — |
| ≥150 mg | 17764 (39.2) | 14029 (37.9) | 3735 (45.1) | — |
| Maximum daily dose, mg | | | | |
| Mean (SD) | 127.8 (87.0) | 123.6 (82.5) | 146.2 (102.5) | <0.001 |
| N (%) | | | | |
| <150 mg | 21468 (47.4) | 18162 (49.0) | 3306 (39.9) | — |
| ≥150 mg, <300 mg | 19763 (43.6) | 15913 (43.0) | 3850 (46.5) | — |
| ≥300 mg | 4100 (9.0) | 2970 (8.0) | 1130 (13.6) | — |
| Prescription period, day | | | | |
| Mean (SD) | 111.9 (124.2) | 118.5 (126.8) | 82.6 (107.0) | <0.001 |
| Median (25, 75 percentile) | 53 (21, 163) | 56 (21, 182) | 36 (14, 94) | <0.001 |
| Prescription period over 90 days, N (%) | 16762 (37.0) | 14595 (39.4) | 2167 (26.2) | <0.001 |
| Change in dose, N(%) | 12205 (26.9) | 9584 (25.9) | 2621 (31.6) | <0.001 |
| Coprescribed oral drugs, mean (SD) | 4.2 (3.7) | 3.9 (3.6) | 5.7 (4.0) | <0.001 |
| Coprescribed analgesics, N (%) | | | | |
| 1-2-Line drugs | 4698 (10.4) | 4017 (10.8) | 681 (8.2) | <0.001 |
| TCAs | 615 (1.4) | 473 (1.3) | 142 (1.7) | — |
| Gabapentin | 160 (0.4) | 120 (0.3) | 40 (0.5) | — |
| Neurotropin | 3656 (8.1) | 3256 (8.8) | 400 (4.8) | — |
| Duloxetine | 258 (0.6) | 178 (0.5) | 80 (1.0) | — |
| Mexiletine | 217 (0.5) | 162 (0.4) | 55 (0.7) | — |
| Opioids | 3843 (8.5) | 2117 (5.7) | 1726 (20.8) | <0.001 |
| Oral opioids | 3071 (6.8) | 1825 (4.9) | 1246 (15.0) | — |
| Nonoral opioids | 790 (1.7) | 275 (0.7) | 515 (6.2) | — |
| Strong opioids | 2219 (4.9) | 954 (2.6) | 1265 (15.3) | — |
| Weak opioids | 1688 (3.7) | 1184 (3.2) | 504 (6.1) | — |
| NSAIDs | 17303 (38.2) | 13657 (36.9) | 3646 (44.0) | <0.001 |
| Neuropathic pain-related disorders*, N (%) | | | | |
| Spinal disorders | 23502 (51.8) | 21144 (57.1) | 2358 (28.5) | <0.001 |
| Postherpetic neuropathy | 2795 (6.2) | 2435 (6.6) | 360 (4.3) | <0.001 |
| Diabetic neuropathy | 1478 (3.3) | 1244 (3.4) | 234 (2.8) | 0.014 |
| Cancer-related pain | 3933 (8.7) | 2172 (5.9) | 1761 (21.3) | <0.001 |
| Trigeminal neuralgia | 780 (1.7) | 713 (1.9) | 67 (0.8) | <0.001 |
| Entrapment peripheral neuropathy of the upper limb | 1329 (2.9) | 1251 (3.4) | 78 (0.9) | <0.001 |
| Other neuropathic pain disorders | 11564 (25.5) | 9728 (26.3) | 1836 (22.2) | — |
| Fibromyalgia | 153 (0.3) | 127 (0.3) | 26 (0.3) | 0.681 |
| Others | 3178 (7.0) | 1113 (3.0) | 2065 (24.9) | — |

1-2-line drugs: first- and second-line drugs of the Japanese guideline; TCAs: tricyclic antidepressants (amitriptyline hydrochloride, imipramine hydrochloride, and nortriptyline hydrochloride); neurotropin; extract of cutaneous tissue of rabbit inoculated with vaccinia virus. *Patients in these categories are not mutually exclusive. —, statistical analyses not performed.

inpatients, the most frequently coprescribed analgesics were NSAIDs, followed by opioids; strong opioids were more frequently coprescribed than weak ones.

About one half of the outpatients had spinal disorders; other disorders, in descending order of frequency, included postherpetic neuropathy, cancer-related pain, and diabetic neuropathy. About 30% of inpatients had spinal disorders and about 20% had cancer-related pain.

To exclude the effects of short-trial pregabalin use on the results, a subgroup analysis of 12-month continuous users was conducted (Supplementary Table S1). Compared with the results of the main analysis, the mean maximum daily dose increased to 153.5 ± 106.2, 16.4% of the patients were prescribed ≥300 mg as the maximum dose, and 51.7% of them underwent a change in dose. Other parameters were comparable to those in the main analysis.

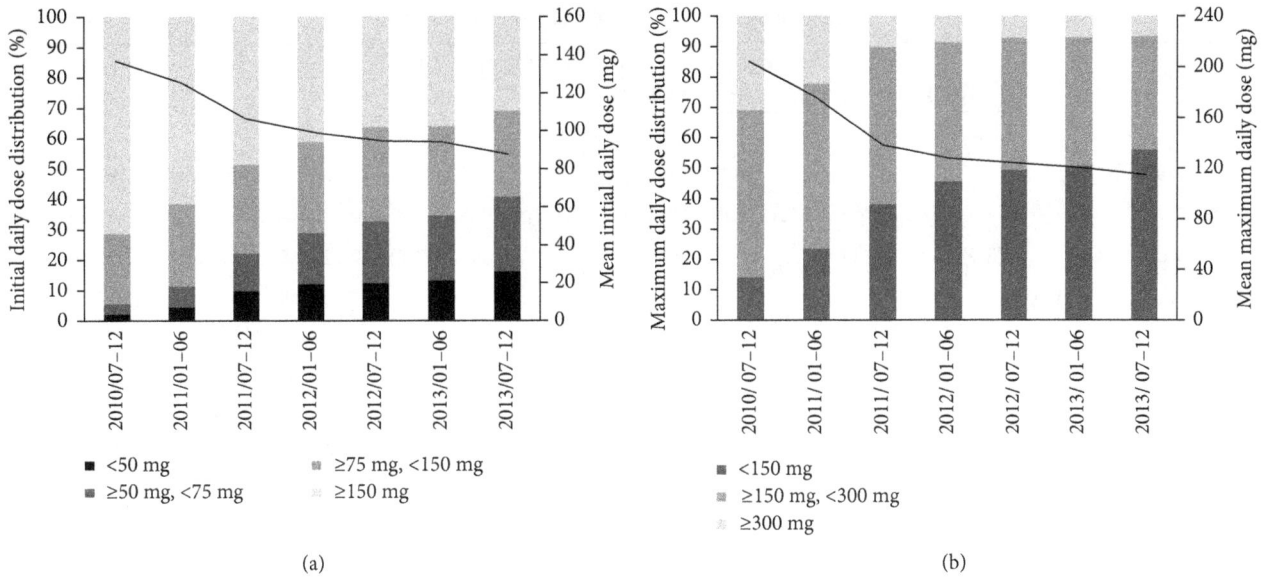

FIGURE 3: The initial (a) and maximum (b) daily doses. Solid columns represent the daily dose distribution. Solid line represents the mean daily dose.

TABLE 2: Prescription patterns according to gender and age.

| | N (%) | | Initial daily dose Mean (SD) | | | Maximum daily dose Mean (SD) | | | Prescription period Mean (SD) | | | Median (25, 75 percentile) | | |
|---|---|---|---|---|---|---|---|---|---|---|---|---|---|---|
| | | | | | | Age | | | | | | | | |
| | <65 | ≥65 | <65a | ≥65 | P value | <65 | ≥65 | P value | <65 | ≥65 | P value | <65 | ≥65 | P value |
| **Sex** | | | | | | | | | | | | | | |
| Male | 8578 (50.8) | 13507 (47.5) | 110.6 (57.8) | 98.0 (58.4) | <0.001 | 149.7 (97.2) | 130.4 (88.9) | <0.001 | 104.7 (118.4) | 118.8 (126.5) | <0.001 | 49 (21,144) | 57 (22,184) | <0.001 |
| Female | 8318 (49.2) | 14928 (52.5) | 101.9 (55.2) | 86.6 (53.2) | <0.001 | 132.3 (85.3) | 110.2 (75.7) | <0.001 | 100.5 (118.0) | 116.2 (128.1) | <0.001 | 43 (16,132) | 54 (21,178) | <0.001 |
| **Initial daily dose** | | | | | | | | | | | | | | |
| <50 mg | 1470 (8.7) | 4267 (15.0) | — | — | — | 55.7 (55.6) | 51.4 (54.7) | 0.001 | 112.4 (124.5) | 130.1 (132.2) | <0.001 | 56 (21,161) | 63 (27,225) | <0.001 |
| ≥50 mg, <75 mg | 2714 (16.1) | 5977 (21.0) | — | — | — | 86.2 (66.7) | 78.8 (54.0) | <0.001 | 113.5 (122.5) | 126.9 (129.1) | <0.001 | 56 (24,164) | 65 (28,205) | <0.001 |
| ≥75 mg, <150 mg | 4886 (28.9) | 8253 (29.0) | — | — | — | 116.2 (71.6) | 109.8 (67.4) | <0.001 | 98.4 (114.7) | 117.3 (127.4) | <0.001 | 44 (20,127) | 56 (21,182) | <0.001 |
| ≥150 mg | 7826 (46.3) | 9938 (34.9) | — | — | — | 191.9 (86.9) | 182.2 (76.4) | <0.001 | 99.7 (117.4) | 106.5 (123.0) | <0.001 | 42 (14,135) | 46 (16,149) | 0.013 |

*3.3. Pregabalin Prescription Patterns according to Gender and Age.* Table 2 shows the pregabalin prescription patterns according to gender and age. The initial and maximum daily doses prescribed for males were higher than those prescribed for females, and were also higher for patients younger than 65 years than for those 65 years or older. On the other hand, there were only small differences in the durations of the prescription period between males and females, while the duration of the prescription period for patients younger than 65 was shorter than that of those 65 years or older. The maximum daily dose tended to increase with increasing first daily doses. The prescription period tended to be shorter for those receiving initial daily doses of more than 75 mg/day.

*3.4. Subgroup Analysis of Individual Disorders.* The use of pregabalin and coprescribed drugs was analyzed in subgroups of the following individual disorders: spinal disorders, postherpetic neuropathy, diabetic neuropathy, cancer-related pain, trigeminal neuralgia, and entrapment peripheral neuropathy of the upper limb (Table 3). The male ratio was higher for diabetic neuropathy and cancer-related pain. The mean age of patients was greater than 60 years for all disorders. The initial and maximum daily doses of pregabalin tended to be slightly lower in outpatients with spinal disorders, diabetic neuropathy, and entrapment neuropathy of the upper limb than in those with other disorders. The maximum daily dose of pregabalin was higher in inpatients than in outpatients with

TABLE 3: Subgroup analysis of individual disorders.

| | Spinal disorders | | P value | Postherpetic neuropathy | | P value | Diabetic neuropathy | | P value |
|---|---|---|---|---|---|---|---|---|---|
| | Outpatient | Inpatient | | Outpatient | Inpatient | | Outpatient | Inpatient | |
| N | 21144 | 2358 | | 2435 | 360 | | 1244 | 234 | |
| Sex (male), N (%) | 10219 (48.3) | 1211 (51.4) | 0.006 | 1142 (46.9) | 168 (46.7) | 0.935 | 745 (59.9) | 146 (62.4) | 0.473 |
| Age, mean (SD) | 67.3 (13.9) | 70.0 (13.1) | <0.001 | 69.1 (13.2) | 70.8 (13.0) | 0.030 | 67.7 (11.7) | 69.1 (11.6) | 0.084 |
| Initial daily dose (mg), mean (SD) | 89.5 (54.1) | 101.4 (56.8) | <0.001 | 108.0 (58.7) | 104.8 (52.6) | 0.321 | 96.9 (54.2) | 99.1 (57.8) | 0.570 |
| Maximum daily dose (mg), mean (SD) | 115.2 (76.4) | 140.0 (92.9) | <0.001 | 146.5 (96.9) | 164.5 (106.2) | 0.002 | 129.9 (85.1) | 139.1 (92.6) | 0.135 |
| Prescription period (day) | | | | | | | | | |
|   Mean (SD) | 123.6 (128.2) | 95.7 (116.1) | <0.001 | 95.2 (116.5) | 94.0 (112.8) | 0.857 | 160.3 (143.6) | 103.2 (124.1) | <.0.001 |
|   Median (25, 75 percentile) | 62 (28, 196) | 43 (15, 122) | <0.001 | 42 (14, 119) | 43.5 (20, 111.5) | 0.600 | 91 (30, 365) | 43 (17, 129) | <0.001 |
| Prescription period over 90 days, N (%) | 8726 (41.3) | 724 (30.7) | <0.001 | 747 (30.7) | 105 (29.2) | 0.562 | 634 (51.0) | 74 (31.6) | <0.001 |
| Coprescribed oral drugs, mean (SD) | 4.0 (3.7) | 5.5 (4.2) | <0.001 | 4.3 (3.7) | 5.4 (4.0) | <0.001 | 7.0 (4.4) | 7.4 (4.6) | 0.232 |
| 1-2-line drugs, N (%) | 2798 (13.2) | 272 (11.5) | 0.021 | 350 (14.4) | 49 (13.6) | 0.670 | 171 (13.7) | 31 (13.2) | 0.839 |
| Opioids, N (%) | 881 (4.2) | 322 (13.7) | <0.001 | 95 (3.9) | 33 (9.2) | <0.001 | 33 (2.7) | 21 (9.0) | <0.001 |
| NSAIDs, N (%) | 8813 (41.7) | 1119 (47.5) | <0.001 | 959 (39.4) | 164 (45.6) | 0.026 | 264 (21.2) | 63 (26.9) | 0.054 |

| | Cancer-related pain | | P value | Trigeminal neuralgia | | P value | Entrapment neuropathy of the upper limb | | P value |
|---|---|---|---|---|---|---|---|---|---|
| | Outpatient | Inpatient | | Outpatient | Inpatient | | Outpatient | Inpatient | |
| N | 2172 | 1761 | | 713 | 67 | | 1251 | 78 | |
| Sex (male), N(%) | 1167 (53.7) | 1089 (61.8) | <0.001 | 320 (44.9) | 31 (46.3) | 0.828 | 499 (39.9) | 37 (47.4) | 0.188 |
| Age, mean (SD) | 64.3 (12.2) | 65.0 (12.6) | 0.060 | 65.9 (13.7) | 68.9 (12.8) | 0.079 | 65.4 (14.2) | 68.7 (12.7) | 0.044 |
| Initial daily dose (mg), mean (SD) | 108.3 (54.2) | 107.1 (58.8) | 0.515 | 109.9 (60.2) | 117.4 (69.8) | 0.337 | 84.4 (52.7) | 93.1 (60.7) | 0.161 |
| Maximum daily dose (mg), mean (SD) | 150.0 (96.4) | 165.1 (116.7) | <0.001 | 148.7 (97.3) | 165.5 (93.2) | 0.176 | 107.8 (74.3) | 142.8 (124.8) | <0.001 |
| Prescription period (day) | | | | | | | | | |
|   Mean (SD) | 118.3 (123.2) | 72.3 (92.4) | <0.001 | 124.0 (135.2) | 76.6 (100.3) | 0.006 | 125.6 (128.4) | 126.9 (137.0) | 0.935 |
|   Median (25, 75 percentile) | 63 (28, 177) | 36 (14, 84) | <0.001 | 51 (14, 220) | 39 (16, 88) | 0.371 | 63 (28, 204) | 54 (21, 228) | 0.631 |
| Prescription period over 90 days, N(%) | 888 (40.9) | 418 (23.7) | <0.001 | 287 (40.3) | 15 (22.4) | 0.005 | 520 | (41.6) | 31 (39.7) |
| Coprescribed oral drugs, mean (SD) | 5.1 (3.4) | 5.7 (3.5) | <0.001 | 4.1 (4.0) | 6.4 (4.3) | <0.001 | 3.8 (3.9) | 5.8 (4.2) | <0.001 |
| 1-2-line drugs, N(%) | 93 (4.3) | 84 (4.8) | 0.463 | 82 (11.5) | 7 (10.4) | 0.796 | 201 (16.1) | 11 (14.1) | 0.646 |
| Opioids, N(%) | 1001 (46.1) | 1127 (64.0) | <0.001 | 25 (3.5) | 8 (11.9) | 0.001 | 28 (2.2) | 7 (9.0) | <0.001 |
| NSAIDs, N(%) | 1111 (51.2) | 1035 (58.8) | <0.001 | 161 (22.6) | 33 (49.3) | <0.001 | 363 (29.0) | 34 (43.6) | 0.007 |

1-2-line drugs: first- and second-line drugs of the Japanese guideline.

spinal disorders, postherpetic neuropathy, cancer-related pain, and entrapment neuropathy of the upper limb. Inpatients tended to have shorter durations of the prescription period than did outpatients with spinal disorders, diabetic neuropathy, cancer-related pain, and trigeminal neuralgia.

Only about 5% of patients with cancer-related pain were coprescribed 1-2-line analgesic drugs, while these were prescribed for 10.4% to 16.1% of the patients with other disorders. By contrast, about half of the patients with cancer-related pain were coprescribed opioids, while at most 15% of the patients with other pain disorders received opioids. More inpatients were coprescribed opioids along with the first prescription than were outpatients. Smaller percentages of diabetic neuropathy patients (both inpatients and outpatients) as well as outpatients with trigeminal neuropathy and entrapment neuropathy of the upper limb were coprescribed NSAIDs.

*3.5. After the Pregabalin Discontinuation Period.* After the pregabalin discontinuation period (Table 4), 10.2% of patients were represcribed pregabalin, and 8.2% and 15.2% of patients were prescribed 1-2-line drugs and opioids, respectively. About 5% of patients continued receiving prescriptions of the same 1-2-line drugs, and 3.4% received new 1-2-line prescriptions, while 4.0% continued previously prescribed opioids, and 7.4% received new opioid prescriptions.

When individual pain disorders were analyzed separately (Supplementary Table S2), pregabalin was represcribed for less than 10% of postherpetic neuralgia and cancer-related pain patients. The frequency of prescribed opioids for cancer-related pain (50.2%) was highest in patients with these disorders, and most were continued prescriptions or changes/additions of the drugs/routes (all greater than 10%).

# 4. Discussion

The data for the 45,331 patients newly prescribed pregabalin included in the MDV database, showed that the number of new users increased considerably from the launch of pregabalin in the second half of 2010 to the second half of 2011, when this increase leveled off. Indications for pregabalin were expanded in 2012 and 2013; however, these expansions were for fibromyalgia and central neuropathic pain and had little affect on the number of pregabalin prescriptions, as there are fewer of these patients than those with the prior indications for peripheral neuropathic pain.

The initial daily dose was lower than the approved initial daily dose in Japan (150 mg), and decreased yearly; 60.8% of patients were prescribed less than the approved dose. The reason for this decrease may be due to the many adverse events observed early in the launch of pregabalin [16]. A notice for elderly patients was released by the Pharmaceuticals and Medical Devices Agency of Japan in July 2012 [30] stating that "In elderly patients, some cases of falls due to dizziness, somnolence, loss of consciousness, etc. leading to fractures have been reported; therefore extra caution should be exercised." The initial daily doses prescribed for males were higher than those for females and were also higher for patients younger than 65 years than for those 65 years or older. Differences in physical status (weight and height) or excretory function and older age being a risk factor for early onset of adverse events, such as somnolence and dizziness [31], were considered possible reasons for these differences. The duration of the prescription period was shorter in those patients who received more than 75 mg/day as an initial daily dose. The incidence of adverse events in those receiving more than 75 mg/day may have increased, resulting in a shorter duration of the prescription period.

The maximum daily dose was lower than both the approved initial (150 mg) and maintenance (≥300 mg) daily

TABLE 4: Analgesic drugs used before and after the pregabalin discontinuation.

| | Before | After |
|---|---|---|
| $N$ | 39249 | 39249 |
| Analgesics ($N$, %) | | |
|   Represcribed pregabalin use | — | 4009 (10.2) |
| 1-2-line drugs | 5416 (13.8) | 3213 (8.2) |
|   Continued use | — | 1761 (4.5) |
|   New use | — | 1348 (3.4) |
|   Changed/added drugs | — | 104 (0.3) |
| TCAs | 837 (2.1) | 448 (1.1) |
| Gabapentin | 355 (0.9) | 197 (0.5) |
| Neurotropin | 3775 (9.6) | 2106 (5.4) |
| Duloxetine | 501 (1.3) | 455 (1.2) |
| Mexiletine | 310 (0.8) | 221 (0.6) |
| Opioids | 8171 (20.8) | 5954 (15.2) |
|   Continued use | — | 1580 (4.0) |
|   New use | — | 2894 (7.4) |
|   Changed/additions of drugs/route | — | 1480 (3.8) |
| Oral opioids | 5008 (12.8) | 3350 (8.5) |
|   Continued use | — | 1358 (3.5) |
|   New use | — | 1649 (4.2) |
|   Changed/added drugs | — | 160 (0.4) |
|   Changed/additions of route | — | 183 (0.5) |
| Nonoral opioids | 4737 (12.1) | 3368 (8.6) |
|   Continued use | — | 702 (1.8) |
|   New use | — | 1465 (3.7) |
|   Changed/added drugs | — | 527 (1.3) |
|   Changed/additions of route | — | 674 (1.7) |
| Weak opioids | 3238 (8.2) | 2377 (6.1) |
|   Continued use | — | 710 (1.8) |
|   New use | — | 1444 (3.7) |
|   Changed/added drugs | — | 76 (0.2) |
|   Changed/additions of the strength | — | 147 (0.4) |
| Strong opioids | 5928 (15.1) | 3963 (10.1) |
|   Continued use | — | 1010 (2.6) |
|   New use | — | 1644 (4.2) |
|   Changed/added drugs | — | 1062 (2.7) |
|   Changed/additions of the strength | — | 247 (0.6) |

1-2-line drugs:, first- and second-line drugs of the Japanese guideline; TCAs: tricyclic antidepressants (amitriptyline hydrochloride, imipramine hydrochloride, and nortriptyline hydrochloride); neurotropin: extract of cutaneous tissue of rabbit inoculated with vaccinia virus.

doses in Japan; the proportions of patients prescribed less than approved doses were 47.4% and 91.0%, respectively. In the subgroup analysis of 12-month continuous users, the maximum daily dose (153.5 mg) was comparable to the approved initial daily dose in Japan, and the proportions of patients prescribed less than the approved doses were 38.6% and 83.6%, respectively. Such low doses were also reported in another Japanese study (134.9 mg) [16]. In USA and European studies, the maximum or average daily doses (about 170–280 mg) [18–24] were less than 300 mg and although not many patients were prescribed more than 300 mg (about 20–30%) [18, 19, 21, 23, 25], these numbers were still higher than those in Japan. In randomized control trials, the efficacy of 150 mg/day was inconsistent [14–16]. Especially in those conducted in Japan [32–34], only one study for postherpetic neuralgia had a 150 mg group as the maintenance dose, but significant effects were not shown

[32]. The maximum daily dose in Japan was considered much lower, this might be associated with differences in age; the patients in this study (67 years old) were older than those in other studies (45–67 years old). There were also differences in physical status; Japanese people are generally less heavy and shorter than Westerners. Prescribing doctors may also have had anxiety about the reported adverse events; the initial daily dose was being decreased and many patients were prescribed the same daily dose during the prescription period.

The ratio of males, initial daily dose, maximum daily dose, and number of coprescribed opioids were higher in inpatients than in outpatients. The high ratio of males was considered to result from the high ratio of cancer-related pain patients and a low ratio of spinal disorders because there was a higher ratio of cancer-related pain in males and a lower ratio of males with spinal disorders. The higher ratio of coprescribed opioids in inpatients was observed for all disorders, including cancer-related pain. This may be because severer pain patients may more often be inpatients than outpatients.

The 1-2-line drugs were coprescribed for about 15% patients with all disorders except cancer-related pain, and NSAIDs were coprescribed for 20% to 40% of patients. The high frequency of coprescribed NSAIDs may be due to many patients also having nociceptive pain, another component of pain. Approximately half of the patients with cancer-related pain were coprescribed opioids, and one half of the patients were coprescribed NSAIDs. NSAIDs and opioids were recommended for cancer pain, and pregabalin was coprescribed for adjuvant analgesics or relief of neuropathic pain from cancer or cancer treatment and/or the coexistence of these pains.

This study had several strengths. First, a large population of patients who were prescribed pregabalin was analyzed about 10 times that of other drug-use investigations in Japan [15], and the maximum follow-up period was 4 times longer. Second, the database contained the data of patients who visited hospitals regardless of their kind of insurance. There were patients of a variety of ages, including later-stage elderly (75 or older) and a variety of jobs. Third, pregabalin was only approved in Japan for pain disorder, neuropathic pain, and fibromyalgia, and unapproved for other symptoms, such as seizure and generalized anxiety disorder; therefore, the analysis in this study was able to specialize in its use for pain.

There were also some limitations. First, the follow-up of patients was limited because this was a database of hospital-based data. After discontinuation of pregabalin, other analgesics were prescribed for about 30% of patients. When there were no data of analgesic prescriptions, it was not possible to know whether no analgesics had been prescribed or the patients had consulted a different hospital. However, these patients were considered to be unsatisfied with the effectiveness of pregabalin. Second, the reasons for discontinuation were not confirmed because the effects and the most adverse drug reactions of pregabalin, such as dizziness and somnolence, were not collected for this database. Third, there is a possibility of bias in the patient population because

many small scale hospitals have not introduced the DPC/PDPS [29]. Moreover, as the DPC/PDPS is a system for hospitalization, this database has no data from hospitals without inpatient facilities and little data from small scale hospitals. Forth, the disorders for which pregabalin was prescribed were not confirmed. In this database, prescribed drugs and the disorders for which they were prescribed were not combined; therefore, for example, the neuropathic pain-related disorders were categorized from those treated in the same month of the first prescription date.

## 5. Conclusion

In Japan, the number of patients being newly prescribed pregabalin increased over the course of the study period, but the initial and maximum daily doses decreased yearly after pregabalin went on the market. The maximum daily dose in Japan was lower than those reported in the USA and Europe, which may be associated with differences in age and physical status and anxiety about possible adverse events.

## Authors' Contributions

Mikito Hirakata contributed to conception and design, acquisition of data, analysis and interpretation of data, and drafting the manuscript, Satomi Yoshida contributed to analysis and interpretation of data, and the other authors contributed to conception and design and analysis and interpretation of the data. All authors contributed to critically revising the article for important intellectual content and had final approval of the version to be published.

## Acknowledgments

The authors thank Dr. Sei Fukui, Clinical Professor of Pain Management Clinic, Interdisciplinary Pain Management Center, Shiga University of Medical Science Hospital, for helpful discussions. The authors also thank Dr. Yoshika Onishi, Dr. Isao Nahara, Dr. Chikashi Takeda, and Dr. Hiroshi Yonekura, Department of Pharmacoepidemiology, Graduate School of Medicine and Public Health, Kyoto University, for helpful considerations.

## References

[1] J. D. Loeser and R. D. Treede, "The Kyoto protocol of IASP basic pain terminology," *Pain*, vol. 137, no. 3, pp. 473–477, 2008.

[2] T. S. Jensen, R. Baron, M. Haanpää et al., "A new definition of neuropathic pain," *Pain*, vol. 152, no. 10, pp. 2204-2205, 2011.

[3] O. van Hecke, S. K. Austin, R. A. Khan, B. H. Smith, and N. Torrance, "Neuropathic pain in the general population: a systematic review of epidemiological studies," *Pain*, vol. 155, no. 4, pp. 654–662, 2014.

[4] D. J. Wallace and D. S. Hallegua, "Fibromyalgia: the gastrointestinal link," *Current Pain and Headache Report*, vol. 8, no. 5, pp. 364–368, 2004.

[5] J. H. Chung, S. A. Kim, B. Y. Choi et al., "The association between overactive bladder and fibromyalgia syndrome: a community survey," *Neurourology and Urodynamics*, vol. 32, no. 1, pp. 66–69, 2013.

[6] L. P. Queiroz, "Worldwide epidemiology of fibromyalgia," *Current Pain and Headache Report*, vol. 17, no. 8, p. 356, 2013.

[7] M. Matsumoto, "Epidemiology of fibromyalgia," *Pharma Medica*, vol. 24, no. 6, pp. 35–39, 2006, in Japanese.

[8] I. Nakamura, K. Nishioka, C. Usui et al., "An epidemiologic internet survey of fibromyalgia and chronic pain in Japan," *Arthritis Care and Research*, vol. 66, no. 7, pp. 1093–1101, 2014.

[9] N. Attal, G. Cruccu, R. Baron et al., "European federation of neurological societies. EFNS guidelines on the pharmacological treatment of neuropathic pain: 2010 revision," *European Journal of Neurology*, vol. 17, no. 9, pp. 1113–1123, 2010.

[10] NICE, *Neuropathic Pain—Pharmacological Management: The Pharmacological Management of Neuropathic Pain in Adults in Nonspecialist Settings*, 2016, http://www.nice.org.uk/guidance/cg173.

[11] N. B. Finnerup, N. Attal, S. Haroutounian et al., "Pharmacotherapy for neuropathic pain in adults: a systematic review and meta-analysis," *The Lancet Neurology*, vol. 14, no. 2, pp. 162–173, 2015.

[12] D. Ziegler and V. Fonseca, "From guideline to patient: a review of recent recommendations for pharmacotherapy of painful diabetic neuropathy," *Journal of Diabetes and its Complications*, vol. 29, no. 1, pp. 146–156, 2015.

[13] The Committee for the Guidelines for the Pharmacologic Management of Neuropathic Pain of JSPC, *Guidelines for the Pharmacologic Management of Neuropathic Pain*, Publishing Department, Shinko Trading Co. Ltd., Hyogo, Japan, 2011.

[14] R. Freeman, E. Durso-Decruz, and B. Emir, "Efficacy, safety and tolerability of pregabalin treatment for painful diabetic peripheral neuropathy; findings from seven randomized controlled trials across a range of doses," *Diabetes Care*, vol. 31, no. 7, pp. 1448–1454, 2008.

[15] R. A. Moore, S. Straube, P. J. Wiffen, S. Derry, and H. J. McQuay, "Pregabalin for acute and chronic pain in adults," *Cochrane Database of Systematic Reviews*, vol. 3, p. CD007076, 2009.

[16] N. B. Finnerup, S. H. Sindrup, and T. S. Jensen, "The evidence for pharmacological treatment of neuropathic pain," *Pain*, vol. 150, no. 3, pp. 573–581, 2010.

[17] A. Navarro, M. T. Saldaña, C. Pérez, S. Torrades, and J. Rejas, "Patient-reported outcomes in subjects with neuropathic pain receiving pregabalin: evidence from medical practice in primary care settings," *Pain Medicine*, vol. 11, no. 5, pp. 719–731, 2010.

[18] P. Sun, Y. Zhao, Z. Zhao, M. Bernauer, and P. Watson, "Dosing pattern comparison between duloxetine and pregabalin among patients with diabetic peripheral neuropathic pain," *Pain Practice*, vol. 12, no. 8, pp. 641–648, 2012.

[19] P. Johnson, L. Becker, R. Halpern, and M. Sweeney, "Real-world treatment of post-herpetic neuralgia with gabapentin or pregabalin," *Clinical Drug Investigation*, vol. 33, no. 1, pp. 35–44, 2013.

[20] B. Wettermark, L. Brandt, H. Kieler, and R. Bodén, "Pregabalin is increasingly prescribed for neuropathic pain, generalised anxiety disorder and epilepsy but many patients discontinue treatment," *International Journal of Clinical Practice*, vol. 68, no. 1, pp. 104–110, 2014.

[21] M. Happich, E. Schneider, F. G. Boess et al., "Effectiveness of duloxetine compared with pregabalin and gabapentin in diabetic peripheral neuropathic pain: results from a German observational study," *Clinical Journal of Pain*, vol. 30, no. 10, pp. 875–885, 2014.

[22] K. Asomaning, S. Abramsky, Q. Liu, X. Zhou, R. E. Sobe, and S. Watt, "Pregabalin prescriptions in the United Kingdom: a drug utilisation study of The Health Improvement Network (THIN) primary care database," *International Journal of Clinical Practice*, vol. 70, no. 5, pp. 380–388, 2016.

[23] M. Gore, A. B. Sadosky, G. Zlateva, and D. J. Clauw, "Clinical characteristics, pharmacotherapy and healthcare resource use among patients with fibromyalgia newly prescribed gabapentin or pregabalin," *Pain Practice*, vol. 9, no. 5, pp. 363–374, 2009.

[24] P. Sun, Y. Zhao, Z. Zhao, and P. Watson, "Medication dosing patterns associated with duloxetine and pregabalin among patients with fibromyalgia," *Current Medical Research and Opinion*, vol. 27, no. 9, pp. 1793–1801, 2011.

[25] Y. Liu, C. Qian, and M. Yang, "Treatment patterns associated with ACR-recommended medications in the management of fibromyalgia in the United States," *Journal of Managed Care and Specialty Pharmacy*, vol. 22, no. 3, pp. 263–271, 2016.

[26] S. Ogawa, M. Komatsu, S. Ohno, H. Yamane, and K. Hayakawa, "Interim report of drug use investigation of pregabalin (Lyrica®)," *Progress in Medicine*, vol. 33, no. 10, pp. 2159–2171, 2013, in Japanese.

[27] S. Tanaka, K. Seto, and K. Kawakami, "Pharmacoepidemiology in Japan: medical databases and research achievements," *Journal of Pharmaceutical Health Care and Sciences*, vol. 1, no. 1, p. 16, 2015.

[28] H. Ueyama, S. Hinotsu, S. Tanaka et al., "Application of a self-controlled case series study to a database study in children," *Drug Safety*, vol. 37, no. 4, pp. 259–268, 2014.

[29] Ministry of Health, Labour and Welfare of Japan, 2016, http://www.mhlw.go.jp/file/05-Shingikai-12404000-Hokenkyoku-Iryouka/0000121094.pdf, in Japanese.

[30] *Pharmaceuticals and Medical Devices Agency*, 2017, http://www.pmda.go.jp/files/000153585.pdf.

[31] H. Kato, M. Miyazaki, M. Takeuchi et al., "A retrospective study to identify risk factors for somnolence and dizziness in patients treated with pregabalin," *Journal of Pharmaceutical Health Care and Sciences*, vol. 1, no. 1, p. 22, 2015.

[32] S. Ogawa, M. Suzuki, A. Arakawa, S. Araki, and T. Yoshiyama, "Efficacy and tolerability for postherpetic neuralgia: a multicenter, randomized, double-blind, placebo-controlled clinical trial," *Journal of the Japan Society of Pain Clinicians*, vol. 17, no. 2, pp. 141–152, 2010, in Japanese.

# 11

# Sensory Function and Chronic Pain in Multiple Sclerosis

Rogier J. Scherder,[1] Neeltje Kant,[2] Evelien T. Wolf,[1] Bas C. M. Pijnenburg,[3] and Erik J. A. Scherder ⓘ[1]

[1]Department of Clinical Neuropsychology, Vrije Universiteit, Amsterdam, Netherlands
[2]Department of Neuropsychology, Reade, Amsterdam, Netherlands
[3]Acibadem International Medical Center, Amsterdam, Netherlands

Correspondence should be addressed to Erik J. A. Scherder; e.j.a.scherder@vu.nl

Academic Editor: Anna Maria Aloisi

*Objective.* To examine whether hypoesthesia and chronic pain are related in patients with MS. *Methods.* Sixty-seven MS patients with pain and 80 persons without MS were included. Sensory functioning was tested by bedside neurological examination. Touch, joint position (dorsal column-medial lemniscus pathway), temperature sense, and pain (spinothalamic tract) were tested. Pain intensity was measured by the Colored Analogue Scale (CAS Intensity) and the Faces Pain Scale (FPS); pain affect was also measured by CAS Affect and Number of Words Chosen-Affective (NWC-A). Mood was assessed with the SCL-90 anxiety and depression subscales and the Beck Depression Inventory (BDI). *Results.* A significant negative relationship was found between pain intensity and the function of the dorsal column-medial lemniscal pathway, but not with the spinothalamic tract. *Conclusion.* In addition to the already known relation between hyperesthesia and pain, hypoesthesia for touch and joint position also seems to be related to chronic pain in MS patients.

## 1. Introduction

Chronic pain is a common symptom in multiple sclerosis (MS) [1]. Between 29 and 86 percent of all MS patients suffer from chronic pain [2]. This pain has been described in MS as both nociceptive and neuropathic [1, 3]. Nociceptive pain occurs when nociceptors are activated in response, for example, to tissue damage [4]. In MS, nociceptive pain can be provoked by abnormalities in the musculoskeletal system, for example, spasms [1]. Neuropathic pain may include both central and peripheral neuropathic pain and can be caused by lesions in the brain or spinal cord [5, 6].

A lesion in the brain or spinal cord may express itself in sensory disturbances. It is well known that MS is characterized by sensory disturbances reflected in both hyper- and hypoesthesia [5]. Hyperesthesia is often expressed in allodynia, a painful response to a nonpainful stimulus [7]. Allodynia is also a characteristic of central neuropathic pain [8]. There is thus a direct relationship between sensory disturbances, like allodynia, and pain, that is, central

neuropathic pain, in MS. However, patients with chronic pain conditions (e.g., osteoarthritis, musculoskeletal pain, and peripheral and central neuropathy) may show a *decline* in sensory functions, for example, hypoesthesia to touch [9–11]. The question arises as to whether a decline in sensory functions and chronic pain is also interrelated phenomena in MS. Support for a relationship between hypoesthesia and chronic pain emerges from a study investigating sensory functions of MS patients with and without chronic pain [12]. Compared with MS patients without pain, the group of MS patients with pain, irrespective of its nature, showed a decreased sensitivity for, among others, vibration, joint position, and touch assessed by bedside sensory testing. In that study, the functioning of the dorsal column-medial lemniscal pathway was assessed using vibration, joint position, and touch and the functioning of the spinothalamic pathway using pain and temperature [12]. However, the results of that remain obscure as to whether hypoesthesia was related to pain.

Compared with the role of the spinothalamic pathway in pain, little is known about the role of the dorsal column-medial lemniscal pathway in chronic pain in MS [13]. In examining the role of both the spinothalamic pathway and the dorsal column-medial lemniscal pathway in the relationship between sensory functions and pain, a distinction between pain intensity and pain affect was made in the present study. Such a distinction is known in pain research. A brain region that plays a crucial role in the processing of pain intensity is the somatosensory cortex [14], which is the target area of the dorsal column-medial lemniscal pathway [15]. Pain affect is processed by the spinothalamic tract, projecting to the prefrontal cortex, among others [14]. In other words, distinguishing between pain intensity and pain affect may provide more insight into the functioning of the dorsal column-medial lemniscal pathway and the spinothalamic tract.

The cumulative goal of the present study was thus to examine a possible relationship between chronic pain intensity and affect, and a decline in sensory functioning in patients with MS. Such a relationship may be clinically relevant as it implies that the presence of chronic pain in MS may be reflected by both hypo- and hyperesthesia. This study hypothesizes that, depending on the types of sensory dysfunction, that is, temperature, pain, light touch, and position sense, hypoesthesia may also be indicative of chronic pain intensity, pain affect, or both.

## 2. Materials and Methods

*2.1. Study Design.* The present cross-sectional study was part of a larger study examining the relationship between pain and cognition in patients with multiple sclerosis [16, 17].

*2.2. Participants.* From the larger study, we included in the present study 67 MS patients who suffered from chronic pain. MS patients were recruited from a center, specialized in MS and other neurodegenerative disorders in the Netherlands, or enrolled from the personal environment of the researchers. In each case, an official diagnosis of MS was made by a neurologist, according to the criteria of Poser or McDonald criteria [18, 19]. We also included 80 persons without MS (control group). Well-instructed and trained medical and psychology students tested the MS patients and the controls.

*2.3. Education.* Both the MS patients and the control participants were screened for education. Education was divided into five categories: elementary school not finished (score = 1), elementary school (score = 2), lower secondary school (score = 3), higher secondary school (score = 4), and higher vocational training for 18+/university (score = 5).

*2.4. Chronic Painful Conditions.* Both groups suffered from arthrosis/rheumatoid arthritis, musculoskeletal disorders (e.g. neck-shoulder pain), migraine, osteoporosis, and peripheral neuropathic pain. Peripheral neuropathic pain was due to metatarsalgia, carpal tunnel syndrome, low back pain with irradiation, and meralgia paresthetica. Probably, our participants did not suffer from central neuropathic pain

reflected in an absence of allodynia. Chronic pain was defined as pain occurred during a period of 3 months or longer [20].

*2.5. Medication.* Within the scope of the present study, we listed analgesics (baclofen, paracetamol, diclofenac, naproxen, ibuprofen, and cannabis) and medication that might be related to sensory disturbances: sedatives (e.g., temazepam), antipsychotics (e.g., Fluanxol), antidepressives (e.g., citalopram), anxiolytics (e.g., Rivotril), and neurological disorders (e.g., epilepsy: Depakine).

*2.6. Comorbidities.* Comorbidities that might cause sensory disturbances, that is, diabetes, transient ischemic attack (TIA), migraine, and epilepsy, were listed (for a full list of comorbidities see [17]).

*2.7. Exclusion Criteria.* Participants (patients and controls) were excluded if they had a history of neoplasms, cerebral traumata, alcoholism, normal pressure hydrocephalus, disorders of the central nervous system other than MS, or disturbances of consciousness.

*2.8. Informed Consent.* The local medical ethical committee gave their approval for the present study (NL 19801.029.07, 2007.211). The patients were asked to give oral and written consent after they had been extensively informed about the aim and procedure of the study. After permission, the neuropsychological, the sensory function, and the pain perception tests were obtained. The patients were able to discontinue their participation at any time during the current study.

*2.9. Sensory Function.* Sensory function was tested by a bedside neurological examination. In particular, it was tested whether the sensory function of the MS patient was normal (score = 2) or decreased (score = 1) on two levels: dorsal column-medial lemniscal function (by testing joint position and touch) and function of the spinothalamic cortical pathway (by testing temperature sense and pain). The classification from Svendsen and colleagues was used to assess the spinothalamic cortical pathway and dorsal column-medial lemniscal pathway [12].

*2.9.1. Dorsal Column-Medial Lemniscal Pathway.* This pathway mediates fine touch and joint position. Fine touch was tested by applying a cotton wool on the dorsal side of the right and left hand, forearm, and upper arm. Joint position was tested by passively stretching or bending one finger of the patient. The patient was asked which finger has been stretched or bended. Three fingers of each hand were moved. Fine touch or joint position were considered to be disturbed if the participant failed, by giving one or more incorrect answers, to indicate whether they were touched or gave an incorrect answer concerning the position of the joint. During all of these tests the patients kept their eyes closed [21].

### 2.9.2. Spinothalamic Cortical Pathway.
This pathway mediates pain and temperature. Pain was tested by applying a pinprick with a needle with either a sharp or blunt end on the dorsal side of the participant's right and left hand, forearm, and upper arm. Temperature sense was evaluated by making a distinction between warm and cold. The investigator touches the dorsal side of the right and left hand, forearm, and upper arm with a small plastic bottle filled with either cold or hot water. The patient kept their eyes closed during the test. If the participant gave one or more incorrect answers, sensory function was considered to be disturbed [21].

### 2.10. Pain

#### 2.10.1. Colored Analogue Scale (CAS).
Two CAS scales were applied: one measures the intensity of pain (CAS Intensity) and the other measures the affective/emotional components of pain (CAS Affect) [22]. The CAS is a visual analogue scale with a plastic slide, which can be moved by the patient from the bottom ("no pain," light pink) to the top ("maximum pain," dark red). To measure the intensity or affective/emotional aspects of pain adequately, a scale from 0 to 10 has been drawn (score: 0 = no pain; score: 10 = severe pain) on the back.

#### 2.10.2. Number of Words Chosen-Affective (NWC-A).
This is the affective part of the McGill Pain Questionnaire (Dutch version) and is composed of 5 groups [23]. Each group consists of 3 affective words, for example, alarming, frightening, and terrifying. The patient was asked to choose one word of each group that levels their pain experience (maximum score: 15).

#### 2.10.3. Faces Pain Scale (FPS).
This scale consists of seven different faces with different expressions. Each face represents an increased feeling of pain [24, 25]. The patient was asked to choose one face that matches their pain experience (score: 0 = no pain; score: 6 = severe pain).

Two pain domains were composed: (1) pain intensity, which is composed of the CAS Intensity and the FPS, and (2) pain affect, which is composed of CAS Affect and the NWCA. The MS patients were asked to indicate their level of pain during the last week. This way of measuring the level of pain is reliable, according to a study of Forouzanfar and colleagues [26].

The extent to which patients were suffering from pain is presented in the Results section.

### 2.11. Mood.
As pain may be associated with depression and anxiety [27], three questionnaires were used to assess depression and anxiety: the Beck Depression Inventory (BDI) (minimum score = 0; maximum score = 63) [28, 29], the SCL-90 anxiety subscale (minimum score = 0; maximum score = 40) [30], and the SCL-90 depression subscale (minimum score = 0; maximum score = 52) [31].

The scores of these three scales were first converted into z-scores. Subsequently, a reliability analysis resulted in a Cronbach's alpha of 0.84. Next, we made a composite domain score "mood."

### 2.12. Procedure.
The pain scales (CAS Intensity, CAS Affect, NWC-A, and FPS) and sensory tests (touch, joint position, pinprick, and temperature sense) were administered in one session. First, the pain scales were conducted from the patient, after which the sensory functions were assessed.

### 2.13. Data Analysis.
We used the SPSS-PC program for the data analyses. Chi-square tests, $t$-tests, and Mann–Whitney $U$ tests were applied to analyze data between groups. As some cells had a low cell count, statistical significance was established by means of Fischer's exact tests (two-tailed). The relationships between chronic pain, the dorsal column-lemniscal pathway, and the spinothalamic tract were analyzed by hierarchical linear regression analyses: one model predicting pain intensity and one predicting pain affect. In the first step, mood was added as a predictor; in the second step, the dorsal column-medial lemniscal pathway; and in the third step, the spinothalamic tract was entered. Adjusted $R^2$ and $R^2$ are reported as measures of model fit and $\Delta R^2$ as a measure of the effect of sensory functioning (dorsal column-medial lemniscal pathway and the spinothalamic tract) on pain while controlling for mood. The level of significance was set at $p < 0.05$.

## 3. Results

### 3.1. Demographics

#### 3.1.1. Age.
The mean age of the MS patients (M = 51.25 years; SD = 9.84) did not differ significantly from the mean age of the control group (M = 48.79 years; SD = 10.49) ($t$ (145) = 1.46; $p = 0.15$).

#### 3.1.2. Gender.
The distribution of gender within the group of MS patients is as follows: 66.2% women and 33.8% men. Within the control group, the distribution of gender was 66.3% women and 33.8% men (chi square: 0.99, $df = 1$, and $p = 0.99$).

#### 3.1.3. Education.
The mean level of education of the MS patients is 3.57 (SD = 0.76). The mean level of education of the control group was 3.50 ($t$ (141) = 0.55; $p < 0.59$).

### 3.2. Mood.
With respect to depression and anxiety, MS patients showed significant higher scores than the controls (for means, standard deviations, and Mann–Whitney $U$ tests see Table 1). Consequently, concerning the mood domain, the group with MS patients (mean rank: 91.64) differed significantly from the control group (mean rank: 58.11) (Mann–Whitney $U$ test: $Z = 4.78$; $p < 0.001$).

TABLE 1: Means, standard deviations, and Mann–Whitney $U$ tests concerning the scores on the Beck Depression Inventory and the SCL-90 anxiety and depression scale of persons with and without multiple sclerosis (MS).

| | MS patients | | Controls | | Mann–Whitney $U$ tests | |
|---|---|---|---|---|---|---|
| | M | SD | M | SD | Z | $p <$ |
| Beck Depression Inventory | 7.42 | 5.04 | 4.75 | 4.39 | 4.02 | 0.001 |
| SCL-90 depression | 22.35 | 7.01 | 18.74 | 4.47 | 4.00 | 0.001 |
| SCL-90 anxiety | 13.89 | 4.73 | 11.89 | 2.47 | 3.06 | 0.003 |

SCL-90: symptom checklist.

TABLE 2: Means (M), standard deviations (SD), and Mann–Whitney $U$ tests concerning the various sensory functions in persons with and without multiple sclerosis (MS).

| | MS patients | | Controls | | Mann–Whitney $U$ tests | |
|---|---|---|---|---|---|---|
| | M | SD | M | SD | Z | $p <$ |
| *Dorsal column-medial lemniscal pathway* | | | | | | |
| Light touch | 1.73 | 0.48 | 1.96 | 0.19 | 3.80 | 0.001 |
| Position sense | 1.71 | 0.49 | 1.99 | 0.11 | 4.64 | 0.001 |
| *Spinothalamic tract* | | | | | | |
| Temperature | 1.79 | 0.41 | 1.91 | 0.33 | 2.27 | 0.03 |
| Pain | 1.54 | 0.56 | 1.79 | 0.54 | 3.47 | 0.001 |

### 3.3. Sensory Function

*3.3.1. Dorsal Column-Medial Lemniscal Pathway.* 23.9% of the MS patients had decreased sensibility to touch. Disturbances in joint position were found in 25.8% of the MS patients. Both sensory functions were significantly more disturbed in MS patients than in the control group (see Table 2 for means, standard deviations, and Mann–Whitney $U$ tests).

*3.3.2. Spinothalamic Tract.* When pain experience was tested by applying a pinprick, 40.3% had sensory disturbances. Disturbances in temperature were found in 20.9% of the cases. Compared to the control group, MS patients showed significantly more disturbances in both sensory functions (see Table 1 for means, standard deviations, and Mann–Whitney $U$ tests; Figures 1 and 2).

*3.4. Sensory Function in Relation to Comorbidity.* The group of MS patients was divided into a group of patients with sensory disturbances (either dorsal column-medial lemniscal pathway or spinothalamic tract or both) and a group of patients without sensory disturbances. We were interested whether, compared to MS patients without sensory disturbances, those with sensory disturbances suffered more from comorbidities that might have caused those sensory disturbances. As can be seen in Table 3, comorbidities such as diabetes mellitus, transient ischemic attack (TIA), migraine, and epilepsy did not differ significantly between both groups. Arteriosclerosis, stroke, and traumatic brain injury appeared not to be present in our patients.

*3.5. Pain Experience.* Data analyses by means of Mann–Whitney $U$ tests show that MS patients suffer significantly

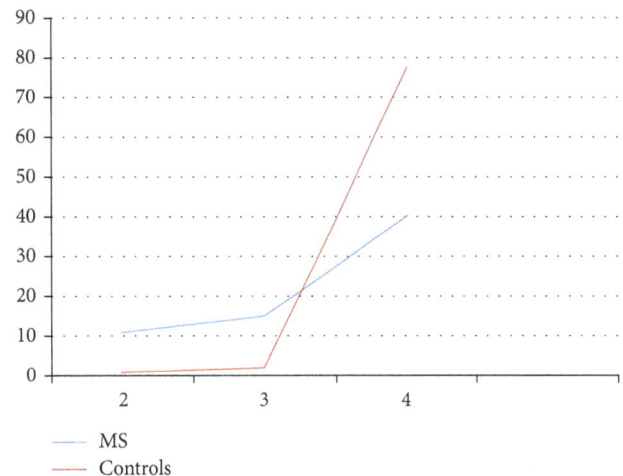

FIGURE 1: Scores of the patients with multiple sclerosis (MS) and controls on position sense and light touch (dorsal column-medial lemniscal pathway). The lower the score, the more disturbances in sensory functioning.

more from pain intensity and pain affect, compared to controls (for means, standard deviations, and Mann–Whitney $U$ tests see Table 4).

*3.6. Pain Medication.* MS patients used significantly more baclofen, paracetamol, and cannabis than the controls (see Table 5 for percentages, chi-square, and Fisher's exact tests).

*3.7. Sensory Function in Relation to Medication.* The use of analgesics and the use of medication prescribed for disorders that might affect sensory functioning (sedatives, antipsychotics, antidepressives, anxiolytics, and medication for neurological disorders, e.g., epilepsy) were examined by

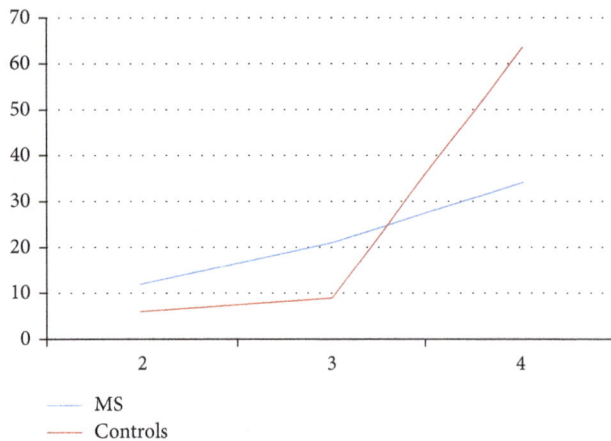

FIGURE 2: Scores of the patients with multiple sclerosis (MS) and controls on temperature and pain (spinothalamic tract). The lower the score, the more disturbances in sensory functioning.

means of chi-square test and Fisher's exact test. The results show that concerning analgesics, only cannabis differed significantly between both groups; MS patients with sensory disturbances used significantly more cannabis than those without sensory disturbances. No significant differences between both groups were observed concerning the other medications that might be related to sensory disturbances (see Table 6 for percentages, chi-square test and Fisher's exact test).

### 3.8. Relationship between Pain, Sensory Function, and Mood

*3.8.1. The Relationship between Pain Intensity and Sensory Function.* The results of a hierarchical regression analysis show a significant relationship between mood and pain intensity, thereby explaining 9% of its variance (Model 1). Adding the functioning of the dorsal column-medial lemniscal pathway explained an additional 10% of variance in pain intensity (Model 2). There was no significant change in explained variance in pain intensity, after adding the function of the spinothalamic tract (Model 3) (Table 7).

*3.8.2. The Relationship between Pain Affect and Sensory Function.* The results of a hierarchical regression analysis show a significant relationship between mood and pain affect, explaining 9% of the variance in pain affect (Model 1). No significant relationships were found between pain affect and the function of the dorsal column-medial lemniscal pathway (Model 2) and between pain affect and the function of the spinothalamic tract (Model 3) (Table 8).

## 4. Discussion

The goal of the present study was to examine a possible relationship between hypoesthesia and chronic pain in MS patients. The main finding relates to our observation of a significant negative relationship between pain intensity and hyposensitivity concerning light touch and joint position (dorsal column-medial lemniscal pathway) (Table 7).

This finding implies that the larger the decline in the perception of light touch and joint position, the higher the pain intensity, and higher the patient suffers. This finding has not previously been described in the MS literature, where there are descriptions of the relationship between hyperesthesia and chronic pain, in particular central neuropathic pain [12, 32]. The lack of a relationship between hypoesthesia and pain affect (Table 8) may be due to the fact that the MS patients indicated less pain affect (NWC-A, CAS Affect) than pain intensity (FPS, CAS Intensity).

The rationale is that chronic pain, known to be present in MS [33], may be due to a dysfunction of the dorsal column-medial lemniscal pathway expressed in hypoesthesia. Alternatively, as has previously been described in the literature, chronic pain such as complex regional pain syndromes and chronic arthropathies may cause hypoesthesia, for example, for touch [34]. One of the underlying mechanisms is that nociceptive activation of the unmyelinated C-fibers may inhibit the processing of nonnociceptive information (e.g., light touch) transmitted by beta fibers, for example, [34]. This might occur at both a spinal and cortical level. Geber and colleagues [34] further suggest that if pain experience decreases through more adequate treatment, the hypoesthesia should diminish.

The main finding yielded related questions. One of these include whether MS patients with sensory disturbances differed from those without sensory disturbances concerning comorbidities that might provoke sensory disturbances. This appeared not to be the case (Table 3). A similar question concerned the use of analgesics and other medications that could be related to sensory disturbances (Table 6). There were no significant differences between MS patients with and without sensory disturbances concerning analgesic medication, except for cannabis. Cannabis is often prescribed for chronic pain and for spasm in MS patients, although its effectiveness is not consistent [35]. Häuser and colleagues [35] also mention possible side effects of cannabis in their review, and disturbances in sensory functioning are not among them. To our knowledge, a negative effect of cannabis on the functioning of the dorsal column-medial lemniscal pathway or on the functioning of the spinothalamic pathway has not yet been reported in literature. Despite the lack of significant differences (except for cannabis) between MS patients with and without sensory disturbances, we analyzed whether there was a relationship between (analgesic) medication and sensory dysfunction; this appeared not to be the case (data not shown).

Compared with controls, the use of baclofen, paracetamol, and cannabis was significantly higher in our MS patients (Table 5). The higher usage of analgesics by MS patients fits the higher level of pain intensity and pain affect in this group, compared with the controls (Table 4).

Our finding concerning the relationship between hypoesthesia and pain intensity in MS patients may be clinically relevant. In cases of hyperesthesia, a patient may respond quite vividly to light touch, for example, due to a considerable increase in pain [36], even when the patient is not able to communicate about pain. However, if the patient hardly responds to light touch, for example, at least two explanations

TABLE 3: Comorbidities that might be related to sensory disturbances in MS patients with and without sensory disturbances.

| Comorbidities | MS group with sensory disturbances | | MS group without sensory disturbances | | Statistics | |
|---|---|---|---|---|---|---|
| | $n$ | % | $n$ | % | $\chi^2(1)$ | Fisher's exact test |
| Diabetes | 1 | 3.3 | 2 | 8.0 | 0.58 | 0.59 |
| TIA | 0 | 0 | 1 | 4.0 | 1.22 | 0.46 |
| Migraine | 1 | 3.3 | 0 | 0 | 0.85 | 1.00 |
| Epilepsy | 2 | 6.7 | 0 | 0 | 1.73 | 0.50 |

MS: multiple sclerosis; TIA: transient ischemic attack.

TABLE 4: Pain experience in patients with multiple sclerosis (MS) and controls.

| Pain scales | MS patients | | Controls | | Mann-Whitney $U$ tests | |
|---|---|---|---|---|---|---|
| | M | SD | M | SD | Z | $p <$ |
| NWC-A | 4.76 | 4.09 | 1.05 | 1.98 | 6.75 | 0.001 |
| CAS Pain Intensity | 4.09 | 2.51 | 0.97 | 1.80 | 8.06 | 0.001 |
| CAS Pain Affect | 3.47 | 2.76 | 0.84 | 1.82 | 7.41 | 0.001 |
| FPS | 2.34 | 1.77 | 0.62 | 1.15 | 6.45 | 0.001 |

NWC-A: Number of Words Chosen-Affective; CAS: Colored Analogue Scale; FPS: Faces Pain Scale.

TABLE 5: Analysis of the pain medication of the patients with multiple sclerosis (MS) and controls by means of chi-square and Fisher's exact tests.

| Pain medication | MS group | | Controls | | Statistics | |
|---|---|---|---|---|---|---|
| | $n$ | % | $n$ | % | $\chi^2(1)$ | Fisher's exact test |
| Baclofen | 19 | 33.9 | 0 | 0 | 27.25 | 0.000 |
| Paracetamol | 16 | 28.6 | 1 | 1.5 | 19.07 | 0.000 |
| Diclofenac | 2 | 3.5 | 2 | 2.9 | 0.03 | 1.00 |
| Naproxen | 1 | 1.8 | 0 | 0 | 1.22 | 0.45 |
| Ibuprofen | 3 | 5.4 | 0 | 0 | 3.73 | 0.09 |
| Cannabis | 4 | 19.0 | 0 | 0 | 15.10 | 0.002 |

are possible: the first is that the patient experiences the light touch as normal but cannot express his or her feelings clearly enough, and the second is that the patient is actually impaired in processing light touch. Not knowing which of the two is applicable to the patient, the clinician may want to opt for the "worst case scenario," that is an impairment in processing light touch. In the latter case, the clinician will be motivated to search for the presence of chronic pain.

Our results further show that compared with controls, MS patients had higher scores on scales measuring mood, more specifically depression and anxiety (Table 1). The relatively low mean scores suggest that MS patients suffer from depressive *symptoms* instead of major depressive disorders [37]. We observed a significant relationship between mood and pain intensity and between mood and pain affect in MS patients (Tables 7 and 8). These findings are congruent with previous studies in which depression and pain coincided in MS patients [37]. Feistein and colleagues [37] emphasize the importance of focusing treatment on both symptoms simultaneously [37]. They also state that anxiety disorders may occur even more frequently in MS but do not receive as much attention as depression. Treatment of anxiety is the more important as, untreated, it may further aggravate cognitive decline [37].

The present study has several limitations. Firstly, we were unable to perform quantitative sensory testing (QST) to examine sensory function in MS patients in an objective way. This is because our study was based partly on Svendsen and colleagues' study [12], which examined the sensory functions belonging to the dorsal column-medial lemniscal pathway and the spinothalamic tract by both bedside sensory testing and quantitative sensory testing (QST). Only the bedside sensory testing method appeared to be sensitive for differences in sensory functioning between MS patients with and without pain. MS patients with pain showed a decrease in sensibility in touch, among others [12]. Nevertheless, to assess the perception threshold for touch, vibration, and temperatures [5], QST should be applied in studies examining pain in MS.

In addition to QST, a neurophysiological examination in a study on pain in MS could be conducted, for example, by measuring somatosensory-evoked potentials that are transmitted by thick-myelinated A$\beta$ fibers (nonnociceptive; dorsal column-medial lemniscal pathway) or by laser-evoked potentials that are transmitted by A$\delta$ fibers (nociceptive) [38].

Another limitation of the present study is that we did not observe central neuropathic pain in our patients. Central

TABLE 6: Use of analgesics and medication that might be related to sensory disturbances (medication "sensory") between MS patients with and without sensory disturbances.

| Analgesics/medication related to sensory disturbances | MS group with sensory disturbances | | MS group without sensory disturbances | | Statistics | |
|---|---|---|---|---|---|---|
| | $n$ | % | $n$ | % | $\chi^2(1)$ | Fisher's exact test |
| *Analgesics* | | | | | | |
| Baclofen | 9 | 30 | 9 | 36 | 0.22 | 0.77 |
| Paracetamol | 8 | 26.7 | 7 | 28 | 0.01 | 1.00 |
| Diclofenac | 2 | 6.5 | 0 | 0 | 1.67 | 0.50 |
| Naproxen | 1 | 3.3 | 0 | 0 | 0.85 | 1.00 |
| Ibuprofen | 0 | 0 | 3 | 12 | 3.81 | 0.09 |
| Cannabis | 4 | 40 | 0 | 0 | 5.44 | 0.04 |
| *Medication "sensory"* | | | | | | |
| Sedatives | 15 | 50 | 7 | 28 | 2.75 | 0.17 |
| Antipsychotics | 3 | 10 | 0 | 0 | 2.64 | 0.24 |
| Antidepressives | 5 | 16.7 | 5 | 20 | 0.10 | 1.00 |
| Anxiolytics | 12 | 40 | 4 | 16 | 3.81 | 0.08 |
| Neurological disorders | 16 | 53.3 | 8 | 32 | 2.52 | 0.17 |

TABLE 7: Hierarchical regression analyses with the domain pain intensity as a dependent variable and mood, DCML, STT, and analgesics as predictors in patients with MS ($n = 55$).

| Pain intensity | Beta (SE) | $t$ | $p$ | $F$ | $df$ | $p$ | $R^2_{adj}$ | $R^2$ | $\Delta R^2$ |
|---|---|---|---|---|---|---|---|---|---|
| *Model 1* | | | | 5.10 | 1.54 | 0.03 | 0.07 | 0.09 | n/a |
| Mood | 0.29 (0.03) | 2.26 | 0.03 | | | | | | |
| *Model 2* | | | | 5.92 | 2.51 | 0.005 | 0.16 | 0.19 | 0.10 |
| Mood | 0.29 (0.03) | 2.37 | 0.02 | | | | | | |
| DCML | −0.32 (0.64) | −2.50 | 0.02 | | | | | | |
| *Model 3* | | | | 3.91 | 3.50 | 0.01 | 0.14 | 0.19 | n/a |
| Mood | 0.30 | 2.37 | 0.02 | | | | | | |
| DCML | −0.34 (0.80) | −2.19 | 0.03 | | | | | | |
| STT | 0.05 (0.81) | 0.31 | 0.76 | | | | | | |

DCML, dorsal column-medial lemniscal pathway; STT, spinothalamic tract.

TABLE 8: Hierarchical regression analyses with the domain pain affect as a dependent variable and mood, DCML, STT, and analgesics as predictors in patients with MS ($n = 63$).

| Pain affect | Beta (SE) | $t$ | $p$ | $F$ | $df$ | $p$ | $R^2_{adj}$ | $R^2$ | $\Delta R^2$ |
|---|---|---|---|---|---|---|---|---|---|
| *Model 1* | | | | 5.76 | 1.62 | 0.02 | 0.07 | 0.09 | n/a |
| Mood | 0.29 (0.05) | 2.40 | 0.02 | | | | | | |
| *Model 2* | | | | 3.02 | 2.60 | 0.06 | 0.06 | 0.09 | n/a |
| Mood | 0.28 (0.05) | 2.31 | 0.02 | | | | | | |
| DCML | −0.09 (0.99) | −0.76 | 0.45 | | | | | | |
| *Model 3* | | | | 1.98 | 3.59 | 0.13 | 0.05 | 0.09 | n/a |
| Mood | 0.29 (0.05) | 2.30 | 0.03 | | | | | | |
| DCML | −0.11 (1.24) | −0.68 | 0.50 | | | | | | |
| STT | 0.02 (1.26) | 0.13 | 0.90 | | | | | | |

DCML, dorsal column-medial lemniscal pathway; STT, spinothalamic tract.

neuropathic pain might occur in 50% of the MS patients [4]. Although central neuropathic pain may be present only for a short period of time [39], it may also express itself in a more continuous way [4]. Irrespective of its prevalence and expression, we might have missed central neuropathic pain in our study, as it most often occurs in the legs and feet [6]. We performed our sensory testing on the right and left hand, forearm, and upper arm. On the other hand, the presence of central neuropathic pain would not have violated our main finding, that is, a negative relationship between hypoesthesia for touch and joint position and chronic pain.

A final limitation is that we did not include an MS group *without* chronic pain in the present study. Such a control group would have been appropriate to examine the clinical and neuropathological characteristics of MS patients who do suffer from chronic pain.

# 5. Conclusion

The present study indicated a negative relationship between hypoesthesia, for light touch and joint position, and pain intensity in MS patients who suffer from chronic pain. As a consequence, the clinician should be aware of the fact that, although hypoesthesia need not per se be related to chronic pain, it *could* be an indication of chronic pain in MS patients.

# Authors' Contributions

Rogier J. Scherder was the principal investigator, performed the study, and had a major role in the writing of the paper. Neeltje Kant contributed by selecting the participants and by supervising the assessments. Evelien T. Wolf assisted in analyzing the data and in writing the Results section. Bas C. M. Pijnenburg was responsible for controlling the medical records of the participants and for including those data into the manuscript. Erik J. A. Scherder made the overall plan for the study and assisted in the rewriting of the various versions of the manuscript, including the final version.

# Acknowledgments

This study was supported by a grant from the Arnold Oosterbaan Brain Foundation.

# References

[1] A. Truini, F. Galeotti, and G. Cruccu, "Treating pain in multiple sclerosis," *Expert Opinion on Pharmacotherapy*, vol. 12, no. 15, pp. 2355–2368, 2011.

[2] A. B. O'Connor, S. R. Schwid, D. N. Herrmann, J. D. Markman, and R. H. Dworkin, "Pain associated with multiple sclerosis: systematic review and proposed classification," *Pain*, vol. 137, no. 1, pp. 96–111, 2008.

[3] C. Solaro and M. M. Uccelli, "Management of pain in multiple sclerosis: a pharmacological approach," *Nature Reviews Neurology*, vol. 7, no. 9, pp. 519–527, 2011.

[4] C. Solaro, E. Trabucco, and M. Messmer Uccelli, "Pain and multiple sclerosis: pathophysiology and treatment," *Current Neurology and Neuroscience Reports*, vol. 13, no. 1, p. 320, 2013.

[5] A. Österberg and J. Boivie, "Central pain in multiple sclerosis—sensory abnormalities," *European Journal of Pain*, vol. 14, no. 1, pp. 104–110, 2010.

[6] A. Österberg, J. Boivie, and K. A. Thuomas, "Central pain in multiple sclerosis—prevalence and clinical characteristics," *European Journal of Pain*, vol. 9, no. 5, pp. 531–542, 2005.

[7] G. Moalem and D. J. Tracey, "Immune and inflammatory mechanisms in neuropathic pain," *Brain Research Reviews*, vol. 51, no. 2, pp. 240–264, 2006.

[8] N. Attal and D. Bouhassira, "Neuropathic pain: experimental advances and clinical applications," *Revue Neurologique*, vol. 160, no. 2, pp. 199–203, 2004.

[9] C. Gummesson, I. Atroshi, C. Ekdahl, R. Johnsson, and E. Ornstein, "Chronic upper extremity pain and co-occurring symptoms in a general population," *Arthritis & Rheumatism*, vol. 49, no. 5, pp. 697–702, 2003.

[10] A. Westermann, A. K. Rönnau, E. Krumova et al., "Pain-associated mild sensory deficits without hyperalgesia in chronic non-neuropathic pain," *Clinical Journal of Pain*, vol. 27, no. 9, pp. 782–789, 2011.

[11] C. Maier, R. Baron, T. R. Tölle et al., "Quantitative sensory testing in the German Research Network on Neuropathic Pain (DFNS): somatosensory abnormalities in 1236 patients with different neuropathic pain syndromes," *Pain*, vol. 150, no. 3, pp. 439–450, 2010.

[12] K. B. Svendsen, T. S. Jensen, H. J. Hansen, and F. W. Bach, "Sensory function and quality of life in patients with multiple sclerosis and pain," *Pain*, vol. 114, no. 3, pp. 473–481, 2005.

[13] Y. Cruz-Almeida, E. R. Felix, A. Martinez-Arizala, and E. G. Widerström-Noga, "Decreased spinothalamic and dorsal column medial lemniscus-mediated function is associated with neuropathic pain after spinal cord injury," *Journal of Neurotrauma*, vol. 29, no. 17, pp. 2706–2715, 2012.

[14] E. J. Scherder, J. A. Sergeant, and D. F. Swaab, "Pain processing in dementia and its relation to neuropathology," *The Lancet Neurology*, vol. 2, no. 11, pp. 677–686, 2003.

[15] R. Melzack and K. L. Casey, "Sensory, motivational and central control determinants of pain: a new conceptual model," in *Proceedings of the International Symposium of the Skin Senses*, D. Kenshalo, Eds., C. C. Thomas, Tallahassee, FL, USA, 1968.

[16] R. Scherder, N. Kant, E. Wolf, A. C. M. Pijnenburg, and E. Scherder, "Pain and cognition in multiple sclerosis," *Pain Medicine*, vol. 18, no. 10, pp. 1987–1998, 2017.

[17] R. Scherder, N. Kant, E. Wolf, B. Pijnenburg, and E. Scherder, "Psychiatric and physical comorbidities and pain in patients with multiple sclerosis," *Journal of Pain Research*, vol. 11, pp. 325–334, 2018.

[18] C. M. Poser, D. W. Paty, L. Scheinberg et al., "New diagnostic criteria for multiple sclerosis: guidelines for research protocols," *Annals of Neurology*, vol. 13, no. 3, pp. 227–231, 1983.

[19] W. L. McDonald, A. Compston, G. Edan et al., "Recommended diagnostic criteria for multiple sclerosis: guidelines from the International Panel on the diagnosis of multiple sclerosis," *Annals of Neurology*, vol. 50, no. 1, pp. 121–127, 2001.

[20] J. Young, B. Amatya, M. P. Galea, and F. Khan, "Chronic pain in multiple sclerosis: a 10-year longitudinal study," *Scandinavian Journal of Pain*, vol. 16, no. 1, pp. 98–203, 2017.

[21] E. J. Scherder, N. N. Rommelse, T. Bröring, S. T. Faraone, and J. A. Sergeant, "Somatosensory functioning and experienced pain in ADHD-families: a pilot study," *European Journal of Paediatric Neurology*, vol. 12, no. 6, pp. 461–469, 2008.

[22] P. A. McGrath, C. E. Seifert, K. N. Speechley, J. C. Booth, L. Stitt, and M. C. Gibson, "A new analogue scale for assessing children's pain: an initial validation study," *Pain*, vol. 64, no. 3, pp. 435–443, 1996.

[23] W. A. van der Kloot, R. A. B. Oostendorp, J. van der Meij, and J. van den Heuvel, "De Nederlandse versie van McGill pain questionnaire: een betrouwbare pijnvragenlijst," *Nederlands Tijdschrift voor Geneeskunde*, vol. 139, no. 13, pp. 669–673, 1995.

[24] E. J. Kim and M. T. Buschmann, "Reliability and validity of the Faces Pain Scale with older adults," *International Journal of Nursing Studies*, vol. 43, pp. 447–456, 2006.

[25] D. Bieri, R. A. Reeve, G. D. Champion, L. Addicoat, and J. B. Ziegler, "The faces pain scale for the self-assessment of the severity of pain experienced by children: development, initial validation, and preliminary investigation for ratio scale properties," *Pain*, vol. 41, no. 2, pp. 139–150, 1990.

[26] T. Forouzanfar, M. Kemler, A. G. Kessels, A. J. Koke, M. van Kleef, and W. E. Weber, "Comparison of multiple against single pain intensity measurements in complex regional pain syndrome type I: analysis of 54 patients," *Clinical Journal of Pain*, vol. 18, no. 4, pp. 234–237, 2002.

[27] R. Gorczyca, R. Filip, and E. Walczak, "Psychological aspects of pain," *Annals of Agricultural and Environmental Medicine*, vol. 20, no. 1, pp. 23–27, 2013.

[28] A. T. Beck, C. H. Ward, M. Mendelson, J. Mock, and J. Erbaugh, "An inventory for measuring depression," *Archives of General Psychiatry*, vol. 4, no. 6, pp. 561–571, 1961.

[29] J. E. Aikens, M. A. Reinecke, N. H. Pliskin et al., "Assessing depressive symptoms in multiple sclerosis: is it necessary to omit items from the original beck depression inventory?," *Journal of Behavioral Medicine*, vol. 22, no. 2, pp. 127–142, 1999.

[30] L. R. Derogatis, K. Rickels, and A. F. Rock, "The SCL-90 and the MMPI: a step in the validation of a new self-report scale," *British Journal of Psychiatry*, vol. 128, no. 3, pp. 280–289, 1976.

[31] W. A. Arrindell and J. H. M. Ettema, *SCL-90: Handleiding bij een Multidimensionele Psychopathologie-Indicator*, Swets & Zeitlinger, Lisse, Netherlands, 1986.

[32] K. B. Svendsen, L. Sorensen, T. S. Jensen, H. J. Hansen, and F. W. Bach, "MRI of the central nervous system in MS patients with and without pain," *European Journal of Pain*, vol. 15, no. 4, pp. 395–401, 2011.

[33] A. B. Sullivan, J. Scheman, A. Lopresti, and H. Prayor-Patterson, "Interdisciplinary treatment of patients with multiple sclerosis and chronic pain: a descriptive study," *International Journal of MS Care*, vol. 14, no. 4, pp. 216–220, 2012.

[34] C. Geber, W. Magerl, R. Fondel et al., "Numbness in clinical and experimental pain—a cross-sectional study exploring the mechanisms of reduced tactile function," *Pain*, vol. 139, no. 1, pp. 73–81, 2008.

[35] W. Häuser, F. Petzke, and M. A. Fitzcharles, "Efficacy, tolerability and safety of cannabis-based medicines for chronic pain management-an overview of systematic reviews," *European Journal of Pain*, vol. 22, no. 3, pp. 455–470, 2017.

[36] P. Karmacharya, K. Shah, R. Pathak, S. Ghimire, and R. Alweis, "Touch me not," *Journal of Community Hospital Internal Medicine Perspectives*, vol. 4, no. 1, p. 23148, 2014.

[37] A. Feistein, S. Magalhaes, J. F. Richard, B. Audet, and C. Moore, "The link between multiple sclerosis and depression," *Nature Reviews Neurology*, vol. 10, no. 9, pp. 507–517, 2014.

[38] A. Truini, F. Galeotti, S. La Cesa et al., "Mechanisms of pain in multiple sclerosis: a combined clinical and neurophysiological study," *Pain*, vol. 153, no. 10, pp. 2048–2054, 2012.

[39] W. Brola, K. Mitosek-Szewczyk, and J. Opara, "Symptomatology and pathogenesis of different types of pain in multiple sclerosis," *Neurologia i Neurochirurgia Polska*, vol. 48, no. 4, pp. 272–279, 2014.

# 12

# Temporomandibular Disorders among Dutch Adolescents: Prevalence and Biological, Psychological, and Social Risk Indicators

**Carolina Marpaung** [ID],[1,2] **Frank Lobbezoo** [ID],[1] **and Maurits K. A. van Selms**[1]

[1]*Department of Oral Kinesiology, Academic Centre for Dentistry Amsterdam (ACTA), University of Amsterdam and Vrije Universiteit Amsterdam, Amsterdam, Netherlands*
[2]*Department of Prosthodontics, Faculty of Dentistry, Trisakti University, Jakarta, Indonesia*

Correspondence should be addressed to Carolina Marpaung; carolina@trisakti.ac.id

Academic Editor: Mieszko Wieckiewicz

*Aims.* To assess the prevalence rates of pain-related temporomandibular disorders (TMDs) and temporomandibular joint (TMJ) sounds in a large group of Dutch adolescents, aged between 12 and 18 years and to determine if the same biological, psychological, and social risk indicators are related to both TMD pain and TMJ sounds. *Methods.* In this cross-sectional questionnaire survey, 4,235 questionnaires were analyzed, with an about equal gender distribution. *Results.* The overall prevalence of pain-related TMDs was 21.6% (26.1% for girls and 17.6% for boys) and that of TMJ sounds was 15.5% (19.3% for girls and 11.7% for boys). Logistic regression analyses revealed that the following variables appeared to be the strongest predictors of TMD pain: female gender, increasing age, sleep bruxism, biting on lips and/or cheeks, stress, and feeling sad. Regarding self-reported TMJ sounds, the multiple regression model revealed that female gender, increasing age, awake bruxism, and biting on lips and/or cheeks were the strongest predictors. *Conclusions.* TMDs are a common finding among Dutch adolescents. Except for the psychological factors that appeared to be associated with TMD pain only, pain-related TMDs and TMJ sounds shared similar biological risk indicators.

## 1. Introduction

Temporomandibular disorders (TMDs) is a collective term that embraces a variety of temporomandibular joint (TMJ) disorders, masticatory muscle disorders, headache disorders, and disorders affecting the associated structures [1, 2]. One way of classifying the different types of TMDs is by dividing them into two broad categories: (1) pain-related TMDs and (2) intra-articular TMDs [2]. Regarding the first category, pain can originate from the TMJs, but more frequently, the masticatory muscles are involved [3, 4]. Pain-related TMDs are usually transient over time and resolve without serious long-term effects [5, 6]. Intra-articular TMDs are expressed by biomechanical signs like TMJ sounds (clicking and crepitation), jaw locking, and limited mouth opening [2]. TMJ sounds are the most common expression of intra-articular TMDs [7] and usually occur without pain or jaw

movement limitation [8, 9]. Even though both categories of TMDs are primarily present among young and middle-aged adults [10, 11], studies performed on children and adolescents seem to indicate that the prevalence of pain-related forms of TMDs increases with increasing age in this age group [11–13]. Likewise, several studies on intra-articular TMDs report an increase of TMJ sounds in the young population [8, 14, 15].

It is generally believed that a variety of biological, psychological, and social factors may reduce the adaptive capacity of the masticatory system, thus resulting in TMDs [6, 16]. Since pain-related TMDs and TMJ sounds represent clusters of related disorders in the masticatory system [6], this would imply that overlap exists among the risk indicators for both categories of TMDs. For instance, it is commonly believed that teeth grinding or jaw clenching (i.e., bruxism) causes TMD pain due to overloading of the musculoskeletal structures [17]. At the same time, bruxism-induced overloading of the TMJs that exceeds the normal adaptive capacity might result in more TMJ sounds due to degenerative changes of the anatomical structures, or a tendency of the disc to be dislodged off the condyle [18, 19]. Surprisingly, many risk assessment studies on TMDs in the young population focused on one category of TMDs only (e.g., [8, 13, 20]), whereas in others, the various signs and symptoms of TMDs were merged into one overall TMD diagnosis (e.g., [21–23]). As it is, however, generally agreed that TMDs represent a nonspecific umbrella term, it is essential to differentiate pain-related TMDs from intra-articular TMDs. The aims of the present study, therefore, were (1) to assess the prevalence rates of self-reported pain-related TMDs and TMJ sounds in a large group of adolescents aged between 12 and 18 years, (2) to determine their associations with biological, psychological, and social risk indicators, and (3) to determine if the same risk indicators are related to both categories of TMDs.

## 2. Materials and Methods

*2.1. Data Collection.* This investigation was designed as a cross-sectional, population-based study. During three subsequent semesters, participants were drawn from among adolescents attending nine Dutch secondary schools that were willing to participate in this investigation. Because of time demand or other priorities at that time, 23 schools declined participation. All approached schools were dispersed over the southern and western parts of Netherlands and were situated in urban areas. Prior to the data collection, the parents/legal representatives received an information letter about the study. The children and/or the parents/legal representatives had the right to refuse participation.

On the day of data collection, a questionnaire was handed over to the schools' pupils and collected several minutes later, before the lessons started. This questionnaire contained 17 items that covered demographic items, sleep and awake bruxism, signs and symptoms of TMDs, and psychosocial and behavioural factors [24]. Most questions were derived from already existing questionnaires, like the Dutch translation of the Research Diagnostic Criteria for Temporomandibular Disorders (RDC/TMD) [25] and an oral habits questionnaire [26]. During the time the questionnaires were completed, the pupils were supervised by the class teacher and the investigators to ensure that the questionnaires were completed individually. Due to this approach, the participation rate was 100%. The institutional review board of the Academic Centre for Dentistry Amsterdam (ACTA) and the school boards of the participating schools approved the data collection procedures. Prior to the investigation, the feasibility of the research process was field-tested in a pilot study. In addition, the test-retest reliability of the employed questionnaire was assessed, yielding fair-to-good to excellent reliability scores. For detailed information about the data collection methods, see van Selms et al. [24].

*2.2. Outcome Variables*
   (i) Orofacial pain, indicative of TMD pain, was assessed by means of the following question: "Have you had

pain in the face, jaw, temple, in front of the ear or in the ear?" (no, yes). The question referred to the presence of pain within the last month.

   (ii) The presence of TMJ sounds was assessed using the question "Does your jaw make a clicking or popping sound when you open or close your mouth, or while chewing?" (no, yes). The question referred to the presence of TMJ sounds within the last month.

Since no clinical diagnoses were established in this study, the term "pain-related TMDs" has to be interpreted as "pains indicative of TMD pain" and "TMJ sounds" as "self-perceived TMJ sounds."

*2.3. Independent Variables*

*2.3.1. Biological Items*
   (i) Age (years) and sex (0, "male"; 1, "female").

   (ii) The presence of sleep bruxism was assessed using the question "Have you been told, or did you notice yourself, that you grind your teeth or clench your jaws when you are asleep?" The presence of awake bruxism was assessed using the question "Do you grind your teeth or clench your jaws during the day?" These questions referred to the last month, and the pupils could choose between no, yes, or unknown. Other oral activities that may be stressful to the masticatory system were asked by the following four questions: Do you chew on chewing gum? Do you bite your nails? Do you bite on pens/pencils? Do you bite your lips/cheeks? Again, these questions referred to the last month, and the answer possibilities were no, occasionally, regularly, often, and very often.

   (iii) The following exogenous aspects were assessed: "Do you smoke cigarettes?" and "Do you drink alcohol?" (both questions: no, occasionally, regularly, often, and very often).

*2.3.2. Psychological Items*
   (i) An impression of the psychological status was assessed by means of the following two questions "Are you stressed?" and "Are you feeling sad?" (both questions referred to the last month: no, occasionally, regularly, often, and very often).

*2.3.3. Social Items*
   (i) Ethnic background was classified following the method of Statistics Netherlands (CBS), using the country of birth from both parents. This procedure resulted in a classification into two subgroups, namely, native Dutch (i.e., both parents were born in Netherlands, regardless of the country of birth of the subject; coded "0") and nonnative Dutch (i.e., all other subjects; coded "1").

   (ii) Educational level was characterized by the type of the secondary educational system that was followed. Depending on their abilities, Dutch children around the age of 12 can choose for either vmbo, vmbo/havo, havo, havo/vwo, or vwo. The vmbo diploma gives access to advanced vocational education, the havo diploma to polytechnic education, and the vwo diploma to university education. The 5-point Likert scale item educational level was recoded into a dichotomous variable (vwo (1) versus the other levels (0)).

*2.4. Data Analysis.* Descriptive statistics included frequency distributions of each of the independent variables. In order to determine the prevalence rates of TMD pain and TMJ sounds, the prevalence data were stratified by gender and age and ratios were calculated. The chi-square test was performed to test the association between TMD pain and TMJ sounds as depicted in a $2 \times 2$ contingency table. To determine the association between the outcome variables and each of the independent variables, hierarchical logistic regression analyses were performed. First, single regression analyses were executed to determine the associations between each of the various predictors and the outcome variable. Regarding the ordinal variables, initial analyses were based on the full range of the 5-point Likert response options, and linearity of their effect on the presence of TMD pain was checked by analysis of dummy variables. When the regression coefficients of the dummy variables consistently increased or decreased, linearity was considered present. In case of a nonlinear association, the variable was dichotomized. Second, independent variables that showed at least a moderate association with the outcome measure were entered in a multiple regression model. Due to the fact that the large sample size may impact the corresponding $P$ values, a more conservative level of significance was chosen (i.e., $P$ value $< 0.05$ instead of $P$ value $< 0.1$). Subsequently, the variables with the weakest association with the outcome variable were removed from the multiple regression model. This was repeated in a backward stepwise manner until all variables that were retained in the model showed a $P$ value $< 0.01$; for each removed independent variable, the P-to-Exit is reported. Of the independent variables included in the final model, the odds ratios and their confidence intervals are reported. All analyses were conducted using the IBM SPSS Statistics 24 software package (IBM Corp., Armonk, NY). The data in the multiple regression model were checked for multicollinearity, using a tolerance value $< 0.10$ and a variance inflation factor $> 10$.

# 3. Results

Initially, a total of 4,285 pupils, with ages ranging from 10 to 22 years, completed the questionnaire. Since the present study focuses on TMD pain during adolescence, the data of pupils under twelve years (children) and above eighteen years (adults) were excluded ($n = 42$; $<1\%$ of the total number). An additional eyeball verification of the paper questionnaires was performed in order to check the face validity of the data. In case a pupil deliberately had noted only extremes on all single items, this questionnaire was removed from further analysis ($n = 8$). Therefore, the final

TABLE 1: Descriptive statistics of the predictor variables.

| Independent variable | |
| --- | --- |
| Age (years) | 14.5 ($\pm 1.6$) |
| Gender | |
| Male | 1,974 (50.1%) |
| Female | 1,966 (49.9%) |
| Sleep bruxism | |
| No | 2,874 (82.0%) |
| Yes | 633 (18.0%) |
| Awake bruxism | |
| No | 3,334 (90.0%) |
| Yes | 372 (10.0%) |
| Chewing gum | |
| No | 261 (6.2%) |
| Yes | 3,943 (93.8%) |
| Biting nails | |
| No | 2,105 (50.0%) |
| Yes | 2,104 (50.0%) |
| Biting pens and pencils | |
| No | 2,397 (56.9%) |
| Yes | 1,819 (43.1%) |
| Biting lips and/or cheeks | |
| No | 1,793 (42.6%) |
| Yes | 2,414 (57.4%) |
| Smoking cigarettes | |
| No | 3,658 (86.7%) |
| Yes | 559 (13.3%) |
| Alcohol consumption | |
| No | 2,166 (51.4%) |
| Yes | 2,046 (48.6%) |
| Being stressed | |
| No | 1,680 (39.9%) |
| Yes | 2,534 (60.1%) |
| Feeling sad | |
| No | 2,183 (51.8%) |
| Yes | 2,030 (48.2%) |
| School type | |
| Lower levels | 2,386 (56.3%) |
| Highest level | 1,849 (43.7%) |
| Ethnic background | |
| Native Dutch | 3,368 (82.0%) |
| Nonnative Dutch | 740 (18.0%) |

The dichotomized categorical variables are presented as absolute numbers (ratio); age is presented as mean value ($\pm$standard deviation).

sample consisted of 4,235 adolescents with a mean age of 14.5 ($\pm 1.6$) years (Table 1). Of the 3,940 adolescents who completed the question about gender, 1,966 (49.9%) were girls. In addition, 82.0% of the adolescents were classified as native Dutch, and 43.7% of the pupils followed the highest educational level (vwo).

Of the 3,935 adolescents who completed the questions about gender and TMDs, the overall prevalence of pain-related TMDs was 21.6% (26.1% for girls and 17.6% for boys). The overall prevalence of TMJ sounds was 15.5% ($n = 3,920$; 19.3% for girls and 11.7% for boys). The prevalence rates of both TMD pain and TMJ sounds, stratified by age and gender, revealed that girls had higher rates at all ages studied and that the prevalence tended to increase with age for both genders (Figure 1). TMD pain and TMJ sounds appeared to be highly associated ($\chi^2(1) = 176.6$; $P < 0.001$).

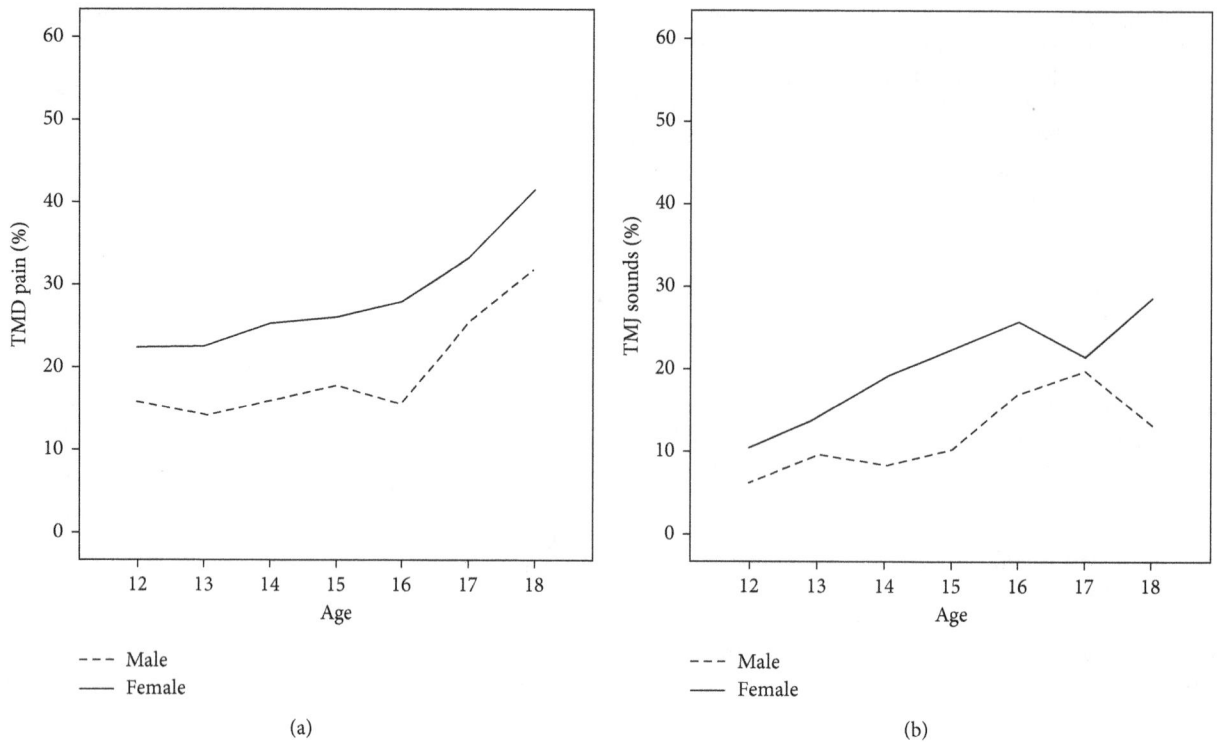

FIGURE 1: Age- and gender-specific prevalence of TMD pain (a) and TMJ sounds (b) among Dutch adolescents.

TABLE 2: Single and multiple logistic regression models for the prediction of TMD pain among Dutch adolescents.

| | | Single regression | | | P-to-Exit | Multiple regression ($n = 3,131$) | | |
| --- | --- | --- | --- | --- | --- | --- | --- | --- |
| | $n$ | $P$ value | OR | 95% CI | | $P$ value | OR | 95% CI |
| Biological items | | | | | | | | |
| Female gender | 1,964 | <0.001 | 1.66 | 1.42–1.94 | | 0.008 | 1.29 | 1.07–1.55 |
| Age (years) | 4,106 | <0.001 | 1.12 | 1.06–1.17 | | <0.001 | 1.11 | 1.05–1.17 |
| Smoking cigarettes (positive) | 559 | <0.001 | 1.60 | 1.31–1.95 | 0.467 | — | — | — |
| Drinking alcohol (positive) | 2,044 | <0.001 | 1.49 | 1.29–1.73 | 0.097 | — | — | — |
| Sleep bruxism (positive) | 631 | <0.001 | 1.76 | 1.45–2.14 | | <0.001 | 1.60 | 1.29–1.98 |
| Awake bruxism (positive) | 372 | <0.001 | 1.93 | 1.53–2.44 | 0.262 | — | — | — |
| Chewing gum (positive) | 3,938 | n.s. | 1.00 | 0.74–1.36 | | | | |
| Biting nails (positive) | 2,100 | n.s. | 0.95 | 0.82–1.10 | | | | |
| Biting pencils (positive) | 1,816 | <0.001 | 1.34 | 1.16–1.55 | 0.435 | — | — | — |
| Biting lips and/or cheeks (positive) | 2,409 | <0.001 | 1.69 | 1.45–1.97 | | 0.003 | 1.33 | 1.10–1.61 |
| Psychological items | | | | | | | | |
| Being stressed (positive) | 1,679 | <0.001 | 2.33 | 1.97–2.74 | | <0.001 | 1.60 | 1.28–1.99 |
| Feeling sad (positive) | 2,025 | <0.001 | 2.14 | 1.84–2.48 | | <0.001 | 1.55 | 1.27–1.88 |
| Social items | | | | | | | | |
| Non-Dutch ethnicity | 738 | n.s. | 0.97 | 0.80–1.18 | | | | |
| Highest educational level | 1,848 | n.s. | 1.03 | 0.88–1.19 | | | | |

Associations are expressed as odds ratio (OR) and 95% confidence interval (CI). For each removed predictor variable, the P-to-Exit is reported; n.s. = not significant. Significance levels are 0.05 and 0.01, respectively.

In order to find out which biological, psychological, or social factors had the strongest association with the presence of pain-related TMDs, logistic regression analyses were performed. In the first step, all variables were entered consecutively in a single regression model in order to determine their unadjusted association with the TMD pain. Regarding the included 5-point ordinal variables, inspection of the regression coefficients of the dummy variables revealed that perfect linearity of their effect on the presence of TMD pain was present only for the predictor "biting lips and/or cheeks." All ordinal variables were therefore dichotomized (no = 0; all other categories = 1). Table 2 shows the results of the single and multiple regression models. Except for the biological items gum chewing and nail biting and the social items ethnic background and educational level, all variables had a significant association with TMD pain in the single regression model. According to the multiple regression model, the following variables appeared

TABLE 3: Single and multiple logistic regression models for the prediction of TMJ sounds among Dutch adolescents.

| | Single regression | | | | P-to-Exit | Multiple regression ($n = 3,337$) | | |
|---|---|---|---|---|---|---|---|---|
| | $n$ | P value | OR | 95% CI | | P value | OR | 95% CI |
| Biological items | | | | | | | | |
| Female gender | 1,959 | <0.001 | 1.81 | 1.51–2.16 | | <0.001 | 1.77 | 1.45–2.16 |
| Age (years) | 4,090 | <0.001 | 1.19 | 1.13–1.26 | | <0.001 | 1.21 | 1.14–1.29 |
| Smoking cigarettes (positive) | 557 | <0.001 | 1.55 | 1.23–1.94 | 0.156 | — | — | — |
| Drinking alcohol (positive) | 2,040 | <0.001 | 1.53 | 1.29–1.82 | 0.406 | — | — | — |
| Sleep bruxism (positive) | 633 | <0.001 | 1.62 | 1.30–2.02 | 0.045 | — | — | — |
| Awake bruxism (positive) | 369 | <0.001 | 1.98 | 1.53–2.56 | 0.262 | <0.001 | 1.79 | 1.36–2.36 |
| Chewing gum (positive) | 3,922 | 0.046 | 1.50 | 1.01–2.22 | 0.011 | — | — | — |
| Biting nails (positive) | 2,093 | n.s. | 1.14 | 0.96–1.34 | | | | |
| Biting pencils (positive) | 1,811 | n.s. | 1.34 | 0.96–1.35 | 0.435 | — | — | — |
| Biting lips and/or cheeks (positive) | 2,406 | <0.001 | 1.66 | 1.39–1.98 | | <0.001 | 1.46 | 1.19–1.80 |
| Psychological items | | | | | | | | |
| Being stressed (positive) | 1,668 | <0.001 | 1.81 | 1.50–2.17 | 0.042 | — | — | — |
| Feeling sad (positive) | 2,019 | 0.001 | 1.31 | 1.12–1.56 | 0.123 | — | — | — |
| Social items | | | | | | | | |
| Non-Dutch ethnicity | 732 | n.s. | 0.81 | 0.64–1.02 | | | | |
| Highest educational level | 1,846 | n.s. | 0.86 | 0.73–1.02 | | | | |

Associations are expressed as odds ratio (OR) and 95% confidence interval (CI). For each removed predictor variable, the P-to-Exit is reported; n.s. = not significant. Significance levels are 0.05 and 0.01, respectively.

to be the strongest predictors of TMD pain: female gender, increasing age, sleep bruxism, biting on lips and/or cheeks, stress, and feeling blue. There were no signs of multicollinearity among the predictor variables in the final model.

Table 3 shows the results of the regression analyses with the presence of self-reported TMJ sounds as an outcome variable. Again, most biological items were associated with joint sounds in the single regression model. In addition, feeling stressed and feeling sad had a significant association with TMJ sounds. The multiple regression model revealed that female gender, increasing age, awake bruxism, and biting on lips and/or cheeks were the strongest predictors of TMJ sounds.

## 4. Discussion

The present questionnaire study aimed to assess the prevalence rates of two categories of temporomandibular disorders (TMDs), namely, pain-related manifestations of TMDs and TMJ sounds, in a large group of Dutch adolescents aged between 12 and 18 years. In addition, we examined which biological, psychological, or social risk indicators were associated with them and if both categories of TMDs yielded similar risk indicators. The results demonstrated that self-reported TMD pain is relatively common among 12- to 18-year-old Dutch adolescents, with an overall prevalence of about 20%. Besides the fact that the occurrence of TMD pain was highly associated with that of TMJ sounds, this pain was correlated to female gender, increasing age, reports of sleep bruxism, biting on lips and/or cheeks, stress, and feeling sad. The overall prevalence of TMJ sounds was about 15%; female gender, increasing age, awake bruxism, and biting on lips and/or cheeks were the best predictors. Except for the psychological factors that appeared to be associated with TMD pain only, pain-related TMDs and TMJ sounds shared similar biological risk indicators.

*4.1. Prevalence of TMD Pain.* It is generally acknowledged that depending on the study, the prevalence of TMD pain in children and adolescents varies widely [27]. In 2007, a large-scale study was published that focused on TMD pain among adolescents aged 12–19 years [13]. Of the 28,899 adolescents that participated, 4.2% reported TMD pain during their annual routine examination in Public Dental Service (PDS) clinics. In another Swedish study, seven percent of the 862 adolescents from a public dental clinic were diagnosed with TMD pain [28]. This rate was also found in a recent study on Norwegian adolescents [29]. The most likely explanations for the fact that the present study yielded a higher prevalence rate (namely, 21.6%) are differences in diagnostic criteria and the method of data collection. In the present study, orofacial pain had to be present within the last month, whereas in the study by Nilsson, a time span of one week was used. In the studies by List et al. and Ostensjo et al., a clinical pain diagnosis according to the Research Diagnostic Criteria for Temporomandibular Disorders (RDC/TMD) was set, which may have resulted in a lower prevalence. On the other hand, when these clinical criteria were applied in two Brazilian studies performed on young adolescents, it was concluded that about 25% of the schoolchildren could be diagnosed with painful TMDs [20, 30]. As long as no uniform diagnostic criteria are available to obtain a reliable diagnosis of TMDs in the young population, studies on this topic will continue to present a multitude of different results. Future studies must therefore aim to develop a standardized assessment tool for the young population. Unfortunately, the recently published Diagnostic Criteria for TMD (DC/TMD) [2] have not yet been validated for usage among children and adolescents.

*4.2. Risk Indicators for Pain-Related TMDs.* Regarding the role of biological risk indicators on pain-related forms of TMDs, we demonstrated that the prevalence of TMD pain increases with increasing age in the period of adolescence. This is in line with several other studies (e.g., [11, 13, 31, 32]) and coincides with the suggestion that pubertal development increases the probability of self-reported TMD pain [12, 31]. Moreover, girls had higher rates of TMD pain at all ages studied compared to boys (namely, 26.1% and 17.6%, resp.), which corroborates with most studies on this topic (e.g., [12, 13, 28, 33]). Even though it is likely that sex differences exist in basic pain mechanisms and in associated psychosocial factors, the mechanisms underlying this difference are still not well understood [34]. Another biological factor that is frequently suggested to be associated with TMD pain in adolescents is overloading of the masticatory system due to oral habits (e.g., [20, 35]). As a result, it was not surprising that the final regression model included sleep bruxism and the adverse oral habit "biting on lips and/or cheeks."

Based on the present findings, it appeared that the two included psychological factors (namely, being stressed and feeling sad) contributed significantly to the presence of TMD pain among adolescents. Again, this is not surprising as both factors are frequently mentioned in relation to this pain (e.g., [31, 36–38]). The same neurotransmitters, especially serotonin and norepinephrine, are involved in both pain and mood regulation [39]. An increase of cortisol secretion in people with high psychological load has also been shown to be related with chronic pain development [40]. However, caution has to be paid to this assumption, as causal links have not been clearly defined. Do these factors increase the risk of TMD pain or are they the result of this pain because such persons have become more stressed and less cheerful by their pain condition?

Finally, the social factors ethnic background and educational level were not associated with the presence of TMD pain. The negative findings in this study might show that differences in ethnicity and educational level in Dutch adolescents do not necessarily represent different social environments in relation to the report of pain. Out of a vast range of social factors that have been considered to influence an individual's pain behaviour, parent emotions, behaviours, and health seem to play an important role in a child's pain experience [41]. This topic might be an interesting avenue for future research.

*4.3. Prevalence of TMJ Sounds.* The overall prevalence of self-reported TMJ sounds was 15.5%, which is in line with approximately 14% as reported in a recent meta-analysis on the prevalence of TMJ sounds (click or crepitation) in children and adolescents [42]. Unfortunately, the authors of that systematic review did not differentiate between boys and girls. The gender-specific prevalence rates that we found in the present study (19.3% for girls and 11.7% for boys) seem to corroborate with those presented in earlier studies [12, 43]. On the other hand, even though a lower overall prevalence was found in a study of Feteih (8.7% of the participants reported joint sounds), they still observed a higher prevalence in girls [44]. It is generally acknowledged that differences in methodology lead to considerable variation in prevalence of TMJ sounds [42]. However, it can still

be concluded that TMJ sounds are a commonly reported sign of TMDs in the adolescent population.

*4.4. Risk Indicators for TMJ Sounds.* As for TMD pain, four biological factors appeared to be associated with TMJ sounds. Consistent with other studies on the young population, the prevalence of TMJ sounds increased considerably with age [14, 15, 45], especially during adolescence. Until now, there is no explanation for this trend. It has been suggested that increasing age leads to a temporary space insufficiency within the TMJ [14]. During the period of adolescence, the articular eminence gets its more prominent anatomical shape [46], which can cause a lack of space within the TMJ complex [14]. As a result, this insufficient space forces the disc to be pushed from its normal position on top of the condyle to the anterior or anterolateral side during the closing movement of the mouth. The disc only resumes its normal position during the opening movement, during which TMJ sounds are produced [47, 48]. As for TMD pain, female gender was found to be associated with TMJ sounds. However, conflicting evidence exists regarding this association [14, 15, 49]. As the current study utilized self-reported data, the finding that prevalence rates are higher among girls might also be due to the fact that female adolescents report physical symptoms more often than their male counterparts [50–52]. Finally, the associations found in this study between daytime clenching and/or grinding and TMJ sounds and between biting on lips and/or cheeks and TMJ sounds corroborate with other studies [53–55]. A possible explanation for these associations is that adverse oral activities cause compression of the articular disc as was shown in a finite element model study [56]. The occurring stresses may facilitate the disc to be dislodged off the head of the condyle to the anterior or anterolateral side, thus creating clicking sounds upon condyle translation movements [18, 47].

*4.5. Methodology.* This study has several limitations. First of all, pain-related TMDs and TMJ sounds were obtained by a questionnaire with no objective confirmation of signs and symptoms, thus being at risk of recall bias. However, high validity can exist between self-reported pain questions and the outcome of a clinical examination in adolescents [13]. Likewise, in a longitudinal study on signs and symptoms of TMDs in Finnish adolescents by Könönen and Nystrom, reported and clinically examined TMJ clicking sounds correlated significantly with each other [45]. Second, for an indication of TMJ sounds, all pupils had to note if they experienced any clicking or popping sound when opening or closing the mouth. The presence of crepitation was, however, not asked for. Even though crepitation has a much lower occurrence in the adolescent population, if present at all [15, 42], other results might have been obtained in case this type of TMJ sound was included. Third, the present study was conducted in an adolescent population composed of nonpatients. However, to fulfill the objective of determining associations with biological, psychological, and social risk indicators, different results might have been obtained in case a group of symptomatic patients was included. Therefore, further studies should be performed with representative samples of patients with TMD pain and TMJ sounds as well. The fourth aspect that should be mentioned is that, with increasing age, larger cognitive capacity, and better recall, older adolescents might remember and therefore report any physical symptoms better than younger ones [50]. This might have influenced the obtained results with respect to prevalence and associations.

## 5. Conclusions

This study indicates that both pain-related manifestations of TMDs and TMJ sounds are a common finding in the adolescent population. Both categories share similar biological risk indicators, whereas psychological factors were only associated with pain-related TMDs.

## Acknowledgments

The authors would like to thank the participating schools for their willingness to invest time and effort in this study. The authors would especially like to acknowledge the following dental students, bachelor students at the time, for their contributions: M. D. Kwehandjaja, R. N. van Minnen, F. K. M. ten Berge, E. M. de Bakker, L. M. M. Kes, I. A. M. Veerman, M. Hessling, and F. Peereboom. The study was partly funded by Trisakti University and Gesere Foundation, a private foundation to support young scientists from North Sumatra, Indonesia.

## References

[1] C. C. Peck, J. P. Goulet, F. Lobbezoo et al., "Expanding the taxonomy of the diagnostic criteria for temporomandibular disorders," *Journal of Oral Rehabilitation*, vol. 41, no. 1, pp. 2–23, 2014.

[2] E. Schiffman, R. Ohrbach, E. Truelove et al., "Diagnostic criteria for temporomandibular disorders (DC/TMD) for clinical and research applications: recommendations of the international RDC/TMD consortium network and orofacial pain special interest group," *Journal of Oral and Facial Pain and Headache*, vol. 28, no. 1, pp. 6–27, 2014.

[3] J. P. Okeson and R. de Leeuw, "Differential diagnosis of temporomandibular disorders and other orofacial pain disorders," *Dental Clinics of North America*, vol. 55, no. 1, pp. 105–120, 2011.

[4] J. M. Zakrzewska, "Differential diagnosis of facial pain and guidelines for management," *British Journal of Anaesthesia*, vol. 111, no. 1, pp. 95–104, 2013.

[5] S. F. Dworkin and D. L. Massoth, "Temporomandibular disorders and chronic pain: disease or illness?," *Journal of Prosthetic Dentistry*, vol. 72, no. 1, pp. 29–38, 1994.

[6] R. de Leeuw and G. D. Klasser, "Diagnosis and management of TMDs," in *Orofacial Pain: Guidelines for Assessment, Di-agnosis, and Management*, R. de Leeuw, Ed., pp. 127–186, Quintessence Publishing Co., Chicago, IL, USA, 2013.

[7] W. B. Farrar and W. L. MacCarty, *Diseases of the TMJ in a Clinical Outline of Temporomandibular Joint Diagnosis and Treatment*, Normandie Study Group for TMJ Dysfunction, Montgomery, AL, USA, 1982.

[8] M. Könönen, A. Waltimo, and M. Nystrom, "Does clicking in adolescence lead to painful temporomandibular joint locking?," *The Lancet*, vol. 347, no. 9008, pp. 1080-1081, 1996.

[9] C. S. Greene and D. M. Laskin, "Long-term status of TMJ clicking in patients with myofascial pain and dysfunction," *Journal of the American Dental Association*, vol. 117, no. 3, pp. 461–465, 1988.

[10] L. LeResche, "Epidemiology of temporomandibular disorders: implications for the investigation of etiologic factors," *Critical Reviews in Oral Biology & Medicine*, vol. 8, no. 3, pp. 291–305, 1997.

[11] A. A. Köhler, A. N. Helkimo, T. Magnusson, and A. Hugoson, "Prevalence of symptoms and signs indicative of temporomandibular disorders in children and adolescents. A cross-sectional epidemiological investigation covering two decades," *European Archives of Paediatric Dentistry*, vol. 10, no. 1, pp. 16–25, 2009.

[12] C. Hirsch, J. Hoffmann, and J. C. Turp, "Are temporomandibular disorder symptoms and diagnoses associated with pubertal development in adolescents? An epidemiological study," *Journal of Orofacial Orthopedics*, vol. 73, no. 1, pp. 6–8, 2012.

[13] I. M. Nilsson, "Reliability, validity, incidence and impact of temporomandibular pain disorders in adolescents," *Swedish Dental Journal*, vol. 183, pp. 7–86, 2007.

[14] J. J. Huddleston Slater, F. Lobbezoo, N. C. Onland-Moret, and M. Naeije, "Anterior disc displacement with reduction and symptomatic hypermobility in the human temporomandibular joint: prevalence rates and risk factors in children and teenagers," *Journal of Orofacial Pain*, vol. 21, no. 1, pp. 55–62, 2007.

[15] A. Wänman and G. Agerberg, "Temporomandibular joint sounds in adolescents: a longitudinal study," *Oral Surgery, Oral Medicine, Oral Pathology*, vol. 69, no. 1, pp. 2–9, 1990.

[16] T. I. Suvinen, P. C. Reade, P. Kemppainen, M. Kononen, and S. F. Dworkin, "Review of aetiological concepts of temporomandibular pain disorders: towards a biopsychosocial model for integration of physical disorder factors with psychological and psychosocial illness impact factors," *European Journal of Pain*, vol. 9, no. 6, pp. 613–633, 2005.

[17] P. Svensson and T. Graven-Nielsen, "Craniofacial muscle pain: review of mechanisms and clinical manifestations," *Journal of Orofacial Pain*, vol. 15, no. 2, pp. 117–145, 2001.

[18] M. Naeije, A. H. Te Veldhuis, E. C. Te Veldhuis, C. M. Visscher, and F. Lobbezoo, "Disc displacement within the human temporomandibular joint: a systematic review of a 'noisy annoyance'," *Journal of Oral Rehabilitation*, vol. 40, no. 2, pp. 139–158, 2013.

[19] E. Tanaka, M. S. Detamore, and L. G. Mercuri, "Degenerative disorders of the temporomandibular joint: etiology, diagnosis, and treatment," *Journal of Dental Research*, vol. 87, no. 4, pp. 296–307, 2008.

[20] G. Fernandes, M. K. van Selms, D. A. Goncalves, F. Lobbezoo, and C. M. Camparis, "Factors associated with temporomandibular disorders pain in adolescents," *Journal of Oral Rehabilitation*, vol. 42, no. 2, pp. 113–119, 2015.

[21] L. J. Pereira, T. Pereira-Cenci, S. M. Pereira et al., "Psychological factors and the incidence of temporomandibular disorders in early adolescence," *Brazilian Oral Research*, vol. 23, no. 2, pp. 155–160, 2009.

[22] U. Sermet Elbay, H. Demirturk Kocasarac, M. Elbay, C. Kaya, C. Ugurluel, and C. Baydemir, "Temporomandibular disorders and oral parafunction in children living with their parents and children living in institutional protective care: a comparative study," *International Dental Journal*, vol. 67, no. 1, pp. 20–28, 2017.

[23] H. Karibe, K. Shimazu, A. Okamoto, T. Kawakami, Y. Kato, and S. Warita-Naoi, "Prevalence and association of self-reported anxiety, pain, and oral parafunctional habits with temporomandibular disorders in Japanese children and adolescents: a cross-sectional survey," *BMC Oral Health*, vol. 15, no. 1, p. 8, 2015.

[24] M. K. van Selms, C. M. Visscher, M. Naeije, and F. Lobbezoo, "Bruxism and associated factors among Dutch adolescents," *Community Dentistry and Oral Epidemiology*, vol. 41, no. 4, pp. 353–363, 2013.

[25] F. Lobbezoo, M. K. van Selms, M. T. John et al., "Use of the Research Diagnostic Criteria for Temporomandibular Disorders for multinational research: translation efforts and reliability assessments in the Netherlands," *Journal of Orofacial Pain*, vol. 19, no. 4, pp. 301–308, 2005.

[26] M. J. van der Meulen, F. Lobbezoo, I. H. Aartman, and M. Naeije, "Self-reported oral parafunctions and pain intensity in temporomandibular disorder patients," *Journal of Orofacial Pain*, vol. 20, no. 1, pp. 31–35, 2006.

[27] P. Toscano and P. Defabianis, "Clinical evaluation of temporomandibular disorders in children and adolescents: a review of the literature," *European Journal of Paediatric Dentistry*, vol. 10, no. 4, pp. 188–192, 2009.

[28] T. List, K. Wahlund, B. Wenneberg, and S. F. Dworkin, "TMD in children and adolescents: prevalence of pain, gender differences, and perceived treatment need," *Journal of Orofacial Pain*, vol. 13, no. 1, pp. 9–20, 1999.

[29] V. Ostensjo, K. Moen, T. Storesund, and A. Rosen, "Prevalence of painful temporomandibular disorders and correlation to lifestyle factors among adolescents in Norway," *Pain Research and Management*, vol. 2017, Article ID 2164825, 10 pages, 2017.

[30] A. L. Franco-Micheloni, G. Fernandes, D. A. de Godoi Goncalves, and C. M. Camparis, "Temporomandibular disorders in a young adolescent Brazilian population: epidemiologic characterization and associated factors," *Journal of Oral & Facial Pain and Headache*, vol. 29, no. 3, pp. 242–249, 2015.

[31] L. LeResche, L. A. Mancl, M. T. Drangsholt, K. Saunders, and M. V. Korff, "Relationship of pain and symptoms to pubertal development in adolescents," *Pain*, vol. 118, no. 1, pp. 201–209, 2005.

[32] T. Magnusson, I. Egermarki, and G. E. Carlsson, "A prospective investigation over two decades on signs and symptoms of temporomandibular disorders and associated variables. A final summary," *Acta Odontologica Scandinavica*, vol. 63, no. 2, pp. 99–109, 2005.

[33] L. J. Pereira, T. Pereira-Cenci, A. A. Del Bel Cury et al., "Risk indicators of temporomandibular disorder incidences in early adolescence," *Pediatric Dentistry*, vol. 32, no. 4, pp. 324–328, 2010.

[34] L. Leresche, "Defining gender disparities in pain management," *Clinical Orthopaedics and Related Research*, vol. 469, no. 7, pp. 1871–1877, 2011.

[35] E. Winocur, D. Littner, I. Adams, and A. Gavish, "Oral habits and their association with signs and symptoms of temporomandibular disorders in adolescents: a gender comparison," *Oral Surgery, Oral Medicine, Oral Pathology, Oral Radiology, and Endodontology*, vol. 102, no. 4, pp. 482–487, 2006.

[36] T. List, K. Wahlund, and B. Larsson, "Psychosocial functioning and dental factors in adolescents with temporomandibular disorders: a case-control study," *Journal of Orofacial Pain*, vol. 15, no. 3, pp. 218–227, 2001.

[37] K. Wahlund, "Temporomandibular disorders in adolescents. Epidemiological and methodological studies and a randomized controlled trial," *Swedish Dental Journal*, vol. 164, pp. 2–64, 2003.

[38] L. R. Bonjardim, M. B. Gaviao, L. J. Pereira, and P. M. Castelo, "Anxiety and depression in adolescents and their relationship with signs and symptoms of temporomandibular disorders," *International Journal of Prosthodontics*, vol. 18, no. 4, pp. 347–352, 2005.

[39] M. H. Trivedi, "The link between depression and physical symptoms," *Primary Care Companion to The Journal of Clinical Psychiatry*, vol. 6, no. 1, pp. 12–16, 2004.

[40] R. J. Gatchel, Y. B. Peng, M. L. Peters, P. N. Fuchs, and D. C. Turk, "The biopsychosocial approach to chronic pain: scientific advances and future directions," *Psychological Bulletin*, vol. 133, no. 4, pp. 581–624, 2007.

[41] T. M. Palermo, C. R. Valrie, and C. W. Karlson, "Family and parent influences on pediatric chronic pain: a developmental perspective," *American Psychologist*, vol. 69, no. 2, pp. 142–152, 2014.

[42] C. G. da Silva, C. Pacheco-Pereira, A. L. Porporatti et al., "Prevalence of clinical signs of intra-articular temporomandibular disorders in children and adolescents: a systematic review and meta-analysis," *Journal of the American Dental Association*, vol. 147, no. 1, pp. 10–18.e18, 2016.

[43] A. Michelotti, G. Iodice, M. Piergentili, M. Farella, and R. Martina, "Incidence of temporomandibular joint clicking in adolescents with and without unilateral posterior crossbite: a 10-year follow-up study," *Journal of Oral Rehabilitation*, vol. 43, no. 1, pp. 16–22, 2016.

[44] R. M. Feteih, "Signs and symptoms of temporomandibular disorders and oral parafunctions in urban Saudi Arabian adolescents: a research report," *Head & Face Medicine*, vol. 2, no. 1, p. 25, 2006.

[45] M. Kononen and M. Nystrom, "A longitudinal study of craniomandibular disorders in Finnish adolescents," *Journal of Orofacial Pain*, vol. 7, no. 4, pp. 329–336, 1993.

[46] J. M. Dibbets and G. E. Dijkman, "The postnatal development of the temporal part of the human temporomandibular joint. A quantitative study on skulls," *Annals of Anatomy*, vol. 179, no. 6, pp. 569–572, 1997.

[47] J. W. Osborn, "The disc of the human temporomandibular joint: design, function and failure," *Journal of Oral Rehabilitation*, vol. 12, no. 4, pp. 279–293, 1985.

[48] S. Kalaykova, F. Lobbezoo, and M. Naeije, "Effect of chewing upon disc reduction in the temporomandibular joint," *Journal of Orofacial Pain*, vol. 25, no. 1, pp. 49–55, 2011.

[49] M. L. Riolo, D. Brandt, and T. R. TenHave, "Associations between occlusal characteristics and signs and symptoms of TMJ dysfunction in children and young adults," *American Journal of Orthodontics and Dentofacial Orthopedics*, vol. 92, no. 6, pp. 467–477, 1987.

[50] M. Eminson, S. Benjamin, A. Shortall, T. Woods, and B. Faragher, "Physical symptoms and illness attitudes in adolescents: an epidemiological study," *Journal of Child Psychology and Psychiatry*, vol. 37, no. 5, pp. 519–528, 1996.

[51] S. W. Powers, D. K. Gilman, and A. D. Hershey, "Headache and psychological functioning in children and adolescents," *Headache: The Journal of Head and Face Pain*, vol. 46, no. 9, pp. 1404–1415, 2006.

[52] B. S. Larsson, "Somatic complaints and their relationship to depressive symptoms in Swedish adolescents," *Journal of Child Psychology and Psychiatry*, vol. 32, no. 5, pp. 821–832, 1991.

[53] A. M. Velly, M. Gornitsky, and P. Philippe, "A case-control study of temporomandibular disorders: symptomatic disc displacement," *Journal of Oral Rehabilitation*, vol. 29, no. 5, pp. 408–416, 2002.

[54] A. Michelotti, I. Cioffi, P. Festa, G. Scala, and M. Farella, "Oral parafunctions as risk factors for diagnostic TMD subgroups," *Journal of Oral Rehabilitation*, vol. 37, no. 3, pp. 157–162, 2010.

[55] A. Emodi-Perlman, F. Lobbezoo, A. Zar, P. Friedman Rubin, M. K. van Selms, and E. Winocur, "Self-reported bruxism and associated factors in Israeli adolescents," *Journal of Oral Rehabilitation*, vol. 43, no. 6, pp. 443–450, 2016.

[56] M. Hirose, E. Tanaka, M. Tanaka et al., "Three-dimensional finite-element model of the human temporomandibular joint disc during prolonged clenching," *European Journal of Oral Sciences*, vol. 114, no. 5, pp. 441–448, 2006.

# 13

# The Effect of Mulligan Mobilization Technique in Older Adults with Neck Pain: A Randomized Controlled, Double-Blind Study

Oznur Buyukturan ⓘ,[1] Buket Buyukturan,[1] Senem Sas,[2] Caner Karartı,[1] and İsmail Ceylan[1]

[1]School of Physical Therapy and Rehabilitation, Ahi Evran University, Kırşehir, Turkey
[2]Department of Physical Medicine and Rehabilitation, Ahi Evran University Training and Research Hospital, Kırşehir, Turkey

Correspondence should be addressed to Oznur Buyukturan; fzt_oznur@hotmail.com

Academic Editor: Fabio Antonaci

*Background.* The purpose of this study was to examine the effect of Mulligan mobilization technique (MMT) on pain, range of motion (ROM), functional level, kinesiophobia, depression, and quality of life (QoL) in older adults with neck pain (NP). *Methods.* Forty-two older adults with NP were included in the study, and they were randomly divided into two groups: traditional physiotherapy (TP) group and traditional physiotherapy-Mulligan mobilization (TPMM) group. Treatment program was scheduled for 10 sessions. Participants were assessed in terms of pain, ROM, functional level, kinesiophobia, depression, and QoL both pre- and posttreatment. *Results.* Pain, ROM, functional level, kinesiophobia, depression, and QoL improved in both groups following treatment ($p < 0.05$). When comparing effects of these two treatment programs, it was observed that the TPMM group had a better outcome ($p < 0.05$) in terms of ROM, kinesiophobia, depression, and QoL. *Conclusion.* In older adults with NP, MMT has been found to have significant effects on pain, ROM, functional level, kinesiophobia, depression, and QoL as long as it is performed by a specialist. "This trial is registered with NCT03507907".

## 1. Introduction

Neck pain (NP) is one of the common musculoskeletal problems. NP can be caused by the stress over the musculoskeletal system due to postural disorders and may also be associated with other causes such as intervertebral disc herniation, nerve compression, or fracture [1]. The prevalence of NP is reported to range from 43% to 66.7%, which increases along with aging [2]. In a study conducted by March et al., on individuals over 65 years of age, the prevalence of NP was found to be 38.7% [3].

The use of various methods of manual treatments such as exercise, mobilization, and manipulation is supported by recent reviews on conservative treatments for mechanical NP [4]. Mulligan is one of the mobilization techniques that can be applied in case of NP. Being an important treatment tool used by most of the manual physical therapists,

Mulligan mobilization techniques (MMTs) include several methods such as sustained natural epiphyseal glides (SNAGs) and natural epiphyseal glides that target the spine [5]. An immediate improvement in pain-free range of motion (ROM) in the involved joints is reposted as a result of applying this treatment approach [5, 6]. As a successful treatment approach for various orthopedics dysfunctions, a combination of the MMT concept along with several other methods of manual therapy has been suggested by the literature [7]. However, the application of the MMT for nonspecific NP in the older adults has not been investigated.

When the literature is examined, there is no randomized controlled study investigating the effect of the MMT on older adults with NP. This study aims to investigate the effect of Mulligan mobilization technique on pain, range of motion, functional level, kinesiophobia, fear of movement, depression, and quality of life in older adults with neck pain.

## 2. Material and Methods

*2.1. Study Design.* This study was designed as a randomized controlled, double-blinded study. Patients who agreed to participate in the study were divided into two groups—as the traditional physiotherapy (TP) group and traditional physiotherapy-Mulligan mobilization (TPMM) group—using a matched randomization method based on gender and age. Both the researchers performing the assessment (CK) and the treatment (OB) and the participants were blind about the groups. All assessments were made by the same investigator (CK) before and after treatment.

*2.2. Participants.* Individuals older than 65 years of age with NP, who were referred to the Physical Therapy and Rehabilitation Center of Ahi Evran University by a physiatrist (SS), were included in this study. Ongoing NP for at least 3 months having no neurological, rheumatological, or musculoskeletal problems and had not taken any analgesic medication for neck pain for the last 3 months were the inclusion criteria of the study. Exclusion criteria, however, were as follows: NP originating from various pathologies (tumor, rheumatoid arthritis, ankylosing spondylitis, fracture, dislocation, etc.), presence of cord compression, vertebrobasilar artery insufficiency, severe radiculopathy, osteoporosis or osteopenia ($t$ score $> -1$), long-term use of anticoagulant or corticosteroid drugs, and patients who had received any treatment for their NP. In accordance with the guidelines approved by the local ethical committee and the Declaration of Human Rights, Helsinki, written informed consent was obtained from all participants.

*2.3. Evaluation Methods*

*2.3.1. Demographic Data.* All patients were verbally inquired regarding their age, body mass index, and information about when the symptoms onset was. All these data were recorded.

*2.3.2. Pain.* The severity of pain at rest and during activity was assessed by visual analog scale (VAS). Participants were questioned about their average pain over the last 4 weeks. They were asked to mark the severity of their pain on a 10 cm long line, where 0 represented no pain and 10 stood for vicious pain [8]. The results were recorded in cm.

*2.3.3. Neck Disability Index (NDI).* This scale was used to evaluate how the participants' daily life was influenced by their NP. Total score of the scale ranges from 0 to 35, and higher scores indicate higher levels of disability [9].

*2.3.4. Tampa Scale of Kinesiophobia (TSK).* This scale was used to assess the patients' fear of pain or reinjury due to movement. It consists of 17 items and assesses various factors of fear/avoidance and injury/reinjury in several activities. Total score of the scale varies between 17 and 68, and higher scores represent higher levels of kinesiophobia [10].

*2.3.5. Range of Motion.* A universal goniometer was used to assess the ROM of the cervical vertebrae. Cervical flexion, extension, right and left lateral flexion, and right and left rotation movements were measured 3 times in an active manner while the patients were in a comfortable sitting position. The average value of the measurements was recorded as ROM [11]. The pain-free maximum degree of movement for each range was measured in degrees. This method has demonstrated good reliability [12].

*2.3.6. Beck Depression Inventory (BDI).* Participants' level of depression was assessed using BDI that consists of 21 categories with 4 options in each category. Each item has a score between 0 and 3, and total score varies from 0 to 63. Score ranges are interpreted as 0–9 points = minor depression, 10–16 points = mild depression, 17–29 points = moderate depression, and 30–63 points = severe depression [13].

*2.3.7. Short Form-36 (SF-36).* This form was used to assess the QoL of the participants. This questionnaire consisted of 36 questions that are categorized into 8 groups as follows: physical role functioning, emotional role functioning, bodily pain, energy, social role functioning, mental health, and general health perception. Each category is scored on a 0–100 range, and higher scores indicate better QoL [14].

*2.4. Treatment Programs.* Forty-two older adults who agreed to participate in the study were divided into two groups using a matched randomization method. All participants in both the TP group and the TPMM group were included in a treatment program for 10 sessions.

*2.4.1. Traditional Physiotherapy Group.* In this study, traditional physiotherapy includes heat modalities, electrotherapy (transcutaneous electrical nerve stimulation (TENS) and ultrasound therapy), and exercises. Patients were asked to lie down in prone, and a pillow was placed under their abdomen for relaxation. We used the hot pack to induce vasodilitation and reduce muscle spasm in this study. A hot pack wrapped in 4 layers of towel was used for 15 minutes to treat for relaxing muscle spasms and for improving soft tissue elasticity [15]. TENS is a simple noninvasive modality and commonly used in both acute and chronic neck pains. The mechanism of analgesia with TENS is described as the "gate control theory" of pain, which is characterized by the modulation of nociceptive input in the dorsal horn of the spinal cord, by peripheral electrical stimulation of large sensory afferent nerves. Alternatively, electrical stimulation of certain receptor sites in the dorsal horn of the spinal cord may release endorphins and produce analgesia that can be reversed by the naloxone. A 50 Hz conventional TENS with a pulse duration <150 microseconds was used in our study. TENS was applied to the painful area of the neck for 20 minutes [16]. Ultrasound therapy, which is used to heat deep tissues, is one of the most important physical treatment methods. Ultrasound increases local metabolism, circulation, regeneration, and extensibility of connective tissue with its assuming thermal and mechanical effects. Ultrasound device (Chattanooga, USA) was used in the study. Ultrasound's gel was applied circularly with a thickness of 2-3 mm. Then, ultrasound with a $4 \, cm^2$ probe was applied with 1 MHz frequency and $1.5 \, Wt/cm^2$, for 5 min [17]. Furthermore, massage and exercise were suggested to participants. Classic regional massage was performed on the cervical and thoracic regions. Participants were informed and educated about effective ways of performing their daily life activities. In the context of therapeutic exercises, the older adults were trained for ROM exercises (anterior, lateral, and rotational) and posture exercises (shoulder circumduction, scapular adduction, and pectoral stretching). These exercises were repeated 5 times within the treatment program and 10 times after the program.

*2.4.2. Traditional Physiotherapy-Mulligan Mobilization Group.* In this group, the MMT was applied in addition to the treatment program applied to the TP group. For two weeks, participants received SNAGs five days per week. According to the MMT, any minor positional fault at a joint can cause a limitation in its physiological movement. The first intervention of the MMT was the application of the natural apophyseal glides (NAGs) applied between C2 and C7. Patients were asked to sit and rest their back against a chair. The mobilization was reapplied by the oscillatory movements and was less than 6 repeats. SNAGs were a combination of mobilization and active movements for the vertebral column. Load-bearing positions were selected and performed at each spinal level. The technique was done without pain at the end of the joint movement [5]. With patients in a seated position, cervical SNAGs were applied with one thumb supported by the other that was placed—depending on the indication—on either the articular pillar or the spinous process of the upper vertebra of the functional spine unit. The therapist applied a passive intervertebral movement which was in a superoanterior direction along the facet plane. The therapist maintained this "glide" as the patient actively moved in any range of physiological movement and then sustained it at the end-range position for a few seconds. The release of the "glide" was when the patient returned to the starting position of the active movement [5]. For two weeks, this mobilization was repeated 6 times per session by a physiotherapist (OB) who holds a certificate in the MMT with 8 years of experience.

*2.5. Sample Size.* In accordance with the study by Ganesh et al., sample size was based on NDI scores in the patient with NP [4]. Their study was designed to investigate the effects of MMT on NP. Large effect size was calculated for this study. Therefore, with a statistically significant level of 5% ($p = 0.05$), a statistical power of 80%, an effect size of 0.8, and a minimum of 21 participants were required per group. Allowing for a 10% dropout rate, 47 subjects were recruited into the study.

*2.6. Statistical Analysis.* Statistical analyzes of the study were conducted using the "Statistical Package for Social Sciences" (SPSS) Version 18.0 (SPSS Inc. Chicago, IL, USA). Normal distribution of the data was examined using the "Shapiro–Wilk test." All outcome analyses were conducted according to the intention-to-treat principle. The "Wilcoxon paired two sample test" was used to compare pretreatment and posttreatment intragroup differences in the findings obtained as a result of the evaluations. "Mann–Whitney $U$ Test" was used to compare differences between the two groups.

## 3. Results

Among 47 older adults assessed at baseline, 3 were not meeting the inclusion criteria and 4 were lost to follow-up. Finally, the study was completed with 21 older adults in group TPMM, and 19 individuals in group TP (Figure 1). Sociodemographic data of the older adults in both the TP and TPMM groups were similar ($p > 0.05$) (Table 1).

Comparing pretreatment and posttreatment findings indicated that the participants in both groups had a significant decrease in their pain, NDI, BDI, and TSK. They also had significant increase in their ROM and SF-36, except for the physical health condition category for the TPMM group ($p < 0.05$) (Table 2).

Comparing the gains of the participants in the two groups indicated that pain, NDI, right/left neck rotation, left lateral flexion ROM, and mental health subcategory of SF-36 had similar improvement rate in both groups ($p > 0.05$) (Table 3).

However, the two groups were different in terms of ROM (except for right/left neck rotation and left lateral flexion), TSK, BDI, and SF-36 (except for mental health subcategory), in all of which the TPMM group had greater improvements (Table 3).

## 4. Discussion

The results of this randomized, controlled, and double-blinded study showed that all participants had less pain, depression, and kinesiophobia; greater ROM; and better QoL and functional level. It was also found that there was greater improvement in joint ROM (except for right/left rotation and left lateral flexion), kinesiophobia, depression, and QoL (excluding mental health) in the TPMM group compared to the other group.

As in all age groups, NP is a common health problem in the older adults [18]. As a result of the treatment programs of the present study with older adults, NP decreased in a similar way in both groups. In their study on individuals with chronic mechanical NP, Said et al. reported that the MMT had a greater impact on pain reduction compared to the traditional treatment [19]. According to the main explanation provided for the pain-reducing effect of the mobilization, mobilization movements correct positional faults in the bony structure and hence reduce pain [19, 20]. Some studies have reported that spinal manipulative therapy produces a specific hypoalgesic effect. Manipulation-induced hypoalgesia may seem to be nonopioid in nature; that is, it is not reversed by the naloxone and could not improve tolerance to repeated stimulation. It may occur

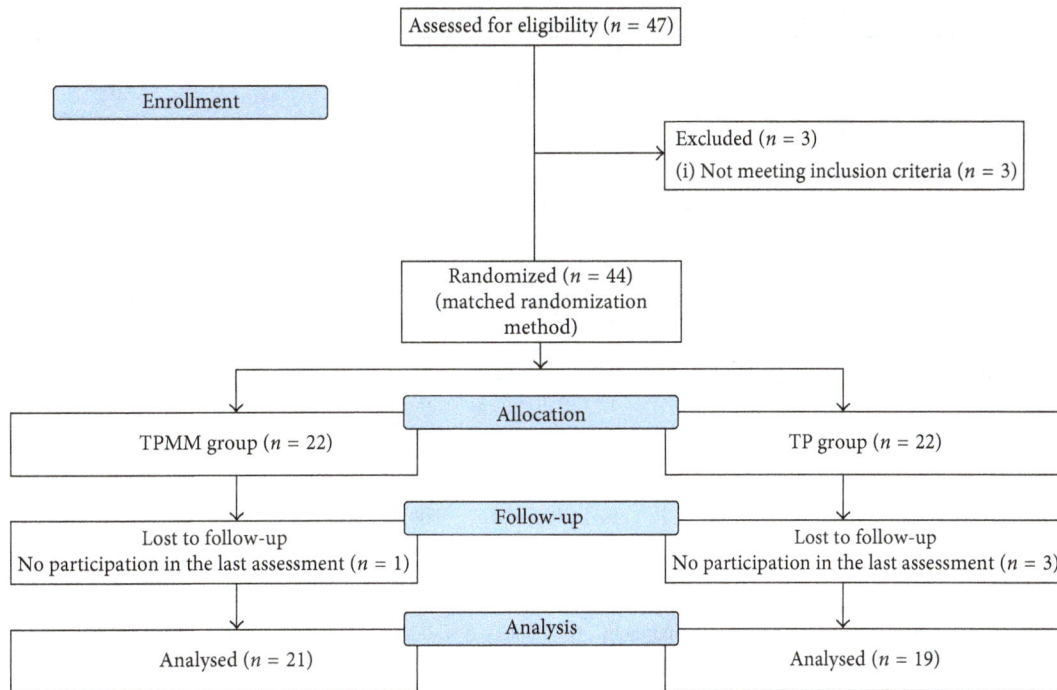

FIGURE 1: Flow chart of the study.

concurrent to changes in sympathetic and motor systems. Furthermore, preliminary evidence indicates that mechanical hypoalgesia is more effective against thermal hypoalgesia in study populations. This specific effect is produced by manipulative therapy [21, 22]. It was believed that the precise mechanism of the sudden development brought about by SNAGs was complex containing many systems including sympathoexcitation and nonopioid hypoalgesia. [23]. El-Sayed et al. was emphasized that the rationale for the technique was initially based on a biomechanical explanation where repositioning of the superior articular facet using a SNAG would cause correction of positional fault, thus resulting in reduced pain and increased ROM in the neck [23]. In accordance with abovementioned studies, results of this study indicated a reduced level of pain in both groups. However, the fact that our participants consisted of older adults suffering NP was an outstanding point of the present study.

One of the most common symptoms of cervical spine problems are restricted ROM [24]. According to the treatment results, there was an increase in the ROM in both groups. However, this increase was found to be greater in the TPMM group except for neck rotation and left lateral flexion. In their randomized controlled study, Gautam et al. divided 30 individuals with NP into 3 groups. They applied the MMT, Maitland technique, and TP to the first, second, and third groups, respectively. They reported that out of the three, the MMT had a greater impact on pain, ROM, and disability [11]. According to Edmonston and Singer, SNAGs are particularly important in painful movement dysfunctions as a result of degenerative changes, as these techniques make pain-free movements possible throughout the available ROM. Furthermore, the potential problems that may occur during passive movements are less likely as the patient

TABLE 1: Demographic information of individuals.

| | TP group median (IQR) | TPMM group median (IQR) | $p$ |
|---|---|---|---|
| Age (years) | 67 (65.5–72) | 69 (65–70.5) | 0.575 |
| BMI (kg/m²) | 27.78 (24.675–28.545) | 28.34 (24.245–30.01) | 0.763 |
| Duration of diagnosis (years) | 10 (6–12) | 9 (7–12) | 0.453 |

IQR: inter quartile range; BMI: body mass index.

is in control of the movement [25]. It is stated that in the MMT, zygapophyseal joints guide the spine, and thus applying NAGs and SNAGs lead to an increase in ROM [26]. The reason for the technique was based on a biomechanical explanation that repositioning the superior articular facet using SNAGs at the beginning would lead to correction of the positional impairment and thus result in pain reduction and increased ROM. Furthermore, normal movement on the articular surface is necessary to maintain the mobility of adjacent nerves that altered biomechanics may affect the nervous outgrowth. Because of this, restoration of normal mechanics in joint space may normalize negative neuron-names that appear as a consequence of limited joint movement [23]. Many studies have indicated a decrease in cervical joint mobility as a result of aging, as well [27–29]. Older adults with neck pain were included in our study, and the MMT were found to improve ROM of the joints. In the literature, however, the MMT seems to be applied to young adults [11, 30]. For this reason, there is a need for studies that investigate the efficacy of the MMT on older adults with NP.

Ganesh et al. divided individuals aged 21–45 years with mechanical neck pain into 3 groups in their studies. They applied Mulligan mobilization to group 1, Maitland

TABLE 2: Comparing pretreatment and posttreatment participants in both groups.

| | | TP group | | | TPMM group | | | p2 |
|---|---|---|---|---|---|---|---|---|
| | | Before median (IQR) | After median (IQR) | p1 | Before median (IQR) | After median (IQR) | p1 | |
| VAS (0–10) | | | | | | | | |
| Rest | | 5 (4–7) | 2 (0–3) | 0.007* | 4 (2–5.5) | 0 | 0.002* | 0.171 |
| Activity | | 7 (4–8.5) | 2 (0–4) | 0.005* | 7 (5–8) | 1 (0–2) | 0.002* | 0.224 |
| ROM | | | | | | | | |
| Cervical flexion | | 34 (32.2–36.3) | 41 (39.2–43.3) | 0.005* | 35 (33.3–36.5) | 46 (40.8–47.5) | 0.003* | 0.165 |
| Cervical extension | | 35 (34.6–36.2) | 40 (35.4–42.3) | 0.005* | 33 (32.5–36.4) | 41 (37.4–45.2) | 0.003* | 0.089 |
| Cervical lateral flexion | Right | 32 (30.2–33.4) | 38 (35.7–39.7) | 0.005* | 33 (30.4–38.5) | 42 (40.2–48.5) | 0.002* | 0.153 |
| | Left | 32 (29.6–34.3) | 37 (34.5–39.6) | 0.005* | 34 (31.6–36.3) | 40 (38.4–45.7) | 0.003* | 0.083 |
| Cervical rotation | Right | 42 (39.2–43.1) | 45 (40.01–44.8) | 0.007* | 45 (39.6–46.5) | 52 (45.7–53.5) | 0.012* | 0.091 |
| | Left | 39 (34.4–42.5) | 42 (39.2–44.03) | 0.008* | 35 (32.7–36.5) | 48 (45.5–52.4) | 0.003* | 0.079 |
| NDI (0–35 points) | | 17 (15–18) | 7 (4–8) | 0.005* | 18 (16–20) | 5 (4–6) | 0.002* | 0.116 |
| TSK (17–68 points) | | 41 (40–41) | 38 (37–41) | 0.005* | 40 (39–42) | 36 (35–40) | 0.003* | 0.057 |
| BDI | | 15 (7–19) | 7 (3–9) | 0.005* | 13 (10–14) | 6 (4–8) | 0.002* | 0.098 |
| Quality of life (SF-36) | Physical component | 35.8 (33–41.2) | 40.4 (40.5–42.7) | 0.005* | 36.4 (34.6–36.9) | 42.3 (41.8–46.5) | 0.182 | 0.091 |
| | Mental component | 39.8 (37.5–43.6) | 43.3 (40.6–46.3) | 0.005* | 38.7 (36.5–40.2) | 45.7 (41.5–48.7) | 0.003* | 0.131 |
| | Total | 70.5 (69.2–76.7) | 80.3 (78–85.5) | 0.005* | 72.4 (70.2–75.9) | 88.2 (85.4–89.1) | 0.002* | 0.052 |

TP: traditional physiotherapy, TPMM: traditional phyisotherapy + Mulligan mobilization, IQR: interquartile range, VAS: visual analog scale, ROM: range of motion, NDI: neck disability index, TSK: Tampa scale of kinesiophobia, BDI: Beck depression inventory, SF-36: Short Form-36. $p1$ denotes the differences between before and after treatment scores for both groups with using "Wilcoxon paired two sample test," and $p2$ denotes the differences between the baseline scores of two groups with using "Mann–Whitney U test." $^*p < 0.05$.

TABLE 3: Comparing the gains of the participants in both groups.

| | | TP group Δ median (IQR) | TPMM group Δ median (IQR) | p |
|---|---|---|---|---|
| VAS (0–10) | | | | |
| Rest | | −3 (−6 to −3) | −4 (−6 to −2) | 0.862 |
| Activity | | −5 (−5 to −4) | −6 (−6 to −3) | 0.083 |
| ROM | | | | |
| Cervical flexion | | 6.4 (4.2–6.9) | 10.2 (8.3–12.4) | ≤0.001* |
| Cervical extension | | 5.3 (3.7–6.4) | 8.4 (5.8–9.7) | ≤0.001* |
| Cervical lateral flexion | Right | 6 (4.4–7.1) | 9 (8.01–11.2) | 0.004* |
| | Left | 5 (3.5–6.8) | 6 (5.4–8.2) | 0.089 |
| Cervical rotation | Right | 3 (2.7–4.7) | 7 (5.6–8.3) | 0.527 |
| | Left | 3 (2.9–4.5) | 13 (10.5–15.6) | 0.354 |
| NDI (0–35 point) | | −10 (−12 to −8) | −13 (−14 to −7) | 0.335 |
| TSK (17–68 point) | | 3 (4–6) | 5 (4–8) | 0.006* |
| BDI | | −8 (−11 to −4) | −7 (−10 to −4) | 0.007* |
| Quality of life (SF-36) | Physical component | 4.5 (2.1–6.2) | 5.9 (4.3–6.7) | 0.002* |
| | Mental component | 4.7 (3.2–10.43) | 7.3 (5.25–9.82) | 0.092 |
| | Total | 10.5 (4.3–12.4) | 16.1 (8.9–20.21) | 0.002* |

TP: traditional physiotherapy, TPMM: traditional phyisotherapy + Mulligan mobilization, VAS: visual analog scale, ROM: range of motion, NDI: neck disability index, TSK: Tampa scale of kinesiophobia, BDI: Beck depression inventory, SF-36: Short Form-36. $^*p < 0.05$.

mobilization to group 2, and exercise therapy only to group 3. At the end of their studies, they found that manual therapy techniques were not as good as pain relief, increase to ROM and neck disability as compared to exercise (level of evidence = 1C) [4]. Shin and Lee designed a single blind and randomized controlled trial in their study and divided randomly forty patients with headache into the SNAGs group and the control group. Shin and Lee were reported that the SNAGs technique can help to relieve headache and cervical pain in middle-aged women suffering from cervical headache (level of evidence = 1B) [31]. El-Sayed et al. divided randomly patients with radiculopathy whose ages were 40–55 years into the SNAGs + conventional physical therapy group and the conventional physical therapy group in their study. They explained that the SNAGs technique combined with TP is more effective in the rehabilitation program (level of evidence = 1B) [23]. Copurgensli et al. designed a single blind and randomized controlled trial. They were randomly placed into three groups: group 1: conventional rehabilitation; group 2: conventional rehabilitation and MMT; and group 3: conventional rehabilitation and kinesio taping. Results of their study showed that the MMT and kinesio taping have no additional effects on neck pain, muscle strength, and neck-related disability. Furthermore, they said that the use of the MMT and kinesio taping in addition to conventional rehabilitation, the gain in cervical ROM, and deep cervical flexor muscle strength may be increased in patients with cervical spondylosis (level of evidence = 1B) [32]. These studies are generally randomized controlled (level of evidence = 1B) studies in the literature. In comparison studies of the MMT with other treatments there are different opinions about whether it is effective or not [4, 23, 31, 32]. In our study, older adults aged 65 years and over were included, and the MMT has been found to have significant effects on pain, ROM, functional level, kinesiophobia, depression, and QoL. Moreover, the studies in young adults in the literature have been designed nonblindness or single blindness. This study was designed as a double-blinded-randomized controlled trial. To the best of our knowledge, there were few studies which compare the effects of the MMT on pain, ROM, functional level, kinesiophobia, depression, and QoL in older adults with chronic neck pain.

It has been shown that there is an important relationship between pain and kinesophobia in individuals suffering NP. As a result of our study, it was determined that fear of movement decreased in both groups. This decrease was more pronounced in the TPMM group. It is also stated that, in case of NP, ROM in the cervical region decreases, movements are slower than normal, and proprioception is impaired [24, 30]. It is thought that any increase in ROM results in an increase in the proprioceptive sensation in the neck region, which may result in reduced kinesophobia in patients.

NDI was used in the present study to assess the patients' disabilities in daily life due to their NP. According to our posttreatment evaluations, NDI results had improved in both TP and TPMM groups in a similar manner. Our results are in agreement with Sudarshan, who applied a simultaneous combination of neurodynamic mobilization and SNAGs and reported immediate improvement in VAS, cervical ROM, and NDI. In our study, similar development was achieved in both groups [33]. This is thought to be due to the fact that older adults are able to perform their daily life activities better as a result of reduced pain.

SF-36 was used to assess the QoL of the participants. This questionnaire was developed specifically to assess QoL in patients with physical illnesses [14]. At the end of our treatment programs, there was an increase in QoL in both the TP and TPMM groups, which was found to be higher in the TPMM group except for the mental health score. Maiers et al. investigated the effects of spinal manual therapy (cervical joint and soft tissue mobilization) and exercises in the older adults with chronic NP. They reported minor improvement in QoL following the treatment; however, this improvement was not statistically significant [18]. Even though the present study is similar to the one by Maiers et al. in terms of patient population, we achieved greater gains in QoL of our participants. The TPMM group showed more pronounced improvement in QoL (except for the mental health scores), and this is thought to be a result of higher ROM and reduced pain, both of which have positive effects on QoL. These two parameters are more significantly gained in the TPMM group.

BDI was used to determine the risk of depression in patients and/or to measure the level of depressive symptoms and the change in its severity [13]. As a result of this study, both the TP and TPMM groups showed a decrease in depression levels, and this decrease was found to be higher in the TPMM group.

The most important outcome of the present study is that the MMT can be safely applied in older adults with NP without harming the patients. In addition, functional limitations in older adults with NP were reduced, and pain-free ROM was obtained. Although there are some studies in the literature evaluating the efficacy of the MMT in individuals suffering NP, there are no studies investigating the efficacy of this technique on older adults. Two strengths of this study are that the patient group consists of older adults and that it is a random-controlled double-blind study.

Long-term effects of the MMT in older adults with NP are not investigated, which is a limitation of the present study. To have more precise results, it is necessary to continue long-term follow-up evaluations of the patients to investigate the rate of recurrence in each group.

## 5. Conclusion

According to the findings of this study, applying the MMT in older adults with NP has positive effects on pain, ROM, functional level, kinesiophobia, fear of movement, ES, and QoL.

## Authors' Contributions

Buket Buyukturan, Oznur Buyukturan, and İd ur Buyuktu contributed to the study concept and design. Oznur Buyukturan applied the treatment. Buket Buyukturan and Oznur Buyukturan drafted the manuscript. Caner Karartı assessed the physical tests. Senem Sas initially diagnosed and referred the patients. All authors discussed the results, commented on, and approved the final manuscript.

## References

[1] T. T. Chiu, E. Y. Law, and T. H. Chiu, "Performance of the craniocervical flexion test in subjects with and without chronic neck pain," *Journal of Orthopaedic and Sports Physical Therapy*, vol. 35, no. 9, pp. 567–571, 2005.

[2] D. Falla, R. Lindstrøm, L. Rechter, S. Boudreau, and F. Petzke, "Effectiveness of an 8-week exercise programme on pain and specificity of neck muscle activity in patients with chronic neck pain: a randomized controlled study," *European Journal of Pain*, vol. 17, no. 10, pp. 1517–1528, 2013.

[3] L. M. March, A. J. Brnabic, J. C. Skinner et al., "Musculoskeletal disability among elderly people in the community," *Medical Journal of Australia*, vol. 168, no. 9, pp. 439–442, 1998.

[4] G. S. Ganesh, P. Mohanty, M Pattnaik, and C. Mishra, "Effectiveness of mobilization therapy and exercises in mechanical neck pain," *Physiotherapy Theory and Practice*, vol. 31, no. 2, pp. 99–106, 2014.

[5] L. Exelby, "The Mulligan concept: its application in the management of spinal conditions," *Manual Therapy*, vol. 7, no. 2, pp. 64–70, 2002.

[6] B. R. Mulligan, *Manual Therapy NAGS SNAGS MWMS etc.*, Plane View Services Ltd., Wellington, New Zealand, 5th edition, 2003.

[7] L. Exelby, "Mobilisation with movement: a personal view," *Physiotherapy*, vol. 81, no. 12, pp. 724–729, 1995.

[8] B. Cagnie, E. Derese, L. Vandamme, K. Verstraete, D. Cambier, and L. Danneels, "Validity and reliability of ultrasonography for the longus colli in asymptomatic subjects," *Manuel Therapy*, vol. 14, no. 4, pp. 421–426, 2009.

[9] A. Bicer, A. Yazici, H. Camdeviren, and C. Erdogan, "Assessment of pain and disability in patients with chronic neck pain: reliability and construct validity of the Turkish version of the neck pain and disability scale," *Disability and Rehabilitation*, vol. 26, no. 16, pp. 959–962, 2004.

[10] O. T. Yılmaz, Y. Yakut, F. Uygur, and N. Ulug, "Tampa Kinezyofobi Ölçeğinin Türkçe versiyonu ve test-tekrar test güvenilirliği," *Fizyoterapi Rehabilitasyon Dergisi*, vol. 22, pp. 44–49, 2011.

[11] R. Gautam, J. K. Dhamija, and A. Puri, "Comparison of Maitland and Mulligan mobilization in improving neck pain, ROM and disability," *International Journal of Physiotherapy and Research*, vol. 2, pp. 482–487, 2014.

[12] K. L. Whitcroft, L. Massouh, R. Amirfeyz, and G. Bannister, "Comparison of methods of measuring active cervical range of motion," *Spine*, vol. 35, no. 19, pp. E976–E980, 2010.

[13] N. Hisli, "Reliability and validity of Beck depression inventory among university students," *Journal of Turkish Psychology*, vol. 7, pp. 3–13, 1989.

[14] H. Koçyiğit, Ö. Aydemir, G. Fişek, N. Ölmez, and A. Memiş, "The reliability and validity of the Turkish version of the Short Form-36," *İlaç ve Tedavi Dergisi*, vol. 12, pp. 102–106, 1999.

[15] G. D. Cramer and S. A. Darby, *Basic and Clinical Anatomy of the Spine, Spinal Cord, and ANS*, Elsevier, Mosby, St. Louis, MO, USA, 3rd edition, 2013.

[16] C. Bedwell, T. Dowswell, J. P. Neilson, and L. T. Midwifery, "The use of transcutaneous electrical nerve stimulation (TENS) for pain relief in labour: a review of the evidence," *Midwifery*, vol. 27, no. 5, pp. 141–148, 2011.

[17] D. Windt, G. Heijden, S. Berg, G. Riet, A. Winter, and L. Bouter, "Ultrasound therapy for musculoskeletal disorders: a systematic review," *Pain*, vol. 81, no. 3, pp. 257–271, 1999.

[18] M. Maiers, G. Bronfort, R. Evans et al., "Spinal manipulative therapy and exercise for seniors with chronic neck pain," *The Spine Journal*, vol. 14, no. 9, pp. 1879–1889, 2014.

[19] M. S. Said, O. I. Ali, S. N. A. Elazm, and N. A. Abdelraoof, "Mulligan self mobilization versus Mulligan snags on cervical position sense," *International Journal of Physiotherapy*, vol. 4, no. 2, pp. 93–100, 2017.

[20] B. Vicenzino, A. Paungmali, and P. Teys, "Mulligan's mobilization-with-movement, positional faults and pain relief: current concepts from a critical review of literature," *Manual Therapy*, vol. 12, no. 2, pp. 98–108, 2007.

[21] B. Vicenzino, A. Paungmali, S. Buratowski, and A. Wright, "Specific manipulative therapy treatment for chronic lateral epicondylalgia produces uniquely characteristic hypoalgesia," *Manual Therapy*, vol. 6, no. 4, pp. 205–212, 2001.

[22] M. Sterling, G. Jull, and A. Wright, "Cervical mobilisation: concurrent effects on pain, sympathetic nervous system activity and motor activity," *Manual Therapy*, vol. 6, no. 2, pp. 72–81, 2001.

[23] W. El-Sayed, A. F. E. Mohamed, G. El-Monem, and H. H. Ahmed, "Effect of SNAGS Mulligan technique on chronic cervical radiculopathy: a randomized clinical trial," *Medical Journal of Cairo University*, vol. 85, no. 2, pp. 787–793, 2017.

[24] P. Sjölander, P. Michaelson, S. Jaric, and M. Djupsjöbacka, "Sensorimotor disturbances in chronic neck pain range of motion of movement, and repositioning acuity," *Manual Therapy*, vol. 13, no. 2, pp. 122–131, 2008.

[25] S. J. Edmonston and K. P. Singer, "Anatomical and biomechanical consideration for manual therapy," *Manual Therapy*, vol. 2, no. 3, pp. 123–131, 1997.

[26] L. Exelby, "Peripheral mobilisation with movement," *Manual Therapy*, vol. 1, no. 3, pp. 118–126, 1996.

[27] D. Ferlic, "The range of motion of the "normal" cervical spine," *Bulletin of the Johns Hopkins Hospital*, vol. 110, pp. 59–65, 1962.

[28] H. Hayashi, K. Okada, M. Hamada, K. Tada, and R. Ueno, "Etiologic factors of myelopathy: a radiographic evaluation of the aging changes in the cervical spine," *Clinical Orthopaedics and Related Research*, vol. 214, pp. 200–209, 1987.

[29] F. J. Kottke and R. S. Blanchard, "A study of degenerative changes of the cervical spine in relation to age: a preliminary report," *Bulletin of the University of Minnesota Hospital*, vol. 24, pp. 470–479, 1953.

[30] T. Hall, H. T. Chan, L. Christensen, B. Odenthal, C. Wells, and K. Robinson, "Efficacy of a C1-C2 self sustained natural apophyseal glide (SNAG) in the management of cervicogenic headache," *Journal of Orthopaedic Sports Physical Therapy*, vol. 37, no. 3, pp. 100–107, 2007.

[31] E. J. Shin and B. H. Lee, "The effect of sustained natural apophyseal glides on headache, duration and cervical function in women with cervicogenic headache," *Journal of Exercise Rehabilitation*, vol. 10, no. 2, pp. 131–135, 2014.

[32] C. Copurgensli, G. Gur, and V. B. Tunay, "A comparison of the effects of Mulligan's mobilization and Kinesio taping on pain, range of motion, muscle strength, and neck disability in patients with cervical spondylosis: a randomized controlled study," *Journal of Back and Musculoskeletal Rehabilitation*, vol. 30, no. 1, pp. 51–62, 2016.

[33] A. Sudarshan, "The effect of sustained natural apophyseal glide (SNAG) combined with neuro-dynamics in the management of a patient with cervical radiculopathy: a case report," *Physiotherapy Theory and Practice*, vol. 31, no. 2, pp. 140–145, 2015.

# 14

# Effects of Exercise Training Combined with Increased Physical Activity to Prevent Chronic Pain in Community-Dwelling Older Adults: A Preliminary Randomized Controlled Trial

**Tatsuya Hirase** [ID],[1] **Hideki Kataoka,**[2,3] **Shigeru Inokuchi,**[1] **Jiro Nakano,**[1] **Junya Sakamoto** [ID],[1] **and Minoru Okita**[2]

[1]*Department of Physical Therapy Science, Nagasaki University Graduate School of Biomedical Sciences, 1-7-1 Sakamoto, Nagasaki 852-8520, Japan*
[2]*Department of Locomotive Rehabilitation Science, Nagasaki University Graduate School of Biomedical Sciences, 1-7-1 Sakamoto, Nagasaki 852-8520, Japan*
[3]*Department of Rehabilitation, Nagasaki Memorial Hospital, 11-54 Fukahori, Nagasaki 851-0301, Japan*

Correspondence should be addressed to Tatsuya Hirase; htatsuya@nagasaki-u.ac.jp

Academic Editor: Parisa Gazerani

*Objective.* With the aim of developing a chronic pain prevention program, this randomized controlled trial examined whether exercise training combined with increased physical activity more effectively improves pain and physical activity than exercise training alone in community-dwelling older adults without chronic pain. *Methods.* We randomized 76 older adults without chronic pain into an intervention group ($n = 38$) involving exercise training combined with increased physical activity and a control group ($n = 38$) involving exercise training alone. The exercise training comprised weekly 60-min sessions for 12 weeks. The program to increase physical activity required participants to record their daily step counts using pedometers. Pain intensity, total number of pain sites, and physical activity were assessed before and 12 weeks after the intervention. *Results.* A time-by-group interaction was found for physical activity, with the intervention group showing significant improvement ($p < 0.05$). The intervention group also showed greater improvement in pain intensity and total number of pain sites at 12 weeks after intervention than the control group ($p < 0.05$). *Conclusions.* In older adults without chronic pain, exercise training combined with increased physical activity improves key outcome indicators more effectively than exercise training alone. "This trial is registered with UMIN000018503."

## 1. Introduction

Chronic pain causes increased health-care costs as well as deterioration in quality of life and is common among community-dwelling older adults [1]. Our previous study revealed that 54.4% of community-dwelling older adults had chronic pain, associated with declining physical function, poor psychological status, and low physical activity levels [2]. Kaiho et al. [3] reported that chronic pain is a risk factor for the need for long-term care. Therefore, an effective approach to the prevention of chronic pain in community-dwelling older adults needs to be developed urgently.

In Japan, the number of community-dwelling older adults who require long-term care has increased because of the rapidly aging population. In addition, the average healthy life expectancy is approximately 10 years lower than the mean life expectancy [4]. In 2006, the Japanese Government revised its long-term care insurance system, which provides client-centered services to older adults who are certified as requiring support or care according to their disability levels and introduced new preventive care services to extend the healthy life expectancy of its residents [5]. These care services involve a community-based prevention program to delay the need for long-term care, with exercise classes often provided to older adults assessed as being at risk for requiring long-term care in the near future. Such classes have effectively improved physical function [6], psychological status [7], and physical activity levels [8]. However, in Japan, full assessments of pain, including pain intensity and duration, are not routinely performed during exercise classes because of a lack of recognition that chronic pain is a serious social issue that results in higher health care costs and a declining quality of life [9, 10]. Therefore, the nature of an effective intervention focused on preventing chronic pain in older adults who participate in these classes remains unclear. The development of a community-based intervention program aimed at preventing increased pain intensity in older adults without chronic pain is needed to extend healthy life expectancy in Japan, as the number of older adults with pain is projected to increase over the next 50 years [11].

Park and Hughes [12] reviewed empirical evidence and revealed that exercise training is an effective nonpharmacological approach for managing chronic pain in community-dwelling older adults. In a previous study that used an animal model, Sluka et al. [13] reported that physical inactivity is a risk factor for the development of chronic pain, and that regular physical activity prevents chronic pain. Our previous study revealed that a psychosocial intervention that involved self-management education and increased physical activity, combined with exercise training, more effectively decreased pain intensity than exercise training alone in older adults with chronic pain who participated in community-based exercise classes [14]. Therefore, an intervention program to increase physical activity, combined with exercise training, may be beneficial to preventing chronic pain in older adults.

On the basis of the findings of previous studies [12–14], we hypothesized that a community-based intervention to increase physical activity combined with exercise training, with the aim of developing of a chronic pain prevention program, would more effectively decrease pain intensity and improve physical activity in older adults without chronic pain than exercise training without increased physical activity. The aim of this study was to investigate that hypothesis.

## 2. Materials and Methods

*2.1. Participants.* We enrolled older adults participating in community exercise classes once a week in the Japanese city of Unzen, selecting seven exercise classes supported by physical therapists. Physical therapists were asked to choose potential participants aged ≥65 years who were living at home, able to walk outdoors without a cane, and able to independently perform activities of daily living. We excluded older adults who had chronic pain, defined as the presence of related symptoms within the past month that continued for at least 6 months and corresponded to a Numerical Rating Scale (NRS) of at five or more at the maximum pain site [9]. We also excluded older adults who had exercised at least four times during the month before the initial interview and those who had musculoskeletal, neurological, or cardiovascular conditions that may be aggravated by exercise, according to the judgments of their primary care doctors. Moreover, we excluded older adults who were

unable to respond to interview questions because of cognitive impairment.

Each participant provided written informed consent in accordance with the guidelines of the Nagasaki University Graduate School of Medicine and the 2008 Helsinki Declaration of Human Rights. The Ethics Review Board of Nagasaki University Graduate School of Biomedical Sciences approved this study.

*2.2. Design and Randomization.* This randomized controlled trial was performed from August 2015 to November 2016. Participants who met the inclusion criteria were randomized into two groups (1 : 1) using computer-generated randomization lists. The groups comprised an intervention group that involved increased physical activity combined with exercise training and a control group that involved exercise training alone. An independent investigator performed the randomization after baseline assessment. Physical therapists who supported the community exercise classes assessed the participants and implemented the intervention program.

*2.3. Interventions.* We asked participants in both groups to attend a 60 min weekly exercise class for 12 weeks. The class comprised 10 min of warm-up, 20 min of strength training, 20 min of balance training, and 10 min of cool-down, as described in our previous study [14]. All classes involved approximately 10 participants. The intensity of the strength and balance training during the 40 min was constant over the course of the intervention period and included a total 10 min of breaks, depending on the participants' physical capacity. As a participant resource, and to ensure the consistency of the training, we provided a videotape of the correct executions of the exercises, and instructors were supervised by the physical therapists who supported each class.

The intervention group also participated in a program to increase physical activity during the 12-week intervention period. Only participants in this group were given pedometers (Yamax Digiwalker SW-200; Yamasa Tokei Keiki Co., Ltd., Tokyo, Japan), which they wore at all times they were awake, and daily diaries to record their daily step counts. Yamada et al. [15] reported that an intervention followed by goal setting to progressively increase daily step counts, self-monitoring, and feedback is a useful method for increasing the physical activity of community-dwelling older adults. On the basis of these findings, the physical therapists supporting the community exercise classes checked participants' diaries once a week and advised them to increase their daily step counts by approximately 10% relative to their baseline during the first month. During the second and third months, we advised participants in the intervention group to increase their step counts by approximately 20% and 30%, respectively, relative to their baseline. Participants in this group were asked to record their daily step counts at the end of each day; written activity logs were averaged weekly to determine whether the participants were achieving their step goal. Physical therapists checked the participants' daily step counts during their weekly exercise class and provided feedback and encouragement for 10 minutes during the class, so that the participants could achieve their step goal.

*2.4. Assessment.* The primary outcome of this study was pain intensity, and the secondary outcomes were physical function, psychological status, and physical activity level. Before the study began, the physical therapists received training from one of the authors (Tatsuya Hirase) on the assessment protocols.

Pain was assessed by determining the total number of pain sites and intensity at the maximum pain site, using NRS. Participants used a body chart to identify their pain sites and scored their pain intensity according to NRS.

Physical function was assessed using the Chair Stand Test (CST) [16] and the Timed Up-and-Go (TUG) test [17]. These tests were conducted twice, and the best value from the two tests was recorded.

The psychological status was evaluated using the 15-item version of the Geriatric Depression Scale (GDS-15) [18] and the Pain Catastrophizing Scale (PCS) [19]. The PCS includes the same 13 items reported by Sullivan et al. [20] and comprises three categories: rumination (five items), helplessness (five items), and magnification (three items). Each item is assessed on a five-point scale ranging from zero ("not at all") to four ("all the time"), with a total score ranging from 0 to 52, and higher scores indicating greater catastrophizing. Pain, physical function, and the psychological status in both groups were evaluated before and within 7 days of the end of the 12-week program.

Participants in both groups wore a pedometer with an accelerometer (Kenz Lifecorder GS; Suzuken Co., Ltd., Nagoya, Japan) to assess their physical activity levels during the same 2-week periods—the first week of the study and the final week of the study—to evaluate the preintervention and postintervention effects. Participants were instructed to wear the pedometer on their belt or waistband, above the right midline of the thigh, from the moment they got out of bed in the morning until they went to bed in the evening, except while bathing or swimming. Based on a previous report by Matsubara et al. [21], we calculated the participants' mean daily step counts and activity times for mild (1–3 metabolic equivalents (METS)), moderate (4–6 METS), and heavy (7–9 METS) exercise during each period with the Lifecorder GS (Suzuken Co., Ltd.) pedometer.

*2.5. Required Sample Size.* We designed this study to detect an effect size of 0.61, according to the results of our previous study [14]. With a statistical significance level of 5% ($p \leq 0.05$), a statistical power of 80%, and allowance for a 5% dropout rate, we required a minimum of 36 participants in each group.

*2.6. Statistical Analysis.* Statistical analyses were performed using SPSS 22.0 for Windows (IBM Corp., Armonk, NY, USA). We used unpaired *t*-tests to evaluate significant differences in age, height, body weight, and outcome measures between the two groups before the intervention, and chi-square tests for group comparisons of sex distribution and proportion of dropouts. We analyzed the effects of the intervention program on the outcome measures using a $2 \times 2$ (time (baseline and 12-week postintervention) × group (intervention and control groups)) analysis of variance. We used post hoc Bonferroni tests for specific comparisons, and significance was two-sided.

# 3. Results

Figure 1, a flow chart, outlines the study's recruitment of participants and randomization into the two study groups. A total of 225 older adults were screened as potential participants; 149 either declined to participate ($n = 20$) or failed to meet the inclusion criteria ($n = 129$). Of those who did not meet the inclusion criteria, 120 had chronic pain, five were unable to respond to interview questions because of cognitive impairment, and four had exercised four or more times in the month before the initial interview. We enrolled the remaining 76 older adults into the study, and randomly allocated each of them to either the intervention group ($n = 38$) or the control group ($n = 38$). Three participants in the intervention group (3.9% of the sample) withdrew from the trial; they were admitted to hospital because of serious illness (pneumonia ($n = 2$) and heart disease ($n = 1$)). There were no significant group differences in study withdrawal ($p = 0.240$), and no participants dropped out for reasons relating to the intervention program itself. Seventy-three participants completed the 12-week intervention: 35 in the intervention group and 38 in the control group.

During the intervention period, participants in the intervention and control groups who completed the study attended 91.2% and 90.6% of the classes, respectively. This difference in class attendance was not significant between the groups ($p = 0.817$).

*3.1. Baseline Characteristics.* Table 1 summarizes the participants' baseline characteristics. There were no significant differences in age, sex, pain, physical function, psychological status, or physical activity between the two groups ($p \geq 0.157$ for all comparisons).

*3.2. Effects of the Interventions on Pain, Physical Function, Psychological Status, and Physical Activity.* Table 2 shows the effects of the interventions on the outcome measures in the preintervention and postintervention periods. There was a significant time-by-group interaction for daily step counts ($p = 0.022$).

*3.2.1. Effects of the Interventions on the Primary Outcome for Both Groups.* The mean number of total pain sites and NRS score at the maximum pain site at 12 weeks after intervention in the intervention group were significantly better than the values in the control group ($p = 0.016$ and $p = 0.002$, resp.). Within the control group, the mean NRS score at the maximum pain site at 12 weeks after intervention was significantly worse than that before intervention

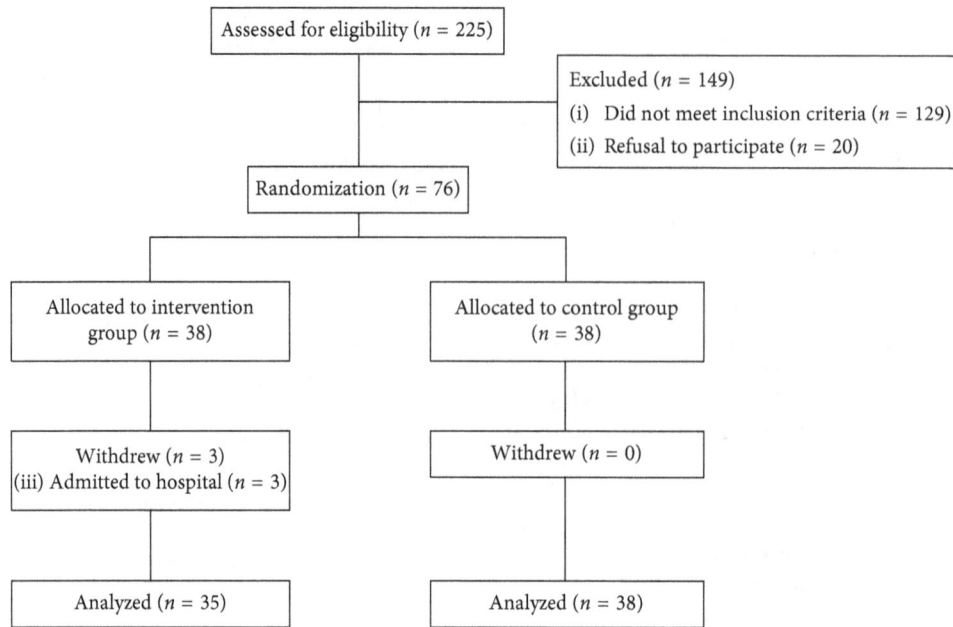

FIGURE 1: Flowchart outlining the study's participant recruitment process and randomization into the two study groups.

TABLE 1: Participants' baseline characteristics.

| Characteristics | Intervention group ($n = 38$) | Control group ($n = 38$) | $p$ value |
|---|---|---|---|
| Age (years) | $78.3 \pm 5.8$ | $78.3 \pm 6.5$ | 0.956 |
| Female, $n$ (%) | 29 (76.3) | 29 (76.3) | 0.999 |
| Height (cm) | $150.7 \pm 7.6$ | $152.5 \pm 7.0$ | 0.303 |
| Weight (kg) | $50.3 \pm 9.0$ | $52.6 \pm 8.9$ | 0.252 |
| Total number of pain sites | $1.7 \pm 1.5$ | $2.0 \pm 2.0$ | 0.566 |
| NRS at the site of maximum pain | $2.4 \pm 2.2$ | $2.7 \pm 2.4$ | 0.555 |
| CST (s) | $7.7 \pm 2.7$ | $7.4 \pm 2.0$ | 0.544 |
| TUG (s) | $7.6 \pm 1.6$ | $7.6 \pm 1.6$ | 0.938 |
| GDS-15 score (points) | $3.2 \pm 3.5$ | $2.7 \pm 2.9$ | 0.497 |
| PCS total score (points) | $23.3 \pm 13.1$ | $23.4 \pm 11.1$ | 0.963 |
| Rumination score (points) | $11.0 \pm 6.1$ | $10.8 \pm 4.7$ | 0.850 |
| Helplessness score (points) | $7.2 \pm 4.7$ | $7.6 \pm 4.3$ | 0.704 |
| Magnification score (points) | $5.1 \pm 3.7$ | $5.2 \pm 3.3$ | 0.974 |
| Daily step counts (steps) | $4533.1 \pm 2515.8$ | $4030.2 \pm 2266.5$ | 0.363 |
| Mild activity times (s) | $2471.7 \pm 1368.2$ | $2382.8 \pm 1158.3$ | 0.762 |
| Moderate activity times (s) | $484.9 \pm 683.0$ | $303.0 \pm 442.0$ | 0.157 |
| Heavy activity times (s) | $17.2 \pm 26.0$ | $20.0 \pm 49.7$ | 0.761 |

Values are expressed as mean ± standard deviation (SD). NRS: Numerical Rating Scale; CST: Chair Stand Test; TUG: Timed Up-and-Go test; GDS-15: 15-item version of the Geriatric Depression Scale; PCS: Pain Catastrophizing Scale.

($p = 0.027$). We found no significant difference in the pre-intervention and postintervention mean values within the intervention group.

### 3.2.2. Effects of the Interventions on the Secondary Outcomes for Both Groups.

The mean daily step count in the intervention group increased by 20.0% (from $4312.9 \pm 2392.5$ to $5175.7 \pm 3126.1$) and that in the control group decreased by 3.1% (from $4030.2 \pm 2266.5$ to $3918.6 \pm 1870.3$). The mean daily step count and moderate activity time at 12 weeks after intervention in the intervention group were significantly better than those in the control group ($p = 0.039$ and $p = 0.017$,

resp.). Within the intervention group, the mean daily step count and mild activity time at 12 weeks after intervention improved significantly compared with the preintervention values ($p = 0.006$ and $p = 0.015$, resp.). No similar improvement was seen in the control group values.

We found no significant differences in mean CST and TUG scores at 12 weeks after intervention between the two groups. Within both groups, the mean at 12 weeks after intervention had improved significantly compared with the preintervention values ($p < 0.001$).

We found no significant differences in mean values at 12 weeks after intervention for GDS-15, total PCS, rumination, helplessness, and magnification scores between the two

TABLE 2: Group comparisons of outcome measures during the intervention period.

| Item | Intervention group (n = 35) | | | Control group (n = 35) | | | Time-by-group interaction | |
|---|---|---|---|---|---|---|---|---|
| | Preintervention | After 12 weeks | Mean difference | Preintervention | After 12 weeks | Mean difference | F value | p value |
| Total number of pain sites | $1.7 \pm 1.4$ | $1.3 \pm 1.1^a$ | $-0.3 \pm 1.0$ | $2.0 \pm 2.0$ | $2.2 \pm 1.6$ | $0.2 \pm 1.7$ | 2.622 | 0.110 |
| NRS at the site of maximum pain | $2.3 \pm 2.1$ | $2.1 \pm 1.6^a$ | $-0.2 \pm 1.5$ | $2.7 \pm 2.4$ | $3.6 \pm 2.4^b$ | $0.9 \pm 3.2$ | 3.642 | 0.060 |
| CST (s) | $7.7 \pm 2.8$ | $7.0 \pm 2.5^b$ | $-0.7 \pm 1.4$ | $7.4 \pm 2.0$ | $6.7 \pm 1.8^b$ | $-0.7 \pm 1.0$ | 0.012 | 0.913 |
| TUG (s) | $7.6 \pm 1.7$ | $7.0 \pm 1.3^b$ | $-0.6 \pm 1.0$ | $7.6 \pm 1.6$ | $7.2 \pm 1.7^b$ | $-0.5 \pm 0.7$ | 0.529 | 0.469 |
| GDS-15 score (points) | $3.0 \pm 3.3$ | $2.5 \pm 3.1$ | $-0.5 \pm 2.0$ | $2.7 \pm 2.9$ | $2.6 \pm 2.4$ | $-0.1 \pm 2.3$ | 0.490 | 0.486 |
| PCS total score (points) | $23.0 \pm 13.3$ | $20.8 \pm 11.5$ | $-2.2 \pm 8.1$ | $23.4 \pm 11.1$ | $23.6 \pm 12.9$ | $0.2 \pm 10.2$ | 1.200 | 0.277 |
| Rumination score (points) | $10.7 \pm 6.2$ | $9.6 \pm 5.4$ | $-1.1 \pm 3.8$ | $10.8 \pm 4.7$ | $11.3 \pm 5.4$ | $0.5 \pm 4.9$ | 2.271 | 0.136 |
| Helplessness score (points) | $7.2 \pm 4.8$ | $7.0 \pm 4.1$ | $-0.2 \pm 3.8$ | $7.6 \pm 4.3$ | $7.5 \pm 4.9$ | $-0.1 \pm 4.5$ | 0.005 | 0.947 |
| Magnification score (points) | $4.9 \pm 3.6$ | $4.2 \pm 2.9$ | $-0.7 \pm 2.2$ | $5.2 \pm 3.3$ | $4.9 \pm 3.2$ | $-0.3 \pm 2.5$ | 0.660 | 0.419 |
| Daily step counts (steps) | $4312.9 \pm 2392.5$ | $5175.7 \pm 3126.1^{ab}$ | $862.8 \pm 1933.9$ | $4030.2 \pm 2266.5$ | $3918.6 \pm 1870.3$ | $-111.6 \pm 1630.9$ | 5.445 | 0.022 |
| Mild activity times (s) | $2394.2 \pm 1399.9$ | $2774.8 \pm 1550.8^b$ | $457.7 \pm 1037.3$ | $2382.8 \pm 1158.3$ | $2385.0 \pm 1049.1$ | $2.2 \pm 844.2$ | 3.218 | 0.077 |
| Moderate activity times (s) | $428.1 \pm 545.1$ | $555.3 \pm 689.8^a$ | $143.9 \pm 422.9$ | $303.0 \pm 442.0$ | $255.7 \pm 286.0$ | $-47.3 \pm 341.4$ | 3.801 | 0.055 |
| Heavy activity times (s) | $16.6 \pm 26.9$ | $18.1 \pm 29.4$ | $1.6 \pm 31.2$ | $20.0 \pm 49.7$ | $20.5 \pm 40.8$ | $0.5 \pm 35.1$ | 0.016 | 0.900 |

Values are expressed as mean ± standard deviation (SD). NRS: Numerical Rating Scale; CST: Chair Stand Test; TUG: Timed Up-and-Go test; GDS-15: 15-item version of the Geriatric Depression Scale; PCS: Pain Catastrophizing Scale. [a]Significant group difference ($p < 0.05$), [b]Significant preintervention to postintervention difference ($p < 0.05$).

groups. There were also no significant within-group differences in the mean values between the preintervention and postintervention time points.

## 4. Discussion

This randomized controlled trial revealed that a community-based intervention program that combined exercise training with increased physical activity effectively improved physical activity and prevented worsening of pain intensity in older adults without chronic pain. In Japan, the front-runner of "super-aged societies," efforts to extend healthy life expectancy are needed because the number of community-dwelling older adults who require long-term care has increased because of rapid population aging. In addition, the development of an effective intervention to prevent chronic pain is urgently needed because the proportion of older adults with chronic pain is high, and chronic pain is associated with the need for long-term care. Our data suggest that exercise training in combination with increased physical activity is beneficial in preventing chronic pain in older adults who have not yet experienced chronic pain. Consequently, this study is both novel and important, because, to the best of our knowledge, it is the first to test the efficacy of a community-based intervention program for preventing chronic pain in older adults.

Again, to the best of our knowledge, no previous studies have investigated the preventive effects of a community-based intervention program on pain in community-dwelling older adults without chronic pain, as most studies have targeted individuals with chronic pain [1, 12, 14]. In previous animal model studies that used mice, Sluka et al. [13]

reported that an 8-week wheel-running activity intervention effectively prevented decreases in muscle withdrawal thresholds and increased responses to mechanical stimulation of the paw for up to 72 hours after the noninflammatory pain model was induced with two injections of unbuffered pH 4.0 saline into one gastrocnemius muscle 5 days apart, compared with sedentary controls. Grace et al. [22] showed that a 6-week voluntary wheel-running intervention with mice before chronic constriction injury prevented the full development of allodynia for up to 3 months duration of the injury. These studies suggest that increased physical activity is beneficial for preventing chronic pain. In the current study, to increase physical activity, participants in the intervention group were given pedometers and daily diaries and asked to record their daily step counts. Additionally, physical therapists who supported the community exercise classes checked participants' diaries once a week and advised them to progressively increase their daily step counts during the 12-week intervention period. As a result, we found a time-by-group interaction for daily step counts, with participants in the intervention group showing significant improvement and moderate activity times 12 weeks after intervention compared with the control group. Moreover, the total number of pain sites and maximum pain site scores improved significantly compared with the control group 12 weeks after intervention in the intervention group. Consequently, our results suggest that exercise training combined with increased physical activity effectively improves physical activity levels, which leads to a relatively low number of total pain sites and decreased pain intensity, ultimately preventing the development of chronic pain in older adults. In the control group, pain scores at the maximum pain site 12 weeks after intervention significantly worsened compared with the equivalent preintervention value, and no significant difference was observed in the preintervention and postintervention within the intervention group. These results may suggest that only exercise intervention once a week is insufficient to decrease pain intensity and to prevent the development of chronic pain; however, exercise training combined with increased physical activity can prevent the development of chronic pain. Although the detailed mechanism is unclear, increasing physical activity would be important in preventing chronic pain, because participants' physical activity levels did not change in the control group, but it increased in the intervention group.

Within both groups, CST and TUG scores, as markers of lower extremity muscle strength [16] and walking ability [17], improved significantly during the 12-week intervention period, and there were no significant differences in the mean values at 12 weeks after intervention between the two groups. Previous studies have reported that exercise programs that involve muscle strength and balance training significantly improve physical function in community-dwelling older adults, according to CST and TUG scores [6, 23]. Our results were similar to those of previous studies and suggested that exercise training leads to improved physical function in community-dwelling older adults without chronic pain.

Regarding the psychological status, there were no significant differences in the mean GDS-15 and PCS values at 12 weeks after intervention between the two groups. Vlaeyen and Linton [24] showed that pain-related catastrophizing is an important factor in the development of chronic pain, which can cause disability, depression, and low physical activity levels. Our previous study [14] revealed that a psychosocial intervention that leads to improved PCS scores effectively decreases pain intensity and improves physical activity levels in older adults with chronic pain. The findings of the abovementioned studies suggest that intervention programs that modify the cognitive aspects of pain are beneficial in older adults suffering from chronic pain. In the present study, the participants' psychological status may not have changed because our study targeted older adults without chronic pain, and as such the provision of an intervention program to modify the cognitive aspects of pain was out of scope.

During this study, no study-related adverse events occurred. The intervention and control groups had similarly low withdrawal rates and high rates of participation in the exercise sessions. These findings suggest that exercise training combined with increased physical activity was widely embraced by the participants and is a safe and feasible intervention during community-based exercise classes.

Our study has several limitations. The first limitation is that the physical therapists who assessed the participants also conducted the intervention programs. Therefore, our results may have been influenced by the physical therapists' expertise and/or reporting bias during the community exercise classes. In saying this, all the physical therapists who participated in the study received the same level of training from a senior physical therapist before the trial began, and we videotaped the exercise program to ensure consistency. Therefore, we believe that the physical therapists' expertise had only minimal effects on the study results. The second limitation is that our 12-week intervention period was relatively short. Therefore, further study is needed to evaluate the long-term benefits of this preliminary randomized controlled trial.

## 5. Conclusions

An intervention program that involved exercise training combined with increased physical activity, with the aim of developing a chronic pain prevention program to extend healthy life expectancy, improved pain and physical activity levels more effectively than exercise training alone in a sample of older adults without chronic pain. The intervention program was widely embraced by these older adults. Therefore, we believe that exercise training combined with increased physical activity is an effective and feasible intervention program to prevent the development of chronic pain in community-dwelling older adults.

## Acknowledgments

This work was supported by the Japan Society for the Promotion of Science KAKENHI (Grant no. JP17H06959). The authors acknowledge Mr. Tatsuya Jinnouchi, Mr. Kengo Shibahara, Mr. Shohei Sakai, Mr. Tomohide Matsumoto, and Miss. Kanami Sakuta for their contributions to data collection. The authors also acknowledge Takako Matsubara, Ph.D., for guidance in this research.

## References

[1] M. C. Reid, C. Eccleston, and K. Pillemer, "Management of chronic pain in older adults," *BMJ*, vol. 350, p. h532, 2015.
[2] T. Hirase, H. Kataoka, S. Inokuchi, J. Nakano, J. Sakamoto, and M. Okita, "Factors associated with chronic musculoskeletal pain in Japanese community-dwelling older adults: a cross-sectional study," *Medicine*, vol. 96, no. 23, p. e7069, 2017.
[3] Y. Kaiho, Y. Sugawara, K. Sugiyama et al., "Impact of pain on incident risk of disability in elderly Japanese: cause-specific analysis," *Anesthesiology*, vol. 126, no. 4, pp. 688–696, 2017.
[4] S. Tokudome, S. Hashimoto, and A. Igata, "Life expectancy and healthy life expectancy of Japan: the fastest graying society in the world," *BMC Research Notes*, vol. 9, no. 1, p. 482, 2016.
[5] T. Tsutsui and N. Muramatsu, "Japan's universal long-term care system reform of 2005: containing costs and realizing a vision," *Journal of the American Geriatrics Society*, vol. 55, no. 9, pp. 1458–1463, 2007.
[6] M. Hasegawa, S. Yamazaki, M. Kimura, K. Nakano, and S. Yasumura, "Community-based exercise program reduces chronic knee pain in elderly Japanese women at high risk of requiring long-term care: a non-randomized controlled trial," *Geriatrics and Gerontolology International*, vol. 13, no. 1, pp. 167–174, 2013.
[7] S. Inokuchi, N. Matsusaka, T. Hayashi, and H. Shindo, "Feasibility and effectiveness of a nurse-led community exercise programme for prevention of falls among frail elderly people: a multi-centre controlled trial," *Journal of Rehabilitation Medicine*, vol. 39, no. 6, pp. 479–485, 2007.

[8] S. Nishiguchi, M. Yamada, T. Tanigawa et al., "A 12-week physical and cognitive exercise program can improve cognitive function and neural efficiency in community-dwelling older adults: a randomized controlled trial," *Journal of the American Geriatrics Society*, vol. 63, no. 7, pp. 1355–1367, 2015.

[9] M. Nakamura, Y. Nishiwaki, T. Ushida, and Y. Toyama, "Prevalence and characteristics of chronic musculoskeletal pain in Japan," *Journal of Orthopaedic Science*, vol. 16, no. 4, pp. 424–432, 2011.

[10] S. Inoue, F. Kobayashi, M. Nishihara et al., "Chronic pain in the Japanese community-prevalence, characteristics and impact on quality of life," *PLoS One*, vol. 10, no. 6, article e0129262, 2015.

[11] M. Suka and K. Yoshida, "The national burden of musculoskeletal pain in Japan: projection to the year 2055," *Clinical Journal of Pain*, vol. 25, no. 4, pp. 313–319, 2009.

[12] J. Park and A. K. Hughes, "Nonpharmacological approaches to the management of chronic pain in community-dwelling older adults: a review of empirical evidence," *Journal of the American Geriatrics Society*, vol. 60, no. 3, pp. 558–568, 2012.

[13] K. A. Sluka, J. M. O'Donnell, J. Danielson, and L. A. Rasmussen, "Regular physical activity prevents development of chronic pain and activation of central neurons," *Journal of Applied Physiology*, vol. 114, no. 6, pp. 725–733, 2013.

[14] T. Hirase, H. Kataoka, J. Nakano, S. Inokushi, J. Sakamoto, and M. Okita, "Effects of a psychosocial intervention programme combined with exercise in community-dwelling older adults with chronic pain: a randomized controlled trial," *European Journal of Pain*, vol. 22, no. 3, pp. 592–600, 2018.

[15] M. Yamada, S. Nishiguchi, N. Fukutani, T. Aoyama, and H. Arai, "Mail-based intervention for sarcopenia prevention increased anabolic hormone and skeletal muscle mass in community-dwelling Japanese older adults: the INE study," *Journal of the American Medical Directors Association*, vol. 16, no. 8, pp. 654–660, 2015.

[16] M. M. Gardner, D. M. Buchner, M. C. Robertson, and A. J. Campbell, "Practical implementation of an exercise-based falls prevention programme," *Age and Ageing*, vol. 30, no. 1, pp. 77–83, 2001.

[17] D. Podsiadlo and S. Richardson, "The timed up-and-go: a test of basic functional mobility for frail elderly persons," *Journal of the American Geriatrics Society*, vol. 39, no. 2, pp. 142–148, 1991.

[18] J. I. Sheikh and J. A. Yesavage, "Geriatric Depression Scale (GDS): recent findings and development of a shorter version," in *Clinical Gerontology: A Guide to Assessment and Intervention*, T. Brink, Ed., pp. 165–173, Haworth Press, New York, NY, USA, 1986.

[19] R. Iwaki, T. Arimura, M. P. Jensen, and H. Hosoi, "Global catastrophizing vs catastrophizing subdomains: assessment and associations with patient functioning," *Pain Medicine*, vol. 13, no. 5, pp. 677–687, 2012.

[20] M. J. Sullivan, S. R. Bishop, and J. Pivik, "The pain catastrophizing scale: development and validation," *Psychological Assessment*, vol. 7, no. 4, pp. 524–532, 1995.

[21] T. Matsubara, Y. C. Arai, K. Shimo et al., "Effects of cognitive-behavioral therapy on pain intensity and level of physical activity in Japanese patients with chronic pain: a preliminary quasi-experimental study," *Journal of Physical Therapy*, vol. 1, no. 2, pp. 49–57, 2010.

[22] P. M. Grace, T. J. Fabisiak, S. M. Green-Fulgham et al., "Prior voluntary wheel running attenuates neuropathic pain," *Pain*, vol. 157, no. 9, pp. 2012–2023, 2016.

[23] T. Hirase, S. Inokuchi, N. Matsusaka, and M. Okita, "Effects of a balance training program using a foam rubber pad in community-based older adults," *Journal of Geriatric Physical Therapy*, vol. 38, no. 2, pp. 62–70, 2015.

[24] J. W. S. Vlaeyen and S. J. Linton, "Fear-avoidance and its consequences in chronic musculoskeletal pain: a state of the art," *Pain*, vol. 85, no. 3, pp. 317–323, 2000.

# 15

# Pain Reconceptualisation after Pain Neurophysiology Education in Adults with Chronic Low Back Pain: A Qualitative Study

Richard King,[1] Victoria Robinson,[1] Helene L. Elliott-Button,[2] James A. Watson,[2] Cormac G. Ryan (iD),[2] and Denis J. Martin[2]

[1]The Pain Clinic, South Tees Hospitals NHS Foundation Trust, Middlesbrough TS3 4BW, UK
[2]Health and Social Care Institute, Teesside University, Middlesbrough TS1 3BA, UK

Correspondence should be addressed to Cormac G. Ryan; c.ryan@tees.ac.uk

Academic Editor: Federica Galli

Pain neurophysiology education (PNE) is an educational intervention for patients with chronic pain. PNE purports to assist patients to reconceptualise their pain away from the biomedical model towards a more biopsychosocial understanding by explaining pain biology. This study aimed to explore the extent, and nature, of patients' reconceptualisation of their chronic low back pain (CLBP) following PNE. Eleven adults with CLBP underwent semistructured interviews before and three weeks after receiving PNE. Interviews were transcribed verbatim and thematically analysed in a framework approach using four a priori themes identified from our previous research: (1) degrees of reconceptualisation, (2) personal relevance, (3) importance of prior beliefs, and (4) perceived benefit of PNE. We observed varying degrees of reconceptualisation from zero to almost complete, with most participants showing partial reconceptualisation. Personal relevance of the information to participants and their prior beliefs were associated with the degree of benefit they perceived from PNE. Where benefits were found, they manifested as improved understanding, coping, and function. Findings map closely to our previous studies in more disparate chronic pain groups. The phenomenon of reconceptualisation is applicable to CLBP and the sufficiency of the themes from our previous studies increases confidence in the certainty of the findings.

## 1. Introduction

Pain neurophysiology education (PNE) has become a commonly used educational intervention for patients with chronic pain. PNE is a cognitive behavioural-based intervention in that it aims to reduce inappropriate beliefs and maladaptive behaviours, in order to decrease pain and disability, by explaining the biology of pain to the patient [1]. A growing body of literature supports its effectiveness [2–10].

Patients with chronic pain, fuelled by health care professionals, often hold strong biomedical model beliefs that their pain is due to tissue damage [11–14]. A number of conceptual models have proposed that such inappropriate beliefs can lead to the development/ maintenance of chronic pain. Within the fear-avoidance model, when pain is perceived as threatening, catastrophic thinking can result in pain-related fear and anxiety, leading to avoidance behaviour, disability, and a vicious cycle of chronic pain [15]. Additionally, as proposed within the model of misdirected problem-solving, inappropriate beliefs about tissue damage housed within a medical model framework can lead patients with chronic pain to repetitively seek solutions to remove their pain, moving from one treatment to the next, stuck within a *perseverance loop*. Each unsuccessful solution amplifies the condition and can prevent the patient from reframing their efforts away from an arguably unachievable goal of pain cessation to one of pursuing a *valued life in the presence of pain* [16].

A primary mechanism by which PNE purports to work is by helping patients better understand their pain and issues around its causes, correcting inappropriate beliefs—reconceptualising their pain [17]. Reconceptualisation can be defined by four key concepts: *(i) pain does not provide a measure of the state of the tissues; (ii) pain is modulated by many factors across somatic, psychological, and social domains; (iii) the relationship between pain and tissue becomes less predictable as pain persists; and (iv) pain can be conceptualised as a conscious correlate of the implicit perception that tissue is in danger* [17]. In theory, pain reconceptualisation should reduce the commonly perceived fear that pain is a clear signal of tissue damage by dispelling the notion that pain is an accurate indication of the state of tissue. Reduction of this fear may lead to reduced pain-related fear, distress, and disability; improved physical and mental health [15, 18]; an escape from the perseverance loop identified within the misdirected problem-solving model [16]; and potentially reduced levels of pain [8].

Only a few studies have been carried out exploring the phenomenon of reconceptualisation as a key mechanism of PNE. Evidence that PNE improves participants' knowledge of pain neurophysiology and reduces fear avoidance and pain catastrophising has been used to imply that reconceptualisation is a key factor [3, 4, 19, 20]. However, the narrow scope of the outcome measures (using structured questionnaires) in these studies provides limited insight into the complex phenomenon of pain reconceptualisation, and a validated questionnaire for the measurement of reconceptualisation has not been developed. At this stage of the development of evidence, qualitative methodology is better suited to studying pain reconceptualisation as it allows for an indepth exploration of multifaceted phenomenon [21] such as reconceptualisation. Our previous studies have found that patients with chronic pain often hold conflicting views about the cause/nature of their pain. Qualitative methods can help to reveal and explore these conflicting complex beliefs to an extent that quantitative methods cannot [22].

Two recent qualitative studies completed by our group identified the level of pain reconceptualisation following a single 2-hour session of PNE in patients with chronic pain as "partial and patchy" [23, 24]. However, where degrees of reconceptualisation were evident, we also saw clinical improvements, supporting the idea that reconceptualisation is a central mechanism of PNE's effect. A notable finding was the importance of relevance of PNE to the individual's specific experience as opposed to being relevant to a more general experience of living with pain [23, 24]. The participants included in these two studies were from a range of pain conditions including multisite pain, lower back pain (with and without leg pain), thoracic pain, throat pain, complex regional pain syndrome, neck pain, and upper limb pain. A key factor which may impact upon relevance to the patient is their pain condition and how they perceive PNE fits with their symptoms. Poor perceived fit between symptoms and PNE may reduce perceived relevance for the patient. "*For me personally I didn't think it was any good for the symptoms that I have... it was for more for people with different parts of the body pain and not the one I have*" [24].

Thus, looking at the experience of PNE for specific pain populations may be important.

In Robinson et al. [23], four participants out of a total of 10 demonstrated some evidence of reconceptualisation following PNE. All four had multisite pain. In contrast, two of the four participants with chronic low back pain (CLBP) reported that PNE was not relevant to them, they perceived no benefit, and showed no signs of reconceptualisation. Within educational theory, conceptual change requires a dissatisfaction with one's current understanding of a concept [25]. For many, perhaps most people, there is a strong belief that back pain can be readily aligned with the medical/tissue injury model [26]. This gives rise to the possibility that they may be more accepting of a biomedical explanation and thus less open to reconceptualisation than people with multisite pain or painful conditions that defy the logic of a medical model explanation. It may also be that they are less likely to have encountered an alternative explanation for their pain beyond the medical model. This corresponds with observations we made from previous work [24], where a participant with CRPS, a condition that fits poorly with the medical model, demonstrated pain reconceptualisation following PNE and showed clear signs of an awareness and understanding of pain hypersensitivity before receiving PNE.

Chronic low back pain (CLBP) is a particularly important pain subgroup to focus upon as it is one of the most common pain conditions globally and it is the largest single cause of disability-adjusted life years (2,313 per 100,000 population) in the UK [27]. The National Institute for Health and Care Excellence (NICE) estimates that back pain costs the UK economy over 2.1 billion annually [28]. Considering the potential importance of the person's pain condition with respect to perceived relevance, reconceptualisation, and ultimately the effectiveness of PNE, there is a need to explore pain reconceptualisation in people with CLBP following PNE. In doing so, new approaches to tailoring and enhancing this education specifically for patients with CLBP may be identified. Thus, the aim of this study was to investigate the extent, and nature, of people's reconceptualisation of their CLBP following PNE.

## 2. Materials and Methods

*2.1. Design.* We used the approach of theoretical thematic analysis [29] with a focus towards deductive analysis to explore the applicability of the themes we had found in our previous work on people with chronic pain in general [23, 24] to a group with CLBP only. Due to the heterogeneity of this study sample, we felt that it was important to be open to exploring the data for any additional/new themes that may emerge. To reflect this, we also used inductive analysis.

*2.2. Recruitment and Sample.* Participants were recruited from a single site—an NHS pain clinic in the North East of England. We aimed to recruit a convenience sample of 10–12 participants. While no formal guidelines exist with respect to sample size estimation for qualitative studies, it has been proposed that in studies where the aim is to understand common perceptions and experiences, twelve interviews should be sufficient [30]. Patients were eligible for inclusion if they had been referred to PNE as part of their usual care, were ≥18 years of age, and if their primary complaint was chronic (>6 months duration) lower back pain (±leg symptoms) of a neuro/musculoskeletal origin. All referrals were made by consultants in pain management following assessment. None of the participants required spinal or orthopaedic surgery.

Patients were excluded from the study if their level of English was not judged suitable enough to take part in an interview or if their pain was not primarily associated with the musculoskeletal system such as neurological conditions. To limit any feeling of coercion, patients of the interviewer (RK) were also excluded from taking part in the study. Patients with the primary complaint of LBP who had been referred to PNE as part of their usual care were sent a brief information sheet regarding the study. Following this, the patient was contacted by a research assistant and asked if they would like to receive more information regarding the study. If they did, this information was sent to them and they were contacted to see if they would like to participate. Data were collected between September and November 2014. This study was approved by NRES Committee Yorkshire and The Humber – Sheffield (REC Reference number: 14/YH/0153). Written informed consent was obtained from all participants before they entered the study. On completion of data collection, all data were fully anonymised.

*2.3. Intervention.* All participants in this study received PNE as part of their routine usual NHS care. The PNE session was heavily based upon the manual *Explain pain* [1]. The PNE session was delivered in a group setting of 10–12 patients with chronic pain. The patients within the groups were heterogeneous with respect to their clinical condition; however, only people with CLBP were recruited into this study. Thus, the PNE delivered was not back pain specific. The intervention was delivered by two experienced, pain specialist physiotherapists who have worked within the pain setting for >5 years each, had undertaken postgraduate training in pain, and attended *Explain Pain* courses delivered by the Neuro Orthopaedic Institute. Published service evaluation data have shown that patients with chronic pain who receive PNE at this clinic demonstrate average increases in pain knowledge in keeping with increases reported in the literature [31, 32].

*2.4. Data Collection.* Participants underwent a semi-structured interview one week prior to PNE. The interview script is provided in Supplementary Material (available here). The pre-PNE interview focused on beliefs about the nature, cause, and experiences of their pain. Three weeks after PNE, participants were reinterviewed by the same researcher using the same semi-structured approach. Participants were asked the same questions as in the first interview but were also asked to reflect on any change in their

understanding of their pain. All interviews took place in the hospital in a private room lasting approximately one hour, with only the interviewer and participant present. They were audio recorded and transcribed verbatim for thematic analysis.

*2.5. Analysis.* The primary analysis of the data was conducted by RK using NVivo software (version 10), following the guidelines for theoretical thematic analysis outlined by Braun and Clarke [29]. Each transcript was read multiple times and statements were coded according to their meaning. Coded statements were grouped together into four a priori themes that we found in our previous work [23, 24]—degrees of reconceptualisation, personal relevance, importance of prior beliefs, and perceived benefit of PNE. We also provided for the emergence of themes that did not fit with the above.

To ensure dependability, all views were treated equally. Three weeks following the second interview, RK telephoned all participants to verify that he had an accurate interpretation of the participants account. Only 8 participants could be contacted. During the telephone conversation, extracts from the interview were described to the participant to assess/verify if the researcher had made an appropriate interpretation of the interview comments. In all cases, the participants agreed with the interpretation of the account. Therefore, no amendments were made. The average duration of the telephone conversation was 12 minutes. Following this process, a second researcher (HE) read all the transcripts to ensure the themes were logical and rooted in the data. To increase credibility, the results were circulated throughout the rest of the research team for further refinement and to be collected into a coherent account.

Evidence for or against the a priori themes was sought from participants' subjective accounts and changes were explored by comparing participants' pre- and post-PNE interviews.

*2.6. Reflexivity.* Reflexivity relates to the amount of influence the researcher—consciously or unconsciously—has on the outcome of the study and can be defined as *"a continuous process of reflection by the researcher on their values, preconceptions, behaviour, or presence and those of the participant which can affect interpretation of responses"* [33]. Therefore, disclosure of the researchers' standpoints allows the reader to consider how this might have impacted on the findings. To this end, four of the researchers (RK, VR, JW, and CR) have experience of delivering PNE. RK and VR have extensive experience in pain management (6 and 11 years' full-time physiotherapists in pain management, resp.), regularly deliver PNE as part of their clinical practice, and have undertaken professional training to do so. It is their (RK, VR, JW, and CR) belief that PNE is a clinically useful intervention; however, they have no vested interest in the outcome of this study. DM and HE do not have experience of delivering PNE clinically. Their involvement is from a research method's perspective. They support the potential

TABLE 1: Participant demographics and thematic analysis for each of the four a priori themes.

| Id | Age (yrs) | Sex | Duration of pain (yrs) | Work status | Pre | | Post | | | |
|----|-----------|-----|------------------------|-------------|-----|-----|------|-----|-----|-----|
| | | | | | Belief that pain may not be due to tissue damage | Awareness of an emotion-pain relationship | Tissue damage reconceptualisation | Role of emotion reconceptualisation | Personal relevance | Perceived benefit |
| P1 | 42 | F | 22.0 | Unemployed | No | No | Partial | Yes | Yes | Yes |
| P2 | 51 | M | 26.0 | Unemployed | No | Partial | Partial | No | Yes | Yes |
| P3 | 44 | F | 6.0 | Employed | No | Yes | Partial | Partial | Yes | Yes |
| P4 | 29 | M | 3.0 | Employed | Yes | Yes | Yes | Yes | Yes | Yes |
| P6 | 25 | F | 4.5 | Employed | | | | | | |
| P7 | 46 | F | 10.0 | Unemployed | Yes | Yes | Partial | Yes | Yes | Yes |
| P8 | 55 | M | 8.0 | Retired | No | Partial | Partial | No | No | No |
| P9 | 72 | F | 5.0 | Retired | No | Yes | No | No | Unclear | No |
| P10 | 40 | F | 22 .0 | Employed | No | No | Partial | No | Unclear | — |
| P11 | 62 | F | 0.7 | Retired | No | Partial | No | No | No | No |
| P12 | 56 | M | 7.0 | Employed | No | No | No | No | No | — |
| P14 | 58 | M | 3.0 | Employed | Yes | Partial | Yes | — | Yes | Yes |

Participant's prior beliefs, degree of reconceptualisation, perceived relevance of PNE, and perceptions of benefit are shown. The tissue damage reconceptualisation and role of emotion reconceptualisation categories looked at change from pre-PNE. Blank (—) spaces indicate that the issue was not discussed. "Yes" and "No" are used when there was clear evidence related to the theme and partial when there was tentative evidence. Unclear is used when the issue was discussed, but it could not be determined whether the evidence supported or refuted the issue. P6 did not provide a second interview. F = females, M = male.

underlying theory of reconceptualisation and remain open to the theories being shaped by evidence.

## 3. Results

Out of 12 participants initially recruited, only 11 provided a pre- and postinterview. One participant did not provide a postinterview (Participant 6). This individual did not supply a reason for this and we did not have ethical approval to approach her to find out why she did not attend (Table 1). Of the 12 participants, 7 were female and 5 were male. All participants were diagnosed with low back pain of greater than 6 months duration. The average (range) duration of pain was 10 years and 4 months (8 months–26 years). The average (range) age of participants was 48 years (25–72 years). Of the 12 participants, 3 were unemployed, 6 were employed, and 3 were retired. Participants ranged from having no qualifications to holding a BSc (Hons) degree. A summary of how each participant was analysed against the a priori themes is shown in Table 1. Additional themes, beyond those identified a priori, did not emerge from the data.

*3.1. Theme 1: Degrees of Reconceptualisation.* No evidence for reconceptualisation was found in the accounts of Participants 9, 11, and 12. Following PNE, their explanations of the current cause of their pain were expressed exclusively in biomedical language, as was the case before PNE.

*"When they done the MRI, when they done that, they discovered I had this impingement in my spine."* (P9 pre)

*"The reason why I'm in pain? Because of my impingement..."* (P9 post)

We observed evidence of reconceptualisation in the accounts of P1, 2, 3, 4, 7, 8, and 10. This evidence took various forms: language that no longer discussed pain in purely biomedical terms, the use of neurophysiological terms in a way that was not evident in the interviews before PNE, new language about the links between pain and emotions.

P10's shift from an entirely biomedical view of her pain to becoming open to the idea that such an explanation may not be sufficient is illustrative.

*"...I won't have that made as an excuse for this because there's something real happening in my back. I think there's something wrong with my discs."* (P10 pre)

*"...there might not be [a structural] explanation for it...as it was explained in the session last week, it might not be structural."* (P10 post)

For P1, 2, 3, 7, and 8, we considered the evidence for reconceptualisation as *partial and patchy* because the language consistent with reconceptualisation was accompanied by the language that was consistent with a biomedical understanding of pain. For example, in her interview before PNE, P1's response to being asked about the cause of her back pain was

*"Sclerosis...I know I've got disc degeneration."* (P1 pre)

After PNE, she introduced neurophysiological language using the phrase "new nerve" in relation to neuroplasticity.

*"...it is the new nerve in sending the messages up..."* (P1 post)

while still describing the current cause of her pain in structural terms as before PNE.

*"I know I've got sclerosis of my lower back...whether the arthritis is starting to affect it more I don't know."* (P1 post)

Participant 4, however, showed strong signs of reconceptualisation that exceeded partial reconceptualisation. He demonstrated the clearest change from pre- to post-PNE with respect to his explanation of his pain and his appreciation of the role of psychosocial factors on his pain. Both showed a clear shift away from the medical model. Prior to PNE, the participant believed that the most likely cause of his back pain was a fracture that had shown up in an MRI scan based on consultations with two different health care professionals.

*"He showed me on the thing (MRI scan) with his finger, that looks like a stress fracture to your back."* (P4 pre)

*"He (the health care professional) said, and he believed that I've probably like fractured a couple of bones in my body."* (P4 pre)

After PNE, P4's explanation of his current pain was uniformly expressed in neurophysiological language with an absence of the biomedical language that had dominated the interview before PNE.

*"...any slight jarring, or anything like that, and it sends my back into spasm, which is like just basically creating a protective shell and it's so used to doing it it's on hypersensitive and I think that's generally why my pain is, and it's just not switching off...(Interviewer: What causes that hypersensitivity?) ...I think that's all those too much chemicals in my body."* (P4 post)

Also, he showed a clear change in understanding of the link between pain and mood from tenuous

*"...I won't completely reject it..."* (P4 pre)

to a full acceptance of the links.

*"...the psychology...and stuff like that is massive and knowing how your brain works and stuff like that is huge..."* (P4 post)

Participant 14 was a unique case. With a university-level educational background in biology, P14 had developed a clear understanding of pain mechanisms consistent with reconceptualisation as seen in his interview before PNE.

*"...I've had possibly a few back problems...and my back has picked up on this, if you like the nerve has picked up on this, it's sent the signals to the brain, the brain's sent it back down and it probably happens over two or three months."* (P14 pre)

That understanding did not change after PNE but was reinforced.

*3.2. Theme 2: Personal Relevance.* Even though he already had a clear understanding of pain mechanisms, P14 did find the session relevant to his own condition.

*"it all it did was to completely reaffirm the way that I was actually going or the way I'd actually thought before I came but you did it did help to if you like allay any I was going to say fears but it's not so much fears it's more concerns that I had in many ways, I'm going round the twist."* (P14 post)

Of the 7 participants in whose accounts we observed evidence of reconceptualisation, we counted 5 as having applied that reconceptualisation to their own particular circumstances—P1, 2, 3, 4, and 7. In other words, their new understanding had personal relevance. Typically, this was noted by clear use of the first person singular such as

*"...basically the cause of my pain, my pain is sort of constant..."* (P4 post)

and by clear statements discussing the relevance of the session.

*"...at the time things that she was explaining did make sense and how, you know, things just triggered and how it all moves around your body and your mind and everything...I could relate to it, I could relate to it."* (P7 post)

In contrast P8's account of reconceptualisation was more theoretical and related to a more general experience of living with pain, and when he described his own condition, the language was explicitly biomedical. Participants 9, 11, and 12 showed no clear evidence of relevance and indeed Participant 11 made it clear that she saw PNE as just another of the many things she was open to trying to help with her pain.

*"If you offered another session to me I'd still go, whether it was 100% relevant to me or not, I'll take anything that's going, I won't knock anything."* (P11 post)

Participant 12 also reported a lack of relevance. His problems were pain and numbness in his legs following back surgery that had reduced pain in his back and he lamented the lack of a particular focus on his personal circumstances in the session.

*"...I didn't get the chance to explain what my problems were...it was about pain in general but it wasn't targeted at myself or anybody specific, it was just like everybody."* (P12 post)

*3.3. Theme 3: Importance of Prior Beliefs.* Before PNE, all three participants in whom we found no reconceptualisation (P9, 11, and 12) believed that their current pain was caused by biomechanical factors and did not show any signs of dissatisfaction with this belief. The beliefs of Participants 9 and 12 were passive in that they had not really given other potential causative factors consideration while Participant 11 was actively opposed to any alternative explanation—indeed, she had walked out of a previous consultation when the clinician enquired about social issues.

*"...all she wanted to know about was my personal life and I walked out because I said I'm not here about anything other than a crash..."* (P11 pre)

Participant 8, whose reconceptualisation was general rather than personal, had a steadfast belief that his current pain was caused by damage to his facet joints. For the other six participants in whom we did find some reconceptualisation and relevance (P1, 2, 3, 4, 7, and 10), all apart from Participant 1 stated prior beliefs which demonstrated either a dissatisfaction with their existing biomedical explanation of the current pain.

*"...the only thing I've been told as well it's probably mechanical...I'm not convinced that it is mechanical, it's not the same kind of pain as on the left side..."* (P3 pre)

and/or an openness to a more biopsychosocial/ neurophysiological sensitisation explanation consistent with PNE.

*"I think I've got a lot of nerve, I know I've got a lot nerve damage...I think it's just those nerve endings suddenly coming alive again...I presume it's just that message going to my brain saying you're in pain, that's all I'm thinking you know, I don't know if that's correct."* (P7 pre)

*3.4. Theme 4: Perceived Benefit of PNE.*  Neither Participant 8 nor Participant 10 described any clinical benefit from their PNE session. In the case of P8, rather than showing a clinical benefit after PNE, he discussed scenarios that were at odds with the aims of PNE. Most marked were statements about restricting movement and activity because of the potential damage to structures in his back.

While he offered an explanation for back pain linked to neurophysiology following PNE,

*"... a build-up of the gateways being open permanently...allowing sensation to override..."*

he clearly continued to link his pain with tissue damage.

*"I think it's telling me be careful...because you don't want to aggravate an injury or a potential injury or something's going to happen if you continue with that activity."* (P8 post)

The context of this was that he was comfortable with the facet joint diagnosis that he had received and its plausibility was enhanced because he had experienced benefit from a stretching regime that he could rationalise in terms of that diagnosis. That ties in with his general rather than personal reconceptualisation.

P14 reported clinical benefit mainly in terms of reinforcement of his current understanding

*"...all it did was to completely reaffirm the way that I was actually going or the way that I'd actually thought before I came to you..."* (P14 post)

and clarification of some concerns that were causing him confusion.

*"...it did help to, if you like, allay any, I was going to say fears, but it's not so much fears, it's more concerns that I had in many ways, I'm going round the twist."* (P14 post)

The remaining participants who we considered to have showed various degrees of partial reconceptualisation (P1, 2, 3, 4, and 7) all spoke about benefits from PNE. These described improved understanding about their pain and its management;

*"It made a lot of sense as to why even though especially over the last three or four years and all they've been doing is upping the painkillers why I'm not getting the relief that I thought I would be getting off them."* (P3 post)

an increased ability to cope with pain;

*"...I suppose it's the acceptance what I've got out from this session is like to trying to accept the fact that you've got the pain for life and it's how that pain is managed is what makes life more manageable in itself."* (P2 post)

and functional improvements.

*"...when I was walking quite briskly I just slowed down. I thought, oh calm down you've got plenty of time to get there...where before I would have just carried on..."* (P7 post)

Here, P7 describes how her new understanding of her pain influenced her walking in a form of activity pacing to carry on functioning while still experiencing pain.

Those who did not show signs of reconceptualisation under our criteria (Participants 9, 11, and 12) showed neither personal relevance nor clinical benefit.

*"It was more interesting than useful."* (P11 post)

Participant 2 provided the first example in the literature of evidence of an adverse effect from PNE in that she found the session to be upsetting. She explained how the PNE instructor had given an example of someone who injured his back falling off a ladder and then found his pain triggered when he saw a ladder. From that example, Participant 2 recognised how she associated her back pain with childbirth and that now the presence of her child was acting as a trigger for her pain.

*"They made a reference to a person who had chronic back pain after having fallen off a ladder and every time they saw a ladder or had to go anywhere near a ladder it triggered the pain, made it worse, and although that's nothing like my situation it made me worry because my back pain is related to childbirth that the effects my pain was having on my family... I was upset to think that my pain was sometimes worse when my daughter was being more demanding and although that scenario that was given that person could spend a good quality of their life avoiding the situation, avoiding using a ladder, avoiding going near a ladder, I don't want to and couldn't even if I did want to avoid the situation of being a parent...I mean it was just that the pain could be associated to the cause and knowing the cause of my pain was my daughter initially though it wasn't her fault."* (P2 post)

## 4. Discussion

This study aimed to explore the extent, and nature, of patients' reconceptualisation of their CLBP following PNE. The study investigated if the findings from our previous studies on reconceptualisation with PNE for people with chronic pain were sufficient to describe the experience of people specifically with CLBP. We found that the a priori themes—degrees of reconceptualisation, personal relevance, importance of prior beliefs, and perceived benefit of PNE—were all clearly identifiable within the data and did indeed provide a good description of participants' accounts.

Our finding of partial and patchy reconceptualisation, whereby participants showed a range of degrees of reconceptualisation including none, is similar to what we found previously [23, 24]. Our earlier observation of the importance of prior beliefs applies here as well. This time, however, we found strong signs of reconceptualisation in one participant, P4. What was interesting was that his prior beliefs were not notably dissimilar to that of others.

The role of prior beliefs of participants within our study were in keeping with the four steps to accommodate a new scientific concept outlined by Posner et al. [25]: (1) dissatisfaction with current beliefs, (2) the new concept making sense to the person, (3) plausibility of the new concept, and (4) a belief that the new concept will be of practical help to the person. Broadly, those who showed no signs of reconceptualisation showed no signs of dissatisfaction with their existing biomedical explanation for their pain while the majority of those who did show signs of reconceptualisation were open to the neural sensitisation explanation of pain within PNE as plausible/relevant/potentially helpful.

P4 shows that it is possible to achieve advanced reconceptualisation after one session. However, for most, it seems that more sessions would be required. P14's report of clinical benefit further highlights the importance of the availability of follow-up education. This was someone who had already acquired a high level of reconceptualisation and was functioning at a high level but was suitably troubled to seek help from a pain clinic. His expressed need was clarification of some issues that were causing him problems.

Another finding in this study that we had not come across before was the distress experienced by P2. She reported the distress as happening during the session and it was evident at the time of the interview three weeks after. We do not have any insight into how long if at all the distress continued into the longer term. This is the first reporting of an adverse event associated with PNE in the literature. The participant was offered the opportunity to discuss their feelings with a clinical psychologist; however, they did not think this was necessary and therefore declined the offer.

The lack of long-term follow-up is a limitation of this study. Pain management is an ongoing process and this is an important gap in knowledge. As highlighted by the needs expressed by P14 for education despite having a long history of managing his pain successfully, it would be foolish to think that people would never need further education and advice. The lack of data saturation could also be viewed as a limitation of this study [34]. However, this study did not attempt to achieve data saturation. The need for data saturation in all qualitative studies has not been established and it has been proposed that using saturation as a generic marker of qualitative research quality is misplaced [35]. The sample size employed in this study is in keeping with previous recommendations for studies which aim to *understand common perceptions and experiences* within a homogenous group [30].

As we have previously demonstrated [23, 24], relevance was once again seen as catalytic in the clinical impact of PNE. Interestingly, in Participant 8, we found an example of a participant who had misinterpreted the information to reinforce their maladaptive beliefs and behaviour having come across this in one of our previous studies [24]. This may reflect a form of confirmation bias that has been noted in the learning of scientific concepts [36]. Again, this reinforces the need for follow-up education and support.

A strength of the study was the use of interviews before and after the PNE session, which allows greater insight into changes in beliefs than would be obtained by only interviewing people after PNE. The coherence of the themes between our previous work and the current findings lends confidence to the certainty of this evidence [37]. That said, at this stage, the findings are still subject to the limitations of qualitative research as outlined in our last study [24] with the findings being illustrative rather than representative with limitations determined by the delivery of PNE by way of a single session, the close proximity between the post-PNE interviews and the delivery of the session, and the restriction of the sample to people whose first language is English.

*4.1. Recommendations for Future Research.* Important further work is needed to develop a method, probably using a questionnaire, to allow quantification of reconceptualisation so that a statistical approach can be used to produce more representative findings. This would require careful preliminary work to develop such a questionnaire with appropriate validity and reliability of a potentially mercurial construct. A useful starting point could be the pain neurophysiology quiz which has been developed and revised as a method of assessing change in knowledge of pain physiology information [38]. Also, further work is required to extend the qualitative approach used here to explore the delivery issues stated above.

Given the importance of the personal relevance of the information provided to the patient in PNE identified in this study and our previous work [23, 24], PNE may be most effective when the information is tailored to the individual. This would be in keeping with Moseley who found that PNE was clinically more effective, though less cost-effective, when delivered in a one-to-one compared to a group setting [19]. Future work should explore if PNE delivered in a homogenous patient group setting (e.g., a group of patients with CLBP) facilitating a more tailored group approach would maximise both clinical and cost-effectiveness. Patient group-specific PNE curricula are already available for a range of specific pain groups including people with CLBP [39]. Another clinical approach to facilitate tailoring of the material, to enhance relevance, could be to have the educating therapist undertake a thorough examination of the patient prior to delivering PNE. The examination could be used as a way of identifying individual patient issues (e.g., anxieties, fears, and misconceptions) that could be specifically targeted during the education session. Again, future work should explore if this would enhance the effectiveness of PNE.

PNE may be most effective when delivered in combination with other interventions, such as exercise, compared with when it is delivered in isolation [8, 10] as in this study. It would be interesting to explore qualitatively the extent and nature of patients' pain reconceptualisation following PNE delivered as part of a comprehensive multimodal package of care. Finally, health care professional's beliefs about pain can influence their clinical management of their patients. PNE has been shown to enhance health care students' understanding of pain and increase their likelihood of making appropriate recommendations for patients in practice. [40, 41]. However, that work has been of a quantitative nature and there is a need to further explore health care professional student's experience of PNE and the extent and nature of their pain reconceptualisation qualitatively.

## 5. Conclusion

This study aimed to explore the extent, and nature, of patients' reconceptualisation of their CLBP following PNE using a set of a priori themes developed from previous research with heterogeneous samples of pain patients. We found that patients with CLBP who received PNE underwent varying levels of reconceptualisation, that the degree of reconceptualisation was influenced by previous beliefs and how relevant the information was deemed by the patient. Furthermore, the degree of reconceptualisation appeared to be related to the perceived benefit reported by the patient. No new themes beyond the a priori themes emerged. The findings were in keeping with our previous work, which included chronic pain participants from a range of clinical groups including multisite pain, back pain, and complex

regional pain syndrome. The applicability of the four a priori themes, developed in previous heterogeneous pain samples, indicates that the key experiences of PNE for those with back pain are similar to those identified within samples of patients consisting of heterogeneous pain groups.

## Acknowledgments

The study was funded by a Scheme B grant from the UK Chartered Society of Physiotherapy. The authors would like to thank all staff and participants who facilitated this study.

## References

[1] G. L. Moseley and D. S. Butler, *Explain Pain*, Noigroup Publications, Adelaide, Australia, 2003.

[2] G. L. Moseley, "Combining physiotherapy and education is efficacious for chronic low back pain," *Australian Journal of Physiotherapy*, vol. 48, no. 4, pp. 297–302, 2002.

[3] G. L. Moseley, "Unravelling the barriers to reconceptualization of the problem in chronic pain: the actual and perceived ability of patients and health professionals to understand the neurophysiology," *Journal of Pain*, vol. 4, no. 4, pp. 184–189, 2003.

[4] G. L. Moseley, M. Nicholas, and P. Hodges, "A randomised controlled trial of intensive neurophysiology education in chronic low back pain," *Clinical Journal of Pain*, vol. 20, no. 5, pp. 324–330, 2004.

[5] C. G. Ryan, H. G. Gray, M. Newton, and M. H. Granat, "Pain biology education and exercise classes compared to pain biology education alone for individuals with chronic low back pain: a pilot randomised controlled trial," *Manual Therapy*, vol. 15, no. 4, pp. 382–387, 2010.

[6] C. L. Clarke, C. G. Ryan, and D. J. Martin, "Pain neurophysiology education for the management of individuals with chronic low back pain: a systematic review and meta-analysis," *Manual Therapy*, vol. 16, no. 6, pp. 544–549, 2011.

[7] J. Van Oosterwijck, M. Meeus, L. Paul et al., "Pain physiology education improves health status and endogenous pain inhibition in fibromyalgia: a double-blind randomized controlled trial," *Clinical Journal of Pain*, vol. 29, no. 10, pp. 873–882, 2013.

[8] G. L. Moseley and D. S. Butler, "15 years of explaining pain–the past, present and future," *Journal of Pain*, vol. 16, no. 9, pp. 807–813, 2015.

[9] L. J. Geneen, D. J. Martin, N. Adams et al., "Effects of education to facilitate knowledge about chronic pain for adults: a systematic review with meta-analysis," *Systematic Reviews*, vol. 4, no. 1, p. 132, 2015.

[10] A. Louw, K. Zimney, E. J. Puentedura, and I. Diener, "The efficacy of pain neuroscience education on musculoskeletal pain: a systematic review of the literature," *Physiotherapy Theory and Practice*, vol. 32, no. 5, pp. 332–355, 2016.

[11] B. Darlow, M. Fullen, S. Dean, D. A. Hurley, G. D. Baxter, and A. Dowell, "The association between health care professional attitudes and beliefs and the attitudes and beliefs, clinical management, and outcomes of patients with low back pain: a systematic review," *European Journal of Pain*, vol. 16, no. 1, pp. 3–17, 2012.

[12] B. Darlow, A. Dowell, G. D. Baxter, F. Mathieson, M. Perry, and S. Dean, "The enduring impact of what clinicians say to people with low back pain," *Annals of Family Medicine*, vol. 11, no. 6, pp. 527–534, 2013.

[13] S. Bunzli, R. Watkins, A. Smith, R. Schütze, and P. O'Sullivan, "Lives on hold: a qualitative synthesis exploring the experience of chronic low-back pain," *Clinical Journal of Pain*, vol. 29, no. 10, pp. 907–916, 2013.

[14] I. B. Lin, P. B. O'Sullivan, J. A. Coffin, D. B. Mak, S. Toussaint, and L. M. Straker, "Disabling chronic low back pain as an iatrogenic disorder: a qualitative study in Aboriginal Australians," *BMJ Open*, vol. 3, no. 4, article e002654, 2013.

[15] M. Leeuw, M. E. Goossens, S. J. Linton, G. Crombez, K. Boersma, and J. W. Vlaeyen, "The fear-avoidance model of musculoskeletal pain: current state of scientific evidence," *Journal of Behavioral Medicine*, vol. 30, no. 1, pp. 77–94, 2007.

[16] C. Eccleston and G. Crombez, "Worry and chronic pain: a misdirected problem solving model," *Pain*, vol. 132, no. 3, pp. 233–236, 2007.

[17] G. L. Moseley, "Reconceptualising pain according to modern pain science," *Physical Therapy Reviews*, vol. 12, no. 3, pp. 169–178, 2007.

[18] C. Fletcher, L. Bradnam, and C. Barr, "The relationship between knowledge of pain neurophysiology and fear avoidance in people with chronic pain: a point in time, observational study," *Physiotherapy Theory and Practice*, vol. 32, pp. 271–276, 2016.

[19] G. L. Moseley, "Joining forces-combining cognition-targeted motor control training with group or individual pain physiology education: a successful treatment for chronic lower back pain," *Journal of Manual and Manipulative Therapy*, vol. 11, pp. 88–94, 2003.

[20] G. L. Moseley, "Evidence for a direct relationship between cognitive and physical change during an education intervention in people with chronic low back pain," *European Journal of Pain*, vol. 8, pp. 39–45, 2004.

[21] J. K. Magilvy and E. Thomas, "A first qualitative project. Qualitative descriptive design for novice researchers," *Journal for Specialists in Pediatric Nursing*, vol. 14, no. 4, pp. 298–300, 2009.

[22] C. Pope and N. Mays, "Researching the parts other methods cannot reach: an introduction to qualitative methods in health and health services research," *BMJ*, vol. 311, no. 6996, pp. 42–45, 1995.

[23] V. Robinson, R. King, C. G. Ryan, and D. J. Martin, "A qualitative exploration of people's experiences of pain neurophysiological education for chronic pain: the importance of relevance for the individual," *Manual Therapy*, vol. 22, pp. 56–61, 2016.

[24] R. King, V. Robinson, C. G. Ryan, and D. J. Martin, "An exploration of the extent and nature of reconceptualisation of pain following pain neurophysiology education: a qualitative study of experiences of people with chronic musculoskeletal pain," *Patient Education and Counseling*, vol. 99, no. 8, pp. 1389–1393, 2016.

[25] J. G. Posner, K. A. Strike, P. W. Hewson, and W. A. Gertzog, "Accommodation of a scientific conception: toward a theory of conceptual change," *Science Education*, vol. 66, no. 2, pp. 211–227, 1982.

[26] P. O'Sullivan, "It's time for change with the management of non-specific chronic low back pain," *British Journal of Sports Medicine*, vol. 46, no. 4, pp. 224–227, 2012.

[27] C. J. Murray, M. A. Richards, J. N. Newton et al., "UK health performance: findings of the Global Burden of Disease Study 2010," *The Lancet*, vol. 381, pp. 997–1020, 2013.

[28] NICE, *Low Back Pain: The Early Management of Persistent non-Specific Low Back Pain. NICE Clinical Guideline 88*, 2009, http://guidance.nice.org.uk/cg88.

[29] V. Braun and V. Clarke, "Using thematic analysis in psychology," *Qualitative Research in Psychology*, vol. 3, no. 2, pp. 77–101, 2006.

[30] G. Guest, A. Bunce, and L. Johnson, "How many interviews are enough? An experiment with data saturation and variability," *Field Methods*, vol. 18, no. 1, pp. 59–82, 2006.

[31] V. Robinson and R. King, ""Explain pain" as part of a pain management service improves patient's understanding of the neurophysiology of chronic pain," *Pain and Rehabilitation-The Journal of Physiotherapy Pain Association*, vol. 32, pp. 27–30, 2012.

[32] V. Robinson, R. King, and C. G. Ryan, "Pain neurophysiology education" as part of a pain management service decreases fear avoidance and improves patient's understanding of the neurophysiology of chronic pain at four months follow up," *Pain and Rehabilitation-The Journal of Physiotherapy Pain Association*, vol. 34, pp. 30–33, 2013.

[33] D. Jootun, G. McGhee, and G. R. Marland, "Reflexivity: promoting rigour in qualitative research," *Nurs Stand*, vol. 23, pp. 42–46, 2009.

[34] J. M. Morse, "The significance of saturation," *Qualitative Health Research*, vol. 5, no. 2, pp. 147–149, 1995.

[35] M. O'Reilly and N. Parker, ""Unsatisfactory saturation": a critical exploration of the notion of saturated sample sizes in qualitative research," *Qualitative Research*, vol. 13, no. 2, pp. 190–197, 2013.

[36] C. A. Chinn and W. F. Brewer, "The role of anomalous data in knowledge acquisition: A theoretical framework and implications for science instruction," *Review of Educational Research*, vol. 63, no. 1, pp. 1–49, 1993.

[37] S. Lewin, C. Glenton, H. Munthe-Kaas et al., "Using qualitative evidence in decision making for health and social interventions: an approach to assess confidence in findings from qualitative evidence syntheses (GRADE-CERQual)," *PLoS Medicine*, vol. 12, no. 10, article e1001895, 2015.

[38] M. J. Catley, N. E. O'Connell, and G. L. Moseley, "How good is the neurophysiology of pain questionnaire? A rasch analysis of psychometric properties," *Journal of Pain*, vol. 14, no. 8, pp. 818–827, 2013.

[39] G. L. Moseley and D. S. Butler, *Explain Pain Supercharged*, Noigroup Publications, Adelaide, Australia, 2017.

[40] G. Colleary, K. O'Sullivan, D. Griffin, C. G. Ryan, and D. J. Martin, "Effect of pain neurophysiology education on physiotherapy students' understanding of chronic pain, clinical recommendations and attitudes towards people with chronic pain: a randomised controlled trial," *Physiotherapy*, vol. 103, no. 4, pp. 423–429, 2017.

[41] N. Maguire, P. Chesterton, and C. G. Ryan, "The effect of pain neurophysiology education on sports therapy and rehabilitation students' knowledge, attitudes and clinical recommendations towards athletes with chronic pain," *Journal of Sport Rehabilitation*, pp. 1–19, 2018.

# 16

# An Assessment of Clinically Important Differences on the Worst Pain Severity Item of the Modified Brief Pain Inventory in Patients with Diabetic Peripheral Neuropathic Pain

**James Marcus®,[1] Kathryn Lasch ®,[2] Yin Wan,[1] Mei Yang,[3] Ching Hsu,[3] and Domenico Merante[4]**

[1]*Pharmerit International, Bethesda, MD, USA*
[2]*Pharmerit International, Boston, MA, USA*
[3]*Daiichi Sankyo, Inc., Basking Ridge, NJ, USA*
[4]*Daiichi Sankyo Development Ltd., Gerrards Cross, Buckinghamshire, UK*

Correspondence should be addressed to Kathryn Lasch; klasch@pharmerit.com

Academic Editor: Parisa Gazerani

*Objectives.* Using patient global impression of change (PGIC) as an anchor, an approximately 30% reduction on an 11-point numeric pain intensity rating scale (PI-NRS) is considered a clinically important difference (CID) in pain. Our objective was to define the CID for another pain measure, the worst pain severity (WPS) item of the modified Brief Pain Inventory (m-BPI). *Methods.* In this post hoc analysis of a double-blind, placebo-controlled, phase 2 study, 452 randomized patients with diabetic peripheral neuropathic pain (DPNP) were followed over 5 weeks, with m-BPI data collected weekly and PGIC at treatment conclusion. Receiver operating characteristic (ROC) curves (via logistic regression) were used to determine the changes in the m-BPI-WPS score that best predicted ordinal clinical improvement thresholds (i.e., "minimally improved" or better) on the PGIC. *Results.* Similar to the PI-NRS, a change of −3 (raw) or −33.3% from the baseline on the m-BPI-WPS optimized prediction for the "much improved" or better PGIC threshold and represents a CID. There was a high correspondence between observed and predicted PGIC categories at each PGIC threshold (ROC AUCs were 0.78–0.82). *Conclusions.* Worst pain on the m-BPI may be used to assess clinically important improvements in DPNP studies. Findings require validation in larger studies.

## 1. Introduction

Distal symmetric sensorimotor polyneuropathy, a significant complication of diabetes, is often associated with chronic neuropathic pain [1, 2]. Diabetic peripheral neuropathic pain (DPNP) affects approximately 50% of patients with diabetic neuropathy (16% of all diabetic patients) [3, 4] and has a substantial negative impact on patient functional status, work productivity, and quality of life [5–8]. Pain-related anxiety, depression, and sleep impairment and frequent comorbidity in patients with DPNP further exacerbate the patient burden [6–10].

Alleviation of pain is the cornerstone of patient management. A number of medications are approved or recommended

for treatment of DPNP [11–16]; however, pain relief is elusive because of issues of suboptimal effectiveness or tolerability [17, 18]. Although simple analgesics provide partial, short-term relief, sustained control of neuropathic pain requires therapies that are are more specifically targeted, better tolerated, and more effective over time [19].

Demonstrated effectiveness in terms of pain reduction, assessed using a patient-reported outcomes (PRO) measure, is essential for the approval of new pain treatments. However, the interpretability of an improvement in pain scores and whether they are truly meaningful and clinically relevant is equally important [20]. The emphasis on patient-centered care is highlighted in guidance issued by the US Food and Drug Administration (FDA) outlining the psychometric attributes (reliability, validity, and clinically meaningful score changes) that should be considered in the development of a PRO measure [21].

Pain rating scales, assessed using several different instruments, are widely used PRO measures [22]. In studies of chronic pain conditions, an 11-point pain intensity numeric rating scale (PI-NRS), ranging from 0 = no pain to 10 = worst possible pain, is the gold standard [20]. Farrar et al. [20] conducted an oft-cited study of the clinically important difference (CID) in pain improvement in which each morning, before taking study medication, the patients were asked to circle the number that best described their pain over the preceding 24 hours. An average daily pain score (ADPS) was calculated based on the responses. Farrar et al. recognized the importance of defining the level of changes on the PI-NRS that best reflects what patients consider to be a clinically important improvement. Data from 10 studies of pregabalin for the treatment of various chronic pain conditions ($N = 2879$) were used to determine numeric changes in the PI-NRS (e.g., −1 or −2) that were most closely associated with an improvement on the patient global impression of change (PGIC), a commonly used validated measure of patient global self-assessment of the health status [23]. The results suggested that a reduction of approximately 2 points on the PI-NRS (or 30% change) represented a CID.

The PI-NRS does not qualify the patient pain experience beyond its anchors 0 = "no pain" and 11 = "worst possible pain." Pain thresholds may differ among patients, and their largely subjective interpretation of the measurement scale may lead them to report on different facets of pain (e.g., average pain or worst pain) when responding to the PI-NRS—limiting the intrinsic meaning of its associated CID [24]. The Brief Pain Inventory (BPI), originally developed for assessment of cancer pain, is another commonly used PRO measure in chronic pain studies [25]. While the PI-NRS is typically used to assess average pain over the last 24 hours, the BPI characterizes an additional 3 dimensions of pain intensity (pain at its worst in the last 24 hours, pain at its least in the last 24 hours, and pain right now) measured using an 11-point NRS ranging from 0 = "no pain" to 10 = "pain as bad as you can imagine." By distinguishing between different types of pain, the BPI increases the likelihood that different patients will interpret a given question in a similar way. The BPI has been modified for use in other pain conditions, validated in numerous pain studies [26–32], and Farrar et al. [33] have defined a CID (change of 34%) on the worst pain item of the BPI based on data from duloxetine clinical trials of patients with DPNP and fibromyalgia. Since CID can vary depending on patient population and clinical context [34], it is important to show similar results for multiple pain indications.

The worst pain severity item of the BPI (BPI-WPS) has consistently demonstrated the highest reliability (internal consistency) across the BPI validation studies, and the psychometric properties of the worst pain item meet the standards set forth in the FDA guidance for PRO measures [35]. Moreover, in a recently issued draft guidance, the FDA recommended the use of an instrument that assesses worst pain over a relatively short period (no longer than 24 hours)

to measure the primary efficacy endpoint in clinical trials [36], making the BPI-WPS an optimal candidate for use in pivotal studies of chronic pain treatment.

In this post hoc analysis, our main objective was to evaluate the association of the worst pain severity item of the BPI, modified for use in patients with DPNP (m-BPI-WPS) [30], with improvements on the PGIC and to quantify numeric changes in worst pain scores that constitute a CID. A secondary objective was to evaluate the association of the worst and average pain severity items of the m-BPI with the ADPS derived from the standard PI-NRS.

## 2. Materials and Methods

*2.1. Patients and Study Design.* This post hoc analysis was based on data from a randomized, double-blind, placebo-controlled, active comparator-controlled, adaptive, proof-of-concept, phase 2 study of the efficacy and safety of mirogabalin monobenzenesulfonate (DS-5565, Daiichi Sankyo Co., Ltd., Tokyo, Japan, herein referred to as mirogabalin) for the treatment of DPNP (Clinicaltrials.gov identifier NCT01496365) [37–39]. The adaptive trial design enabled efficient determination of the optimal dosing for safety, while reducing safety risks for patients. A total of 452 adults with type 1 or 2 diabetes who met the study eligibility criteria were randomly assigned (the 2 : 1 : 1 : 1 : 1 : 1 : 1 ratio) to 1 of 7 treatment groups: placebo, dose-ranging mirogabalin (5, 10, 15, 20, and 30 mg/day), or pregabalin (300 mg/day) for 5 weeks. The study duration comprised approximately 9 weeks, reflecting an approximate 3-week screening/baseline period, a 5-week treatment period, and a 1-week follow-up period after the last dose of study medication or the end-of-treatment visit.

This study was conducted in accordance with the Declaration of Helsinki, the International Conference on Harmonisation (ICH) consolidated Guideline E6 for Good Clinical Practice, and all other applicable regulatory requirements. All patients provided written informed consent prior to participating in the study.

*2.2. Measures.* The study's primary efficacy measure was the change in the pain score from the baseline to week 5 or the end of study measured using the ADPS on the 11-point PI-NRS (0 = "no pain" to 10 = "worst possible pain"). The ADPS was calculated as the mean of the last 7 entries in the patients' daily diaries prior to randomization (baseline) and the last 7 entries while taking study medication (endpoint). Weekly change in ADPS was included as a secondary efficacy measure.

The m-BPI, the focus of this paper, was also included in the study as a secondary efficacy measure: its 4-item pain severity scale (pain at its worst in the past 24 hours, pain at its least in the past 24 hours, pain on the average, and pain right now) was assessed weekly from randomization through the end of treatment. A PGIC was assessed at the end of treatment on a 7-point PGIC categorical scale: "Since the start of the study, my overall status is . . ." 1 = very much improved, 2 = much improved, 3 = minimally improved,

4 = no change, 5 = minimally worse, 6 = much worse, and 7 = very much worse.

*2.3. Statistical Analyses.* The SAS software system (PC version 9.4, SAS Institute Inc., Cary, NC) was used to complete all data analyses. Following the methodology outlined by Farrar et al. [20], ordinal logistic regression analyses were used to evaluate the relationship between the worst pain (m-BPI-WPS) item and the PGIC. PGIC categories served as the dependent variable, and either the raw or the percentage change in m-BPI-WPS scores served as the independent variable.

The ordinal logistic regression, using raw or percent change in worst pain as a predictor, compares the cumulative odds of appearing in a given PGIC category or better: "very much improved" (i.e., PGIC scale 1 versus 2–7), "much improved" or better (i.e., PGIC scales 1–2 versus 3–7), and "minimally improved" or better (i.e., PGIC scales 1–3 versus 4–7). The predicted probabilities of appearing on a given side of discretized PGIC categories are compared against a range of cutoff thresholds to construct receiver operating characteristic (ROC) curves that plot the rate of correct predictions (observed PGIC matches prediction; sensitivity) versus false alarms (predicted to be in the higher category, but actually observed in the lower category; 1–specificity). The area under the ROC curve (AUC), reported as the *c* statistic from the logistic regression, represents the total overall association between the m-BPI-WPS score and the discretized PGIC category used to construct the specific curve (AUC/*c* is bounded from 0.50 to 1.00, where a value of 0.50 (i.e., the ROC diagonal) would indicate that worst pain has no ability to predict PGIC). Assuming equal importance of sensitivity and specificity, the probability cutoff that maximizes prediction using change in worst pain is located at the point at which sensitivity and specificity are the closest to being equal; this occurs at the intersection of a 45° tangent line with the ROC curve (the steepest rate of change) [20]. The probability cutoff that resulted in this intersection (i.e., point of sensitivity/specificity equality) can be recovered and compared to the predicted probabilities at each change score to find the change score with the closest match between its predicted probability and the optimal cutoff. In addition, the raw change of the m-BPI-WPS score was graphically displayed by PGIC categories using a box plot.

To address our secondary objective, polyserial correlations were used to understand the relationships among the various items of the m-BPI pain severity scale and the ADPS at study endpoint (week 5). Polyserial correlations are appropriate when examining the relationship between continuous (ADPS) and ordinal variables (individual items of the m-BPI) when it is assumed that the ordinal variable has an underlying continuous dimension [40]. A scale proposed by Chung [41] was used to describe the strength of the correlation coefficients, specifically 0.8 to 1.0 (very strong relationship), 0.6 to 0.8 (strong relationship), 0.4 to 0.6 (moderate relationship), 0.2 to 0.4 (weak relationship), and 0.0 to 0.2 (weak or no relationship). For items that had a strong correlation with the ADPS, regression analyses were

performed to better understand the direction of the correlation (i.e., the slope of the relationship) with the ADPS at week 5 as the dependent variable and the individual items of the m-BPI as independent variables.

# 3. Results

*3.1. ROC Curves for PGIC and Changes in the m-BPI-WPS Scores.* A total of 424 patients had nonmissing PGIC data. The box plot in Figure 1 shows the full distribution of the change in the m-BPI-WPS score for each PGIC category. This figure illustrates that almost all patients who considered themselves "minimally improved or better" (73%), "much improved or better" (44%), or "very much improved" (13%) had at least some decrease in the m-BPI-WPS score, and most of the patients had a decrease of 2 points or more.

Via ordinal logistic regression, a change in the m-BPI-WPS score was an effective predictor of the cumulative PGIC category, satisfying the proportional odds assumption $\chi^2(2) = 2.49$, $p = 0.29$, and achieving a proportional reduction in the error in predicting PGIC of $R^2_{\mathrm{Nag}} = 0.37$. Each 1-point reduction in worst pain increased the odds of advancing to a higher PGIC category by 1.69 (95% confidence interval: 1.55, 1.84).

While the m-BPI has 3 other pain measures—least, average, and pain now—they are not discussed further in the manuscript, either as separately or multivariately modeled predictors. Beyond the reasons cited at the end of Introduction for the primacy of worst pain, empirical evidence was collected for its primacy as well. There was compelling evidence for multicollinearity, with the correlations between the measures at the end of treatment ranging from 0.77 to 0.90. Additionally, when all 4 were included in the model, the 3 others regressed toward 0, and worst pain remained the dominant predictor when it was paired with any 1 or 2 of the other pain measures (models without it had average pain take its place, with a similar regression coefficient). When fitting each pain as the sole predictor in separate models, their regression coefficients were not significantly different ($\beta = 0.47$–$0.56$, $\mathrm{SE}[\beta] = 0.05$), indicating little benefit to exploring them further.

Table 1 provides specific values generated from the ROC analyses for both raw change and percentage change in the m-BPI-WPS score best associated with several definitions of clinically important improvement (i.e., "minimally improved" or better, "much improved" or better, and "very much improved" only). The areas under the ROC curves for the m-BPI-WPS raw score change and percentage change (Figures 2 and 3) are nearly identical for each definition of improvement. A raw change of −3 (70.3% sensitivity and 77.8% specificity) and a percentage change of −33.3% (76.2% sensitivity and 72.8% specificity) were best associated with the PGIC category "much or very much improved" (Table 1).

While not the focus of the paper, we also assessed the impact of the study's treatment conditions using an ordinal logistic model that fit the PGIC cumulative category as a function of change in worst pain score, treatment, and their interaction. Overall model fit improved slightly, with the proportional reduction in the error in predicting the PGIC

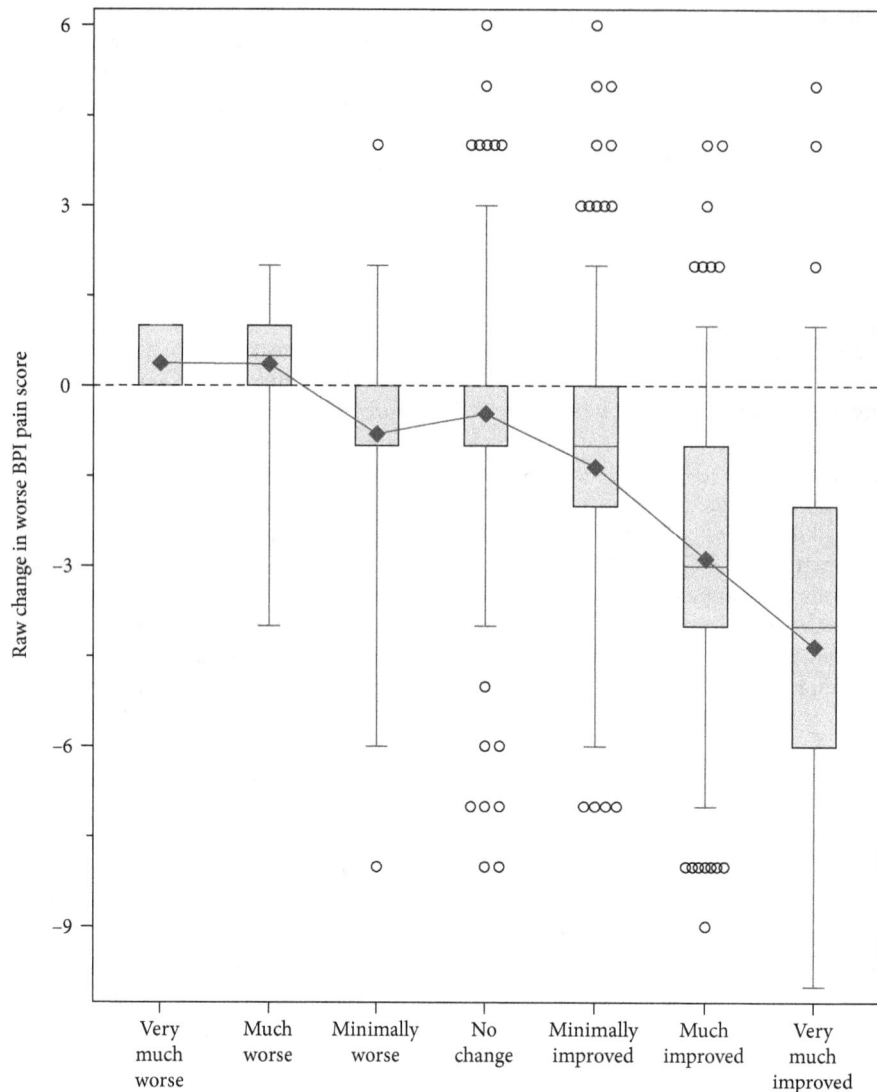

FIGURE 1: Box plot of raw change in the m-BPI score from the baseline to week 5/end of study by PGIC categories. The center line inside the box represents the median, the box's hinges are the 25th and 75th percentile, the whiskers bound the central 95 percent of the distribution, the circles beyond the whiskers are outliers, and the diamond represents the mean. BPI, Brief Pain Inventory; m-BPI, modified Brief Pain Inventory; PGIC, patient global impression of change.

TABLE 1: ROC analyses: model statistics at a tangent for the change in the m-BPI-WPS score.

| Pain score change (type) | PGIC | AUC | Sensitivity (%) | Specificity (%) | Value (change in the pain score)* | Total accuracy (%) |
|---|---|---|---|---|---|---|
| Raw change | Very much improved | 0.801 | 73.7 | 77.7 | −4 | 77.1 |
| Raw change | Much or very much improved | 0.814 | 70.3 | 77.8 | −3 | 74.5 |
| Raw change | Minimally, much, or very much improved | 0.784 | 69.2 | 74.1 | −2 | 70.5 |
| Percentage change* | Very much improved | 0.820 | 75.4 | 74.9 | −50.0 | 75.0 |
| Percentage change* | Much or very much improved | 0.823 | 76.2 | 72.8 | −33.3 | 74.3 |
| Percentage change* | Minimally, much, or very much improved | 0.790 | 72.7 | 73.3 | −20.0 | 72.9 |

Percentage change = raw change in the BPI worst pain score/baseline pain score. *The value of change in the pain score is defined by the intersection of a 45° tangent line with each ROC curve, which is mathematically equivalent to choosing the point at which sensitivity and specificity are the closest to being equal. AUC, area under the curve; m-BPI-WPS, modified Brief Pain Inventory-worst pain severity; PGIC, patient global impression of change; ROC, receiver operating characteristic.

increasing from $R^2_{Nag} = 0.37$ to $R^2_{Nag} = 0.40$ and global AUC slightly increasing from $c = 0.77$ to $c = 0.78$. There was no statistically significant interaction between worst pain and treatment, $F(6407) = 1.20$, $p = 0.30$, but there were statistically significant main effects for both worst pain, $F(1407) = 133.91$, $p < 0.0001$, and for treatment, $F(6407) = 2.62$,

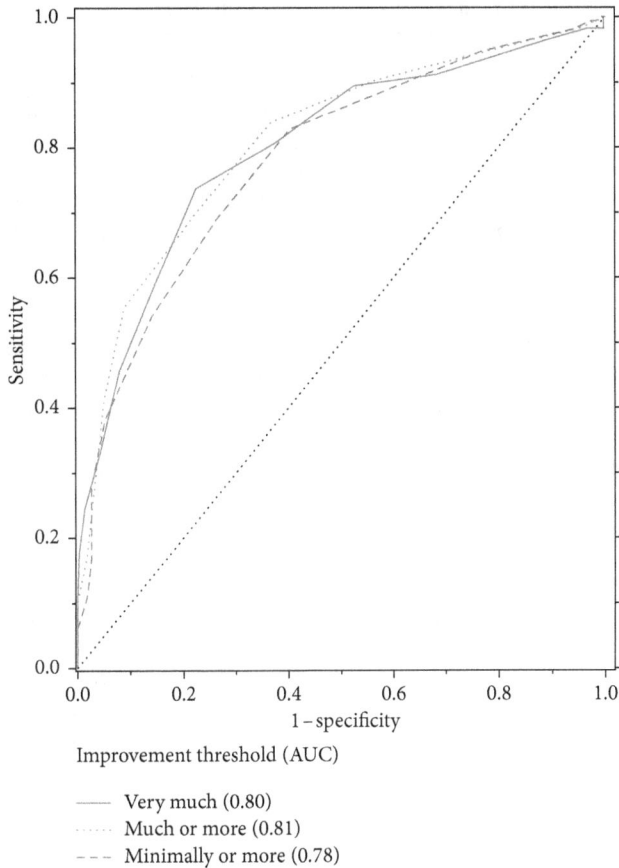

Improvement threshold (AUC)

— Very much (0.80)
...... Much or more (0.81)
- - - Minimally or more (0.78)

FIGURE 2: ROC curve of raw change in the m-BPI-WPS score from the baseline to week 5/end of the study and PGIC. AUC, area under the curve; m-BPI-WPS, modified Brief Pain Inventory-worst pain severity; ROC, receiver operating characteristic.

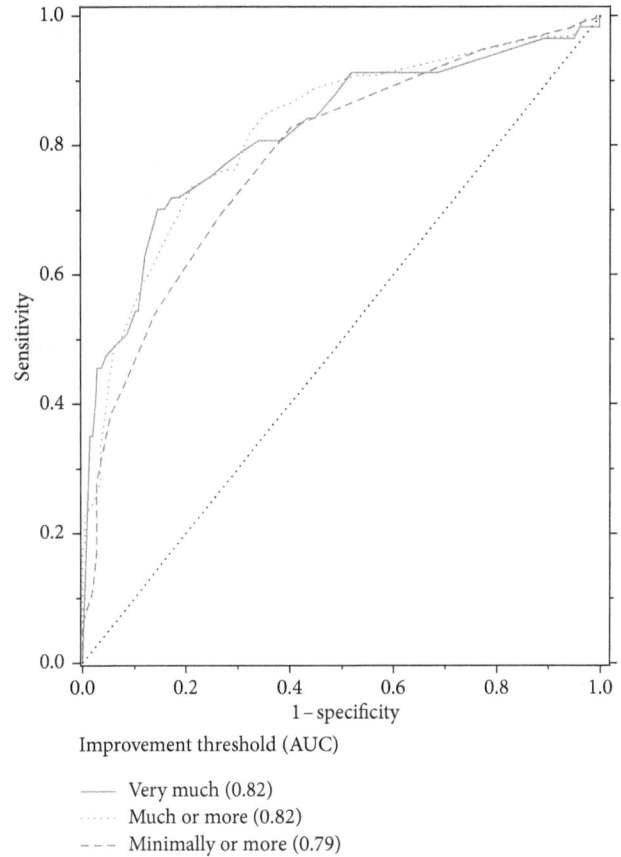

Improvement threshold (AUC)

— Very much (0.82)
...... Much or more (0.82)
- - - Minimally or more (0.79)

FIGURE 3: ROC curve of percentage change in the m-BPI-WPS score from the baseline to week 5/end of the study and PGIC. AUC, area under the curve; m-BPI-WPS, modified Brief Pain Inventory-worst pain severity; PGIC, patient global impression of change; ROC, receiver operating characteristic.

$p = 0.02$. For worst pain, the odds ratio improved from 1.69 to 1.87. As the treatment conditions were largely aimed at examining dose response of mirogabalin, the main effect of treatment was analyzed via Helmert contrasts. Compared with a placebo, mirogabalin doses ≥5 mg increased the odds of advancing PGIC categories by 1.63, $z = 3.18$, $p_{Holm-Sidak} = 0.01$; there was no significant difference in the odds when comparing 5 mg to higher doses. In addition, model results were very similar when worst pain was expressed as the percent change instead of the raw change.

*3.2. Correlation Analysis.* The ADPS was highly correlated (i.e., very strong relationships) with all the items of the m-BPI pain severity scale, including "pain at its worst in the past 24 hours," "pain at its least in the past 24 hours," "pain on the average," and "pain right now." The correlation coefficient was the highest for the worst pain item (0.87) and lowest for the least pain item (0.81). The correlations and regression slopes are presented in Table 2. The regression slopes represent the unit change in the ADPS associated with every 1-point change in the predictor variables (individual items of the m-BPI pain severity scale). Consistent with the correlation analysis, the regression slopes indicate that all

items of the m-BPI had a significant association with the ADPS, with the association being the highest for the average pain item (slope = 0.89) and lowest for the pain right now item (slope = 0.80).

## 4. Discussion

This post hoc analysis demonstrates that the m-BPI-WPS is closely associated with the PGIC and may be used to describe clinically meaningful changes in patient assessment of DPNP. The results also suggest that a 3-point or 33.3% reduction in the m-BPI-WPS score represents a clinically important difference. Our findings are consistent with previous research [20] and reiterate the CID on the BPI worst, least, and average pain severity scales established by Farrar et al. [33]. Although the Farrar et al. study established CID based on associations of the BPI items with patient-perceived improvements at endpoint as measured by the 7-point patient global impression of improvement scale, our finding of a 33.3% reduction representing a CID is almost identical to the 34% reduction reported in that study [33]. Our analyses also describe changes in m-BPI-WPS scores associated with the various categories of global

TABLE 2: Polyserial correlations and regression slopes of the m-BPI pain severity scale items with ADPS.

| m-BPI pain severity scale | n | Correlation coefficient | Slope of items as a predictor for ADPS | p value |
|---|---|---|---|---|
| Pain right now | 385 | 0.834 | 0.800 | <0.001 |
| Pain at its least in the last 24 hours | 385 | 0.811 | 0.845 | <0.001 |
| Pain at its worst in the last 24 hours | 385 | 0.874 | 0.820 | <0.001 |
| Pain on the average | 384 | 0.842 | 0.890 | <0.001 |

Patients with missing data on the BPI pain scales or ADPS at the endpoint were excluded from the correlation analysis. ADPS, average daily pain score; BPI, Brief Pain Inventory; m-BPI, modified Brief Pain Inventory.

improvement, information that could potentially be useful in evaluating the relative effectiveness of chronic pain treatments in clinical practice. For example, a 50% reduction in the m-BPI-WPS score represents the highest level of clinical improvement, whereas a 20% reduction indicates minimal improvement. These benchmarks could be useful to clinicians in guiding prescribing decisions for individual patients.

Although the FDA recently recommended the use of worst pain as a primary endpoint in pain clinical studies [36], the ADPS has historically been used as the gold standard PRO measure. Therefore, to facilitate comparison of our findings with those of previous studies, we wanted to investigate if the m-BPI-WPS item correlated with the ADPS. Our results in DPNP patients indicated a strong correlation of all items of the m-BPI pain severity scale with the ADPS, with the correlations being the strongest for the worst and average pain items. Accordingly, our results suggest that the use of the worst pain score may improve the interpretability of pain measures results in DPNP clinical trials.

Our analyses are subject to several limitations. Data for our study were derived from a single phase 2 study. Therefore, in addition to a small sample size, the homogeneity of the study sample (owing to specific patient recruitment criteria) restricts the generalizability of our findings. It is possible that the CID established in our study may not be relevant for DPNP patients in usual care who present with multiple comorbidities or a disease profile different from those of our trial patients. Although the association of the PGIC with pain scores suggests that a patient's pain experience is closely related to his/her evaluation of the health status, it is possible that patients with more debilitating comorbidities may report global health improvements that are inconsistent with pain reduction.

Our results are based on patients with DPNP who presented with moderate to severe ADPS scores at the baseline (mean ADPS was 7.0 in the placebo arm, 6.7 across all 5 mirogabalin treatment arms, and 6.6 in the pregabalin arm). To facilitate application of our findings in clinical practice, the analysis presented here should be repeated with data collected through observational studies and should include a more representative patient population. In addition, our study sample comprised patients with DPNP, and findings should be applied with caution to patients with other chronic pain conditions.

Finally, the 5-week duration of the treatment period of this clinical trial may not have been long enough to observe possible changes over time in the correspondence between the m-BPI-WPS and the PGIC. However, Farrar et al. showed that a different PRO (the PI-NRS) corresponded well with PGIC regardless of the study length [33]. Therefore, a longer study duration is not expected to impact these results.

## 5. Conclusions

Our results in DPNP patients present preliminary values for raw and percentage changes in scores of the m-BPI-WPS that constitute a CID. Although the generalizability of our findings is limited owing to the small sample size of this adaptive and innovative phase 2 study in DPNP patients, our results not only reinforce previous findings but also add external validity. Researchers have suggested that using a standard definition of CID in studies of chronic pain treatment will simplify comparisons of treatment effects. Our findings provide additional data to support the establishment of such a universal definition of CID.

## Disclosure

The affiliations of Yin Wan and Domenico Merante were their affiliations at the time the study was conducted. Data were presented previously by Dr. Merante at the Annual Congress of the European Pain Federation (EFIC), September 2–5, 2015, Vienna, Austria.

## Authors' Contributions

Drs. Ching Hsu and Domenico Merante participated in the conception, design, and planning of the study. All authors contributed to the data acquisition, analysis, or interpretation of results and drafted the work or revised it critically. All authors approved the final version of the manuscript and agreed to be accountable for all aspects of the work.

## Acknowledgments

The authors thank Dr. Frech-Tamas for assistance with the conduct of the study and helpful discussions and feedback. The authors also thank Mugdha Gore, Ph.D., B.Pharm., and Terri Schochet, Ph.D., and Claire Daniele, Ph.D., of AlphaBioCom, LLC, for editorial assistance in the preparation and submission of this manuscript. Drs. Gore, Schochet, and Daniele were compensated for their services by Daiichi Sankyo, Inc. This research was funded by Daiichi Sankyo, Inc.

# References

[1] B. S. Galer, A. Gianas, and M. P. Jensen, "Painful diabetic polyneuropathy: epidemiology, pain description, and quality of life," *Diabetes Research and Clinical Practice*, vol. 47, no. 2, pp. 123–128, 2000.

[2] S. Morales-Vidal, C. Morgan, M. McCoyd, and A. Hornik, "Diabetic peripheral neuropathy and the management of diabetic peripheral neuropathic pain," *Postgraduate Medicine*, vol. 124, no. 4, pp. 145–153, 2012.

[3] A. Veves, M. Backonja, and R. A. Malik, "Painful diabetic neuropathy: epidemiology, natural history, early diagnosis, and treatment options," *Pain Medicine*, vol. 9, no. 6, pp. 660–674, 2008.

[4] V. Bril, J. D. England, G. M. Franklin et al., "Evidence-based guideline: treatment of painful diabetic neuropathy–report of the American Association of Neuromuscular and Electrodiagnostic Medicine, the American Academy of Neurology, and the American Academy of Physical Medicine & Rehabilitation," *Muscle and Nerve*, vol. 43, no. 6, pp. 910–917, 2011.

[5] A. Sadosky, C. Schaefer, R. Mann et al., "Burden of illness associated with painful diabetic peripheral neuropathy among adults seeking treatment in the US: results from a retrospective chart review and cross-sectional survey," *Diabetes, Metabolic Syndrome and Obesity*, vol. 6, pp. 79–92, 2013.

[6] E. Schneider, D. Ziegler, S. Wilhelm, A. Schacht, and F. Birklein, "Patient expectations in the treatment of painful diabetic polyneuropathy: results from a non-interventional study," *Pain Medicine*, vol. 15, no. 4, pp. 671–681, 2014.

[7] C. J. Alleman, K. Y. Westerhout, M. Hensen et al., "Humanistic and economic burden of painful diabetic peripheral neuropathy in Europe: a review of the literature," *Diabetes Research and Clinical Practice*, vol. 109, no. 2, pp. 215–225, 2015.

[8] M. daCosta DiBonaventura, J. C. Cappelleri, and A. V. Joshi, "A longitudinal assessment of painful diabetic peripheral neuropathy on health status, productivity, and health care utilization and cost," *Pain Medicine*, vol. 12, no. 1, pp. 118–126, 2011.

[9] C. D'Amato, R. Morganti, C. Greco et al., "Diabetic peripheral neuropathic pain is a stronger predictor of depression than other diabetic complications and comorbidities," *Diabetes and Vascular Disease Research*, vol. 13, no. 6, pp. 418–428, 2016.

[10] A. Sadosky, J. Mardekian, B. Parsons, M. Hopps, E. Jay Bienen, and J. Markman, "Healthcare utilization and costs in diabetes relative to the clinical spectrum of painful diabetic peripheral neuropathy," *Journal of Diabetes and its Complications*, vol. 29, no. 2, pp. 212–217, 2015.

[11] C. E. Argoff, B. E. Cole, D. A. Fishbain et al., "Diabetic peripheral neuropathic pain: clinical and quality-of-life issues," *Mayo Clinic Proceedings*, vol. 81, no. 4, pp. S3–S11, 2006.

[12] R. H. Dworkin, A. B. O'Connor, M. Backonja et al., "Pharmacologic management of neuropathic pain: evidence-based recommendations," *Pain*, vol. 132, no. 3, pp. 237–251, 2007.

[13] S. Tesfaye, L. Vileikyte, G. Rayman et al., "Painful diabetic peripheral neuropathy: consensus recommendations on diagnosis, assessment and management," *Diabetes/Metabolism Research and Reviews*, vol. 27, no. 7, pp. 629–638, 2011.

[14] V. Bril, J. England, G. M. Franklin et al., "Evidence-based guideline: treatment of painful diabetic neuropathy: report of the American Academy of Neurology, the American Association of Neuromuscular and Electrodiagnostic Medicine, and the American Academy of Physical Medicine and Rehabilitation," *Neurology*, vol. 76, no. 20, pp. 1758–1765, 2011.

[15] R. H. Dworkin, A. B. O'Connor, J. Audette et al., "Recommendations for the pharmacological management of neuropathic pain: an overview and literature update," *Mayo Clinic Proceedings*, vol. 85, no. 3, pp. S3–S14, 2010.

[16] N. B. Finnerup, N. Attal, S. Haroutounian et al., "Pharmacotherapy for neuropathic pain in adults: a systematic review and meta-analysis," *The Lancet Neurology*, vol. 14, no. 2, pp. 162–173, 2015.

[17] S. Tesfaye, A. J. Boulton, and A. H. Dickenson, "Mechanisms and management of diabetic painful distal symmetrical polyneuropathy," *Diabetes Care*, vol. 36, no. 9, pp. 2456–2465, 2013.

[18] M. Yang, C. Qian, and Y. Liu, "Suboptimal treatment of diabetic peripheral neuropathic pain in the United States," *Pain Medicine*, vol. 16, no. 11, pp. 2075–2083, 2015.

[19] D. Merante, G. Skouteris, and R. Malik, "Developing new molecules for the treatment of painful diabetic peripheral neuropathy: is it feasible given the magnitude of the placebo response in proof of concept clinical studies?," *Journal of Diabetes and Metabolism*, vol. 4, no. 9, 2013.

[20] J. T. Farrar, J. P. Young Jr., L. LaMoreaux, J. L. Werth, and M. R. Poole, "Clinical importance of changes in chronic pain intensity measured on an 11-point numerical pain rating scale," *Pain*, vol. 94, no. 2, pp. 149–158, 2001.

[21] U.S. Food and Drug Administration, "Guidance for industry, patient-reported outcome measures. Use in medical development to support labeling claims," May 2018, http://www.fda.gov/downloads/Drugs/GuidanceComplianceRegulatoryInformation/Guidances/UCM193282.pdf.

[22] D. C. Turk, R. H. Dworkin, M. P. McDermott et al., "Analyzing multiple endpoints in clinical trials of pain treatments: IMMPACT recommendations. Initiative on methods, measurement, and pain assessment in clinical trials," *Pain*, vol. 139, no. 3, pp. 485–493, 2008.

[23] H. Hurst and J. Bolton, "Assessing the clinical significance of change scores recorded on subjective outcome measures," *Journal of Manipulative and Physiological Therapeutics*, vol. 27, no. 1, pp. 26–35, 2004.

[24] J. T. Farrar, "What is clinically meaningful: outcome measures in pain clinical trials," *Clinical Journal of Pain*, vol. 16, no. 2, pp. S106–S112, 2000.

[25] C. Cleeland, "Research in cancer pain. What we know and what we need to know," *Cancer*, vol. 67, no. S3, pp. 823–827, 1991.

[26] C. S. Cleeland and K. M. Ryan, "Pain assessment: global use of the brief pain inventory," *Annals, Academy of Medicine, Singapore*, vol. 23, no. 2, pp. 129–138, 1994.

[27] K. H. Gjeilo, R. Stenseth, A. Wahba et al., "Validation of the brief pain inventory in patients six months after cardiac surgery," *Journal of Pain and Symptom Management*, vol. 34, no. 6, pp. 648–656, 2007.

[28] T. Mendoza, T. Mayne, D. Rublee, and C. Cleeland, "Reliability and validity of a modified brief pain inventory short form in patients with osteoarthritis," *European Journal of Pain*, vol. 10, no. 4, pp. 353–361, 2006.

[29] V. S. Williams, M. Y. Smith, and S. E. Fehnel, "The validity and utility of the BPI interference measures for evaluating the impact of osteoarthritic pain," *Journal of Pain and Symptom Management*, vol. 31, no. 1, pp. 48–57, 2006.

[30] D. C. Zelman, M. Gore, E. Dukes, K. S. Tai, and N. Brandenburg, "Validation of a modified version of the brief pain inventory for painful diabetic peripheral neuropathy," *Journal of Pain and Symptom Management*, vol. 29, no. 4, pp. 401–410, 2005.

[31] D. M. Ehde, K. P. Nitsch, and J. P. Smiley, "Measurement characteristics and clinical utility of the brief pain inventory-short form for individuals with multiple sclerosis," *Rehabilitation Psychology*, vol. 60, no. 4, pp. 365-366, 2015.

[32] L. P. Jelsness-Jorgensen, B. Moum, T. Grimstad et al., "Validity, reliability, and responsiveness of the brief pain inventory in inflammatory bowel disease," *Canadian Journal of Gastroenterology and Hepatology*, vol. 2016, Article ID 5624261, 10 pages, 2016.

[33] J. T. Farrar, Y. L. Pritchett, M. Robinson, A. Prakash, and A. Chappell, "The clinical importance of changes in the 0 to 10 numeric rating scale for worst, least, and average pain intensity: analyses of data from clinical trials of duloxetine in pain disorders," *Journal of Pain*, vol. 11, no. 2, pp. 109–118, 2010.

[34] M. T. King, "A point of minimal important difference (MID): a critique of terminology and methods," *Expert Review of Pharmacoeconomics and Outcomes Research*, vol. 11, no. 2, pp. 171–184, 2011.

[35] T. M. Atkinson, T. R. Mendoza, L. Sit et al., "The brief pain inventory and its "pain at its worst in the last 24 hours" item: clinical trial endpoint considerations," *Pain Medicine*, vol. 11, no. 3, pp. 337–346, 2010.

[36] U.S. Food and Drug Administration, "Guidance for industry. Analgesic indications: developing drugs and biological products," May 2018, http://www.fda.gov/downloads/drugs/guidancecomplianceregulatoryinformation/guidances/ucm384691.pdf.

[37] A. Vinik, J. Rosenstock, U. Sharma, K. Feins, C. Hsu, and D. Merante, "Efficacy and safety of mirogabalin (DS-5565) for the treatment of diabetic peripheral neuropathic pain: a randomized, double-blind, placebo- and active comparator-controlled, adaptive proof-of-concept phase 2 study," *Diabetes Care*, vol. 37, no. 12, pp. 3253–3261, 2014.

[38] D. Merante, K. Truitt, S. Ohwada et al., "Adaptive trial design for chronic pain: a randomized, double-blind, placebo- and active comparator (pregabalin)-controlled adaptive phase 2 study of mirogabalin (DS-5565)," in *Proceedings of the NeuroDiab Annual Meeting*, Neuropathy Study Group of the EASD, Sopron, Hungary, Abstract P-51, September 2014.

[39] D. Merante, J. Rosenstock, U. Sharma, K. Feins, C. Hsu, and A. Vinik, "Efficacy of mirogabalin (DS-5565) on patient-reported pain and sleep interference in patients with diabetic neuropathic pain: secondary outcomes of a phase II proof-of-concept study," *Pain Medicine*, vol. 18, no. 11, pp. 2198–2207, 2017.

[40] T. Gilligan, C. Coon, and L. Nelson, "Let SAS[(R)] do the work: correlation crossroads. SAS Global Forum 2010," May 2018, http://support.sas.com/resources/papers/proceedings10/256-2010.pdf.

[41] M. K. Chung, "Correlation coefficient," in *Encyclopedia of Measurement and Statistics*, N. J. Salkin, Ed., pp. 189–201, Sage Publications, London, UK, 2007.

# 17

# An Analysis of Italian Nurses' Approach to Patients' Pain: A Nationwide Online Survey

Chiara Angeletti [ID],[1] Cristiana Guetti,[2] Martina Paesani,[1] Silvia Colavincenzo,[3] Alessandra Ciccozzi [ID],[3] and Paolo Matteo Angeletti [ID][3]

[1]Operative Unit of Anesthesiology, Intensive Care and Pain Medicine, Civil Hospital G. Mazzini of Teramo, Teramo, Italy
[2]Struttura Operativa Dipartimentale Complessa, Cure Intensive per il Trauma e Supporti Extracorporei, Azienda Ospedaliero-Universitaria Careggi, Firenze, Italy
[3]Department of Life, Health and Environmental Sciences, University of L'Aquila, L'Aquila, Italy

Correspondence should be addressed to Paolo Matteo Angeletti; paolomatteoangeletti@gmail.com

Academic Editor: Jacob Ablin

Healthcare providers play a fundamental role in evaluating pain. Several issues about how nurses are educated remain unsolved. The aim of our study was to address how Italian nurses manage patients suffering from pain in daily practice. A cross-sectional survey was administered among Italian registered nurses. Data were collected using a 34-item questionnaire that had been previously validated during a pilot study. The lowest level of participation/education/information events was observed in the South ($p = 0.0001$). A significant difference among the four areas was found in the department affiliation of responders ($p = 0.0001$). Pain assessment at patients' admission was most frequent in the Northeast (32.9%), whereas the lowest frequency was found in the South (15.1%) ($p = 0.0001$). The prevalence of nurses' knowledge of pain scales and their distribution in usual applications was similar in the Northwest and -east, and Central Italy, but lower in the South ($p = 0.0001$). This study underlines the need for change in the clinical approach to pain treatment in healthcare. Pain assessment is a fundamental step for preparing individualized therapeutic plans, and nurses play a crucial role in improving the quality of life of suffering patients.

## 1. Introduction

Pain is a neurophysiological phenomenon that has affected humans forever; in the last decades, social awareness about its management has improved. In clinical practice, healthcare professionals must deal with the requests of patients in our hypertechnological medical systems.

The prevalence of chronic pain was found to be between 12% in Spain and 30% in Norway [1]. The prevalence recorded for Italy was 26%. At the country level, the percentage range of severe pain carriers ranged from 32% in the UK to 50% in Israel; for Italy, this value was 43% [1]. Pain prevalence was found to be higher in northern regions (32%) than in southern regions (22%) [2].

van Hecke et al. [3] found that chronic noncancer pain affects 20% of the European population and is more frequent in women, the elderly population, and people with sociodemographic, clinical, psychological, and biological risk factors. A recent literature review conducted by Reid et al. [4] showed that the one-month prevalence of chronic noncancer pain of moderate to severe severity can be estimated at 19%.

Pain, as a symptom associated with other pathological conditions, has a prevalence ranging from 40% to 63% in hospitalized patients [5, 6] peaking at 82.3% in oncological patients in advanced or terminal stages of disease [2]. The prevalence of pain in elderly patients not living in institutions ranges from 25% to 50% and from 45 to 80% in those living in elderly care facilities [7].

An Italian study [8] reported an estimated prevalence of chronic pain (more than three months) equal to 21.7% of the entire Italian population (approximately 13 million people). Of these, 41% said they had not received adequate pain control, indicating that in Italy the care response to people in pain is still poor. Pain is undertreated in cancer patients in about 25% of cases; this prevalence may peak up at 64% in some subgroups. In patients who had finished curative treatment, the prevalence of pain was 33% (95% CI 21–46); patients who were being treated with an anticancer therapy experienced a prevalence of 59% (95% CI 44–73); patients characterized by advanced/metastatic or terminal disease experienced a prevalence of 64% (95% CI 58–69); and the majority of patients (at all stages of disease) experienced a prevalence of 53% (95% CI 43–63). In conclusion, the pooled prevalence of pain was >50% for all types of cancer [3].

A fundamental aspect of modern healthcare is the prevention of advanced oncological diseases: many European countries have solid cancer prevention campaigns [9–12]. Elderly residents in health facilities are at highest risk for inadequate pain treatment [7]. Among European countries, Italy ranks first in the clinical use of nonsteroidal anti-inflammatory drugs (NSAIDs) and at the bottom for opiate use [13]. Despite the existence of evidence-based guidelines for the appropriate management of pain, many patients still suffer from inadequate pain treatment [14, 15]. Cultural barriers negatively affect the management of pain [14]; these barriers include the educational training of healthcare professionals, including physicians and nurses, and correct patient information [16]. Healthcare providers also play a fundamental role in the initial evaluation of pain, the short-term control of pain, the analgesic effect of treatment, long-term follow-up, and the satisfaction of patients suffering from pain [17]. Many studies have shown that nurses having inadequate knowledge of pain management may negatively affect the outcomes of suffering patients [16–18]. Several issues regarding the education of nurses remain unsolved; these aspects have been dealt with in Italian law number 38 of March 2010, entitled "Instructions for the access to palliative care and pain therapy."

The aim of this study was to understand how Italian nurses manage patients suffering from pain in daily practice and pain evaluation practices in hospital departments in different regions of the country to investigate the reception of Law 10 and to assess nurses' educational needs.

## 2. Methods

The study was a cross-sectional survey administered online from October 2013 to September 2014 to Italian registered nurses to investigate their approach to pain management. Of the 422,875 nurses in the country, 696 from all regions of Italy took part in the survey. A total of 193 males with a mean age $40.16 \pm 9.5$ years (mean $\pm$ standard deviation) and 503 females with a mean age $41.69 \pm 9.3$ years (ages ranged from 22 to 63 years for both genders) were included. The sample size was estimated using the following parameters: sample error $E = 0.04$, event occurrence proportion $p = 0.5$ (in case of maximum variability), and probability $1 - \alpha = 0.95$.

*2.1. Data Collection.* Data were collected online using a questionnaire drawn by the following scientific societies: the National Federation of Nurses Colleges (IPASVI) and the Italian Association for Pain Study (AISD). The survey

was anonymous, included 34 multiple choice items, and had been previously validated during a pilot study. The members of IPASVI and AISD were invited to participate in the survey via dedicated web pages of their own scientific society web sites (http://www.ipasvi.it, http://www.aisd.it, and http://www.painnursing.it). The survey was promoted by major social networks (Facebook, Twitter, and LinkedIn). The questionnaire included the following sections: (i) demographic data (gender, age, and city), (ii) professional data, department, and qualification (pediatric nurse or head nurse); (iii) participation in training courses focused on pain management, type of course (meetings, symposia, and online courses), and degree of validity/efficacy and appreciation of these courses; (iv) registration and quantification of pain (e.g., pain as the fifth vital sign, knowledge of scales for pain evaluation, frequency of these scales' application and impact on clinical decisions, and the role of nurses in the registration of pain symptoms); and (v) knowledge of Italian laws about pain. Italian regions participating in the study were grouped into four geographical areas according to the Italian National Institute of Statistics (ISTAT): the Northwest, the Northeast, Central Italy, South, and the Islands. Two groups of work departments were defined according to clinical and assistance characteristics: Group 1 included emergency/urgent care departments/wards, general and cardiologic intensive care units, oncology and hematology units, hospice/home-care, and pain treatment division; Group 2 included the remaining surgical and medical departments (pediatric, internal medicine, neurology, obstetrics, and gynecology).

*2.2. Statistical Analysis.* Data were analysed by grouping patients in four geographical areas: the Northwest, the Northeast, Central Italy, and the South. The $\chi^2$ test was used to estimate the association between categorical variables being studied. A $t$-test was used to evaluate continuous variables. Wilcoxon signed-rank and Kruskal–Wallis tests were applied to interval and ordinal variables. A value of $p < 0.05$ was considered statistically significant. SAS software was used for the statistical analyses.

## 3. Results

*3.1. General Data on the Survey's Responders.* The distribution areas of participants are summarized in Table 1. No age differences were found among the areas (the Northwest, the Northeast, Central Italy, and South Italy) ($p = 0.41$). A significant gender difference was noted ($p = 0.004$): Of the 665 people who were interviewed (95.5%), 503 were females (72.3%), as expected in the Italian gender distribution of nurses. An important statistically significant difference between the four areas was found for department affiliation responders ($p < 0.0001$). With reference to Group 1, the greatest concentration of participants was in the South (58.5%), while the lowest was observed in the Northeast (30.5%). Regarding occupation, our results showed that pediatric nurses were the least represented among the responders compared to nurses and head nurse ($p = 0.03$).

*3.2. Education.* A statistically significant difference was detected concerning education (Table 1). In particular, the lowest level of participation in education/information events was

TABLE 1: Distribution of participant features.

| Variable | Total responders | | Northwest | | Northeast | | Central | | South | | p |
|---|---|---|---|---|---|---|---|---|---|---|---|
| | Number | % | Number | % | Number | % | Number | % | Number | % | |
| Gender | | | | | | | | | | | |
| Male | 665 | 95.5 | 44 | 26.0 | 43 | 20.2 | 45 | 36.3 | 53 | 33.3 | |
| Female | | | 125 | 74.0 | 170 | 79.8 | 79 | 63.7 | 106 | 66.7 | 0.004 |
| Age group | | | | | | | | | | | |
| 25–35 | 665 | 95.5 | 27 | 16.0 | 29 | 13.6 | 26 | 21.0 | 14 | 8.8 | |
| 35–45 | | | 52 | 30.8 | 52 | 24.4 | 27 | 21.8 | 49 | 30.8 | 0.41 |
| 45–55 | | | 57 | 33.7 | 93 | 43.7 | 50 | 40.3 | 65 | 40.9 | |
| >55 | | | 33 | 19.5 | 39 | 18.3 | 21 | 16.9 | 31 | 19.5 | |
| Occupational category | | | | | | | | | | | |
| Nurse | 665 | 95.5 | 136 | 80.4 | 178 | 83.6 | 111 | 89.5 | 143 | 89.9 | |
| Head nurse | | | 25 | 14.8 | 34 | 16.0 | 12 | 9.7 | 16 | 10.1 | 0.03 |
| Pediatric nurse | | | 8 | 4.7 | 1 | 0.4 | 1 | 0.8 | 0 | 0.0 | |
| Department of affiliation | | | | | | | | | | | |
| Group 1[a] | 665 | 95.5 | 55 | 32.5 | 65 | 30.5 | 40 | 32.3 | 93 | 58.5 | |
| Group 2[b] | | | 114 | 67.5 | 148 | 69.5 | 84 | 67.7 | 66 | 41.5 | <0.0001 |
| Participation education/information events | | | | | | | | | | | |
| Yes | 665 | 95.5 | 105 | 62.1 | 140 | 65.7 | 66 | 53.2 | 66 | 41.5 | |
| No | | | 64 | 37.9 | 73 | 34.3 | 58 | 46.8 | 93 | 58.5 | <0.0001 |
| Utility of education/information events | | | | | | | | | | | |
| Very good | 380/665 | 57.1 | 75 | 71.4 | 126 | 89.3 | 48 | 71.6 | 49 | 73.1 | |
| Good | | | 19 | 18.1 | 11 | 7.8 | 14 | 20.9 | 16 | 23.9 | 0.002 |
| Poor | | | 11 | 10.5 | 4 | 2.8 | 5 | 7.5 | 2 | 3.0 | |

[a]Department Group 1: surgical departments. [b]Department Group 2: medical departments.

observed in the South, whilst the highest level of education was found in the Northeast ($p \leq 0.0001$) (i.e., these events were deemed most useful in the Northeast ($p = 0.002$)).

3.3. *Pain Evaluation.* Table 2 presents data relating to pain evaluation in the hospital facilities of the four geographic areas. Pain assessment at admission was most frequent in the Northeast (32.9%) and least common in the South (15.1%) ($p = 0.0001$). Prevalence of nurses' knowledge of pain scales was similar in the Northwest (95.9%), the Northeast (95.3%), and Central Italy (92.7%), but lower in the South (69.2%) ($p = 0.0001$). A similar distribution in the usual application of pain evaluation scales was found: the Northwest (81.0%), the Northeast (84.5%), Central Italy (72.6%), and the South (37.1%) ($p = 0.0001$). The most commonly used pain scale was VAS, followed by V-NRS, with a range of 85.2% in the Central region to 77.27% in the South and 18.7% in the Northeast and 7.2% in the South, respectively. The structured questionnaires revealed that instruments such as the McGill Pain Questionnaire/BPI and qualitative scales were poorly applied in clinical situations. Treatment plans including scales of pain assessment were also less frequent in the South (75.5%) compared to the remaining three areas ($p = 0.0009$). Knowledge of devices and invasive procedures for pain treatment had the following frequency distribution: the Northwest (51.5%), the Northeast (55.4%), Central Italy (38.7%), and the South (42.1%) ($p = 0.0007$). The simultaneous presence of a physician and a nurse as referring persons for pain management had the highest frequency in Central Italy (51.6%) compared to the remaining areas ($p < 0.0001$). Thereafter, variables were stratified according to the referring department (Table 3). As expected, Group 1

(emergency/urgent care departments, intensive care, cardiology intensive care, oncology/oncohaematology, and hospice/home care units) had the highest score for dedicated staff compared to other departments or units ($p = 0.0001$), as well as for knowledge of devices and invasive procedures for pain treatment (59.3%) ($p = 0.0001$).

3.4. *Pain as the Fifth Vital Sign and Law Number 38.* A statistically significant difference has been revealed regarding the consideration of pain as the fifth vital sign, with the following frequency distribution: the Northwest (88.1%), the Northeast (81.2%), Central Italy (70.1%), and the South (69.1%) ($p < 0.0001$). It is relevant that the highest percentages of nurses working in places where pain is not considered a vital parameter were found in Central Italy (29.9%) and in the South (30.8%). Nurses from the South were less aware of the existence of a law in Italian legislation which makes the evaluation of pain mandatory (61.4%) ($p = 0.0001$).

Globally, the pain problem is considered sufficiently treated and taken into consideration by nurses following this trend in the different areas evaluated: the Northwest, 57.4%; the Northeast, 60.1%; Central Italy, 58.1%; and the South, 63.5%. A statistically significant difference for this issue was found in the department group responders ($p = 0.001$).

## 4. Discussion

Pain relief is a fundamental right; nurses, as healthcare providers, have a central role in this context [13, 19–22]. From triage in an emergency department to postoperative care, from home care to palliative care at the end of life, the crucial professional figure is the nurse, who today requires specific

TABLE 2: Evaluation of pain according to geographic areas.

| Variable | Total responders | | Northwest | | Northeast | | Central | | South | | p |
|---|---|---|---|---|---|---|---|---|---|---|---|
| | Number | % | Number | % | Number | % | Number | % | Number | % | |
| Pain is seen as the fifth vital parameter. Is this the case in your working place? | | | | | | | | | | | |
| Yes | 665 | 95.5 | 149 | 88.1 | 173 | 81.2 | 87 | 70.1 | 110 | 69.1 | |
| No | | | 20 | 11.8 | 40 | 18.8 | 37 | 29.9 | 49 | 30.8 | <0.0001 |
| How frequently do you assess pain in your hospital? | | | | | | | | | | | |
| When requested by the patient | 664 | 95.4 | 56 | 33.1 | 65 | 30.5 | 53 | 42.7 | 97 | 61.4 | |
| At patient's admission in the ward | | | 46 | 27.2 | 57 | 26.8 | 27 | 21.8 | 26 | 16.5 | <0.0001 |
| Once | | | 15 | 8.9 | 16 | 7.5 | 6 | 4.8 | 2 | 1.2 | |
| Twice | | | 51 | 30.2 | 70 | 32.9 | 31 | 25.0 | 24 | 15.1 | |
| Never | | | 1 | 0.6 | 5 | 2.3 | 7 | 5.7 | 9 | 5.7 | |
| Do you know the scales for pain evaluation? | | | | | | | | | | | |
| Yes | 665 | 95.5 | 162 | 95.9 | 203 | 95.3 | 115 | 92.7 | 110 | 69.2 | |
| No | | | 7 | 4.1 | 10 | 4.7 | 9 | 7.3 | 49 | 30.8 | <0.0001 |
| If yes, which do you know? | | | | | | | | | | | |
| VAS | 590 | | 137 | 84.6 | 161 | 79.3 | 98 | 85.2 | 85 | 77.27 | |
| V-NRS | | | 19 | 11.7 | 38 | 18.7 | 9 | 7.8 | 8 | 7.2 | 0.0002 |
| McGill pain questionnaire | | | 3 | 1.8 | 1 | 0.5 | 3 | 2.6 | 5 | 4.6 | |
| BPI | | | 0 | 0.0 | 0 | 0.0 | 0 | 0.0 | 1 | 0.9 | |
| Qualitative scales | | | 3 | 1.9 | 3 | 1.5 | 5 | 4.3 | 11 | 10.0 | |
| Do you usually apply the scales for pain evaluation? | | | | | | | | | | | |
| Yes | 665 | 95.5 | 137 | 81.0 | 180 | 84.5 | 90 | 72.6 | 59 | 37.1 | |
| No | | | 32 | 18.9 | 33 | 15.5 | 34 | 27.4 | 100 | 62.9 | <0.0001 |
| If no why? | | | | | | | | | | | |
| Do you recognize the complaining patient? | 207 | | 19 | 48.7 | 8 | 24.2 | 7 | 20.6 | 28 | 27.7 | |
| I have no time | | | 4 | 10.3 | 4 | 12.1 | 5 | 14.7 | 15 | 14.8 | 0.005 |
| It is not my job | | | 2 | 5.1 | 2 | 6.1 | 3 | 8.8 | 18 | 17.8 | |
| Nobody asked me to do that | | | 4 | 10.3 | 5 | 15.2 | 3 | 8.8 | 23 | 22.8 | |
| Others | | | 10 | 25.6 | 4 | 42.4 | 16 | 7.1 | 17 | 16.8 | |
| Does the evaluation scale affect the subsequent assistance plans? | | | | | | | | | | | |
| Yes | 665 | 95.5 | 149 | 88.2 | 189 | 88.7 | 110 | 88.7 | 120 | 75.5 | |
| No | | | 20 | 11.8 | 24 | 11.3 | 14 | 11.3 | 39 | 24.5 | 0.0009 |
| Are you aware about devices or invasive procedures for pain treatment? | | | | | | | | | | | |
| Yes | 665 | 95.5 | 87 | 51.5 | 118 | 55.4 | 48 | 38.7 | 67 | 42.1 | |
| No | | | 82 | 48.5 | 95 | 44.6 | 76 | 61.3 | 92 | 57.9 | 0.007 |
| Does a reference person for pain management exist in your hospital ward? | | | | | | | | | | | |
| Yes, a physician | 665 | 95.5 | 49 | 29.0 | 45 | 21.1 | 39 | 31.5 | 73 | 45.9 | |
| Yes, a nurse | | | 12 | 7.1 | 26 | 12.2 | 7 | 5.7 | 2 | 1.3 | <0.0001 |
| Yes, both physician and nurse | | | 24 | 14.2 | 67 | 31.5 | 14 | 11.2 | 8 | 5.0 | |
| No reference person is present | | | 84 | 49.7 | 75 | 35.2 | 64 | 51.6 | 76 | 47.8 | |
| Are you aware about the existence of a law prescribing as mandatory the measurement of pain? | | | | | | | | | | | |
| Yes | 664 | 95.4 | 145 | 85.8 | 187 | 87.8 | 103 | 83.1 | 97 | 61.4 | |
| No | | | 24 | 14.2 | 26 | 2.2 | 21 | 16.9 | 61 | 38.6 | <0.0001 |
| Are, in your opinion, problems related to pain sufficiently taken into account by care providers in your working department? | | | | | | | | | | | |
| Yes | 665 | 95.5 | 97 | 57.4 | 128 | 60.1 | 72 | 58.1 | 101 | 63.5 | |
| No | | | 72 | 42.6 | 85 | 39.9 | 52 | 41.9 | 58 | 36.5 | 0.69 |

VAS, visual analogue scale; V-NRS, verbal numeric rating scale; BPI, brief pain inventor.

knowledge of how to manage pain. The nurse enters fully into the overall care of the patient experiencing pain. Nurses represent an essential component in the patient pain management team: in all healthcare scenarios, they often represent the only daily caregivers who are continually expected to practice symptom management. Nurses spend more time with patients and are able to assess and manage patient pain effectively. They also play a key role in the initial assessment, control, and follow-up of analgesic treatment. However, numerous surveys conducted over the last few years, both nationally and internationally, have shown that nursing staff often lack sufficient knowledge of how to manage pain and the specific skills to treat it [23–28]. Inadequate knowledge and attitudes of nurses with regard to pain management significantly worsen the outcome of suffering patients [28]. The identification of nodes to be solved in terms of the definition of the role of the nurse in pain and the adjustment of standards of care must be a priority for those working in any healthcare environment where the pain is prevalent or even present. These issues, which remain unresolved today, were addressed in Italy by law number 38, "Provisions to ensure access to palliative care and pain therapy," promulgated in March 2010.

TABLE 3: Evaluation of pain according to affiliation of departments considered.

| Variable | Total responders | | Department Group 1[a] | | Department Group 2[b] | | $p$ |
|---|---|---|---|---|---|---|---|
| Pain is seen as the fifth vital sign. Is this true in your working place? | | | | | | | |
| Yes | 696 | 100.0 | 217 | 81.9 | 325 | 75.4 | 0.045 |
| No | | | 48 | 18.1 | 106 | 24.6 | |
| How frequently do you assess pain in your hospital? | | | | | | | |
| When requested by the patient | 695 | 99.9 | 97 | 36.6 | 185 | 43.0 | 0.06 |
| At patient's admission in the ward | | | 63 | 23.8 | 103 | 24.0 | |
| Once | | | 17 | 6.4 | 23 | 5.3 | |
| Twice | | | 80 | 30.2 | 105 | 24.4 | |
| Never | | | 8 | 3.0 | 14 | 3.3 | |
| Do you know the scales for pain evaluation? | | | | | | | |
| Yes | 696 | 100.0 | 228 | 86.0 | 387 | 89.8 | 0.13 |
| No | | | 37 | 14.0 | 44 | 10.2 | |
| Do you usually apply the scales for pain evaluation? | | | | | | | |
| Yes | 696 | 100.0 | 188 | 70.9 | 299 | 69.4 | 0.66 |
| No | | | 77 | 29.1 | 132 | 30.6 | |
| Does the evaluation scale affect the subsequent assistance plans? | | | | | | | |
| Yes | 696 | 100.0 | 230 | 86.8 | 365 | 84.7 | 0.44 |
| No | | | 35 | 13.2 | 66 | 15.3 | |
| Are you aware about devices or invasive procedures for pain treatment? | | | | | | | |
| Yes | 696 | 100.0 | 157 | 59.3 | 174 | 40.4 | <0.0001 |
| No | | | 108 | 40.7 | 257 | 59.6 | |
| Does a reference person for pain management exist in your hospital ward? | | | | | | | |
| Yes, a physician | 696 | 100.0 | 105 | 39.6 | 110 | 25.5 | <0.0001 |
| Yes, a nurse | | | 12 | 4.5 | 38 | 8.8 | |
| Yes, a physician and nurse | | | 48 | 18.1 | 69 | 16.0 | |
| No reference person is present | | | 100 | 37.7 | 214 | 49.7 | |
| Are you aware about the existence of a law prescribing as mandatory the measurement of pain? | | | | | | | |
| Yes | 695 | 99.9 | 217 | 82.2 | 339 | 78.7 | 0.26 |
| No | | | 47 | 17.8 | 92 | 21.3 | |
| Are, in your opinion, problems related to pain sufficiently taken into account by care providers in your working department? | | | | | | | |
| Yes | 696 | 100.0 | 178 | 67.2 | 235 | 54.5 | 0.001 |
| No | | | 87 | 32.8 | 196 | 45.5 | |

[a]Department Group 1: surgical departments. [b]Department Group 2: medical departments.

*4.1. Education in and Knowledge of Pain Management.* Education of nurses and care providers should be seen as a strategic method in order to create an adequate culture of and attract attention to the problem of pain [29]. The present analysis has identified major differences in education, particularly related to the geographic area of the study sample. A higher level of qualification and commitment in nurses' education was present in the Northeast, while a lower commitment was identified in the South of Italy. From this analysis, it appears that differences in the institutional and financial commitment for the persistent education and professional improvement of nurses represent a major issue. In fact, the differences found in the four geographical areas in which ISTAT divides the national territory reflects the diffusion of specific pain therapies and palliative care services, which, according to latest report by the Ministry of Health on the implementation of law number 38, are more common in Northern and Central Italy [30]. Recent studies report that the majority of nurses involved in pain management admit to lacking adequate knowledge and instruments to address this challenge [31, 32]. As reviewed by Mattacola et al. [33], a limited number of studies are available regarding nurses' knowledge of and attitudes toward pain management in Italy

compared to other European, North American, or emerging countries [24–28, 34, 35]. Nurses' education in pain management is badly needed due to the increased awareness on this issue, according to Italian law number 38 and the international community [36]. The existence and diffusion of dedicated services could be a driving force for continuing training and research in pain therapy. However, training in the treatment of pain and the role of the nurse in symptom management should start early in the course of study. A recent review by Chow and Chan [32] shows not only how the knowledge of pain, and of the problems associated with it, is scarce among nursing students but also how it can be optimal after proper training [32]. Not only primary education but also continuous education should be seen as an important investment, because knowledge is not usually automatically transferred in daily assistance; unfortunately, two different attitudes toward this problem have been identified in Italy. Basic knowledge, its application, and attention to the needs of suffering patients are issues of major importance. Basic knowledge and practical expertise alone, however, are not sufficient to change nursing practice unless basic principles of pain evaluation and management in daily practice are concomitantly standardized [37]. Several reports in the literature have analysed the importance of education and demonstrated that education may change nurses' attitudes and improve their knowledge and professional behaviour [28, 38–40]. After attending educational events, indeed, nurses become fully aware of methods of managing pain [38, 41]. This was also a relevant aspect of our survey, and one which reflected a high degree of satisfaction and utility of educational events about pain, although the percentage of nurses attending these courses was very heterogeneous across the country (Table 1).

*4.2. Pain Evaluation.* This study indicates that nurses from the North (-east and -west) correctly use the pain rating scales both at the first physical examination and later on as they register a patient's parameters during the entire time span of assistance, in order to provide reference measurements for planning care and treating pain itself. A negative attitude is still present in a high percentage of nurses operating in the South of Italy, where pain is evaluated only after patients have insistently complained and required care. At this point, pain must be promptly relieved; this misguided attitude causes discomfort for the patient and interrupts the daily activities of nurses, who are often operating in crowded hospital wards with undersized staffs, are underpaid, and burdened with excessive duties. This national situation corresponds with that reported in the literature. A few studies examined the degree of application of a rating scale (numeric, nominal, analogical, or illustrated) [42]; available data from the literature indicate that this scale is used in about 50% of cases [22, 27, 28, 36, 37]. At the national level, a gap in the use of this scale was observed between the northern (95%) and southern regions (69%). Some reports indicated that nurses use a simple interview or nonstandardized methods, or even omit the evaluation [40] in the belief that this duty belongs to the physician rather than to them [35, 42–44]. Pain evaluation is often based on reports obtained by the patient or on alleged levels of pain in patients unable to communicate [25, 43]. As in other international settings, nurses mostly complain about the lack of time for pain evaluation due to assistance duties, particularly during exhausting work shifts [26, 43, 44]. These problems have been widely documented in our survey. Pain should be quantified with a numeric parameter: this crucial aspect of assisting patients has been underlined by law number 38. Pain assessment allows for treatments to be standardized. The analysis of data from South Italy indicates that little attention is paid to pain evaluation at the time a patient is admitted, thereby limiting the subsequent approach to the patient. A direct consequence of this attitude is the poor quality of care perceived by patients and the low level of analgesia achieved. Considering hospital departments and wards, the geographical differences among nurses were less evident. Among nurses working in emergency or surgical departments, oncology hospices, or community care, expertise regarding and knowledge of technical devices and protocols were similar in the different Italian regions.

Our study indicates that nurses from the North (-east and -west) fully understood the rule of law number 38. This North-South gradient was also evident in the results of our survey; in fact, nurses from the Northern and Central Italy showed greater awareness of patients' pain than those in the South. Nurses in the Southern Italy said they were not aware of the existence of a law that requires the measurement of pain as the fifth vital sign, which also affects their familiarity with the instruments used to measure pain. The definition of professional reference figures may guarantee adequate attention to the problem of pain.

Adequate management of pain in healthcare settings may indeed result in shorter hospitalizations, fewer complications and comorbidities, fewer drugs being administered during the rehabilitation phase, fewer analgesic side effects, reduced fear related to opioid use, and an overall shorter time and less expensive rehabilitation. Our investigation indicates that there is no homogeneous treatment of patients with pain from the nursing point of view across the different areas of the country. The nursing staff in many situations does not seem to be in a position to assess pain both in terms of time and internal organization of the departments and in terms of tools and skills to better address the problem of pain management. Emerging problems for nurses seem mainly to concern inadequate knowledge, limited possibilities to assess and manage pain, and finally a reluctance to use pain assessment tools and to consider pain a vital parameter. Nurses must be aware of their central role and responsibility and must be informed about their profession. Appropriate training and continuous updating will enable healthcare personnel to achieve the necessary level of expertise in pain assessment and management needed to bridge the gap between our country and others in Europe and around the world. The most urgent problem to solve is to clearly define the border between the role of nursing and medical competence, a limit that has been overcome in other countries but which is still rather confused in Italy.

## 5. Limitations

The responders to the questionnaire may not be a representative of the Italian nurse population. Indeed, it was a relatively small group of nurses who were strongly motivated or simply were aware of the existence of the survey and were given the opportunity to participate; a possible limitation is therefore that the questionnaire was not submitted to a group of nurses selected according to a specific rule or work setting, and thus the distribution of the responders in the groups analysed could be subject to unknown biases. Drawing any definitive conclusion on differences between geographical areas is also difficult. New cross-sectional studies are needed to investigate the full application of the law, the role of nurses in the regional and national management of pain, and the usefulness of training in this field.

## 6. Conclusion

The present study aimed at emphasizing the need for a change in the clinical approach to pain treatment. Pain as a disease is an emergency that must be faced with a multidisciplinary approach; in this setting, nurses around the world play a central role, as they are directly involved in the care of patients suffering from cancer- or noncancer-related pain. Pain assessment is a fundamental step for preparing individualized therapeutic plans. Thus, pain should be seen a vital parameter and assessed several times in the course of 24 hours. Nowadays, a primary duty of nurses should be to offer personalized assistance and elaborate care and take part in research in order to improve the quality of life of suffering patients.

## Abbreviations

NSAIDs: Nonsteroidal anti-inflammatory drugs
IPASVI: National federation of nurses colleges
AISD: Italian association for pain study
ISTAT: Italian national institute of statistics
VAS: Visual analogue scale
V-NRS: Verbal numeric rating scale
BPI: Brief pain inventory.

## Disclosure

Chiara Angeletti, Cristiana Guetti, Paolo Matteo Angeletti, Alessandra Ciccozzi, Martina Paesani, and Silvia Colavincenzo took responsibility for the paper as a whole.

## Authors' Contributions

Chiara Angeletti, Cristiana Guetti, and Paolo Matteo Angeletti, conceived the study, designed the survey, managed the data (including quality control), provided statistical advice on the study design, analysed the data, and critically revised the manuscript. Chiara Angeletti, Alessandra Ciccozzi, Martina Paesani, and Silvia Colavincenzo supervised the conduct of the study and the data collection. Chiara Angeletti, Cristiana Guetti, and Paolo Matteo Angeletti drafted the manuscript, and all authors interpreted the data and contributed the contents within the discussion section. Chiara Angeletti, Cristiana Guetti, Paolo Matteo Angeletti, and Martina Paesani reviewed the manuscript. All authors read and approved the final manuscript.

## Acknowledgments

The authors wish to acknowledge the assistance of the following organizations and individuals: AISD (Associazione Italiana per lo Studio del Dolore (Italian Association for the Study of Pain)), IPASVI (Federazione Nazionale Collegi Infermieri), and Ms. Lorenza Saini for the web assistance and survey promotion. The authors also wish to offer special thanks with due respect to Ms Anna Ventura for her help in preparing the manuscript.

## References

[1] H. Breivik, B. Collett, V. Ventafridda, R. Cohen, and D. Gallacher, "Survey of chronic pain in Europe: prevalence, impact on daily life, and treatment," *European Journal of Pain*, vol. 10, no. 4, pp. 287–333, 2006.

[2] M. Costantini, P. Viterbori, and G. Flego, "Prevalence of pain in Italian hospitals: results of a regional cross-sectional survey," *Journal of Pain Symptom Management*, vol. 23, no. 3, pp. 221–230, 2002.

[3] O. van Hecke, N. Torrance, and B. H. Smith, "Chronic pain epidemiology and its clinical relevance," *British Journal of Anaesthesia*, vol. 111, no. 1, pp. 13–18, 2013.

[4] K. J. Reid, J. Harker, M. M. Bala et al., "Epidemiology of chronic non-cancer pain in Europe: narrative review of prevalence, pain treatments and pain impact," *Current Medical Research and Opinion*, vol. 27, no. 2, pp. 449–462, 2011.

[5] R. M. Melotti, B. G. Samolsky-Dekel, E. Ricchi et al., "Pain prevalence and predictors among inpatients in a major Italian teaching hospital. A baseline survey towards a pain free hospital," *European Journal of Pain*, vol. 9, no. 5, pp. 485–495, 2005.

[6] W. Gianni, R. A. Madaio, L. Di Ciocco et al., "Prevalence of pain in elderly hospitalized patients," *Archives of Gerontology and Geriatrics*, vol. 51, no. 3, pp. 273–276, 2010.

[7] F. De Conno, C. Ripamonti, and C. Brunelli, "Opioid purchases and expenditure in nine western European countries: 'are we killing off morphine?'," *Palliative Medicine*, vol. 19, no. 3, pp. 179–184, 2005.

[8] G. Fanelli, G. Gensini, P. L. Canonico et al., "Dolore in Italia. Analisi della situazione. Proposte operative," *Recenti Progressi in Medicina*, vol. 103, no. 4, pp. 133–141, 2012.

[9] E. Altobelli, L. Rapacchietta, P. M. Angeletti, L. Barbante, F. V. Profeta, and R. Fagnano, "Breast cancer screening programmes across the WHO European region: differences among countries based on national income level," *International Journal of Environmental Research and Public Health*, vol. 14, no. 4, p. 452, 2017.

[10] E. Altobelli and A. Lattanzi, "Cervical carcinoma in the European Union: an update on disease burden, screening program state of activation, and coverage as of March 2014," *International Journal of Gynecologic Cancer*, vol. 25, no. 3, pp. 474–483, 2015.

[11] E. Altobelli, A. Lattanzi, R. Paduano, G. Varassi, and F. di Orio, "Colorectal cancer prevention in Europe: burden of disease and status of screening programs," *Preventive Medicine*, vol. 62, pp. 132–141, 2014.

[12] E. Altobelli, F. D'Aloisio, and P. M. Angeletti, "Colorectal cancer screening in countries of European Council outside of the EU-28," *World Journal Gastroenterology*, vol. 22, no. 20, pp. 4946–4957, 2016.

[13] Italian Ministry of Health, *Rapporto al Parlamento sullo Stato di Attuazione della Legge n. 38 del 15 Marzo 2010*, January 2016, http://www.salute.gov.it/imgs/C_17_pubblicazioni_2195_allegato.pdf.

[14] S. Ogston-Tuck, "A silent epidemic: community nursing and effective pain management," *British Journal of Community Nursing*, vol. 17, no. 11, pp. 516–518, 2012.

[15] Maryland Board of Nursing, *Pain Management, Nursing Role/Core Competency, A Guide for Nurses*, January 2016, http://www.mbon.org/practice/pain_management.pdf.

[16] K. Mac Lellan, "Postoperative pain: strategy for improving patient experiences," *Journal of Advanced Nursing*, vol. 46, no. 2, pp. 179–185, 2004.

[17] E. Bernhofer, "Ethics: ethics and pain management in hospitalized patients," *Online Journal of Issues Nursing*, vol. 17, no. 1, p. 11, 2011.

[18] B. Wilson, "Nurses' knowledge of pain," *Journal of Clinical Nursing*, vol. 16, no. 6, pp. 1012–1020, 2007.

[19] H. Shahnazi, A. Saryazdi, G. Sharifirad, A. Hasanzadeh, A. Charkazi, and M. Moodi, "The survey of nurse's knowledge

and attitude toward cancer pain management: application of health belief model," *Journal of Education and Health Promotion*, vol. 1, no. 1, p. 15, 2012.

[20] L. Rose, O. Smith, C. Gélinas et al., "Critical care nurses' pain assessment and management practices: a survey in Canada," *American Journal of Critical Care*, vol. 21, no. 4, pp. 251–259, 2012.

[21] B. Ferrell, "Ethical perspectives on pain and suffering," *Pain Management Nursing*, vol. 6, no. 3, pp. 83–90, 2005.

[22] Italian Ministry of Health, *Relazione sull'Attuazione delle Disposizioni per Garantire l'Accesso alle Cure Palliative e alla Terapia del Dolore*, January 2016, http://www.camera.it/dati/leg16/lavori/documentiparlamentari/indiceetesti/238/002_RS/IN TERO_COM.pdf.

[23] B. J. Lewthwaite, K. M. Jabusch, B. J. Wheeler et al., "Nurses' knowledge and attitudes regarding pain management in hospitalized adults," *Journal of Continuing Education in Nursing*, vol. 42, no. 6, pp. 251–259, 2011.

[24] L. J. Ware, P. Bruckenthal, G. C. Davis, and S. K. O'Conner-Von, "Factors that influence patient advocacy by pain management nurses: results of the American society for pain management nursing survey," *Pain Management Nursing*, vol. 12, no. 1, pp. 25–32, 2011.

[25] D. Al-Shaer, P. D. Hill, and M. A. Anderson, "Nurses' knowledge and attitudes regarding pain assessment and intervention," *Medsurg Nursing*, vol. 20, no. 1, pp. 7–11, 2011.

[26] J. Layman Young, F. M. Horton, and R. Davidhizar, "Nursing attitudes and beliefs in pain assessment and management," *Journal of Advanced Nursing*, vol. 53, no. 4, pp. 412–421, 2006.

[27] L. Y. Lui, W. K. So, and D. Y. Fong, "Knowledge and attitudes regarding pain management among nurses in Hong Kong medical units," *Journal of Clinical Nursing*, vol. 17, no. 15, pp. 2014–2021, 2008.

[28] H. J. Jho, Y. Kim, K. A. Kong et al., "Knowledge, practices, and perceived barriers regarding cancer pain management among physicians and nurses in Korea: a nationwide multicenter survey," *PLoS One*, vol. 9 no. 8, article e105900, 2014.

[29] A. Jarrett, T. Church, K. Fancher-Gonzalez, J. Shackelford, and A. Lofton, "Nurses' knowledge and attitudes about pain in hospitalized patients," *Clinical Nurse Specialist*, vol. 27, no. 2, pp. 81–87, 2013.

[30] S. Marchand, "What is pain?," in *The Phenomenon of Pain*, Mission Statement of IASP Press, Seattle, WA, USA, January 2016, http://www.iasppain.org/files/Content/ContentFolders/AboutIASP/IASPAnnualReportPrint2012.pdf.

[31] http://www.salute.gov.it/imgs/C_17_pubblicazioni_2360_allegato.pdf, January 2016.

[32] K. M. Chow and J. C. Y. Chan, "Pain knowledge and attitudes of nursing students: a literature review," *Nurse Education Today*, vol. 35, no. 2, pp. 366–372, 2015.

[33] P. Mattacola, F. Serio, L. Mauro, L. Fabriani, and R. Latina, *Le Conoscenze e le Attitudini degli Infermieri nella Gestione del Dolore: una Revisione Narrativa della Letteratura*, January 2016, http://www.painnursing.it/rassegna/le-conoscenze-e-le-attitudini-degli-infermieri-nella-gestione-del-dolore-una-revisione-narrativa-della-letteratura-2.

[34] M. Bernardi, G. Catania, A. Lambert, G. Tridello, and M. Luzzani, "Knowledge and attitudes about cancer pain management: a national survey of Italian oncology nurses," *European Journal of Oncology Nursing*, vol. 211, no. 3, pp. 272–279, 2007.

[35] M. Di Muzio, D. Barbato, and S. M. Maria, *Pain Management: uno Studio Infermieristico*, 2010, http://www.ipasvi.roma.it/archivio_news/pagine/89/2_10.pdf.

[36] Office of The Army Surgeon General, *Pain Management Task Force Report Providing a Standardized DoD and VHA Vision and Approach to Pain Management to Optimize the Care of Warriors and Their Families*, January 2016, http://www.regenesisbio.com/pdfs/journal/pain_management_task_force_report.pdf.

[37] P. H. Berry and J. L. Dahl, "The new JCAHO pain standards: implications for pain management nurses," *Pain Management Nursing*, vol. 1, no. 1, pp. 3–12, 2000.

[38] M. S. Abdalrahim, S. A. Majali, M. W. Stomberg, and I. Bergbom, "The effect of postoperative pain management program on improving nurses' knowledge and attitudes toward pain," *Nurse Education in Practice*, vol. 11, no. 4, pp. 250–255, 2010.

[39] T. K. Michaels, E. Hubbartt, S. A. Carroll, and D. Hudson-Barr, "Evaluating an educational approach to improve pain assessment in hospitalized patients," *Journal of Nursing Care Quality*, vol. 22, no. 3, pp. 260–265, 2007.

[40] E. I. Patiraki, E. D. Papathanassoglou, C. Tafas et al., "A randomized controlled trial of an educational intervention on Hellenic nursing staff's knowledge and attitudes on cancer pain management," *European Journal of Oncology Nursing*, vol. 10, no. 5, pp. 337–352, 2006.

[41] P. C. Lin, H. W. Chiang, T. T. Chiang, and C. S. Chen, "Pain management: evaluating the effectiveness of an educational programme for surgical nursing staff," *Journal of Clinical Nursing*, vol. 17, no. 15, pp. 2032–2041, 2008.

[42] J. S. Willens, C. DePascale, and J. Penny, "Role delineation study for the American society for pain management nursing," *Pain Management Nursing*, vol. 11, no. 2, pp. 68–75, 2010.

[43] N. Rejeh, F. Ahmadi, E. Mohammadi, M. Anoosheh, and A. Kazemnejad, "Nurses' experiences and perceptions of influencing barriers to postoperative pain management," *International Nursing Review*, vol. 55, no. 4, pp. 468–475, 2008.

[44] B. S. De Silva and C. Rolls, "Attitudes, beliefs, and practices of Sri Lankan nurses toward cancer pain management: an ethnographic study," *Nursing and Health Sciences*, vol. 13, no. 4, pp. 419–424, 2011.

# 18

# Comparison between Collagen and Lidocaine Intramuscular Injections in Terms of Their Efficiency in Decreasing Myofascial Pain within Masseter Muscles: A Randomized, Single-Blind Controlled Trial

**Aleksandra Nitecka-Buchta** (ID),[1] **Karolina Walczynska-Dragon** (ID),[1]
**Jolanta Batko-Kapustecka,**[1] **and Mieszko Wieckiewicz** (ID)[2]

[1]*Department of Temporomandibular Disorders, Unit SMDZ in Zabrze, Medical University of Silesia in Katowice,*
 *Traugutta Sq. 2, 41-800 Zabrze, Poland*
[2]*Department of Experimental Dentistry, Faculty of Dentistry, Wroclaw Medical University,*
 *26 Krakowska St., 50-425 Wroclaw, Poland*

Correspondence should be addressed to Mieszko Wieckiewicz; m.wieckiewicz@onet.pl

Academic Editor: Parisa Gazerani

*Background and Objective.* A novel option for myofascial pain (MFP) management and muscle regeneration is intramuscular collagen injections. The aim of the study was to evaluate the efficiency of intramuscular injections of collagen and lidocaine in decreasing MFP within masseter muscles. *Methods.* Myofascial pain within masseter muscles was diagnosed on the basis of the Diagnostic Criteria for Temporomandibular Disorders (II.1.A. 2 and 3). A total of 43 patients with diagnosed MFP within masseter muscles were enrolled to the study (17 male and 26 female, $40 \pm 3.8$ years old) and randomly divided into three groups. The first group received injections using 2 ml of collagen MD Muscle (Guna), the second group received 2 ml of 2% lidocaine without a vasoconstrictor, and the third group 2 ml of saline as a control (0.9% NaCl). All patients received repeated injections at one-week intervals (days 0 and 7). The visual analogue scale was used to determine pain intensity changes during each follow-up visit (days 0, 7, and 14) in each group. The masseter muscle activity was measured on each visit (days 0, 7, and 14) with surface electromyography (sEMG) (Neurobit Optima 4, Neurobit Systems). *Results.* We found that sEMG masseter muscle activity was significantly decreased in Group I (59.2%), less in Group II (39.3%), and least in Group III (14%). Pain intensity reduction was 53.75% in Group I, 25% in Group II, and 20.1% in Group III. *Conclusions.* The study confirmed that intramuscular injection of collagen is a more efficient method for reducing myofascial pain within masseter muscles than intramuscular injection of lidocaine.

## 1. Introduction

Myofascial pain within masticatory muscles is a popular muscle disorder among patients attending dental practitioners [1–3]. Mental status and bruxism may lead to excessive muscle effort and development of muscle pain [4–7]. The main syndrome of myofascial pain is a trigger point, which is a hard, palpable, localized nodule, painful on compression [8]. Myofascial pain is a symptom of muscle damage. Muscle regeneration is similar to muscle embryonic cell development.

Muscle injury can occur as a result of disease (dystrophy), contact with miotoxins, trauma, contusion, ischemia, temperature, and excessive muscle contraction [9]. Eccentric muscle contraction results in muscle damage and inflammation, resulting in muscle collagen accumulation, and occurs during the repair process of exercise-induced muscle injury [10]. Mechanical stress and cryolesions also induce collagen accumulation and production. During mechanical damage to muscles, sarcomere myofilaments are disrupted, the sarcolemma is damaged and fibers disintegrate [9]. After the muscle damage, interleukin-6 is released, and it induces fibroblasts to produce collagen [11, 12]. During muscle regeneration, stem cells proliferate and undergo differentiation into myoblast cells [13]. Simons' integrated hypothesis postulates energy crisis as the reason for the initial sarcomere contracture, which leads to increased metabolism and decreased capillary blood circulation [14]. The result is local hypoxia, muscle damage, and inflammatory mediators releasing, for example, catecholamines, neuropeptides, and cytokines. Then, muscle inflammation, persistent pain, and myofascial tenderness begin. Contraction knots are formed, as an effect of local injury, ischemia, and fiber lock. The blood flow around and within the trigger point is diminished. High-resistance and retrograde diastolic blood flow in the trigger point have been observed [14]. Vascular resistance is caused by musculature contracture and vessel compression. The effect is pain, tenderness, and nodularity of muscle tissue. Järvholm et al. have found that intramuscular pressure in trigger points decreased local blood flow and caused local ischemia [15]. Many trigger points localized together form myogelosis, where the level of oxygen is extremely low. In this mechanism, the level of ATP (adenosine triphosphate) is decreased. ATP is necessary for breaking the bonds between muscle myofilaments after muscle contracture. A low level of oxygen is a potent factor for bradykinin release [14]. Current approaches for trigger point management are needling, injections, and deep massage.

Lengthening contractions or endurance training may cause skeletal muscle damage, especially to the extracellular matrix (ECM) and muscle fibers. Collagen synthesis in muscle tissue, after damage, is elevated for 3 days [16]. Procollagen is synthesized in the endoplasmic reticulum and is extruded into the ECM. Premature collagen (tropocollagen) is then altered into the matured collagen protein. ECM is essential in muscle cell development and regeneration, and it is an important cell surrounding, which coordinates cell behavior and communication [17]. Interactions between muscle cells and ECM build a very important network in tissues undergoing mechanical stress. The lack of collagen in ECM is a reason for inappropriate muscle regeneration and muscle dystrophies. The lower the number of newly formed microfibers, the fewer the cross-sectional connections and the lower the produced muscle mass [18]. Collagen is strictly needed for proper muscle regeneration. Collagen decreases apoptosis and increases myoblast proliferation [18]. The extracellular matrix is also necessary for growth factors (PDGF and TGF$\beta$s) which regulate the process of stem cell proliferation and differentiation. During healing after injury, ECM is remodeled. Undesired substitutions occur, when fibrotic, connective tissue substitutes for muscle cells. Excessive production of fibrillar collagen can produce a scar, instead of newly formed muscle tissue. In the beginning of the regeneration process, a thick collagen network is formed to locate myogenic cells [18]. Collagen extrusion is mainly performed by interstitial fibroblasts.

Muscle elastic modulus ($E = 12$ kPa) may increase ($E > 18$ kPa) after the muscle injury, during the regeneration phase, because of the higher muscle stiffness and collagen network organization [18]. In chronic temporomandibular disorders, we can observe a reorganization of muscle activity resulting in poor muscle function [19].

Muscle regeneration is performed by stem cells. Myogenic cells are located under the basal lamina surrounding myofibers. Muscle-specific stem cells—satellite cells—precursors of mature myofibers, are responsible for skeletal muscle regeneration after repeated injuries [20]. Stem cells are regulated by collagen VI: biochemical signals, promoting proliferation, and differentiation of newly formed muscle cells.

Collagen is a molecule in ECM that plays an important role in building the base membrane of the myofiber endomysium in skeletal muscles [21]. Collagen is a major protein in ECM of skeletal muscles that builds networks and also present in the nervous system (in endo, peri, and epineurium of Schwann cells) and maintains proper nerve myelination [22, 23]. Collagen is provided to the muscles by interstitial fibroblast cells. Fibroblasts synthetize collagen I and collagen III at different ratios during muscle regeneration. Cultured fibroblasts secrete and deposit collagen VI with beneficial effects on muscle stiffness. Fibroblasts are the main source of collagen and could become an attractive option for medical therapy in the future. Collagen also provides biochemical signals for satellite cells to proliferate into myocells [18]. It is the main component of ECM, needed for muscle regeneration. Excess collagen production can result in cicatrization [24]. Lehto et al. analyzed collagen synthesis in gastrocnemius muscle in rats [25]. 14C-labeled proline was administered intraperitoneally to animal calves. The radioactivity of muscle probes was measured by liquid scintillation spectrophotometry. The uptake of labeled collagen and glycosaminoglycans showed the exact regeneration period: between 10 and 14 days after an injury. The uptake decreased after 21 days post injury. A collagen matrix is injected to guide muscle cell regeneration and differentiation.

There are three phases of muscle regeneration: myofiber breakdown and inflammation; stem cell activation and proliferation; and differentiation into new myofibers [26]. Muscle regeneration can form either a functionally efficient muscle contractile system or a scar [27, 28]. First, necrosis takes place and myofibers are disrupted; the blood level of muscle protein is increased (creatine kinase and troponin). The first inflammatory cells in injured muscle are neutrophils, as soon as 1–6 h after the muscle damage [29, 30]. The next group of inflammatory cells is macrophages that appear in injured tissue after 48 h. The necessary condition for muscle regeneration is blood supply with a bloodstream. Revascularization is modulated by many endocrine factors, for example, the fibroblast growth factor (FGF), which has angiogenic properties. Transforming growth factor-beta (TGF$\beta$s) stimulates collagen production, proteoglycans, fibronectin, and ECM protein production and angiogenesis [25]. The platelet-derived growth factor (PDGF) also influences angiogenesis in vivo.

Lidocainum hydrochloricum 2% is used as a popular analgesic drug in dentistry and cardiology as an antiarrhythmic drug. The mechanism of action is one where sodium channels are blocked causing a decrease in the heart rhythm rate. Neurons cannot send signals to the central nervous system. This was discovered in 1946, and since then, it has been one of the most popular and essential drugs in medicine. It is used for infiltration, blocks, and surface tissue anesthesia. Lidocaine has a very fast onset of action: approximately 1.5 min. It is often used in combination with adrenaline to prolong the effect of anesthesia. In trigger point therapy, it is used without vasoconstrictor agents, because of the risk of ischemic necrosis. The length of analgesia duration is about 30 min to 3 hours. Lidocaine can also be used as an inhalation drug to prevent coughing, especially during intubation. Some patients can be unresponsive to lidocaine, for example, those with Ehlers–Danlos syndrome [31].

The aim of the study was to evaluate the efficiency of intramuscular injections of collagen and lidocaine in reducing MFP within masseter muscles.

## 2. Materials and Methods

*2.1. Study Participants.* Within a group of 102 Caucasian patients who had been referred to the Department of Temporomandibular Disorders at the Medical University of Silesia in Katowice, Poland, the principal investigator (ANB) found 50 with MFP within masseter muscles who were eligible and included in this trial.

The inclusion criteria were the following:

(1) Age ≥18 and ≤80

(2) Presence of myofascial pain and myofascial pain with referral within masseter muscles according to the Diagnostic Criteria for Temporomandibular Disorders (DC/TMD) (II.1.A. 2 and 3) [32]

(3) Presence of trigger points within masseter muscles under palpation (latent or active)

(4) Patients' agreement for taking part into the research study.

The exclusion criteria were the following:

(1) Patients undergoing orthodontic treatment

(2) Patients being treated with or addicted to analgesic drugs and/or drugs that affect muscle function

(3) Patients after traumas to the head and neck region in the previous 2 years

(4) Edentulous patients and patients with unsupported occlusal contacts in the lateral region of the occlusal arches

(5) Patients being treated by neurologist for neurological disorders and/or neuropathic pain and/or headache

(6) Patients after radiotherapy

(7) Pain of dental origin

(8) Pregnancy or lactation

(9) Presence of malignancy

(10) Presence of severe mental disorders

(11) Drug and/or alcohol addiction

(12) Presence of contraindications for injection therapy

(13) Patients with needle phobia

(14) Presence of hypersensitivity to substances to be used in the study.

This study was approved by the Bioethical Committee of the Medical University of Silesia in Katowice, Poland (KNW/0022/KB1/61/I/15), and retrospectively registered at ClinicalTrials.gov NCT03323567 (27 October 2017). The study was performed in accordance with the Declaration of Helsinki as well as the International Conference on Harmonisation: Guidelines for Good Clinical Practice. All included patients gave their consent to participate in the study and received verbal and written information describing the trial.

*2.2. Study Protocol.* This randomized, controlled, single-blind, three-arm trial followed the consolidated standards of reporting trials (CONSORT) statement [33] and was performed between 10 January 2016 and 12 December 2017 in the Department of Temporomandibular Disorders at the Medical University of Silesia in Katowice, Poland. The patients were divided randomly into three groups: Collagen (Group I, $n = 18$), Lidocaine (Group II, $n = 15$), and Saline (Group III, $n = 17$). The randomization was carried out by a researcher who was not involved in the qualification of patients, conduct of interventions, or collection of data (MW). After allocation, 7 patients declined to participate. Consequently, the groups were structured as follows: Group I, $n = 15$, 5 males, 10 females, mean age $37.2 \pm 4.97$; Group II, $n = 13$, 5 males, 8 females, mean age $42.8 \pm 0.98$; and Group III, $n = 15$, 7 males, 8 females, mean age $40.3 \pm 1.18$. Patients were not informed what substance they would be injected. The injections were performed by a principal investigator (ANB) who knew what substance she was administering.

The trial consisted of four visits: (1) screening for study participation and inclusion, (2) first injection of study substances (baseline), (3) 1st follow-up and second injection of study substances, and (4) 2nd follow-up. The period between visits 2, 3, and 4 was one week (0, 7, and 14 days) (Figure 1).

The activities undertaken by the investigators during the trial are presented in Table 1.

*2.3. Treatment.* Group I was injected into the masseter trigger points using 2 ml of Collagen MD Muscle (Guna, Italy), Group II 2 ml of 2% Lidocaine (Lignocainum hydrochloricum WZF, Polfa Warsaw, Poland) without vasoconstrictor, and Group III 2 ml of saline as a control (0.9% NaCl) at 2nd and 3rd visits. In all groups, disposable syringes (2 ml) and needles ($0.4 \times 19$ mm) were used for injections. During the intervention, trigger points within masseter muscles were identified with palpation of the masseter muscle, and each group was injected with the same amount

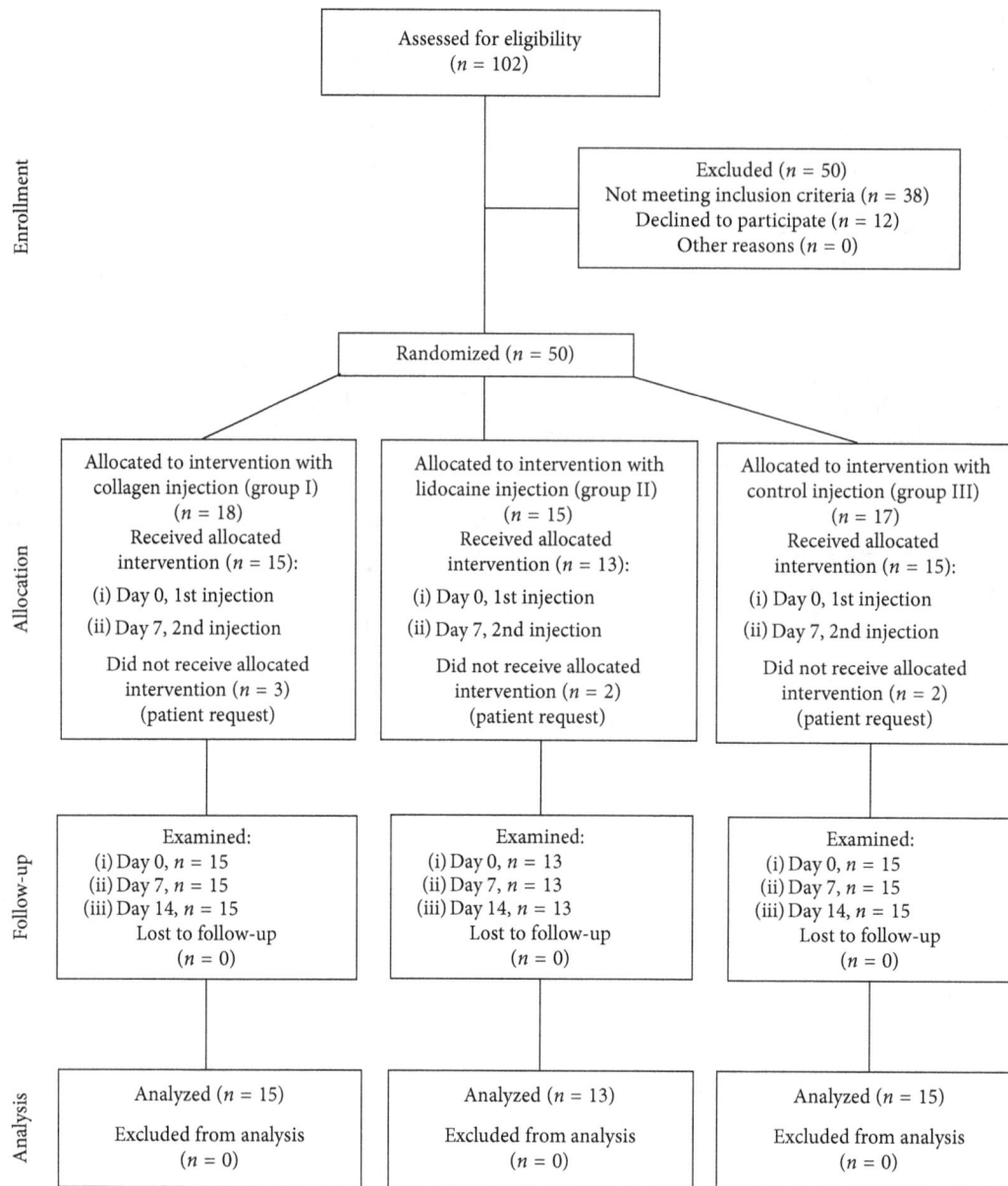

FIGURE 1: CONSORT three-arm diagram showing the flow of participants through each stage of the presented randomized controlled trial.

TABLE 1: Activities of investigators during the trial.

| Visit | 1 (screening and inclusion) | 2 (baseline) | 3 (1st follow-up) | 4 (2nd follow-up) |
|---|---|---|---|---|
| Day of the study | − | Day 0 | Day 7 | Day 14 |
| Injection | − | + | + | − |
| Measure EMG | − | EMG.I.1. EMG.II.1. EMG.III.1. EMG.I.1.NP EMG.II.1.NP EMG.III.1.NP | EMG.I.2. EMG.II.2. EMG.III.2. EMG.I.2.NP EMG.II.2.NP EMG.III.2.NP | EMG.I.3. EMG.II.3. EMG.II.3. EMG.I.3.NP EMG.II.3.NP EMG.II.3.NP |
| Measure VAS | − | VAS.I.1. VAS.II.1. VAS.III.1. | VAS.I.2. VAS.II.2. VAS.III.2. | VAS.I.3. VAS.II.3. VAS.III.3. |

EMG.I.1. = EMG, Group I first measurement; NP = no pain.

of the appropriate substance (2 ml) into the trigger point structure. Injections were deposited approximately 1–1.5 cm under the skin surface. In 40 patients, the injections were unilateral and in 3 patients, bilateral in two masseter muscles with the same substance (2 subjects in Group I and 1 subject in Group II).

*2.4. Treatment Outcome Measures.* To measure treatment outcome, a surface electromyography (sEMG) and visual analogue scale (VAS) were used at the 2nd, 3rd, and 4th visits with one week breaks between visits (0, 7, and 14 days). For the assessment of masseter muscle activity, a surface electromyography was performed with a Neurobit Optima device (Neurobit Systems, Poland). The rest values for masseter muscle were measured for both sides. Muscle activity in the form of surface electromyography data was measured with 5 electrodes positioned bilaterally: in the origin region on the zygomatic arch and maxillary process of the zygomatic bone and in the insertion region on the angle and lateral surface of the mandible ramus. Two electrodes were positioned at each side of the patients head and one, a reference electrode, on the patient's neck. The patient remained seated on a dental chair, keeping his or her mandible in a resting, comfortable, and relaxed position, without tooth contact. The electromyographic evaluation was performed after cleaning the skin surface with cotton pads and an alcohol solution (Octenisept, Schulke, Germany). Electrodes were fixed on the skin covering the masseter muscle and on the patient's neck with a self-adhesive gel. The patient was asked to perform an isometric contraction of the masseter muscles to find the best place for electrode fixation. A 0–10 visual analogue scale with the endpoints marked "no pain" (0) and "worst experienced pain" (10) was used to evaluate the effectiveness in pain reduction of the substances studied. Pain evaluation using VAS and surface electromyography was performed by two investigators (JBK and KWD) and muscle injections were performed by the other investigator (ANB).

*2.5. Sample Size Estimation.* Normal distribution of VAS values was assumed. With the division into three groups, the analysis of variance for repeated measurements was planned, with equal sized groups. The power to achieve was 0.9 with the significance level set to 0.05.

Additional assumptions were the following:

(1) Expected VAS values in individual research groups and subsequent measurements (Table 2).

(2) Standard deviation for all measurements was SD = 1.5.

(3) For the correlation matrix, the LEAR (linear exponent AR (1)) model was adopted, with base correlation set to 0.85 and correlation decay rate equal to 1.

The total number of subjects needed was 36, given the above assumptions; thus, the minimum number of subjects per group was 12. Sample size estimation was performed by using SAS, version 9.4 (SAS Institute Inc., Cary, NC).

TABLE 2: Expected VAS values and measurements.

| Observation | Group | Baseline | 1st follow-up | 2nd follow-up |
| --- | --- | --- | --- | --- |
| 1 | VAS.I | 8 | 5 | 3 |
| 2 | VAS.II | 8 | 6 | 5 |
| 3 | VAS.III | 8 | 7 | 6 |

*2.6. Randomization and Blinding.* Patients who met the inclusion criteria were randomized by computer-generated simple randomization into one of the following groups: Collagen (Group I, $n = 18$), Lidocaine (Group II, $n = 15$), and Saline (Group III, $n = 17$). MW conducted the randomization and prepared the list of interventions by enrolment numbers. ANB administered the injections, according to the list. Patients and members of the study group (ANB, JBK, and KWD, who performed and collected pain intensity using VAS and muscle activity using surface EMG) were blinded for allocation and treatment.

*2.7. Statistical Analysis.* A one-way repeated measures analysis of variance was carried out. To verify the assumptions of the method in all groups, the analysis of the normality of the distribution was performed with Shapiro–Wilk test. The homogeneity of variance was analyzed by Hartley's test, Cochran–Cox test, and Bartlett's chi-square test. Mauchley's sphericity test was also performed. From the analysis of variance, it follows that the assumptions of a one-way repeated measures analysis of variance are met in the analyzed groups. In order to verify statistical hypotheses, the level of significance of alpha = 0.05 was assumed. The calculations were carried out in Statistica 12.0 (StatSoft, Poland).

# 3. Results

*3.1. Demographics and Statistics.* The present study included 43 Caucasian patients (17 males and 26 females). The mean age was $39.97 \pm 3.78$ years. Demographic characteristics of the patients are summarized in Table 3. There were no differences in age or gender between the groups ($p > 0.05$).

Data collected using sEMG and VAS were analyzed using descriptive statistics and briefly presented in Table 4.

Collected values for sEMG masseter muscle activity and pain intensity were normally distributed. The statistical analysis showed that the decreases in the mean values of EMG and VAS over time are statistically significant ($p < 0.001$). The mean values and 95% confidence intervals are shown in the Figures 2 and 3.

*3.2. Primary Treatment Outcome*

*3.2.1. Evaluation of Masseter Muscle Pain Intensity.* Masseter muscle pain intensity was assessed and compared before injection of collagen (VAS.I.1.), lidocaine (VAS.II.1.), and saline (VAS.III.1.) after 7 days (VAS.I.2., VAS. II.2., and VAS. III.2.) and 14 days (VAS.I.3., VAS. II.3., and VAS. III.3.) during baseline and follow-up visits.

TABLE 3: Baseline characteristics of 43 patients with MFP within masseter muscles included in the study.

| | Group I | Group II | Group III |
|---|---|---|---|
| Male/female, $n$ | 5/10 | 5/8 | 7/8 |
| Age (years) | $37.2 \pm 4.97$ | $42.8 \pm 0.98$ | $40.3 \pm 1.18$ |
| Duration of myofascial pain (weeks), mean (SD) | $30.2 \pm 31.48$ | $34.3 \pm 29.26$ | $38.3 \pm 26.47$ |
| Bilateral involvement of myofascial pain (number of patients) | 2 | 1 | 0 |

TABLE 4: Descriptive statistics of sEMG and VAS values.

| | $N$ | Average | Minimum | Maximum | Stand. dev. | One-way repeated measures ANOVA |
|---|---|---|---|---|---|---|
| EMG.I.1. ($\mu$V) | 15 | 56.67 | 47 | 65 | 5.95 | |
| EMG.I.2. ($\mu$V) | 15 | 32.67 | 28 | 41 | 3.85 | $p < 0.001$ |
| EMG.I.3. ($\mu$V) | 15 | 23.73 | 20 | 29 | 2.81 | |
| EMG.I.1.NP ($\mu$V) | 15 | 34.3 | 27 | 45 | 5.17 | |
| EMG.I.2.NP ($\mu$V) | 15 | 34.6 | 27 | 42 | 4.35 | $p = 0.344$ |
| EMG.I.3.NP ($\mu$V) | 15 | 35.2 | 25 | 44 | 5.47 | |
| VAS.I.1. | 15 | 8.07 | 5 | 10 | 1.58 | |
| VAS.I.2. | 15 | 4.67 | 2 | 8 | 1.54 | $p < 0.001$ |
| VAS.I.3. | 15 | 3.73 | 1 | 7 | 1.94 | |
| EMG.II.1. ($\mu$V) | 13 | 59.07 | 49 | 70 | 4.79 | |
| EMG.II.2. ($\mu$V) | 13 | 41.20 | 37 | 49 | 3.36 | $p < 0.001$ |
| EMG.II.3. ($\mu$V) | 13 | 35.07 | 29 | 45 | 4.40 | |
| EMG.II.1.NP ($\mu$V) | 13 | 38.7 | 29 | 60 | 7.3 | |
| EMG.II.2.NP ($\mu$V) | 13 | 39.2 | 31 | 55 | 6.8 | $p = 0.353$ |
| EMG.II.3.NP ($\mu$V) | 13 | 37.7 | 29 | 52 | 6.4 | |
| VAS.II.1. | 13 | 8.33 | 6 | 10 | 1.23 | |
| VAS.II.2. | 13 | 7.40 | 5 | 9 | 1.12 | $p < 0.001$ |
| VAS.II.3. | 13 | 6.07 | 4 | 9 | 1.58 | |
| EMG.III.1. ($\mu$V) | 15 | 64.13 | 56 | 72 | 5.34 | |
| EMG.III.2. ($\mu$V) | 15 | 60.20 | 54 | 69 | 4.41 | $p < 0.001$ |
| EMG.III.3. ($\mu$V) | 15 | 55.27 | 50 | 64 | 4.83 | |
| EMG.III.1.NP ($\mu$V) | 15 | 36.6 | 26 | 43 | 8.3 | |
| EMG.III.2.NP ($\mu$V) | 15 | 34 | 29 | 41 | 4.5 | $p = 0.138$ |
| EMG.III.3.NP ($\mu$V) | 15 | 36.5 | 29 | 42 | 4.3 | |
| VAS.III.1. | 15 | 8.13 | 6 | 10 | 1.19 | |
| VAS.III.2. | 15 | 6.80 | 4 | 9 | 1.57 | $p < 0.001$ |
| VAS.III.3. | 15 | 6.53 | 3 | 9 | 2.03 | |

Pain intensity reduction was observed in all groups: in Group I, the average pain intensity reduction in VAS scale was $4.3 = 53.75\%$; in Group II, the average decrease in pain intensity was $2 = 25\%$; and in Group III, the average value of pain elimination was $1.63 = 20.1\%$ as well (Table 5, Figure 2). Comparing data between measurements performed on days 7 and 14, the authors observed statistically significant pain reduction in all cases, between baseline, 1st follow-up visit, and 2nd follow-up visit (Table 5).

### 3.3. Secondary Treatment Outcome

*3.3.1. Evaluation of the Surface Electromyography.* Masseter muscle activity was assessed and compared before injection of collagen (EMG.I.1.), lidocaine (EMG.II.1.), and saline (EMG.III.1.) after 7 days (EMG.I.2., EMG. II.2., and EMG. III.2.) and 14 days (EMG.I.3., EMG. II.3., and EMG. III.3.)

during follow-up visits. Only rest muscle electromyographic activity was measured in trigger point region on the painful side.

EMG activity of masseter muscles was measured in each group for three times, during baseline and follow-up visits (Figure 3). Mean values for all collected sEMG results are presented in Figure 2. The most significant reduction of sEMG values was observed in Group I ($32.9 \mu$V, $59.2\%$). In Group II, a $23.5 \mu$V ($39.3\%$) reduction was observed. The lowest reduction of sEMG values was noticed in Group III ($8.9 \mu$V, $14\%$) (Table 6). In each group, a statistically significant reduction was observed ($p < 0.001$).

*3.3.2. Evaluation of the Surface Electromyography on the Side without Myofascial Pain.* Masseter muscle activity was also assessed and compared on the asymptomatic side before injections of collagen (EMG.I.1. NP), lidocaine (EMG.II.1.

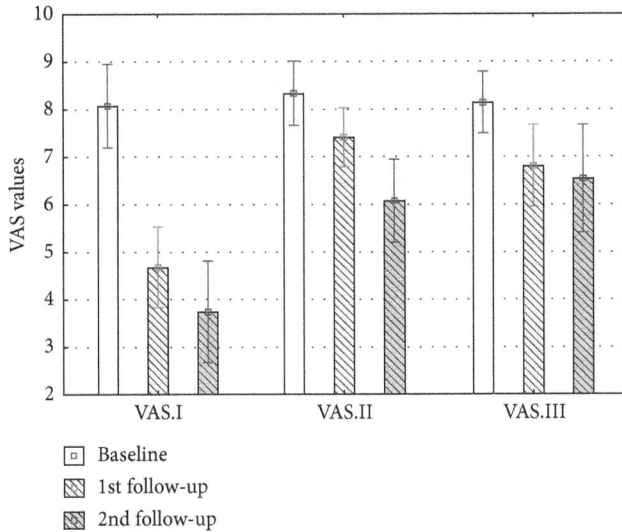

FIGURE 2: VAS mean value changes in Group I, Group II, and Group III during the trial (days 0, 7, and 14).

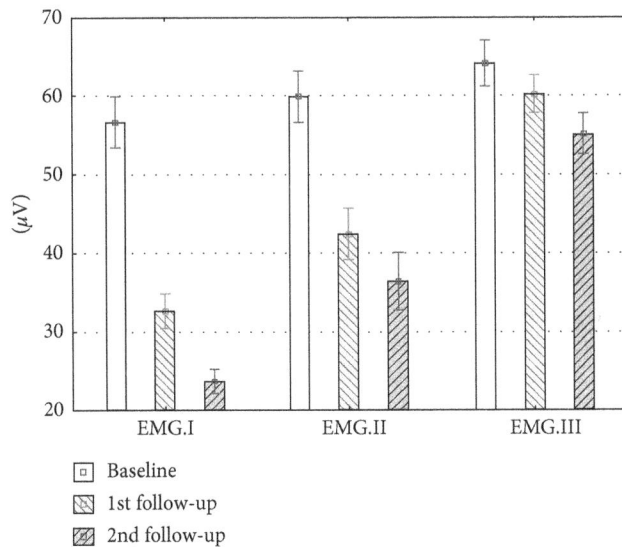

FIGURE 3: Changes in mean values of superficial electromyographic activity of masseter muscles in Group I, Group II, and Group III during the trial (days 0, 7, and 14).

NP), and saline (EMG.III.1. NP) after 7 days (EMG.I.2. NP, EMG. II.2. NP, and EMG. III.2. NP) and 14 days (EMG.I.3. NP, EMG. II.3. NP, and EMG. III.3. NP) during follow-up visits (Table 6). In 3 subjects, pain was observed bilaterally. In each group, no statistically significant changes of sEMG were observed ($p > 0.001$).

*3.4. Adverse Effects.* Approximately 30 minutes after the injection of collagen into the masseter muscle, patients described pain during movement, edema, and muscle stiffness. After approximately 1 hour, pain symptoms were gone. In a few patients (9 subjects), bruises appeared after the injection, directly at the needle insertion points. These

TABLE 5: Changes in VAS mean values in Group I, Group II, and Group III after 14 days.

| Visit | Group I | Group II | Group III |
|---|---|---|---|
| Baseline | 8 | 8.3 | 8.13 |
| 1st follow-up visit | 4.6 | 7.4 | 6.8 |
| 2nd follow-up visit | 3.7 | 6 | 6.5 |
| VAS changes | **−4.3** | **−2** | **−1.63** |
| Percentage VAS changes | **−53.75%** | **−25%** | **−20.1%** |

TABLE 6: Changes in EMG mean values in Group I, Group II, and Group III after 14 days.

| Visit | Group I ($\mu$V) | Group II ($\mu$V) | Group III ($\mu$V) |
|---|---|---|---|
| *Pain side* | | | |
| Baseline | 56.6 | 59.9 | 64.1 |
| 1st follow-up visit | 32.6 | 42.4 | 60.2 |
| 2nd follow-up visit | 23.7 | 36.4 | 55.2 |
| EMG changes | **−32.9** | **−23.5** | **−8.9** |
| Percentage EMG changes | **−59.2%** | **−39.3%** | **−14%** |
| *No pain side* | | | |
| Baseline | 34.3 | 38.7 | 36.6 |
| 1st follow-up visit | 34.6 | 39.2 | 34 |
| 2nd follow-up visit | 35.2 | 37.7 | 36.5 |
| EMG changes | **+0.9** | **−1** | **−0.1** |
| Percentage EMG changes | **+2.6%** | **−2.5%** | **−0.3%** |

adverse effects were temporary and completely reversible. There were no serious adverse effects during the trial.

## 4. Discussion

Intramuscular injections of collagen, lidocaine, and saline into the trigger points of masseter muscles in the treatment of myofascial pain reduction within masseter muscles varied across study groups in terms of their level of success. The best results were achieved in Group I: maximal reduction of sEMG activity (32.9 $\mu$V; 59.2%) and best antinociceptive results (reduction, 4.3; 53.75% on the VAS scale). There are not many research studies analyzing collagen intramuscular injections, besides Milani [34], Yu et al. [35], and Alfieri [36]. These authors stated in their research studies a positive muscle reaction to intramuscular collagen injections, but these studies were not related to orofacial muscle pain.

However, despite the fact that the result is satisfactory, we would like to emphasize that the trial had limitations. The main limitation was the short period of observation of the reduction of pain intensity and the single-blind nature of the trial. Both these limitations resulted in our restricted funding and possibilities of carrying out the trial.

According to the current literature, biomaterial guided regeneration is a new approach for myofascial pain syndrome. This is confirmed by Kuraitis et al. who injected a collagen matrix enhanced with sialyl LewisX (sLeX) to guide skeletal muscle differentiation and regeneration [26]. Muscle tissue damaged by an injected substance has the ability to perform myogenesis and revascularization. We found that satellite cells are active in muscle cell regeneration and collagen VI participates in the activation of satellite cells [17]. The extracellular matrix is a special collagen supply for new myocytes formed in the process of muscle regeneration. The composition of ECM is extremely important for the proper regeneration process to avoid substitution by fibrotic connective tissue, that is, scar production. It is probable that the collagen molecules that were provided by intramuscular injections help to produce an extracellular network that keeps myocytes in their proper positions. The presence of satellite cells in an extracellular matrix is called "a pool" of pluripotential cells for myocyte formation. In this study, the authors noticed better muscle tissue properties and less pathological symptoms after extracellular collagen delivery.

In the clinical trial, we noticed muscle function advancement after collagen intramuscular injections, but Kato et al. found that muscle collagen protein synthesis is not regulated by elevated nutritional or intravenous levels of collagen, but just by mechanical stress [37]. Some authors have observed a better muscle tissue condition and muscle activity decreasing after intramuscular collagen injections. Lawrence and De Luca found a positive correlation between muscle myoelectric signals and the muscle force of the maximal voluntary contraction [38, 39].

In Group II, intramuscular lidocaine injections were performed to decrease pain and to eliminate trigger points. McMillan et al. performed a comparative research between dry needling and procaine injection into the trigger points of masseter muscles in patients with temporomandibular disorders [40]. They concluded that therapy with dry needling and procaine is questionable, because they did not notice any difference in the end point of his study between experimental groups. We found similar results in our study, but in comparison with Group I, lidocaine and dry needling were far less effective.

Antinociceptive results were also observed, but not as successful as in Group I. We can also find some articles about myofascial pain therapy with prolotherapy, which involves the injection of an irritant solution of lidocaine and dextrose into the joint, ligament or painful muscle [41, 42]. Sung et al. identified the correlation between lidocaine concentration and exposure time and tissue cell death [43]. In the future, it would be important to compare anesthetics that are less toxic, for example, ropivacaine. We observed in our research study some effectiveness of injections, with different solutions. We found that we have achieved the best regenerative results with collagen injections, but lidocaine and saline injections also produced pain level decreases as well as sEMG activity decreases. Blasco-Bonora performed a dry-needling technique in masseter muscle trigger points and also achieved an improvement in muscle pain reduction and jaw opening in patients with sleep bruxism [44]. Kalichman and Vulfsons stated in their study that deep dry needling is more effective than superficial dry needling in the therapy of musculoskeletal pain [45]. Masseter muscle lies just underneath the skin, so injections were not very deep (approximately 1.5 cm), but we can call it deep wet needling. Injecting collagen into the trigger point in our opinion may be favorable, not only because of the specific mechanism of action in regenerating muscle tissue, or as a buffer collagen supply, but also as a therapeutic injection. Dry needling and injections into the trigger points have some common points with acupuncture methods [46–49].

It should be noted that a significant effect in terms of reducing sEMG muscle activity and pain intensity was obtained after two injections and the study intervention did not pose a risk of significant adverse effects and high interoperative risk.

## 5. Conclusions

The study confirmed that intramuscular injection of collagen is a more efficient method to reduce myofascial pain within masseter muscles than intramuscular injection of lidocaine. Due to the short observation time, further long-term trials should be conducted.

## Disclosure

The research study was performed as a part of the employment in the Medical University of Silesia in Katowice, Poland, and Wroclaw Medical University, Poland.

## Authors' Contributions

Aleksandra Nitecka-Buchta created trial concept, performed intramuscular injections of collagen, lidocaine, and saline, analyzed the data, and wrote and edited the manuscript. Jolanta Batko-Kapustecka and Karolina Walczynska-Dragon performed and collected pain intensity using VAS and muscle activity using surface electromyography. Mieszko Wieckiewicz conducted the randomization, analyzed data, wrote and edited the manuscript, and finally revised it before submission. All authors read and approved the final manuscript.

## Acknowledgments

Copy-editing service was provided by expert language reviewers from Translmed Publishing Group (PG). The authors would like to thank Michal Skrzypek and Tomasz Halama for statistical analyses and the patients for their participation in the study.

## References

[1] A. Al-Khotani, A. Naimi-Akbar, E. Albadawi, M. Ernberg, B. Hedenberg-Magnusson, and N. Christidis, "Prevalence of diagnosed temporomandibular disorders among Saudi Arabian children and adolescents," *Journal of Headache and Pain*, vol. 17, no. 1, pp. 17–41, 2016.

[2] M. Wieckiewicz, N. Grychowska, K. Wojciechowski et al., "Prevalence and correlation between TMD based on RDC/TMD diagnoses, oral parafunctions and psychoemotional stress in Polish university students," *BioMed Research International*, vol. 2014, Article ID 472346, 7 pages, 2014.

[3] M. A. Osiewicz, F. Lobbezoo, B. W. Loster, J. E. Loster, and D. Manfredini, "Frequency of temporomandibular disorders diagnoses based on RDC/TMD in a Polish patient population," *Cranio®*, pp. 1–7, 2017.

[4] D. R. Reissmann, M. T. John, A. Aigner, G. Schön, I. Sierwald, and E. L. Schiffman, "Interaction between awake and sleep bruxism is associated with increased presence of painful temporomandibular disorder," *Journal of Oral & Facial Pain and Headache*, vol. 31, no. 4, pp. 299–305, 2017.

[5] M. Wieckiewicz, M. Zietek, J. Smardz, D. Zenczak-Wieckiewicz, and N. Grychowska, "Mental status as a common factor for masticatory muscle pain: a systematic review," *Frontiers in Psychology*, vol. 8, p. 646, 2017.

[6] A. Al-Khotani, A. Naimi-Akbar, M. Gjelset et al., "The associations between psychosocial aspects and TMD-pain related aspects in children and adolescents," *Journal of Headache and Pain*, vol. 17, no. 1, p. 30, 2016.

[7] M. Pihut, E. Ferendiuk, M. Szewczyk, K. Kasprzyk, and M. Wieckiewicz, "The efficiency of botulinum toxin type A for the treatment of masseter muscle pain in patients with temporomandibular joint dysfunction and tension-type headache," *Journal of Headache and Pain*, vol. 17, no. 1, p. 29, 2016.

[8] J. Borg-Steina and D. G. Simons, "Myofascial pain," *Archives of Physical Medicine and Rehabilitation*, vol. 83, no. 1, pp. S40–S47, 2002.

[9] M. Karalaki, S. Fili, A. Philippou, and M. Koutsilieris, "Muscle regeneration: cellular and molecular events," *In Vivo*, vol. 23, no. 5, pp. 779–796, 2009.

[10] R. Myllylä, A. Salminen, L. Peltonen, T. E. Takala, and V. Vihko, "Collagen metabolism of mouse skeletal muscle during the repair of exercise injuries," *Pflügers Archiv European Journal of Physiology*, vol. 407, no. 1, pp. 64–70, 1986.

[11] J. Peake, K. Nosaka, and K. Suzuki, "Characterization of inflammatory responses to eccentric exercise in humans," *Exercise Immunology Review*, vol. 11, pp. 64–85, 2005.

[12] M. R. Duncan and B. Berman, "Stimulation of collagen and glycosaminoglycan production in cultured human adult dermal fibroblasts by recombinant human interleukin 6," *Journal of Investigative Dermatology*, vol. 97, no. 4, pp. 686–692, 1991.

[13] F. S. Tedesco, A. Dellavalle, J. Diaz-Manera, G. Messina, and G. Cossu, "Repairing skeletal muscle: regenerative potential of skeletal muscle stem cells," *Journal of Clinical Investigation*, vol. 120, no. 1, pp. 11–19, 2010.

[14] S. Sikdar, J. P. Shah, T. Gebreab et al., "Novel applications of ultrasound technology to visualize and characterize myofascial trigger points and surrounding soft tissue," *Archives of Physical Medicine and Rehabilitation*, vol. 90, no. 11, pp. 1829–1838, 2009.

[15] U. Järvholm, J. Styf, M. Suurkula, and P. Herberts, "Intramuscular pressure and muscle blood flow in supraspinatus," *European Journal of Applied Physiology and Occupational Physiology*, vol. 58, no. 3, pp. 219–224, 1988.

[16] B. F. Miller, J. L. Olesen, M. Hansen et al., "Coordinated collagen and muscle protein synthesis in human patella tendon and quadriceps muscle after exercise," *Journal of Physiology*, vol. 567, no. 3, pp. 1021–1033, 2005.

[17] S. Thorsteinsdóttir, M. Deries, A. S. Cachaço, and F. Bajanca, "The extracellular matrix dimension of skeletal muscle development," *Developmental Biology*, vol. 354, no. 2, pp. 191–207, 2011.

[18] A. Urciuolo, M. Quarta, V. Morbidoni et al., "Collagen VI regulates satellite cell self-renewal and muscle regeneration," *Nature Communications*, vol. 4, no. 1, p. 1964, 2013.

[19] A. Mapelli, B. C. Zanandréa Machado, L. D. Giglio, C. Sforza, and C. M. De Felício, "Reorganization of muscle activity in patients with chronic temporomandibular disorders," *Archives of Oral Biology*, vol. 72, pp. 164–171, 2016.

[20] M. Pihut, M. Szuta, E. Ferendiuk, and D. Zeńczak-Więckiewicz, "Evaluation of pain regression in patients with temporomandibular dysfunction treated by intra-articular platelet-rich plasma injections: a preliminary report," *BioMed Research International*, vol. 2014, Article ID 132369, 7 pages, 2014.

[21] C. G. Bönnemann, "The collagen VI-related myopathies: muscle meets its matrix," *Nature Reviews Neurology*, vol. 7, no. 7, pp. 379–390, 2011.

[22] P. Braghetta, C. Fabbro, S. Piccolo et al., "Distinct regions control transcriptional activation of the alpha1 (VI) collagen promoter in different tissues of transgenic mice," *Journal of Cell Biology*, vol. 135, no. 4, pp. 1163–1177, 1996.

[23] M. Cescon, F. Gattazzo, P. Chen, and P. Bonaldo, "Collagen VI at a glance," *Journal of Cell Science*, vol. 128, no. 19, pp. 3525–3531, 2015.

[24] S. Sorichter, J. Mair, A. Koller et al., "Skeletal troponin I as a marker of exercise-induced muscle damage," *Journal of Applied Physiology*, vol. 83, no. 4, pp. 1076–1082, 1985.

[25] M. Lehto and M. Järvinen, "Collagen and glycosaminoglycan synthesis of injured gastrocnemius muscle in rat," *European Surgical Research*, vol. 17, no. 3, pp. 179–185, 1985.

[26] D. Kuraitis, D. Ebadi, P. Zhang et al., "Injected matrix stimulates myogenesis and regeneration of mouse skeletal muscle after ischaemic injury," *European Cells and Materials*, vol. 24, pp. 175–195, 2012.

[27] D. L. Stocum, *Regenerative Biology and Medicine*, Academic Press, Cambridge, MA, USA, 2012.

[28] F. Mourkioti and N. Rosenthal, "IGF-1, inflammation and stem cells: interactions during muscle regeneration," *Trends in Immunology*, vol. 26, no. 10, pp. 535–542, 2005.

[29] V. Prisk and J. Huard, "Muscle injuries and repair: the role of prostaglandins and inflammation," *Histology and Histopathology*, vol. 18, no. 4, pp. 1243–1256, 2003.

[30] J. M. McClung, J. M. Davis, and J. A. Carson, "Ovarian hormone status and skeletal muscle inflammation during recovery from disuse in rats," *Experimental Physiology*, vol. 92, no. 1, pp. 219–232, 2007.

[31] A. J. Hakim, R. Grahame, P. Norris, and C. Hopper, "Local anaesthetic failure in joint hypermobility syndrome," *Journal of the Royal Society of Medicine*, vol. 98, no. 2, pp. 84-85, 2005.

[32] C. C. Peck, J. P. Goulet, F. Lobbezoo et al., "Expanding the taxonomy of the diagnostic criteria for temporomandibular disorders," *Journal of Oral Rehabilitation*, vol. 41, no. 1, pp. 2–23, 2014.

[33] N. Pandis, B. Chung, R. W. Scherer, D. Elbourne, and D. G. Altman, "CONSORT 2010 statement: extension checklist for reporting within person randomised trials," *BMJ*, vol. 357, p. j2835, 2017.

[34] L. Milani, "A new and refined injectable treatment for musculoskeletal disorders-bioscaffold properties of collagen and its clinical use," *Physiological Regulating Medicine*, vol. 1, pp. 3–15, 2010.

[35] X. J. Yu, G. H. Ding, W. Yao, R. Zhan, and M. Huang, "The role of collagen fiber in "Zusanli" (ST 36) in acupuncture

analgesia in the rat," *Zhongguo Zhen Jiu*, vol. 28, no. 3, pp. 207–213, 2008.

[36] N. Alfieri, "MD-Muscle in the management of myofascial pain syndrome," *Physiological Regulating Medicine*, vol. 17, pp. 23-24, 2016.

[37] M. Pihut, G. Wisniewska, P. Majewski, K. Gronkiewicz, and S. Majewski, "Measurement of occlusal forces in the therapy of functional disorders with the use of botulinum toxin type A," *Journal of Physiology and Pharmacology*, vol. 60, no. 8, pp. 113–116, 2009.

[38] H. Kato, H. Suzuki, Y. Inoue, K. Suzuki, and H. Kobayashi, "Leucine-enriched essential amino acids augment mixed protein synthesis, but not collagen protein synthesis, in rat skeletal muscle after downhill running," *Nutrients*, vol. 8, no. 7, p. 399, 2016.

[39] J. H. Lawrence and C. J. De Luca, "Myoelectric signal versus force relationship in different human muscles," *Journal of Applied Physiology*, vol. 54, no. 6, pp. 1653–1659, 1983.

[40] A. S. McMillan, A. Nolan, and P. J. Kelly, "The efficacy of dry needling and procaine in the treatment of myofascial pain in the jaw muscles," *Journal of Orofacial Pain*, vol. 11, no. 4, pp. 307–314, 1997.

[41] D. Rabago, M. Yelland, J. Patterson, and A. Zgierska, "Prolotherapy for chronic musculoskeletal pain," *American Family Physician*, vol. 84, no. 11, pp. 1208–1210, 2011.

[42] A. R. Daftary and A. S. Karnik, "Perspectives in ultrasound-guided musculoskeletal interventions," *Indian Journal of Radiology and Imaging*, vol. 25, no. 3, pp. 246–260, 2015.

[43] C. M. Sung, Y. S. Hah, J. S. Kim et al., "Cytotoxic effects of ropivacaine, bupivacaine, and lidocaine on rotator cuff tenofibroblasts," *American Journal of Sports Medicine*, vol. 42, no. 12, pp. 2888–2896, 2014.

[44] V. Y. Moraes, M. Lenza, M. J. Tamaoki, F. Faloppa, and J. C. Belloti, "Platelet-rich therapies for musculoskeletal soft tissue injuries," *Cochrane Database of Systematic Reviews*, no. 4, p. CD010071, 2014.

[45] M. S. Hamid, A. Yusof, and M. R. Mohamed Ali, "Platelet-rich plasma (PRP) for acute muscle injury: a systematic review," *PLoS One*, vol. 9, no. 2, article e90538, 2014.

[46] P. M. Blasco-Bonora and A. M. Pintado-Zugasti, "Effects of myofascial trigger point dry needling in patients with sleep bruxism and temporomandibular disorders a prospective case series," *Acupuncture in Medicine*, vol. 35, no. 1, pp. 69–74, 2017.

[47] L. Kalichman and S. Vulfsons, "Dry needling in the management of musculoskeletal pain," *Journal of the American Board of Family Medicine*, vol. 23, no. 5, pp. 640–646, 2010.

[48] X. Li, R. Wang, X. Xing et al., "Acupuncture for myofascial pain syndrome: a network meta-analysis of 33 randomized controlled trials," *Pain Physician*, vol. 20, no. 6, pp. E883–E902, 2017.

[49] J. Fernández-Carnero, R. La Touche, R. Ortega-Santiago et al., "Short-term effects of dry needling of active myofascial trigger points in the masseter muscle in patients with temporomandibular disorders," *Journal of Orofacial Pain*, vol. 24, no. 1, pp. 106–112, 2010.

# 19

# Temporomandibular Disorders Related to Stress and HPA-Axis Regulation

Kordian Staniszewski,[1] Henning Lygre,[1,2] Ersilia Bifulco,[3] Siv Kvinnsland,[1] Lisa Willassen,[1] Espen Helgeland,[1] Trond Berge,[1,4] and Annika Rosén ⓘ[1,4]

[1]Department of Clinical Dentistry, University of Bergen, Bergen, Norway
[2]Oral Health Center of Expertise in Western Norway, Stavanger, Rogaland, Norway
[3]Department of Clinical Science, University of Bergen, Bergen, Norway
[4]Department of Oral and Maxillofacial Surgery, Haukeland University Hospital, Bergen, Norway

Correspondence should be addressed to Annika Rosén; annika.rosen@uib.no

Academic Editor: Shiau Yuh-Yuan

Temporomandibular disorders (TMDs) are characterized by pain and dysfunction in the masticatory apparatus and the temporomandibular joint (TMJ). Previous trauma, stress symptoms, psychosocial impairment, and catastrophizing have been related to TMD. To assess if the hypothalamic-pituitary-adrenal (HPA) axis is upregulated in TMD patients, we performed a cross-sectional study with saliva from 44 TMD patients and 44 healthy sex- and age-matched controls for cortisol ($F$) and cortisone ($E$) with liquid chromatography-tandem mass spectrometry. Furthermore, we calculated the $F/E$ ratio for the evaluation of 11$\beta$-hydroxysteroid dehydrogenase activity. We also assessed anxiety/depression and pain catastrophizing scores from a questionnaire that participants completed prior to the examination. We found that $F$ ($P = 0.01$), $E$ ($P = 0.04$), the $F/E$ ratio ($P = 0.002$), and the sum of glucocorticoids ($E + E$) in saliva ($P = 0.02$) were significantly higher in the TMD group. Anxiety/depression and catastrophizing scores were also significantly higher in the TMD group ($P < 0.0001$). Our findings indicate that patients with TMDs may have an upregulated HPA axis with higher $F$ secretion from the adrenal cortex. Anxiety/depression and pain catastrophizing scores were significantly higher in the TMD group, and psychological factors may contribute to chronic upregulation of the HPA axis.

## 1. Introduction

Temporomandibular disorders (TMDs) are a group of disorders associated with pain and dysfunction affecting the temporomandibular joint (TMJ) and the masticatory apparatus [1, 2]. TMDs occur predominantly in women, who are especially likely to experience more severe symptoms. TMD-associated comorbidities include fibromyalgia, irritable bowel syndrome, and depression, with trauma and stress symptoms frequently present as well [3]. Psychosocial impairment within a TMD, such as somatization and depression, is linked with pain-related disability as well as the duration of pain [4]. The Orofacial Pain Prospective Evaluation and Risk Assessment (OPPERA) study found that psychosocial factors (e.g., somatic awareness, distress, catastrophizing, pain amplification, and

psychosocial stress) had a significantly higher prevalence in subjects with a TMD compared to healthy individuals [2, 5].

During the last few decades, use of physiological markers for assessing psychosocial-related disorders has increased. Stress activates the hypothalamic-pituitary-adrenal (HPA) axis, which results in a cascade of reactions leading to increased secretion of cortisol from the adrenal cortex. Research examining the HPA axis response to stress has yielded contradictory results. A meta-analysis of chronic stress and HPA-axis activity found that HPA response to stress varies with the nature and controllability of stressful stimuli as well as the individual psychiatric response [6]. The role of stress in the etiology and persistence of TMD remains unclear. However, dysregulation of the HPA axis has been correlated with TMD in several studies [7–9]. Accordingly, analysis of cortisol ($F$) levels in saliva may provide a means for examining HPA-axis activity.

Salivary $F$ levels follow circadian fluctuations, and these variations can be used to create a curve depicting unbound free and total cortisol in serum [10]. However, previous analyses of $F$ in saliva from TMD patients have given variable results. Some researchers have found elevated $F$ values in association with TMD [11, 12], while others have not found any significant difference in comparison to a control group [13]. Analyses using immunoassay methods [11–15] have also been undertaken to measure $F$ in saliva from subjects with a TMD. These methods do not separate cortisol ($F$) and cortisone ($E$), which have structural similarities but unequal biological activities. Recent $F$ and $E$ analyses based on liquid chromatography-tandem mass spectrometry (LC-MS/MS) are now available [16].

The primary objective of this study was to assess the stress levels in TMD patients based on an upregulated HPA axis and compare the results with healthy individuals. Secondary objectives were to analyze the saliva for $F$ and $E$ and the scores for self-reported anxiety/depression and catastrophizing from a questionnaire. The hypothesis was that TMD patients have an upregulated HPA axis shown by increased psychological scores and increased level of cortisol in saliva.

## 2. Materials and Methods

*2.1. Study Design.* The present study is a clinical cross-sectional study, which was a part of a multidisciplinary investigation of TMD patients at Haukeland University Hospital, sponsored by the Norwegian Ministry of Health [17]. Ethical approval was granted by the Regional Ethical Review Board South East (2015/930), in accordance with the Helsinki Declaration (1964). A written informed consent was received from all subjects.

*2.2. Participants.* All TMD patients ($n = 60$) were referred by their general practitioner to the National TMD project in Bergen, Norway. The subjects were from all regions in Norway and were consecutively included in the project during the years of 2013–2015. Patients were included, examined, and evaluated based on the severity and duration of symptoms, both for pain and dysfunction and for consequences. Six specialists representing several disciplines, who created an individual treatment proposal for each patient, performed the examination. The investigation included pain intensity and duration, functional impairment (general and jaw-specific), effect on quality of life, and presence of extended periods of sick leave. Inclusion criteria were long-term TMD-related pain. Furthermore, inclusion was based on the examination; thus, patients with and without functional impairment were included. Exclusion criteria were non–TMD-related orofacial pain, relevant drug dependence problems, and obvious psychiatric diagnoses.

A healthy sex- and age-matched control group ($n = 60$) was recruited for comparison with the TMD patients, during 2016. A majority of the control group consisted of employees and students from the Department of Clinical Dentistry at the University of Bergen, who were not affiliated with the study research group. The remaining members of the control group were recruited from the general population in Bergen, Norway. The subjects gave their informed consent to participate in the study. Inclusion criteria for the control group was age 20 years or older and age- and sex-matched with the TMD patient group. Exclusion criteria were TMD symptoms or other musculoskeletal pain and symptoms in the head and neck area. Individuals in the control group were anonymized.

*2.3. Questionnaire.* TMD patients completed a comprehensive questionnaire prior to clinical examination. The questionnaire covered medical history, socioeconomic history, and lifestyle factors and included tools to assess psychosocial factors, specifically the Hospital Anxiety and Depression Scale (HADS) [18] and a 2-item version of the Coping Strategies Questionnaire [19] regarding catastrophizing. The healthy individuals completed a shortened version of the same questionnaire.

*2.4. Saliva Samples and Analyses.* Saliva samples were collected in the morning with the Salivette Cortisol Code Blue test kit (Sarstedt Darmstadt, Germany) and stored at −80°C until analysis. $F$ and $E$ were determined by liquid chromatography-tandem mass spectrometry (LC-MS/MS) at the Core Facility for Metabolomics, University of Bergen. Sample processing was completely robotized (Hamilton Robotics, Inc., Reno, NV, USA). Briefly, $20\,\mu L$ of internal standard (Cortisol-2,3,4-$^{13}C_3$) was added to $100\,\mu L$ of human saliva, which was subjected to liquid-liquid extraction with $480\,\mu L$ of ethylacetate-heptane (80 : 20, v/v). The supernatant ($380\,\mu L$) was subsequently washed with $50\,\mu L$ of sodium hydroxide (0.1 M). Next, $280\,\mu L$ of supernatant was removed and evaporated to dryness under nitrogen flow and then reconstituted in $100\,\mu L$ of a 0.01% aqueous solution of formic acid : methanol (50 : 50, v/v). Samples were then analyzed on a Waters ACQUITY UPLC system connected to a Waters Xevo TQ-S tandem mass spectrometer (Waters, Milford, MA, USA). The compounds were separated on a C-18 BEH phenyl column from Waters ($100 \times 2.1$ mm column, 1.7 mm particle size), which was developed by gradient elution over 5.5 min, using an aqueous solution of formic acid and acetonitrile as mobile phases. Formic acid adducts were detected in negative multiple reaction-monitoring mode. A potential source of bias is that the TMD patients likely experienced more stress prior to the examination compared to the controls because the majority of the controls were examined at their ordinary workplace.

*2.5. Statistical Analyses.* All statistical analyses were performed in STATA. Mean, median, range, and standard deviation (SD) for all variables in both groups were calculated. A paired $t$-test was used to calculate the $P$ value of no difference in $F$, $E$, $F/E$ ratio, and $F + E$ between the TMD group and the control group. A Wilcoxon signed rank test was used to calculate the $P$ value of no difference in HADS and catastrophizing scores between the TMD group and the

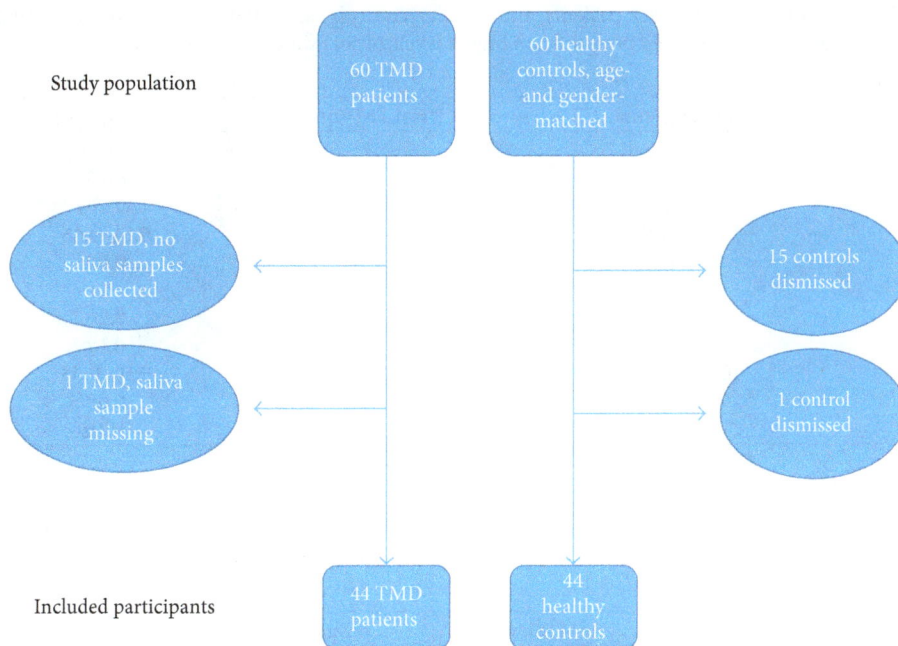

FIGURE 1: Flow chart of the study population: TMD patients and healthy controls.

control group. A linear multiregression between $F$ and psychosocial factors in both groups was performed as well as a linear correlation ($R$) with associated $P$ values between GC levels and psychosocial factors.

## 3. Results

*3.1. Demographic Data.* The multidisciplinary investigation [17] consisted of 60 patients, all experiencing severe TMD symptoms, and 60 healthy control subjects. Because no saliva sampling was done for the first 15 TMD patients and one saliva sample was missing from the patient group, the population in the present study ended up with 44 TMD patients and 44 healthy controls (Figure 1). The patients were aged 20–69 years, with a mean age of 44 years. The control subjects were aged 23–71 years with a mean age of 46 years. Both groups consisted of 38 women and 6 men.

*3.2. Saliva Samples and Analyses.* The TMD patient group had a mean saliva-sampling time point of 2 h, 52 min after awakening. The saliva samples were mostly collected at 9:00 AM but a few were collected at 11:00 AM owing to logistic factors. All subjects in the control group collected saliva 2 h, 45 min after awakening, matching the mean sampling time of the TMD patient group. Saliva samples from the control group were collected between 8:00 AM and 10:00 AM.

The transitions monitored under LC-MS/MS analyses were 405.22→329.24 for $E$ and 407.24→331.26 for $F$. The linearity range was 0.7–100 nmol/L for $E$ and 0.3–50 nmol/L for $F$. Accuracy was between 87% and 110%, and total imprecision was <10%.

*3.3. Stress Scores and Glucocorticoids in Saliva.* Our most important finding was that $F$ in saliva was significantly higher in the TMD group compared to the control group

($P = 0.01$) (Table 1). $E$ ($P = 0.04$), the $F/E$ ratio ($P = 0.002$), and the sum of GC ($F + E$) in saliva ($P = 0.02$) were also significantly higher in the TMD group. Stress scores from questionnaires were significantly higher in the TMD group, including pain catastrophizing ($P < 0.0001$) and HADS ($P < 0.0001$) (Table 2). Pain catastrophizing score in the TMD group was negatively correlated with $E$ and $F + E$ ($P = 0.033$ and $P = 0.047$, resp.); however, no association between $F$ and pain catastrophizing was found (Table 3). In the control group, we observed a significant correlation between depression score and $F + E$ ($P = 0.045$). No other associations between the GC levels in saliva and psychosocial factors were found in the control group (Table 4).

## 4. Discussion

In this study, we found that $F$ and $E$ levels in saliva are significantly higher in TMD patients compared to healthy individuals. Our results were obtained by LC-MS/MS analysis. Compared with immunoassays, LC-MS/MS has much higher specificity and thus permits identification and quantification of $F$ and $E$ [16, 20, 21]. To our knowledge, this study is the first to determine $F$ in TMD by LC-MS/MS and the first to investigate the sum and ratios of different GCs in TMD patients. However, the LC-MS/MS indicates significantly lower $F$ levels than immunoassays due to a lower incidence of cross-reactions [22]. The correlation between LC-MS/MS and immunoassays is poor [16], and the $F$ and $E$ levels measured in this study are consequently not directly comparable to those from previous studies of TMD patients using immunoassays. Accordingly, our study may also contribute to the general assessment of salivary levels of $F$ and $E$ in healthy and diseased subjects.

$F$ levels in healthy individuals follow circadian fluctuations. The lowest value occurs during early sleep and levels

TABLE 1: Glucocorticoid levels in saliva of TMD patients and healthy controls, analyzed with liquid chromatography-tandem mass spectrometry (LC-MS/MS). A paired $t$-test resulted in significant higher levels of cortisone ($E$) and cortisol ($F$), as well as the ratio of $F/E$ and the sum of $F + E$, in TMD patients.

| Glucocorticoids | Cortisone ($E$) (nmol/L) | Cortisol ($F$) (nmol/L) | $F/E$ (ratio) | $F + E$ (nmol/L) |
|---|---|---|---|---|
| TMD ($n = 44$) | | | | |
| Mean | 26.31 | 7.17 | 0.26 | 33.48 |
| Median | 24.83 | 6.29 | 0.26 | 31.37 |
| Range | 13.17–47.05 | 2.24–27.04 | 0.14–0.66 | 15.41–67.77 |
| SD | 8.61 | 4.56 | 0.09 | 12.49 |
| Control ($n = 44$) | | | | |
| Mean | 22.91 | 4.90 | 0.20 | 27.81 |
| Median | 21.56 | 3.81 | 0.18 | 25.35 |
| Range | 10.54–74.38 | 1.42–28.21 | 0.10–0.53 | 15.68–102.59 |
| SD | 9.74 | 4.37 | 0.09 | 13.91 |
| $P$ value (paired $t$-test) | 0.041 | 0.01 | 0.002 | 0.02 |

TABLE 2: Results from the questionnaires Hospital Anxiety and Depression Scale (HADS) and Coping Strategies Questionnaire regarding catastrophizing, assessed in the TMD patients and controls. A signed rank test resulted in significant higher score on all parameters in the TMD patient group.

| Psychosocial scores | Mean | Median | Range | SD | $P$ value (signed rank) |
|---|---|---|---|---|---|
| Catastrophizing (0–12) | | | | | <0.0001 |
| TMD | 7.88 | 8.0 | 1–12 | 2.95 | |
| Control | 1.39 | 0.0 | 0–11 | 2.64 | |
| Anxiety ($A$) (0–21) | | | | | 0.0002 |
| TMD | 7.73 | 7.0 | 0–20 | 5.11 | |
| Control | 3.35 | 2.0 | 0–12 | 3.22 | |
| Depression ($D$) (0–21) | | | | | <0.0001 |
| TMD | 6.28 | 5.0 | 0–19 | 5.07 | |
| Control | 1.70 | 1.0 | 0–9 | 2.32 | |
| $A + D$ (HADS) (0–42) | | | | | <0.0001 |
| TMD | 14.25 | 13.0 | 0–39 | 9.76 | |
| Control | 5.05 | 3.5 | 0–19 | 4.85 | |

rise until awakening and then rise even faster in the cortisol awakening response. The peak value occurs approximately 30–45 min after awakening [23, 24]. Our saliva samples had a mean sampling time 2 h, 52 min after awakening in the TMD group and 2 h, 45 min in the control group. Accordingly, $F$ levels from our patients and controls were not directly comparable to previous TMD studies because of the diurnal decrease in $F$ levels after peaking in addition to lower $F$ levels being expected from LC-MS/MS compared with immunoassays.

Many studies have reported elevated $F$ levels in TMD patients compared to healthy individuals. A significantly higher daytime $F$ value in plasma was reported in subjects with TMD compared to healthy controls [14]. Analysis of saliva from TMD patients also revealed elevated $F$ levels [11, 12]. Significant higher $F$ levels as a response to experimental stress in subjects with TMD has also been reported [15]. In contrast, some researchers have not found significant differences in salivary $F$ levels related to TMD [13]. In a study examining hair $F$ concentration, even lower values of $F$ were found in subjects with TMD [7].

Elevated or lowered basal $F$ levels may reflect changes in the regulation of the HPA axis, which is discussed in other TMD studies and in several studies of stress-related and chronic pain disorders [7, 9, 14, 15, 25–32]. A significantly higher rise in salivary $F$ in response to experimental stress has been reported in a TMD group compared to a healthy control group [15]. An opposite finding within a subgroup separate from the TMD group in the same study showed slightly lower, but nonsignificant, salivary $F$ levels compared to the control group at all measuring points. No significant differences in basal $F$ levels existed between the TMD and control groups before the stress exposure [15]. However, no difference in salivary $F$ levels was reported as a response to experimental pain in a TMD group compared to a control group. Nevertheless, an association between high pain-catastrophizing scores and high $F$ response to pain was observed although basal morning $F$ was lower in association with high pain catastrophizing in both TMD and controls [25]. In our study, we showed that not only $F$, but also $E$ and the sum of both GCs ($F + E$), was significantly higher in the TMD group. This finding means that the total sum of GCs is higher in the TMD group and supports the theory of an upregulated HPA axis, with higher $F$ secretion from adrenal cortex. The high level of the inactive hormone $E$ may be the result of enzymatic conversion of $F$ by 11$\beta$-hydroxysteroid dehydrogenase type 1 (11$\beta$-HSD-1) in the glandula parotis.

TABLE 3: Linear correlation ($R$) with associated $P$ values between glucocorticoid levels and psychosocial factors in the TMD group. Pain-catastrophizing score was significant, negatively correlated with $E$ and the sum of glucocorticoids ($F + E$) ($P = 0.033$ and $P = 0.047$, resp.). No significant association between $F$ and pain catastrophizing was found, neither any significant associations between the other parameters of glucocorticoid levels in saliva and psychosocial factors.

| TMD group | Cortisone ($E$) | Cortisol ($F$) | $F/E$-ratio | $F + E$ |
|---|---|---|---|---|
| Catastrophizing score | | | | |
| $R$ | −0.323 | −0.230 | −0.080 | −0.305 |
| $P$ value | 0.033 | 0.138 | 0.611 | 0.047 |
| Anxiety ($A$) score | | | | |
| $R$ | −0.089 | 0.125 | 0.247 | −0.016 |
| $P$ value | 0.566 | 0.420 | 0.107 | 0.919 |
| Depression ($D$) score | | | | |
| $R$ | −0.091 | 0.036 | 0.128 | −0.049 |
| $P$ value | 0.563 | 0.821 | 0.415 | 0.753 |
| $A + D$ (HADS) score | | | | |
| $R$ | −0.042 | 0.123 | 0.211 | 0.016 |
| $P$ value | 0.785 | 0.426 | 0.169 | 0.919 |

TABLE 4: Linear correlation ($R$) with associated $P$ values between glucocorticoid levels and psychosocial factors in the control group. Depression score was significantly associated with the sum of glucocorticoids ($F + E$) ($P = 0.045$). No significant associations between the other parameters of glucocorticoid levels in saliva and psychosocial factors were observed.

| Control group | Cortisone ($E$) | Cortisol ($F$) | $F/E$-ratio | $F+E$ |
|---|---|---|---|---|
| Catastrophizing score | | | | |
| $R$ | 0.111 | 0.147 | 0.175 | 0.124 |
| $P$ value | 0.473 | 0.340 | 0.256 | 0.422 |
| Anxiety ($A$) score | | | | |
| $R$ | 0.187 | 0.171 | 0.044 | 0.185 |
| $P$ value | 0.225 | 0.266 | 0.778 | 0.231 |
| Depression ($D$) score | | | | |
| $R$ | 0.313 | 0.269 | 0.010 | 0.304 |
| $P$ value | 0.039 | 0.077 | 0.519 | 0.045 |
| $A + D$ (HADS) score | | | | |
| $R$ | 0.273 | 0.242 | 0.077 | 0.268 |
| $P$ value | 0.073 | 0.113 | 0.620 | 0.079 |

Another possible explanation of higher $F$ levels in TMD patients may arise from suppressed negative feedback of the HPA axis, as seen in major depression [27]. An exaggerated $F$ response to CRH as well as higher basal $F$ levels has been reported for patients with irritable bowel syndrome [28]. Since we did not perform any suppression tests in our study, we could not evaluate the negative feedback of the HPA axis for comparison.

The $F/E$ ratio is an indicator of 11$\beta$-HSD activity, which has previously been measured in early morning saliva sample and found to be 0.24 [33], 0.15 [34], and 0.20 [35]. The active molecule $F$ is converted to an inactive form $E$ in parotid tissue by the enzyme 11$\beta$-HSD-1 and a reverse conversion by 11$\beta$-HSD-2. Our calculations resulted in a $F/E$ ratio of 0.26 in TMD patients compared to 0.2 in controls. The difference may be explained by decreased activity of 11$\beta$-HSD-2 in TMD patients or 11$\beta$-HSD-2 saturation at a high substrate concentration [35]. Enzyme saturation has previously been indicated by scatter plots with curve fitting [33, 35], showing that the increase in salivary $E$ is nonlinear with the increase of salivary $F$ at high $F$ concentrations. For example, an elevated $F/E$ ratio was reported in a study of apparent mineralocorticoid excess [36], and $F/E$ ratios in urine were reported to be significantly higher in depressed patients compared to healthy individuals [37]. In fetoplacental tissue, 11$\beta$-HSD-2 has a key function in neurobehavioral development, and loss of its function has resulted in lifelong anxiety in mice [38]. Given that 11$\beta$-HSD-2 is supposed to protect the mineralocorticoid receptor from GC binding [39], examining blood pressure in TMD patients in future studies could be interesting.

Psychosocial factors such as stress, anxiety, and depression may influence the HPA axis as well, although the response seems unclear and inconsistent. Stress may potentially be an important factor in the etiology of TMD [11]. The prevalence of physical and psychological stressors in TMD is high, and they may contribute to dysregulation of the HPA axis [8]. However, no significant differences in salivary morning $F$ were reported from a study of 30 young women with TMD, although the TMD subjects appeared more psychologically distressed compared to healthy individuals [13]. Subjects with TMD also had a significantly higher stress score, despite apparently lower $F$ levels, which were measured through hair analysis [7]. However, $F$ levels in hair may reflect stress and $F$ output over time, while salivary $F$ reflects the same variables at the point of measurement. The TMD patients in our study scored significantly higher on HADS and pain-catastrophizing questionnaires, which could reflect higher stress levels that potentially contribute to an upregulation of the HPA axis. Still, we did not find any significant correlation between anxiety, depression, or catastrophizing scores and $F$ levels. This outcome may be due to the presence of many other factors influencing $F$ levels. Nevertheless, we found a significantly negative association between pain-catastrophizing score and both $E$ and the sum of GCs ($F + E$). $F$ was also lower with higher pain catastrophizing in the TMD group, but the association was nonsignificant. Nevertheless, the findings from our study are comparable with a previous study in which lower basal $F$ was associated with high pain catastrophizing [25]. Nonsignificantly higher catastrophizing scores in a subgroup of TMD patients with low $F$ levels have also been reported [15]. However, we did not see lower $F$ levels correlated to anxiety or depression in the TMD group. In the control group, we observed a significant correlation between depression score and $F + E$, though the majority in the control group had a depression score that ranged zero to very low, and the association has probably low scientific value. We could not find any other correlations between GC levels and any psychological factor in the control group. A recent review on stress in chronic pain patients highlighted that several types of HPA-axis dysregulation can occur in chronic stress and pain conditions, leading to a HPA-axis stress response that cannot be determined by basal $F$ levels only [40].

The role of stress in the etiology of TMD remains unclear. The effect of stress in TMD patients may result in a complex and multifactorial response by biological systems, including neuroendocrine function and psychosocial and physical adjustments [9].

## 5. Conclusion

In summary, we report that a group of TMD patients had significantly higher $F$ and $E$ levels compared to a healthy control group. This finding may indicate that TMD patients have an upregulated HPA axis. Anxiety/depression and pain-catastrophizing scores were significantly higher in the TMD group, and they may potentially indicate chronic upregulation of the HPA axis. Based on these results, the hypothesis that TMD patients have an upregulated HPA axis may be approved. More research is needed to confirm the activity of the HPA axis in TMD patients. In future studies, it would be interesting to collect samples at several time points to compare their diurnal $F$ rhythm. Examination of the $F$ response to experimental stress would be expedient, as would suppression by dexamethasone and further investigation of $11\beta$-HSD; blood pressure would be of great interest.

## Acknowledgments

The authors thank Dr. Rae Bell, psychologist Borrik Schjødt, and physiotherapist Anne Grethe Paulsberg at the Pain Clinic, part of the TMD team, for support and advice in analyzing the data. The authors thank Professor Steinar Hustad for support and feedback on the LC-MS/MS-analyses. Finally, the authors extend our appreciation to the Norwegian Ministry of Health for funding this study.

## References

[1] S. J. Scrivani, D. A. Keith, and L. B. Kaban, "Temporomandibular disorders," New England Journal of Medicine, vol. 359, no. 25, pp. 2693–2705, 2008.

[2] G. D. Slade, R. Ohrbach, J. D. Greenspan et al., "Painful temporomandibular disorder: decade of discovery from OPPERA studies," Journal of Dental Research, vol. 95, no. 10, pp. 1084–1092, 2016.

[3] R. G. Hoffmann, J. M. Kotchen, T. A. Kotchen, T. Cowley, M. Dasgupta, and A. W. Cowley, "Temporomandibular disorders and associated clinical comorbidities," Clinical Journal of Pain, vol. 27, no. 3, pp. 268–274, 2011.

[4] D. Manfredini, E. Winocur, J. Ahlberg, L. Guarda-Nardini, and F. J. Lobbezoo, "Psychosocial impairment in temporomandibular disorders patients. RDC/TMD axis II findings from a multicentre study," Journal of Dentistry, vol. 38, no. 10, pp. 765–772, 2010.

[5] R. B. Fillingim, G. D. Slade, L. Diatchenco et al., "Summary of findings from the OPPERA baseline case-control study: implications and future directions," Journal of Pain, vol. 12, no. 11, pp. 102–107, 2011.

[6] G. E. Miller, E. Chen, and E. S. Zhou, "If it goes up, must it come down? Chronic stress and the hypothalamic-pituitary-adrenocortical axis in humans," Psychological Bulletin, vol. 133, no. 1, pp. 25–45, 2007.

[7] C. A. Lambert, A. Sanders, R. S. Wilder et al., "Chronic HPA axis response to stress in temporomandibular disorder," Journal of Dental Hygiene, vol. 87, no. 1, pp. 73–81, 2013.

[8] R. de Leeuw, D. Bertoli, J. E. Schmidt, and C. R. Carlson, "Prevalence of traumatic stressors in patients with temporomandibular disorders," Journal of Oral and Maxillofacial Surgery, vol. 63, no. 1, pp. 42–50, 2005.

[9] G. H. Gameiro, A. S. Andrade, D. F. Nouer, and M. C. F. A. Veiga, "How may stressful experiences contribute to the development of temporomandibular disorders," Clinical Oral Investigations, vol. 10, no. 4, pp. 261–268, 2006.

[10] T. Umeda, R. Hiramatsu, T. Iwaoka, T. Shimada, F. Miura, and T. Sato, "Use of saliva for monitoring unbound free cortisol levels in serum," Clinica Chimica Acta, vol. 110, no. 2-3, pp. 245–253, 1981.

[11] E. Salameh, F. Alshaarani, H. A. Hamed, and J. A. Nassar, "Investigation of the relationship between psychosocial stress and temporomandibular disorder in adults by measuring salivary cortisol concentration: a case-control study," Journal of Indian Prosthodontic Society, vol. 15, no. 2, pp. 148–152, 2015.

[12] A. Da Silva Andrade, G. H. Gamero, L. J. Pereira, I. C. Junqueira Zanin, and M. B. Gavião, "Salivary cortisol levels in young adults with temporomandibular disorders," Minerva Stomatologica, vol. 57, no. 3, pp. 109–116, 2008.

[13] A. M. Nilsson and L. Dahlström, "Perceived symptoms of psychological distress and salivary cortisol levels in young women with muscular or disk-related temporomandibular disorders," Acta Odontologica Scandinavica, vol. 68, no. 5, pp. 284–288, 2010.

[14] A. Korszun, E. A. Young, K. Singer, N. E. Carlson, M. B. Brown, and L. Crofford, "Basal circadian cortisol secretion in women with temporomandibular disorders," Journal of Dental Research, vol. 81, no. 4, pp. 279–283, 2002.

[15] D. A. Jones, G. B. Rollman, and R. I. Brooke, "The cortisol response to psychological stress in temporomandibular dysfunction," Pain, vol. 72, no. 1, pp. 171–182, 1997.

[16] U. Turpeinen and E. Hämäläinen, "Determination of cortisol in serum, saliva and urine," Best Practice and Research Clinical Endocrinology and Metabolism, vol. 27, no. 6, pp. 795–801, 2013.

[17] T. Berge, B. Schjødt, R. F. Bell et al., "Assessment of patients with severe temporomandibular disorder in Norway—a multidisciplinary approach," Den Norske Tannlegeforeningens Tidene, vol. 126, no. 2, pp. 114–121, 2016.

[18] A. S. Zigmond and R. P. Snaith, "The hospital anxiety and depression scale," Acta Psychiatrica Scandinavica, vol. 67, no. 6, pp. 361–370, 1983.

[19] M. P. Jensen, F. J. Keefe, J. C. Lefebvre, J. M. Romano, and J. A. Turner, "One- and two-item measures of pain beliefs and coping strategies," *Pain*, vol. 104, no. 3, pp. 453–469, 2003.

[20] G. Antonelli, F. Ceccato, C. Artusi, M. Marinova, and M. Plebani, "Salivary cortisol and cortisone by LC-MS/MS: validation, reference intervals and diagnostic accuracy in Cushing's syndrome," *Clinica Chimica Acta*, vol. 451, pp. 247–251, 2015.

[21] U. Turpeinen, H. Markkanen, T. Sane, and E. Hämäläinen, "Determination of free tetrahydrocortisol and tetrahydrocortisone ratio in urine by liquid chromatography-tandem mass spectrometry," *Scandinavian Journal of Clinical and Laboratory Investigation*, vol. 66, no. 2, pp. 147–160, 2006.

[22] R. Miller, F. Plessow, M. Rauh, M. Gröschl, and C. Kirschbaum, "Comparison of salivary cortisol as measured by different immunoassays and tandem mass spectrometry," *Psychoneuroendocrinology*, vol. 38, no. 1, pp. 50–57, 2013.

[23] N. Smyth, A. Clow, L. Thorn, F. Hucklebridge, and P. Evans, "Delays of 5-15 min between awakening and the start of saliva sampling matter in assessment of the cortisol awakening response," *Psychoneuroendocrinology*, vol. 38, no. 9, pp. 1476–1483, 2013.

[24] I. Wilhelm, J. Born, B. M. Kudielka, W. Schlotz, and S. Wust, "Is the cortisol awakening rise a response to awakening?," *Psychoneuroendocrinology*, vol. 32, no. 4, pp. 358–366, 2007.

[25] P. J. Quartana, L. F. Buenaver, R. R. Edwards, B. Klick, J. A. Haythornthwaite, and M. T. Smith, "Pain catastrophizing and salivary cortisol responses to laboratory pain testing in temporomandibular disorder and healthy participants," *Journal of Pain*, vol. 11, no. 2, pp. 186–194, 2010.

[26] P. J. Kennedy, J. F. Cryan, E. M. Quigley, T. G. Dinan, and G. Clarke, "A sustained hypothalamic-pituitary-adrenal axis response to acute psychosocial stress in irritable bowel syndrome," *Psychological Medicine*, vol. 44, no. 14, pp. 3123–3134, 2014.

[27] J. Herbert, "Cortisol and depression: three questions for psychiatry," *Psychological Medicine*, vol. 43, no. 3, pp. 449–469, 2013.

[28] T. G. Dinan, E. M. M. Quigley, S. M. M. Ahmed et al., "Hypothalamic-pituitary-gut axis dysregulation in irritable bowel syndrome: plasma cytokines as a potential biomarker?," *Gastroenterology*, vol. 130, no. 2, pp. 304–311, 2006.

[29] U. Galli, J. Gaab, D. A. Ettlin, F. Ruggia, U. Ehlert, and S. Palla, "Enhanced negative feedback sensitivity of the hypothalamus-pituitary-adrenal axis in chronic myogenous facial pain," *European Journal of Pain*, vol. 13, no. 6, pp. 600–605, 2009.

[30] R. Yehuda, S. M. Southwick, J. H. Krystal, D. Bremner, D. S. Charney, and J. W. Mason, "Enhanced suppression of cortisol following dexamethasone administration in post-traumatic stress disorder," *American Journal of Psychiatry*, vol. 150, no. 1, pp. 83–86, 1993.

[31] M. Bonifazi, A. L. Suman, C. Cambiaggi et al., "Changes in salivary cortisol and corticosteroid receptor-α mRNA expression following a 3-week multidisciplinary treatment program in patients with fibromyalgia," *Psychoneuroendocrinology*, vol. 31, no. 9, pp. 1076–1086, 2006.

[32] S. A. Vreeburg, W. J. G. Hoogendijk, R. H. DeRijk et al., "Salivary cortisol levels and the 2-year course of depressive and anxiety disorders," *Psychoneuroendocrinology*, vol. 38, no. 9, pp. 1494–1502, 2013.

[33] M. Mezzullo, F. Fanelli, A. Fazzini et al., "Validation of an LC-MS/MS salivary assay for glucocorticoid status assessment: evaluation of the diurnal fluctuation of cortisol and cortisone and of their association within and between serum and saliva,"

[34] B. C. McWhinney, S. E. Briscoe, J. P. J. Ungerer, and C. J. Pretorius, "Measurement of cortisol, cortisone, prednisolone, dexamethasone and 11-deoxycortisol with ultra high performance liquid chromatography-tandem mass spectrometry: application for plasma, plasma ultrafiltrate, urine and saliva in a routine laboratory," *Journal of Chromatography B*, vol. 878, no. 28, pp. 2863–2869, 2010.

[35] I. Perogamvros, L. J. Owen, J. Newell-Price, D. W. Ray, P. J. Trainer, and B. G. Keevil, "Simultaneous measurement of cortisol and cortisone in human saliva using liquid chromatography-tandem mass spectrometry: application in basal and stimulated conditions," *Journal of Chromatography B*, vol. 877, no. 29, pp. 3771–3775, 2009.

[36] J. Dötsch, H. G. Dorr, G. K. Stalla, and W. G. Sippel, "Effect of glucocorticoid excess on the cortisol/cortisone ratio," *Steroids*, vol. 66, no. 11, pp. 817–820, 2001.

[37] Z. Xuejia, C. Fen, Z. Chaoran, and L. Yongning, "A simple LC-MS/MS method for determination of cortisol, cortisone and tetrahydro-metabolites in human urine: assay development, validation and application in depression patients," *Journal of Pharmaceutical and Biomedical Analysis*, vol. 107, pp. 450–455, 2015.

[38] C. S. Wyrwoll, M. C. Holmes, and J. R. Seckl, "11β-Hydroxysteroid dehydrogenases and the brain: from zero to hero, a decade of progress," *Frontiers in Neuroendocrinology*, vol. 32, no. 3, pp. 265–286, 2011.

[39] J. R. Seckl and B. R. Walker, "Minireview: 11β-Hydroxysteroid dehydrogenase type 1—a tissue-specific amplifier of glucocorticoid action," *Endocrinology*, vol. 142, no. 4, pp. 1371–1376, 2001.

[40] A. Woda, P. Picard, and F. Dutheil, "Dysfunctional stress responses in chronic pain," *Psychoneuroendocrinology*, vol. 71, pp. 127–135, 2016.

*Journal of Steroid Biochemistry and Molecular Biology*, vol. 163, pp. 103–112, 2016.

# 20

# Patient-Controlled Intravenous Analgesia for Advanced Cancer Patients with Pain: A Retrospective Series Study

**Zhiyou Peng, Yanfeng Zhang, Jianguo Guo, Xuejiao Guo, and Zhiying Feng** (iD)

*Department of Pain Medicine, First Affiliated Hospital, School of Medicine, Zhejiang University, Hangzhou 310003, China*

Correspondence should be addressed to Zhiying Feng; fzy1972@zju.edu.cn

Academic Editor: Wojciech Leppert

*Objective.* To compare the efficacy and side effects of patient-controlled intravenous analgesia (PCIA) with hydromorphone, sufentanil, and oxycodone on the management of advanced cancer patients with pain. *Methods.* Patients allocated to receive PCIA between January 2015 and December 2016 were chosen for this study. After reviewing medical records, we verified if hydromorphone, sufentanil, or oxycodone for PCIA could equally provide effective pain relief. A numeric rating scale (NRS) of cancer pain was applied before PCIA, at 4 hours after PCIA, and at the discontinuation of PCIA. Secondary, the incidence of clinical side effects attributed to PCIA was observed. *Results.* A total of 85 medical records were reviewed. PCIA with hydromorphone ($n = 30$), sufentanil ($n = 34$), and oxycodone ($n = 21$) was used for cancer pain management. PCIA successfully improved pain control in 97.6% of the patients. The most common side effects were constipation (11.8%), nausea (8.2%), and sedation (5.9%). Drug addiction, delirium, or respiratory depression associated with PCIA was not reported in this case series study. No significant intergroup difference was observed in NRS at any of the abovementioned time points. There was no significant difference of analgesic effect among the hydromorphone, sufentanil, or oxycodone. *Conclusion.* PCIA provided timely, safe, and satisfactory analgesia for advanced cancer patients with pain and may be useful for titration of opioids, management of severe breakthrough pain, and conversion to oral analgesia. There was no significant difference of analgesic effect and side effect among the hydromorphone, sufentanil, and oxycodone.

## 1. Introduction

With the increasing number of cancer patients, cancer pain has grown up to be a major public health problem all over the world. Despite recent advances in diagnosis and treatment, cancer pain continues to present a significant challenge to cope with. The World Health Organization (WHO) analgesic ladder is now the preferred protocol of choice all over the world. In clinical practice, this protocol works effectively and is prompt in controlling mild-to-moderate cancer pain initially.

As the disease progresses, alternate routes of administration are frequently used for advanced cancer patients with pain. Although primarily used in the treatment of acute postoperative pain, PCIA has been applied to advanced cancer patients with pain which allows the patient to individualize therapy by self-administrating predetermined doses of opioid analgesics. It was shown that PCIA can decrease the delayed opioid administration from the time requested, accompanied by rapidity and ease of dose titration and adaptability to the variable analgesic dosing needs [1]. Another advantage is that it helps to indicate whether the particular pain was opioid responsive or not. It was well known that many centers now offer PCIA for cancer patients to manage chronic pain [1, 2]. However, evidence of safety and efficacy of PCIA devices was limited to advanced cancer patients with pain.

The goal of this study was to retrospectively review the safety and the analgesic efficacy of hydromorphone, sufentanil, and oxycodone by PCIA in advanced cancer patients with pain.

## 2. Method

The study was approved by the ethics committee of the First Affiliated Hospital, School of Medicine, Zhejiang University.

Patients who used PCIA for cancer pain management with sufentanil, hydromorphone, and oxycodone between January 2015 and December 2016 at the First Affiliated Hospital of the School of Medicine, Zhejiang University, were recruited in the retrospective cohort study. Criteria for exclusion include patient chart not available, discontinuation of PCIA therapy for more than 4 hours, and data not available. A total of 85 patients were identified and collected.

Information gathered from their electronic medical record included general demographic data, cancer diagnosis, date of PCIA pump used, 11-point (0 to 10) NRS before and after PCIA, times of breakthrough pain, the medications placed in the pump for basal and patient-controlled dosing, and opioid medications before and after pump placement.

Hospitalized cancer patients are usually treated by oncologists according to the National Comprehensive Cancer Network (NCCN) guidelines for opioid prescription. Whenever adequate pain control was not achieved with an amount of daily morphine equivalents $\geq 120$ mg, they should get help from the department of pain medicine.

The decision criteria to install a PCIA were that the patient presented with severe breakthrough pain requiring at least five daily doses of systemic opioid rescue medication, unable to take oral medication, or pain control still not satisfied after oral drug titration in the last 24 h. The patient should not have a history of drug or alcohol abuse.

When using different forms of opioid drugs, the opioid equivalence dosage was compared using oral morphine equivalent dose [3–5]. The administration of opioid was launched with the basal infusion and a demand bolus dose. The bolus dose was fixed at 20% of the daily infusion dose approximately.

Discontinuation of therapy criteria is that pain was satisfactorily controlled for at least 24 hours or patients have clinical complications such as respiratory depression.

When the patient received PCIA as a supplementary rescue technique, their usual systemic medication was still using according to the NCCN guideline-based analgesic administration [6]. After the first 24 hours, opioid consumption in PCIA was added to the daily prescription.

Pain relief was defined as comfortable with subtotal pain relief with desired no increase of morphine dose. After pain relief, the patient took oral oxycodone or fentanyl transdermal patch equal to the intravenous requirement [7].

During the PCIA utilizing, a nurse assessed the baseline blood pressure, heart and respiratory rates, level of consciousness, pain score, and any other adverse effects.

Our primary outcome was to verify if different PCIA opioid-based solutions could effectively provide pain relief in cancer patients. In addition, the incidence of clinical side effects associated with PCIA therapy, including respiratory depression, drowsiness, constipation, and delirium was also observed.

Data were collected and analyzed using SPSS version 16.0 for Windows (SPSS Inc., Chicago, IL, USA). Continuous variables were presented as means ± standard deviation, and categorical data were shown as numbers and percentages.

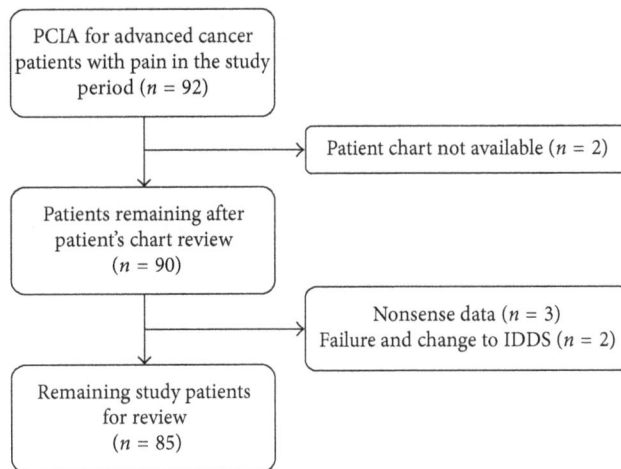

FIGURE 1: Study flowchart.

The independent sample $t$-test, the chi-square test, or the Mann–Whitney $U$ test was utilized to group variables. $P$ value less than 0.05 was considered significant.

## 3. Results

A total of 92 patients' records were included in this retrospective study. Screening of medical records was the first step to select eligible patients. Five were excluded due to missing data. PCIA failed in the remaining 2 patients, and intrathecal drug (morphine) delivery system was implanted for treatment of patients with intractable pain (Figure 1). PCIA with hydromorphone ($n = 30$), sufentanil ($n = 34$), and oxycodone ($n = 21$) was used for cancer pain management. Depending upon the discontinuation criteria for PCIA established, success after PCIA prescription occurred in all of the patients except two patients. PCIA successfully improved pain control in 97.6% of the patients. Baseline characteristics of the patients are shown in Table 1.

A comparison of NRS score was showed before PCIA, at 4 hours after PCIA, and at the discontinuation of PCIA. Mean NRS score before PCIA in group hydromorphone, group sufentanil, and group oxycodone was $5.0 \pm 1.1$, $4.9 \pm 1.0$, and $5.3 \pm 1.1$. At 4 hours after PCIA, these decreased to $2.3 \pm 0.8$, $2.0 \pm 1.0$, and $2.2 \pm 0.7$. When PCIA is discontinued, these decreased to $1.9 \pm 0.7$, $1.7 \pm 0.7$, and $2.0 \pm 0.6$, respectively. No significant intergroup difference was observed in NRS at any of the abovementioned time points (Table 2).

PCIA therapy was employed for an average length of $5.9 \pm 4$ days. The most common side effects were constipation (11.8%), nausea (8.2%), and sedation (5.9%). Drug addiction, delirium, or respiratory depression originated in PCIA was not reported in this case series study (Table 3). There was no significant difference in side effect among hydromorphone, sufentanil, or oxycodone.

## 4. Discussion

The vast majority of advanced cancer patients with pain can obtain satisfactory control by following the WHO analgesic

TABLE 1: Patient characteristics.

| | Hydromorphone | Sufentanil | Oxycodone |
|---|---|---|---|
| Number of patients | 30 | 34 | 21 |
| Male/female | 18/12 | 18/16 | 13/8 |
| Age (years) | $59.8 \pm 9.8$ | $61.8 \pm 9.4$ | $59.9 \pm 10.6$ |
| *Cancer location* | | | |
| Gastrointestinal | 22 | 23 | 14 |
| Bronchopulmonary | 4 | 6 | 1 |
| Urogenital | 1 | 2 | 1 |
| Others | 3 | 3 | 5 |
| Metastases present | 28 | 33 | 19 |
| *Main location of pain* | | | |
| Head/neck/upper extremity | 2 | 2 | 1 |
| Thorax | 4 | 5 | 3 |
| Abdomen-pelvic | 20 | 24 | 14 |
| Hip/lower extremity | 3 | 1 | 2 |
| Multiple sites of pain | 1 | 2 | 1 |

TABLE 2: NRS scores of the two groups at different times in the three groups.

| NRS | Hydromorphone | Sufentanil | Oxycodone |
|---|---|---|---|
| T1 | $5.0 \pm 1.1$ | $4.9 \pm 1.0$ | $5.3 \pm 1.1$ |
| T2 | $2.3 \pm 0.8$ | $2.0 \pm 1.0$ | $2.2 \pm 0.7$ |
| T3 | $1.9 \pm 0.7$ | $1.7 \pm 0.7$ | $2.0 \pm 0.6$ |

T1: before PCIA; T2: at 4 hours after PCIA; T3: at the discontinuation of PCIA.

TABLE 3: The incidences of adverse effect in the three groups.

| | Hydromorphone ($n = 30$) | Sufentanil ($n = 34$) | Oxycodone ($n = 21$) |
|---|---|---|---|
| Nausea/vomiting | 3 | 2 | 2 |
| Sedation | 1 | 3 | 1 |
| Constipation | 5 | 5 | 3 |
| Drug addiction | 0 | 0 | 0 |
| Respiration depression | 0 | 0 | 0 |
| Delirium | 0 | 0 | 0 |

ladder with morphine sustained-release tablets, fentanyl transdermal system, and other noninvasive drug treatments [8]. However, some situations are still difficult to deal with, such as difficulty swallowing, recurrent nausea and vomiting with oral morphine sustained-release tablets, cannot tolerate fentanyl transdermal system, and frequent short bursts of breakthrough pain.

Application of PCIA can maintain the blood drug concentration near the lowest effective plasma concentration. The pharmacological characteristics of PCIA allowed for determining the treatment on needs of the patients. In addition, the effective blood concentration to maintain a stable and minimum effective quantity eliminates the difference to avoid the risk of drug overdose or insufficient. Compared to the conventional analgesic therapy, the PCIA is well accepted as a helpful and effective technique by the cancer patient with being able to control the pain themselves and the minimum delay between request for analgesia and pain relief [9–11].

The breakthrough pain was defined as a rapid onset, short duration, moderate-to-severe intensity, and frequent occurrence. The typical duration of an episode is 15–30 minutes. The frequency of pain episodes can vary from a single time to several times daily or weekly [12, 13]. With growing recognition of the prevalence and potential negative consequences of breakthrough pain, a short-acting drug is usually offered as needed during regular opioid treatment. Although the use of traditional oral opioid formulation and newer transmucosal fentanyl formulation are both valid options, a PCIA with pumps can also be used to allow treatment of breakthrough pain.

An obvious advantage is that PCIA can avoid delays in the administration of analgesics and benefits for patients suffering from frequent breakthrough pain episodes. PCIA has the advantages of immediately releasing the drug whenever the patient demands in low doses, short intervals, short duration of effect, and easy titration of opioids. Another one is that PCIA can ease of dose titration and adaptability to patients need to analgesics [14].

Hydromorphone, sufentanil, and oxycodone are opioid analgesics currently widely used in cancer pain. They are primarily an agonist at $\mu$ receptors which exert potent analgesic effects but also be coupled with adverse effects like nausea, vomiting, constipation, itching, and respiratory depression [3, 15]. The most common adverse reactions following PCIA were constipation (11.8%), nausea (8.2%), and sedation (5.9%), and no life-threatening adverse effects, such as respiratory depression, were recorded, even in older patients or when high doses were administered. Our result indicated that patients administering consistent doses of morphine with rapid modalities showed a minimal risk, if PCIA is done by skilled professionals in an adequate environment. In addition, opiate tolerance in patients who chronically receive relevant opioid doses for the management of cancer pain was considered for another reason.

Our experience suggests that hydromorphone, sufentanil, and oxycodone provides a good safety profile and represents an effective analgesic drug in cancer patient. All cancer patients treated with hydromorphone, sufentanil, and oxycodone of PCIA enjoyed satisfactory analgesia. The pain intensity score and times of breakthrough pain recorded during the treatment with PCIA indicated significant pain relief when compared to the starting time and remained stable for the entire time of treatment.

This study suffered from the limitations of any retrospective design. Some data records were not retrieved. Most detailed pain characteristics data such as movement related, light-dark intervals and sleep quality as was not in a position to be collected. In addition, the data of the effect of PCIA on anxiety, depression, and quality of life were insufficiency. Regardless of the fact that PCIA resulted in shorter length of hospital stay allowing to be available for other patients, the cost of drug and pump increases. The economic aspect of the use of PCIA is a worthwhile topic for further exploration.

In conclusion, PCIA, providing timely, safe, and satisfactory analgesia for advanced cancer patients with pain, may be useful for treating breakthrough pain and titration of opioid to aid weaning to oral analgesia. There was no significant difference of analgesic effect and side effect among the hydromorphone, sufentanil, and oxycodone. Clinicians should be familiar with the benefits and potential risks of PCIA with many kinds of opioids. More prospective, randomized controlled trials of clinical safety and efficacy of PCIA with opioid should be examined in advanced cancer patients with pain.

## Authors' Contributions

Zhiying Feng conceived and designed the experiments. Zhiyou Peng, Yanfeng Zhang, Jianguo Guo, and Xuejiao Guo performed data collection. Zhiyou Peng and Zhiying Feng analyzed the data. Zhiyou Peng wrote the paper.

## Acknowledgments

This research was supported by the Programme of Health and Family Planning Commission of Zhejiang Province (Grant no. 2015113466) to Dr. Zhiyou Peng and by the National Natural Science Foundation, Beijing, China (Grant no. 81603198), to Dr. Zhiyou Peng.

## References

[1] A. M. Sousa, J. de Santana Neto, G. M. Guimaraes, G. M. Cascudo, J. O. Neto, and H. A. Ashmawi, "Safety profile of intravenous patient-controlled analgesia for breakthrough pain in cancer patients: a case series study," *Supportive Care in Cancer*, vol. 22, no. 3, pp. 795–801, 2014.

[2] A. Ruggiero, G. Barone, L. Liotti, A. Chiaretti, I. Lazzareschi, and R. Riccardi, "Safety and efficacy of fentanyl administered by patient controlled analgesia in children with cancer pain," *Supportive Care in Cancer*, vol. 15, no. 5, pp. 569–573, 2007.

[3] R. K. Portenoy, "Treatment of cancer pain," *The Lancet*, vol. 377, no. 9784, pp. 2236–2247, 2011.

[4] G. W. Hanks, F. Conno, N. Cherny et al., "Morphine and alternative opioids in cancer pain: the EAPC recommendations," *British Journal of Cancer*, vol. 84, no. 5, pp. 587–593, 2001.

[5] A. Rennick, T. Atkinson, N. M. Cimino, S. A. Strassels, M. L. McPherson, and J. Fudin, "Variability in opioid equivalence calculations," *Pain Medicine*, vol. 17, no. 5, pp. 892–898, 2016.

[6] N. Janjan, "Improving cancer pain control with NCCN guideline-based analgesic administration: a patient-centered outcome," *Journal of the National Comprehensive Cancer Network*, vol. 12, no. 9, pp. 1243–1249, 2014.

[7] P. G. Fine and R. K. Portenoy, "Establishing "best practices" for opioid rotation: conclusions of an expert panel," *Journal of Pain and Symptom Management*, vol. 38, no. 3, pp. 418–425, 2009.

[8] P. Klepstad, S. Kaasa, and P. C. Borchgrevink, "Starting step III opioids for moderate to severe pain in cancer patients: dose titration: a systematic review," *Palliative Medicine*, vol. 25, no. 5, pp. 424–430, 2011.

[9] M. L. Citron, J. M. Kalra, V. L. Seltzer, S. Chen, M. Hoffman, and M. B. Walczak, "Patient-controlled analgesia for cancer pain: a long-term study of inpatient and outpatient use," *Cancer Investigation*, vol. 10, no. 5, pp. 335–341, 1992.

[10] R. Dev, E. Del Fabbro, and E. Bruera, "Patient-controlled analgesia in patients with advanced cancer. Should patients be in control?," *Journal of Pain and Symptom Management*, vol. 42, no. 2, pp. 296–300, 2011.

[11] C. Schiessl, I. Schestag, R. Sittl, R. Drake, and B. Zernikow, "Rhythmic pattern of PCA opioid demand in adults with cancer pain," *European Journal of Pain*, vol. 14, no. 4, pp. 372–379, 2010.

[12] P. Daeninck, B. Gagnon, R. Gallagher et al., "Canadian recommendations for the management of breakthrough cancer pain," *Current Oncology*, vol. 23, no. 2, pp. 96–108, 2016.

[13] A. Davies, G. Zeppetella, S. Andersen et al., "Multi-centre European study of breakthrough cancer pain: Pain characteristics and patient perceptions of current and potential management strategies," *European Journal of Pain*, vol. 15, no. 7, pp. 756–763, 2011.

[14] J. Hayes, J. J. Dowling, A. Peliowski, M. W. Crawford, and B. Johnston, "Patient-controlled analgesia plus background opioid infusion for postoperative pain in children: a systematic review and meta-analysis of randomized trials," *Anesthesia and Analgesia*, vol. 123, no. 4, pp. 991–1003, 2016.

[15] A. Murray and N. A. Hagen, "Hydromorphone," *Journal of Pain and Symptom Management*, vol. 29, pp. S57–S66, 2005.

# 21

# Clinical and Radiographic Characteristics as Predictive Factors of Swelling and Trismus after Mandibular Third Molar Surgery: A Longitudinal Approach

José Manuel Pérez-González,[1] Vicente Esparza-Villalpando,[2] Ricardo Martínez-Rider,[1] Miguel Ángel Noyola-Frías,[1] and Amaury Pozos-Guillén ⓘD[3]

[1]Department of Oral and Maxillofacial Surgery, Faculty of Dentistry, San Luis Potosi University, San Luis Potosí, SLP, Mexico
[2]Engineering and Materials Science Postgraduate Program, San Luis Potosi University, San Luis Potosí, SLP, Mexico
[3]Basic Sciences Laboratory, Faculty of Dentistry, San Luis Potosi University, San Luis Potosí, SLP, Mexico

Correspondence should be addressed to Amaury Pozos-Guillén; apozos@uaslp.mx

Academic Editor: Eugenio Velasco-Ortega

*Introduction.* Factors that contribute to swelling and trismus are complex, and they are originated by surgical trauma. The aim of the present study was to determine whether clinical and radiographic factors could predict the level of swelling and trismus after lower third molar surgery, through longitudinal approach. *Methodology.* A prospective longitudinal trial was carried out. Forty-five patients of both genders with clinical and radiographic diagnosis of asymptomatic mandibular impacted third molar and with no intake of analgesic or anti-inflammatory drugs 12 h prior to surgery were recruited and evaluated in a 72 h follow-up period. A mixed repeated measures model and backward and restricted maximal likelihood methods were used to analyze the data. *Results.* Male gender, body mass index (BMI), the relation to the lingual and buccal walls, and age were determinants for predicting postoperative swelling and for exerting a significant influence ($P < 0.05$). *Conclusions.* This study suggests the association of male gender, the relation to lingual and buccal walls, BMI, and age with measurement of swelling.

## 1. Introduction

Surgical extraction of mandibular third molars under local anesthesia involves the traumatic manipulation of bone, connective, and muscle tissues. Swelling, pain, and trismus are the principal postoperative signs and symptoms, which are caused mainly by tissue damage [1]. The effect of mandibular third molar surgery on the postoperative period in the majority of patients is marked by pain, swelling, and trismus, either alone or in combination [2]. Control of these conditions comprises an important factor for clinicians, because lower third molar surgery is one of the most common procedures carried out by oral and maxillofacial surgeons [3–7].

Factors that contribute to swelling and trismus are complex, and they are originated by surgical trauma [8, 9].

The control of swelling, pain, and trismus would be based on the understanding of the associated preoperative factors involved on the postoperative results. Previous reports of preoperative conditions related with swelling, pain, and trismus have included clinical and radiological factors [10], the difficulty of the procedure [11, 12], intraoperative factors [13, 14], and patients' characteristics [15]. These studies used a correlation between the different factors and the outcomes; the difficulty of this approach is that the clinical outcomes are dynamic and they change as a function of time. In transversal or punctual measurements, it is not possible to observe changes over time.

Considering a longitudinal approach, the aim of the present pilot study was to determine whether clinical and radiographic factors could predict the level of swelling and trismus after lower third molar surgery.

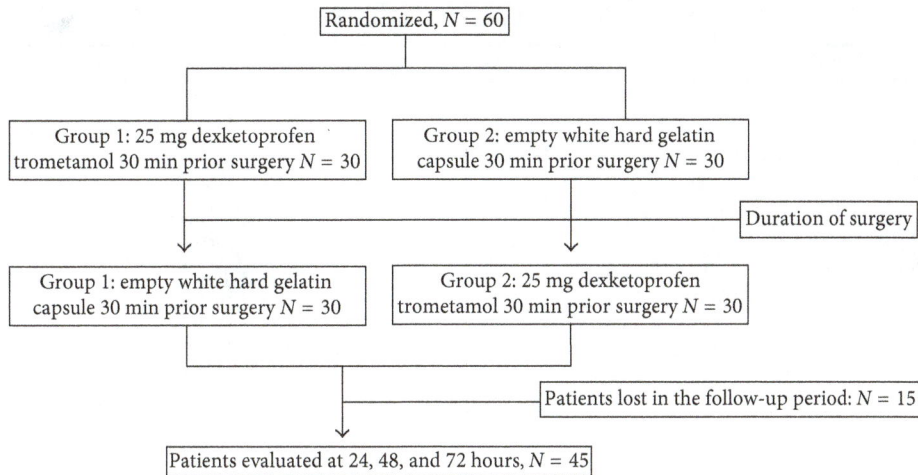

FIGURE 1: Flow chart of patient's distribution.

## 2. Materials and Methods

As part of previous study [4], the present prospective, longitudinal trial recruited 45 patients between 18 and 30 years old from the Department of Oral and Maxillofacial Surgery of the Faculty of Dentistry who had completed the 72-hour follow-up period. Briefly, the patients were assigned to two experimental groups. The first group received 25 mg of dexketoprofen trometamol 30 min before surgery and 1 placebo capsule immediately after the surgery. The second group received the placebo capsule 30 min before surgery and 25 mg of dexketoprofen trometamol immediately after the surgery. The local anesthesia was achieved by inferior alveolar nerve and lingual nerve blockade using lidocaine 2% with epinephrine 1 : 100,000 mL (FD ZEYCO, México), to remove one asymptomatic mandibular third molar. All the surgeries required mucoperiostical flap and osteotomy and were performed by the same surgeon. The patient distribution diagram is shown in Figure 1. The study was conducted in accordance with the Declaration of Helsinki, and the Institutional Ethics Committee approved the study design (CEI-FE-028-014). All participants were informed of the risks of oral surgery, and they signed a consent form.

Inclusion criteria were as follows: patients from both genders, with clinical and radiographic diagnosis of asymptomatic mandibular impacted third molar, and with no intake of analgesic or anti-inflammatory drugs 12 h prior to surgery. Exclusion criteria were the following: pregnant or breast-feeding patients, with the presence of systemic diseases such as diabetes, uncontrolled hypertension, or gastric ulcer, and patients with suspicion or evidence of narcotic or illicit drug use. Elimination criteria were all patients lost in the follow-up period (72 hours).

The facial points pogonion (Pg), labial commissure (Co), gonion (Go), outer eye corner (C), and tragus (T) were marked with indelible ink; measurements of swelling were performed with a millimetric ruler from the facial planes (T-Co, T-Po, C-Go, and Go-Co). The inflammation variable comprised the sum of all of the planes described previously (Figure 2). An independent examiner performed the measurements at the following different times: baseline/time 0

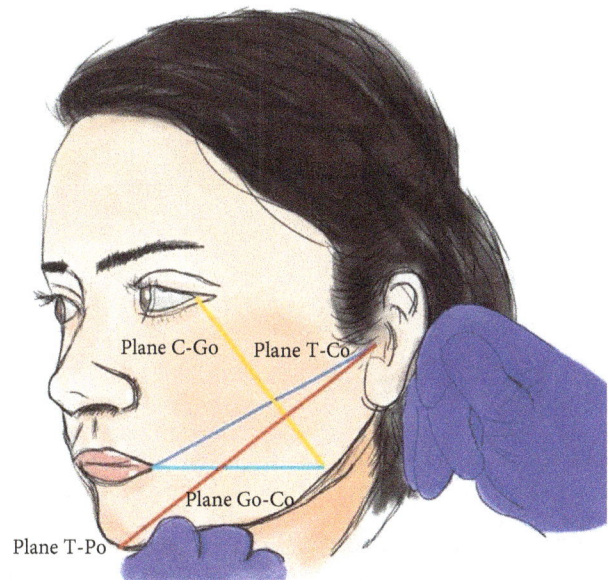

FIGURE 2: Facial planes for swelling measures.

(prior to the surgery); time 24 (24 h after the surgery); time 48 (48 h after the surgery), and time 72 (72 h after the surgery).

Trismus was measured with a millimetric ruler, asking the patient for the maximal oral opening possible and recording the distance from the incisal edge of the upper central incisors to the incisal edge of the lower central incisors. Clinical and radiographic variables recorded prior to the surgery are described in Table 1.

All patients were evaluated at 24, 48, and 72 postoperative hours. For swelling response as a dynamic process, a Mixed Repeated Measures Model (MRMM) analysis was employed. This model included all measurement times (random component), together with different variables (fixed component) (Table 1), and determined which variables result with significance in the swelling and trismus processes during the 72 h follow-up. Statistical software R ver. 3.2.3 was used, with the following packages: BBconRR,

TABLE 1: Variables included in the model (fixed component).

| Code | Variable | Units |
|------|----------|-------|
| Gender | Gender of the patient | F (female) M (male) |
| Baseline | Basal value (time 0) | mm |
| Age | Age of the patient | Years |
| BMI | Body mass index | kg/m$^2$ |
| TQX | Surgical elapsed time | Minutes |
| Total intake | Total consumption of analgesic intake in 72 hours | Number of tablets |
| R2M | Relationship of the third molar to second molar | 0: Crown directed at or above the equator second molar<br>1: Crown directed below the equator second molar<br>2: Crown/roots directed to the middle of the second molar<br>3: Crown/roots directed to the apical third of the second molar |
| RRM | Relation to the mandibular ramus | 0: Sufficient space in the dental arch<br>1: Partially impacted in the ramus<br>2: Completely impacted in the ramus<br>3: Completely impacted in the ramus in distoangular position |
| RRA | Relation to the adjacent alveolar crest (from the uppermost point of the tooth) | 0: Completely erupted<br>1: Partially impacted, but widest part of the crown (equator) is above the bone<br>2: Partially impacted, but widest part of the crown (equator) is below the bone<br>3: Completely impacted |
| RRB | Relation to the lingual and buccal walls | 0: Closer to buccal wall<br>1: In the middle between lingual and buccal walls<br>2: Closer to lingual wall<br>3: Closer to lingual wall, when the tooth is partially/completely impacted |

car, ggplot2, nlme, reshape, and Rcmdr, with 95% confidence intervals (95% CI).

## 3. Results

Forty-five patients were analyzed during a 72 h follow-up period. The baseline characteristics of the sample are described in Table 2.

For the swelling and trismus variables, the multivariate MRMM, restricted maximal likelihood (REML), and backward-stepwise methods were used. The initial model included all of the variables in the fixed component described in Table 1, and, in the random component, all times were included and each patient was measured 3 times, for a total of 135 measurements. For the swelling model, we used a "varIdent" variance structure [16]; this model was compared with the null model (only intercept included) and this comparison showed $p$ value < 0.05. Therefore, and based on the likelihood test, we determined the maximal parsimony model and deleted no significant terms in each iteration; the final model included the significative variables ($p < 0.05$): GENDER, AGE, BMI, and RRB, and the estimates and the significant values are shown in Table 3.

For the trismus variable in the MRMM, the same previous methods were used, and the variance structure utilized was "varPower" [16]; the fixed component included all variables presented in Table 1, and the random component included all trismus measures. The model was compared with the null model (only intercept included), and this comparison showed $p$ value > 0.05. Thus, the variables included in

TABLE 2: Basal characteristics.

| Variable | $n = 45$ | Min-max |
|----------|----------|---------|
| Age (mean (sd)) | 23.58 (3.34) | 18–29 |
| Gender = male (%) | 11 (24.4) | — |
| BMI (mean (sd)) | 23.90 (3.24) | 18.87–32 |
| TQX (mean (sd)) | 19.02 (5.38) | 7–28 |
| Total intake (mean (sd)) | 4.8 (2.61) | 0–9 |
| R2M (%) | | |
| 0 | 3 (6.7) | |
| 1 | 19 (42.2) | |
| 2 | 23 (51.1) | |
| RRM (%) | | |
| 0 | 1 (2.2) | |
| 1 | 31 (68.9) | |
| 2 | 13 (28.9) | |
| RRA (%) | | |
| 1 | 16 (35.6) | |
| 2 | 27 (60.0) | |
| 3 | 2 (4.4) | |
| RRB (%) | | |
| 0 | 2 (4.4) | |
| 1 | 31 (68.9) | |
| 2 | 12 (26.7) | |

TABLE 3: Estimates of the significant variables for swelling response.

| Variable | Slope value | CI 95% | P value | Eta2 |
|----------|-------------|--------|---------|------|
| Gender (male) | 40.99 | 28.6,53.4 | <0.000001 | 0.2613 |
| BMI | 3.06 | 1.4, 4.8 | 0.00027 | 0.0841 |
| RRB | RB1 38.82<br>RB2 44.74 | 14.8,62.8<br>19.7, 69.7 | 0.00143 | 0.0646 |
| Age | −2.57 | −2.6, −1.0 | 0.00068 | 0.0591 |
| Residual | — | — | — | 0.5309 |

the fixed component do not explain the changes in the trismus measures.

## 4. Discussion

To understand clinical and radiographic characteristics as predictor factors of swelling and trismus, after mandibular third molar surgery, it is important to recognize the risk factors associated with clinical complications. Several studies have measured the difficulty of this surgical procedure and clinical and radiological factors [1, 11–14, 17, 18].

Swelling has been determined by different techniques described in the literature; these techniques include visual inspection [6], facial points [19], photographic techniques [20], Computed Tomography (CT) [21], and others [7, 15, 22]. In the present study, swelling was estimated by the sum of the four facial planes. The advantages of this method are its simple implementation and low cost. Trismus was determined by maximal opening of the mouth and the distance between the lower and upper incisors.

Gender, body mass index (BMI), relation to lingual and buccal walls, and age of the patients were determinants in explaining the swelling measurements. The importance of gender in facial swelling was found in the present study, swelling was higher in males than in females, this agreement with that reported by Yuasa and Sigiura [15]. These authors, with a total of 140 patients (153 surgical procedures, 64.7% females), used a sum of two planes (T-Co and C-Go) divided by 2, to measure facial swelling. Measurements were made on postoperative days 1 and 7. The statistical analyses used in their study included logistic regression and correlation without multiple measurements, and the difference between both sexes in the swelling was observed in the first time. This cannot be extended to the dynamic process of swelling. To deal with this issue, we propose the analysis of variables with the MRMM, which is applicable with the longitudinal design in our study [23].

On the other hand, de Santana-Santos et al. [24] reported the influence of the "gender" of the patients in the prediction of swelling. These authors found higher swelling in females than in males, with a sample size of 80 patients (32.5%, females). They employed five measurements of distance between two facial points (the sum of five measurements divided by 5); the measurements were made on postoperative days 2 and 7, and the statistical analysis used was correlation and group differences in one measurement time. Osunde and Saheeb [25] did not find a significant effect of sex on the swelling variable; these authors recruited a total of 150 patients (56%, female). They used the arithmetic mean of two planes (T-Co and C-Go) and the difference between each postoperative measurement at days 1, 2, 3, 5, and 7 and baseline as swelling measurement of the day. However, the authors found a higher mean facial swelling in females than in males, but this result was not significative. The analysis used in their study was one-way ANOVA.

BMI was also reported by de Santana-Santos et al. [24]; they did not find an association with the prediction of swelling. In their study, the authors categorized the BMI value and the swelling measurement. BMI is a measurement of body fat based on height and weight; adipose tissue is a major contributing factor to systemic inflammation, generating approximately one third of the circulating proinflammatory cytokine InterLeukin (IL)-6 [26]. The association of BMI and swelling has been previously explained; people with obesity often experience higher concentrations of inflammatory biomarkers than their normal-weight counterparts [26, 27]. In the present study, the BMI variable had a low weight to explain the swelling in the patients (Table 3).

The relation of lower third molar with lingual and buccal walls has not been, to our knowledge, reported previously as a predictor factor of swelling. Several studies have reported the radiographic classification as a factor contributing to the complexity of the surgery [6, 13, 17, 28, 29]. In the present study, the proximal relation of the lower third molar to the lingual wall, or the relation in the middle position between buccal and lingual walls, corresponded to an increase in the swelling measures in the postoperative evaluation; this can be explained by the hard tissue removed. When the third molar is buccally erupted, the total bone removed for the surgical extraction is lower; on the other hand, when the third molar is in lingual position, the amount of bone removed increases.

The age of the patients has been reported as a predictive factor for swelling. Olmedo Gaya et al. [30] reported increased swelling with increased age. According to a report by Bello et al. [29], there is a positive association between age and swelling and age and trismus. Finally, Osunde et al. [12] did not show a significant association between age and swelling in mandibular third molar surgery. In the present study, the age variable shows an inverse relationship with swelling; this implies that if the patient's age increases, the swelling decreases; however, this relationship shows low weight to explain the swelling (Table 3). This relationship can be explained by the changes involved in the immune system associated with the inflammatory response related to age [31].

One of the advantages of this study is the multiple measurement period. Because the swelling process is dynamic and the main changes are present in the first 72 h [9], the MRMM can be adjusted for multiple measurements and used in a longitudinal approach, and the methods control the intra- and interpatient variability when repeated measures design is used and have a more flexible structure for the analysis [23, 32]. The repeated measures design increased the number of measurements on the same patient; this means we can use more repetitions or measurement values in the model with the same number of patients. However, this type of analysis includes some limitations: the slope values are only valid in the range of the variables included; out of this range, this model cannot be applied. Moreover, the swelling measure was linear and not volumetric and did not involve the volume of the change of tissue. van der Meer et al. [22] and Yamamoto et al. [21] propose new methods to measure facial swelling, and the use of stereophotogrammetry, CT, and laser surface scanning comprises the principal elements in these procedures. The advantages of this include the reproducibility of the measures, in terms of volume and precision; however, cost and implementation must be taken into account in the planning of the clinical trials.

Further studies are necessary to confirm these findings, with a higher sample size and variable ranges. We suggest the use of MRMM to analyze the data with a longitudinal approach and control the follow-up measurements during the first 72 hours. The facial planes method to measure the swelling can be useful; however, this method has some limitations, and other alternatives can be validated to this endpoint.

## 5. Conclusions

This study suggests the association of male gender, the relation to the lingual and buccal walls, BMI, and age with the swelling measurement. The trismus variable did not show any relationship with explanatory variables.

## Acknowledgments

This work was supported partially by PFCE-UASLP 2017 and PRODEP 2018 grants.

## References

[1] R. D. Marciani, "Third molar removal: an overview of indications, imaging, evaluation, and assessment of risk," *Oral and Maxillofacial Surgery Clinics of North America*, vol. 19, no. 1, pp. 1–13, 2007.

[2] M. Colorado-Bonnin, E. Valmaseda-Castellón, L. Berini-Aytés, and C. Gay-Escoda, "Quality of life following lower third molar removal," *International Journal of Oral and Maxillofacial Surgery*, vol. 35, no. 4, pp. 343–347, 2006.

[3] J. Perez-Urizar, R. Martinez-Rider, I. Torres-Roque, A. Garrocho-Rangel, and A. Pozos-Guillen, "Analgesic efficacy of lysine clonixinate plus tramadol versus tramadol in multiple doses following impacted third molar surgery," *International Journal of Oral and Maxillofacial Surgery*, vol. 43, no. 3, pp. 348–354, 2014.

[4] V. Esparza-Villalpando, D. Chavarria-Bolaños, A. Gordillo-Moscoso et al., "Comparison of the analgesic efficacy of preoperative/postoperative oral dexketoprofen trometamol in third molar surgery: a randomized clinical trial," *Journal of Cranio-Maxillo-Facial Surgery*, vol. 44, no. 9, pp. 1350–1355, 2016.

[5] M. Isiordia, A. Pozos-Guillén, R. Martinez, J. Herrera, and J. Perez, "Preemptive analgesic effectiveness of oral ketorolac plus local tramadol after impacted mandibular third molar surgery," *Medicina Oral Patología Oral y Cirugia Bucal*, vol. 16, no. 6, pp. 776–780, 2011.

[6] E. D. Amarillas-Escobar, J. M. Toranzo-Fernández, R. Martínez-Rider et al., "Use of therapeutic laser after surgical removal of impacted lower third molars," *Journal of Oral and Maxillofacial Surgery*, vol. 68, no. 2, pp. 319–324, 2010.

[7] M. Rana, N. C. Gellrich, A. Ghassemi, M. Gerressen, D. Riediger, and A. Modabber, "Three-dimensional evaluation of postoperative swelling after third molar surgery using 2 different cooling therapy methods: a randomized observer-blind prospective study," *Journal of Oral and Maxillofacial Surgery*, vol. 69, no. 8, pp. 2092–2098, 2011.

[8] T. Velnar, T. Baileym, and V. Smrkolj, "The wound healing process: an overview of the cellular and molecular mechanisms," *Journal of International Medical Research*, vol. 37, no. 5, pp. 1528–1542, 2009.

[9] R. A. Seymour, J. G. Meechan, and G. S. Blair, "An investigation into post-operative pain after third molar surgery under local analgesia," *British Journal of Oral and Maxillofacial Surgery*, vol. 23, no. 6, pp. 410–418, 1985.

[10] G. Juodzbalys and P. Daugela, "Mandibular third molar impaction: review of literature and a proposal of a classification," *Journal of Oral and Maxillofacial Research*, vol. 4, no. 2, pp. 1–11, 2013.

[11] F. Blondeau and N. G. Daniel, "Extraction of impacted mandibular third molars: postoperative complications and their risk factors," *Journal-Canadian Dental Association*, vol. 73, no. 4, p. 325, 2007.

[12] O. Osunde, B. Saheeb, and G. Bassey, "Indications and risk factors for complications of lower third molar surgery in a Nigerian teaching hospital," *Annals of Medical and Health Sciences Research*, vol. 4, no. 6, pp. 938–942, 2014.

[13] N. L. Barbosa-Rebellato, A. C. Thomé, C. Costa-Maciel, J. Oliveira, and R. Scariot, "Factors associated with complications of removal of third molars: a transversal study," *Medicina Oral Patología Oral y Cirugia Bucal*, vol. 16, no. 3, pp. 376–380, 2011.

[14] M. A. Pogrel, "What is the effect of timing of removal on the incidence and severity of complications?," *Journal of Oral and Maxillofacial Surgery*, vol. 70, no. 9, pp. 37–40, 2012.

[15] H. Yuasa and M. Sugiura, "Clinical postoperative findings after removal of impacted mandibular third molars: Prediction of postoperative facial swelling and pain based on preoperative variables," *British Journal of Oral and Maxillofacial Surgery*, vol. 42, no. 3, pp. 209–214, 2004.

[16] J. C. Pinheiro and D. M. Bates, "Approximations to the log-likelihood function in the nonlinear mixed-effects model," *Journal of Computational and Graphical Statistics*, vol. 4, pp. 12–35, 1995.

[17] J. Alvira-Gonzalez, R. Figueiredo, E. Valmaseda-Castellon, C. Quesada-Gomez, and C. Gay-Escoda, "Predictive factors of difficulty in lower third molar extraction: A prospective cohort study," *Medicina Oral Patología Oral y Cirugia Bucal*, vol. 22, no. 1, pp. e108–e114, 2017.

[18] P. Coulthard, E. Bailey, M. Esposito, S. Furness, T. F. Renton, and H. V. Worthington, "Surgical techniques for the removal of mandibular wisdom teeth," *Cochrane Database of Systematic Reviews*, vol. 7, p. CD004345, 2014.

[19] C. Gay-Escoda, L. Gómez-Santos, A. Sánchez-Torres, and J. M. Herráez-Vilas, "Effect of the suture technique on postoperative pain, swelling and trismus after removal of lower third molars: A randomized clinical trial," *Medicina Oral Patología Oral y Cirugia Bucal*, vol. 20, no. 3, pp. e372–e377, 2015.

[20] A. V. Van Gool, J. J. Ten Bosch, and G. Boering, "A photographic method of assessing swelling following third molar removal," *International Journal of Oral Surgery*, vol. 4, pp. 121–129, 1975.

[21] S. Yamamoto, H. Miyachi, H. Fujii, S. Ochiai, S. Watanabe, and K. Shimozato, "Intuitive facial imaging method for evaluation of postoperative swelling: A combination of 3-dimensional computed tomography and laser surface

Clinical and Radiographic Characteristics as Predictive Factors of Swelling and Trismus after...

177

scanning in orthognathic surgery," *Journal of Oral and Maxillofacial Surgery*, vol. 74, no. 12, pp. 2506.e1–2506.e10, 2016.

[22] M. J. van der Meer, P. U. Dijkstra, A. Visser, A. Vissink, and Y. Ren, "Reliability and validity of measurements of facial swelling with a stereophotogrammetry optical three-dimensional scanner," *British Journal of Oral and Maxillofacial Surgery*, vol. 52, no. 10, pp. 922–927, 2014.

[23] M. Detry and Y. Ma, "Analyzing repeated measurements using mixed models," *Journal of the American Medical Association*, vol. 315, no. 4, pp. 407-408, 2016.

[24] T. de Santana-Santos, J. de Souza-Santos, P. Martins-Filho, L. da Silva, E. de Oliveira e Silva, and A. Gomes, "Prediction of postoperative facial swelling, pain and trismus following third molar surgery based on preoperative variables," *Medicina Oral Patología Oral y Cirugia Bucal*, vol. 18, no. 1, pp. e65–e70, 2013.

[25] O. D. Osunde and B. D. Saheeb, "Effect of age, sex and level of surgical difficulty on inflammatory complications after third molar surgery," *Journal of Maxillofacial and Oral Surgery*, vol. 14, no. 1, pp. 7–12, 2015.

[26] A. W. Ferrante, "Obesity-induced inflammation: a metabolic dialogue in the language of inflammation," *Journal of Internal Medicine*, vol. 262, no. 4, pp. 408–414, 2007.

[27] E. D. Kantor, J. W. Lampe, M. Kratz, and E. White, "Lifestyle factors and inflammation: associations by body mass index," *PLoS One*, vol. 8, no. 7, article e67833, 2013.

[28] O. A. Akadiri and A. E. Obiechina, "Assessment of difficulty in third molar surgery—A systematic review," *Journal of Oral and Maxillofacial Surgery*, vol. 67, no. 4, pp. 771–774, 2009.

[29] S. A. Bello, W. L. Adeyemo, B. O. Bamgbose, E. V. Obi, and A. A. Adeyinka, "Effect of age, impaction types and operative time on inflammatory tissue reactions following lower third molar surgery," *Head and Face Medicine*, vol. 7, pp. 1–8, 2011.

[30] V. Olmedo Gaya, M. Vallecillo Capilla, and R. Gálvez Mateos, "Relación de las variables del paciente y de la intervención con el dolor y la inflamación postoperatorios en la exodoncia de los terceros molares," *Medicina Oral*, vol. 7, pp. 360–369, 2002.

[31] F. Licastro, G. Candore, D. Lio et al., "Innate immunity and inflammation in ageing: a key for understanding age-related diseases," *Immunity and Ageing*, vol. 2, pp. 338–344, 2005.

[32] A. P. Field and D. B. Wright, "A primer on using multilevel models in clinical and experimental psychopathology research," *Journal of Experimental Psychopathology*, vol. 2, no. 2, pp. 271–293, 2011.

# 22

# Ultrasound-Guided Intervention for Treatment of Trigeminal Neuralgia: An Updated Review of Anatomy and Techniques

Abdallah El-Sayed Allam,[1] Adham Aboul Fotouh Khalil,[2] Basma Aly Eltawab,[3] Wei-Ting Wu,[4] and Ke-Vin Chang[4]

[1]Department of Physical Medicine, Rheumatology and Rehabilitation, Tanta University Hospitals, Faculty of Medicine, Tanta University, Tanta, Egypt
[2]New Kasr El-Aini Teaching Hospital, Cairo, Egypt
[3]Department of Radiology, Tanta University Hospitals, Tanta, Egypt
[4]Department of Physical Medicine and Rehabilitation, National Taiwan University Hospital Bei-Hu Branch, Taipei, Taiwan

Correspondence should be addressed to Ke-Vin Chang; pattap@pchome.com.tw

Academic Editor: Fabiana Ballanti

Orofacial myofascial pain is prevalent and most often results from entrapment of branches of the trigeminal nerves. It is challenging to inject branches of the trigeminal nerve, a large portion of which are shielded by the facial bones. Bony landmarks of the cranium serve as important guides for palpation-guided injections and can be delineated using ultrasound. Ultrasound also provides real-time images of the adjacent muscles and accompanying arteries and can be used to guide the needle to the target region. Most importantly, ultrasound guidance significantly reduces the risk of collateral injury to vital neurovascular structures. In this review, we aimed to summarize the regional anatomy and ultrasound-guided injection techniques for the trigeminal nerve and its branches, including the supraorbital, infraorbital, mental, auriculotemporal, maxillary, and mandibular nerves.

## 1. Introduction

A common cause of chronic facial pain syndrome is trigeminal neuralgia, which can be alleviated by injecting the superficial branches of the nerve, such as the supraorbital, infraorbital, and mental nerves, and deep injection of the maxillary nerve in the pterygopalatine fossa and/or the mandibular nerve posterior to the lateral pterygoid plate [1]. Isolated entrapment of the abovementioned nerves is not rare, but treatments using palpation guidance can be challenging because substantial portions of the nerves lie underneath the skull bone. The use of high-resolution ultrasound facilitates real-time visualization of peripheral nerves and adjacent soft tissue structures, such as tendons, ligaments, muscles, vessels, and subcutaneous fat [2]. Ultrasound-guided intervention allows precise targeting of the affected nerves without collateral damage to the nearby vessels and prevents accidental nerve injury, vascular thrombosis, and postinjection hematoma [3–6]. In this review, we aimed to summarize the regional anatomy and ultrasound-guided injection techniques for the commonly affected branches of the trigeminal nerve, including the supraorbital, infraorbital, mental, auriculotemporal, maxillary, and mandibular nerves.

## 2. Technical Considerations and Regimen for Treatments

All of the sonographic images presented in this review were obtained using MyLab 5 (Esaote Europe B.V., Maastricht, Netherlands). A 10–18 MHz high-frequency linear transducer was used to scan superficial structures. To image deeper structures, such as the lateral pterygoid muscle and plate, a 1–5 MHz curvilinear transducer was used. During the power Doppler examination, the Doppler frequency was set to 6.6 MHz.

To perform the superficial nerve block, 1 to 3 ml of local anesthetic, for example, 0.5% lidocaine, can be injected using a 25-gauge 1.5-inch needle. For deeper nerve blocks, 3 to 5 ml

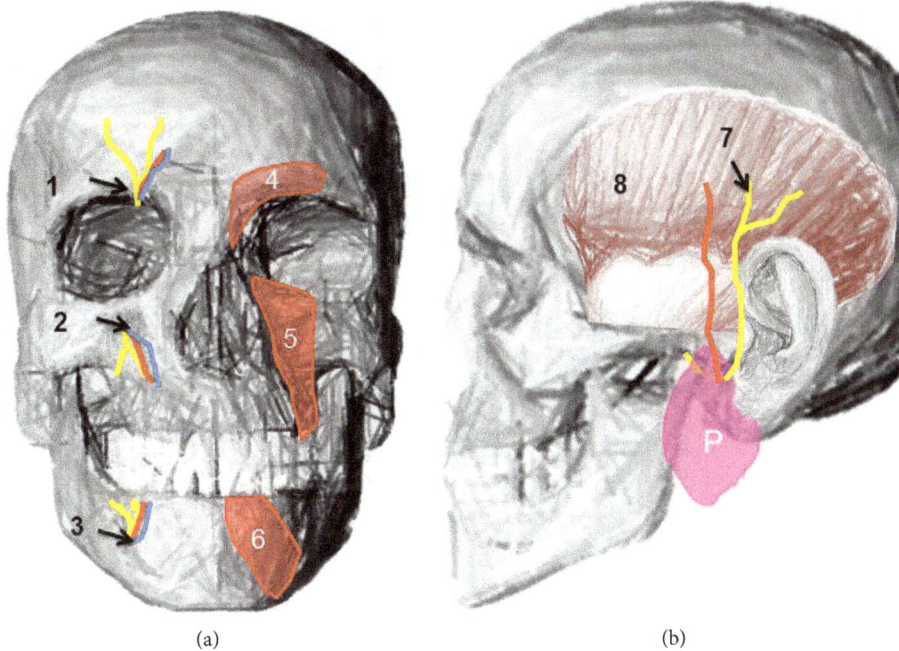

(a)                                              (b)

FIGURE 1: Anatomy of the supraorbital notch, infraorbital foramen, and mental foramen with corresponding neurovascular structures and the course of the auriculotemporal nerve: (a) 1 = supraorbital notch containing the supraorbital nerve and vessels; 2 = infraorbital foramen containing the infraorbital nerve and vessels; 3 = mental foramen containing the mental nerve and vessels; 4 = corrugator supercilii muscle, which is superficial to the supraorbital notch; 5 = levator labii superioris muscle, which is superficial to the infraorbital foramen; 6 = depressor labii inferioris muscle, which is superficial to the mental foramen, and (b) 7 = auriculotemporal nerve; 8 = temporalis muscle; P = parotid gland.

of the anesthetic can be injected using a 22-gauge 3-inch spinal needle. Potential complications include bleeding, hematoma, infection, and hypersensitivity reaction to the injectate. For longer pain relief, the deep injection can be performed using glycerol (100%), alcohol (50–70%), or phenol (5–10%). Because of the serious complications of the abovementioned neurolytic agents, such as permanent sensory deficit, severe allergic reactions, and tissue necrosis, they are gradually replaced by safer and more effective treatments like radiofrequency or cryoablation which may be considered for recalcitrant cases [7, 8].

## 3. Supraorbital Nerve

3.1. Anatomy. The frontal nerve is a branch of the ophthalmic division of the trigeminal nerve. It has two terminal branches: the larger supraorbital and smaller supratrochlear nerves. The supraorbital nerve emerges from the facial bone through the supraorbital notch which lies within the medial one-third of the supraorbital margin, 2 to 3 cm lateral to the midline (Figure 1(a) and Table 1). According to a cadaveric study, bilateral supraorbital notches were present in 49.07% of skulls, bilateral supraorbital foramina were found in 25.93% of skulls, and a notch at one side and a foramen at the contralateral side were seen in 25% of skulls [9]. The supraorbital nerve carries sensory information from the upper eyelid, forehead, and the anterior half of the scalp, except for the area innervated by the supratrochlear nerve, which is close to the midline [10].

3.2. Clinical Symptoms of Nerve Entrapment. Patients with supraorbital neuralgia present with pain, tenderness, hypoesthesia,

and allodynia in the territory supplied by the affected nerve. Fractures of the orbital roof, blunt trauma to the face (in boxers), tumors of the orbit, and tight swimming goggles and motorcycle helmet can cause supraorbital nerve entrapment. Imaging studies using computed tomography or magnetic resonance imaging can be used to diagnose fractures and space-occupying lesions (Figure 2(a)) [4, 11].

3.3. Sonoanatomy and Ultrasound-Guided Injection Technique. During this procedure, the participant lies supine with the head in the neutral position. The eye on the side of examination should be closed to prevent the coupling gel from being smeared into the eye. The transducer is placed over the medial one-third of the supraorbital margin (Figure 3(a)). The supraorbital notch can be identified as an interruption of the hyperechoic bony edge, where the supraorbital nerve and vessels exit (Figure 3(b)). For guided injection, the needle is introduced from the lateral side toward the midline using the in-plane approach to target the supraorbital nerve (Figure 3(c) and Table 1). Turning on the power Doppler mode helps with recognition of the supraorbital vessels (Figure 3(d)). The lateral edge of the transducer can be slightly lifted up to create an opening for advancement of the needle. More sterilized jelly is required to fill the space as a gel bridge (the heel-toe maneuver).

## 4. Infraorbital Nerve

4.1. Anatomy. The infraorbital nerve is the terminal branch of the maxillary division of the trigeminal nerve and carries sensory information from the lower eyelid, one side of the

TABLE 1: Summary of the anatomy and guided injection techniques of the trigeminal nerve and its branches.

| Nerve | Bony landmark | Sensory innervation of the nerve | Accompanying vessel | Adjacent muscle | Transducer selection | Transducer placement | Needle trajectory | Ultrasound-guided technique |
|---|---|---|---|---|---|---|---|---|
| Supraorbital nerve | Supraorbital notch at the medial one-third of the supraorbital margin about 2 to 3 cm lateral to the midline | Upper eyelid, forehead, and the anterior half of the scalp | Supraorbital artery and vein | Corrugator supercilii muscle | Linear transducer | Medial one-third of the supraorbital margin | From lateral to medial | In-plane |
| Infraorbital nerve | Infraorbital foramen 1 cm below the midpoint of the infraorbital margin | Lower eyelid, half side of the nose, and the upper lip | Infraorbital artery and vein | Levator labii superioris muscle | Linear transducer | Body of the maxilla parallel to and 1 cm below the infraorbital margin 3 cm lateral to the midline | From lateral to medial | In-plane |
| Mental nerve | Mental foramen 3 cm lateral to the midline and 1 cm above the lower border of the mandible | Skin of the chin and lower lip and mucosa of the lower lip | Mental artery and vein | Depressor labii inferioris muscle | Linear transducer | 1 cm above and parallel to the lower border of the mandible | From lateral to medial | In-plane |
| Auriculotemporal nerve | Posterior zygomatic arch in front of the tragus | Anterior ear and the posterior part of the skin over the temporalis muscle | Superficial temporal artery | Temporalis muscle | Linear transducer | Parallel to the posterior part of the zygomatic arch just above the level of the tragus | From posterior to anterior | In-plane |
| Maxillary nerve | Pterygopalatine fossa anterior and medial to the lateral pterygoid plate | Lower eyelid, cheek, nose, upper lip, upper teeth and gums, roof of the pharynx, the sphenoid and ethmoid sinuses and meninges | Sphenopalatine artery | Lateral pterygoid muscle | Curvilinear transducer | Distal and parallel to the zygomatic arch to bridge the coronoid and the condylar processes | From posterior to anterior | Out-of-plane |
| Mandibular nerve | Posterior to the lateral pterygoid plate | Anterior two-thirds of the tongue, teeth, and mucosa and periosteum of the mandible, skin of the chin and the lower lip, and the skin over the mandible | Middle meningeal artery | Lateral and medial pterygoid muscles | Curvilinear transducer | Distal and parallel to the zygomatic arch to bridge the coronoid and the condylar processes | From anterior to posterior | Out-of-plane |

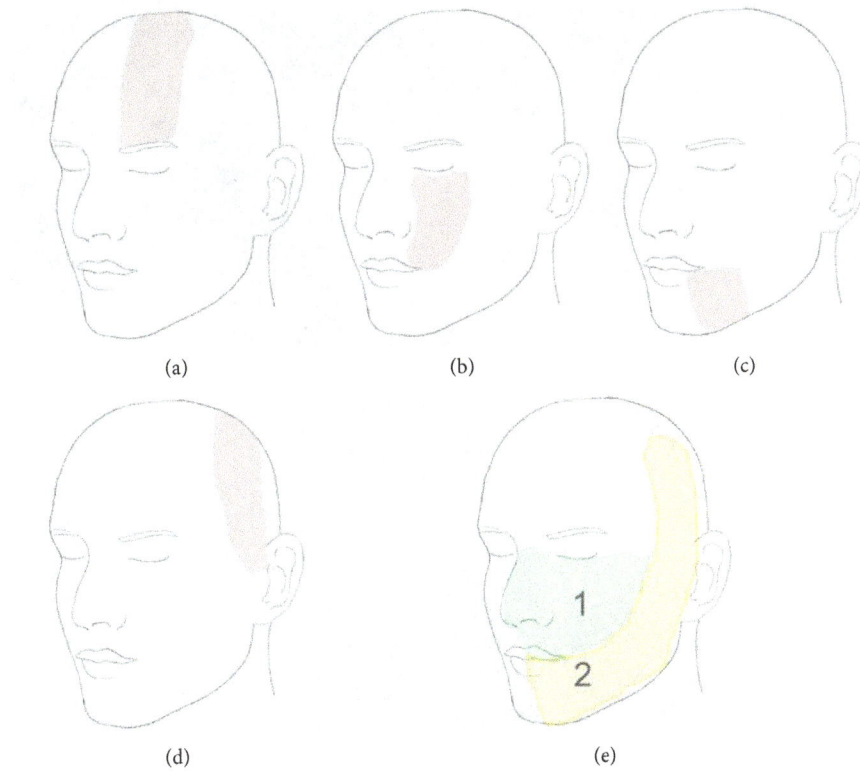

FIGURE 2: Topography of the sensory distribution of the (a) supraorbital nerve, (b) infraorbital nerve, (c) mental nerve, (d) auriculotemporal nerve, and (e) deep branches of the trigeminal nerve; 1 = area supplied by the maxillary nerve and 2 = area supplied by the mandibular nerve.

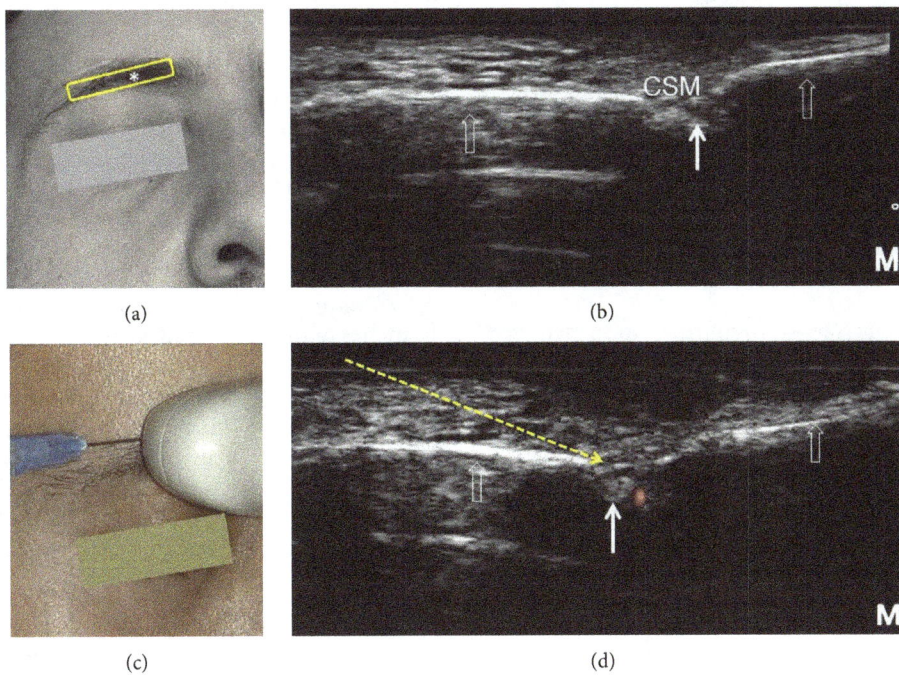

FIGURE 3: Sonoanatomy and ultrasound-guided injection technique for the supraorbital nerve: (a) the position of the transducer (yellow rectangle), (b) ultrasound imaging of the supraorbital nerve emerging from the supraorbital notch, (c) introducing the needle in the lateral-to-medial direction using the in-plane approach to target the supraorbital nerve, and (d) power Doppler image of the supraorbital vessels. The asterisk (*) denotes the supraorbital notch on the face. The empty white arrows denote the supraorbital margin. The solid white arrow denotes the supraorbital nerve. The yellow dashed arrow denotes the needle trajectory. CSM: corrugator supercilii muscle and M: medial side. All the pictures were obtained from the face of the first author.

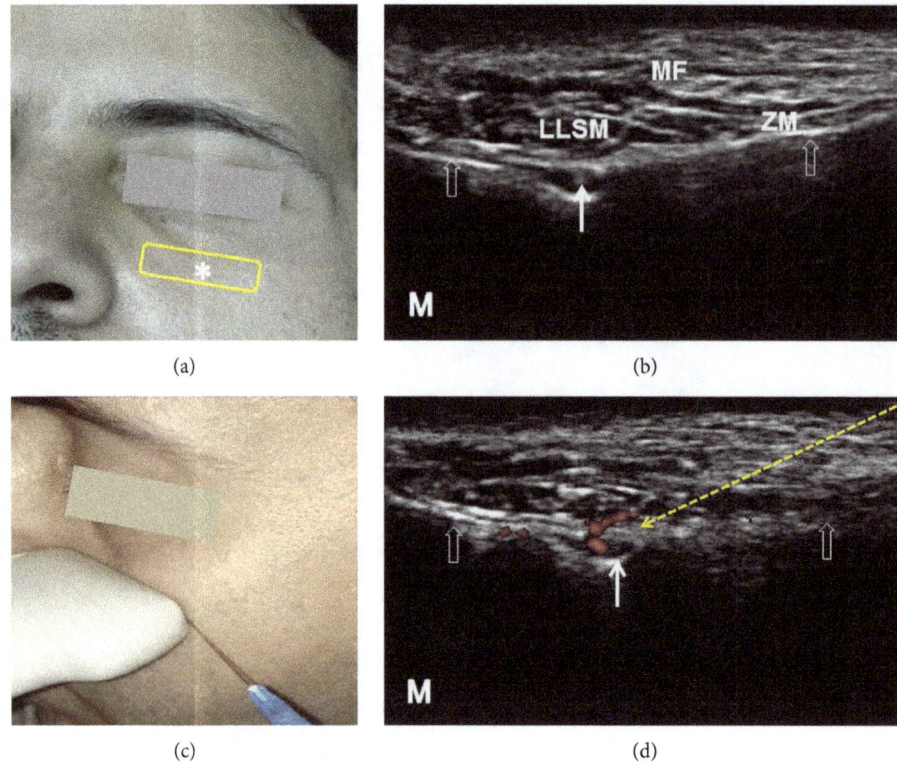

(a)

(b)

(c)

(d)

FIGURE 4: Sonoanatomy and ultrasound-guided injection technique for the infraorbital nerve: (a) the transducer position (yellow rectangle), (b) ultrasound image of the infraorbital nerve (white solid arrow) from the infraorbital foramen, (c) introducing the needle in the lateral-to-medial direction using the in-plane approach to target the infraorbital nerve, and (d) power Doppler image of the infraorbital vessels. The asterisk (*) denotes the infraorbital foramen on the face. The empty white arrows denote the bony cortex of the maxilla. The yellow dashed arrow denotes the needle trajectory. LLSM: levator labii superioris muscle; ZM: zygomaticus minor muscle; MF: malar fat; M: medial side. All the pictures were obtained from the face of the first author.

nose, and the upper lip. It emerges from the infraorbital foramen, extends to the subcutaneous layer, and is accompanied by the infraorbital vessels deep to the levator labii superioris muscle and malar fat. The infraorbital foramen lies on the anterior aspect of the maxilla bone and is approximately 1 cm below the midpoint of the infraorbital margin (Figure 1(a) and Table 1) [10].

4.2. Clinical Symptoms of Nerve Entrapment. The patient may complain of pain, tingling, tenderness, and allodynia in the lower eyelid, one half of the nose, and the upper lip. These symptoms may occur due to fractures of the orbital floor, malignancies of the orbit and maxilla, or blunt trauma (in boxers) which can entrap the nerve. Imaging studies using computed tomography or magnetic resonance imaging should be performed when fractures or hidden malignancies are suspected (Figure 2(b)) [6, 12].

4.3. Sonoanatomy and Ultrasound-Guided Injection Technique. During the procedure, the participant lies supine with the head in the neutral position. The transducer is placed over the body of the maxilla parallel to and 1 cm below the infraorbital margin (Figure 4(a)). The infraorbital foramen can be seen as an opening on the maxillary bone through which the infraorbital nerve and vessels emerge (Figure 4(b)). The needle is introduced from the lateral side toward the midline

using the in-plane approach to target the infraorbital nerve in the infraorbital foramen (Figure 4(c)). The power Doppler mode should be turned on before injection to avoid damaging to the infraorbital vessels (Figure 4(d)).

## 5. Mental Nerve

5.1. Anatomy. The mental nerve is one of two terminal branches of the inferior alveolar nerve, which is rooted in the mandibular division of the trigeminal nerve. It supplies the skin of the chin, as well as the skin and mucous membranes of the lower lip. It emerges to the subcutaneous layer of the face through the mental foramen which lies deep to the depressor labii inferioris muscle. The foramen lies 3 cm lateral to the midline and 1 cm above the lower border of the mandible between the first and second premolar teeth (Figure 1(a) and Table 1) [13].

5.2. Clinical Symptoms of Nerve Entrapment. Patients usually have pain and paresthesia on the skin of the chin, as well as the skin and mucous membrane of the lower lip. The nerve can be entrapped due to fractures of the mandible, blunt trauma to the face (in boxers), dental pathologies, or malignancies of the oral cavity. The computed tomography and magnetic resonance imaging may be required for confirmation of the diagnosis of the underlying cause of entrapment (Figure 2(c)) [3].

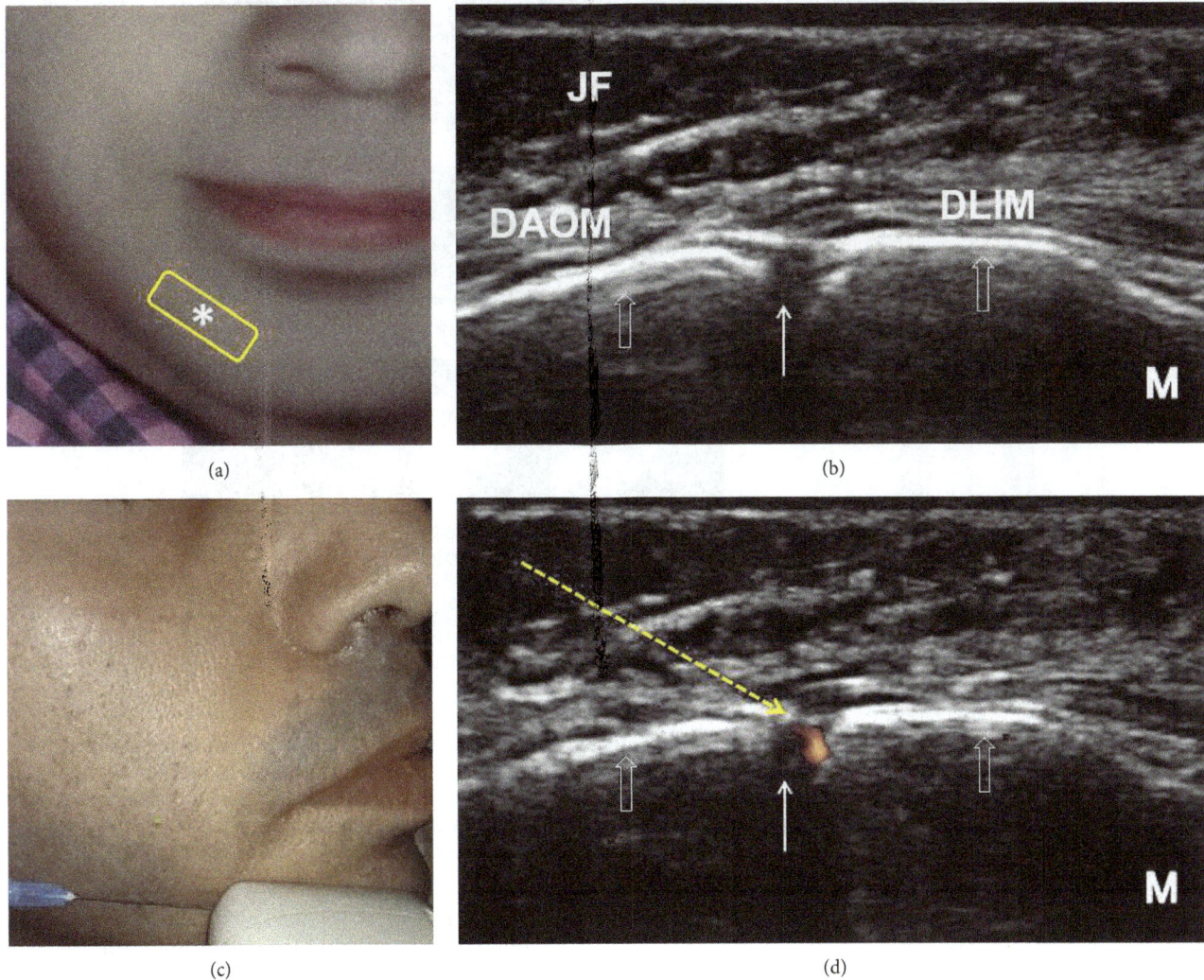

FIGURE 5: Sonoanatomy and ultrasound-guided injection technique for the mental nerve: (a) the transducer position (yellow rectangle), (b) ultrasound imaging of the mental nerve (white solid arrow), (c) introducing the needle from the lateral side toward the midline using the in-plane approach to target the mental nerve, and (d) power Doppler image used to identify the mental vessels. The empty white arrows denote the body of the mandible. The asterisk (*) denotes the mental foramen on the face. The yellow dashed arrow denotes the needle trajectory. DLIM: depressor labii inferioris muscle; DAOM: depressor anguli oris muscle; JF: jowl fat; M: medial side. All the pictures were obtained from the face of the first author.

*5.3. Sonoanatomy and Ultrasound-Guided Injection Technique.* During the procedure, the participant lies supine with the head in the neutral position. The transducer is placed over a point located 3 cm lateral to the midline and 1 cm above and parallel to the lower border of the mandible (between the first and second premolar teeth) (Figures 5(a) and 5(b)). We can identify the mental nerve emerging from the mental foramen based on the accompanying vessel. Using the in-plane approach, the needle can be introduced from the lateral side toward the midline to target the nerve inside the mental foramen (Figures 5(c) and 5(d); Table 1).

## 6. Auriculotemporal Nerve

*6.1. Anatomy.* The auriculotemporal nerve is a branch of the mandibular division of the trigeminal nerve. It runs deep to the condylar process. The nerve courses posterior to the condylar process, pierces the parotid gland, and surfaces at the facial soft tissue. The nerve crosses over the hind part of the zygomatic arch posterior to the superficial temporal artery (Figure 1(b) and Table 1). It carries sensations from the tragus and anterior part of the ear and the posterior part of the skin over the temporalis muscle [14].

*6.2. Clinical Symptoms of Nerve Entrapment.* Patients have unilateral lancinating pain in the tragus and anterior part of the ear, as well as in the posterior part of the temporal bone (Figure 2(d)). Symptoms can be triggered by applying pressure to the area in front of the tragus. Entrapment of the nerve can occur due to tightness of the lateral pterygoid muscle secondary to temporomandibular joint dysfunction [5].

*6.3. Sonoanatomy and Ultrasound-Guided Injection Technique.* In this procedure, the participant lies on his or her side with the affected side of the face facing upward. The

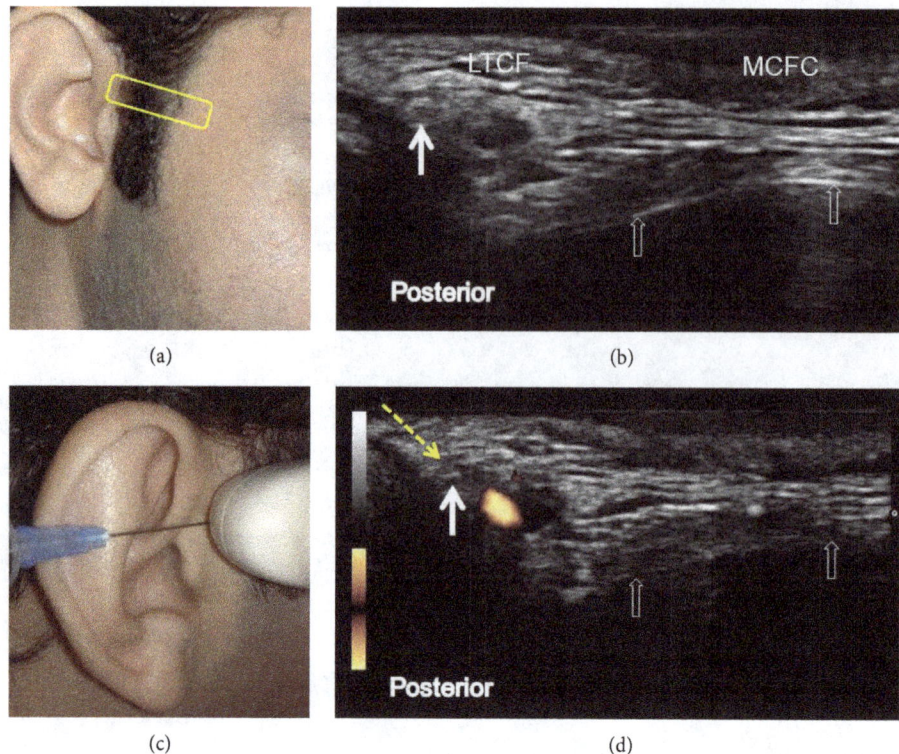

FIGURE 6: Sonoanatomy and ultrasound-guided injection technique for the auriculotemporal nerve: (a) the transducer position (yellow rectangle), (b) ultrasound imaging of the auriculotemporal nerve (white solid arrow), (c) introducing the needle in the posterior-to-anterior direction using the in-plane approach to target the auriculotemporal nerve, and (d) the power Doppler image of the superficial temporal artery. The empty white arrows denote the zygomatic arch. The yellow dashed arrow indicates the needle trajectory. MCFC: middle cheek fat compartment and LTCF: lateral temporal cheek fat. All the pictures were obtained from the face of the first author.

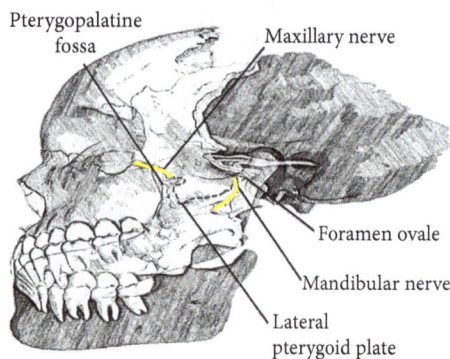

FIGURE 7: Anatomy of the maxillary and mandibular nerves related to the lateral pterygoid plate.

transducer is placed over and parallel to the posterior part of the zygomatic arch just above the level of the tragus (Figure 6(a) and Table 1). The auriculotemporal nerve is seen posterior to the superficial temporal artery. The needle is introduced in the posterior-to-anterior direction using the in-plane approach to target the short axis of the auriculotemporal nerve (Figures 6(b)–6(d)).

## 7. Maxillary and Mandibular Nerves

*7.1. Anatomy.* The Gasserian ganglion of the trigeminal nerve has 3 branches, namely, the ophthalmic and maxillary nerves,

and the sensory root of the mandibular nerve. The maxillary nerve runs through the dura of the lateral wall of the cavernous sinus. It then passes through the foramen rotundum, exits the skull, and enters the pterygopalatine fossa. The maxillary nerve leaves the pterygopalatine fossa through the infraorbital fissure and becomes the infraorbital nerve in the orbital cavity (Figure 7). It carries sensations from the lower eyelid, cheek, nose, upper lip, upper teeth and gums, palate, roof of the pharynx, and the maxillary, sphenoid, and ethmoid sinuses and meninges [15]. The mandibular nerve leaves the middle cranial fossa through the foramen ovale and descends posterior to the lateral pterygoid plate (Figure 7) between the lateral and the medial pterygoid muscles. It provides motor innervation to the mylohyoid, tensor tympani, and tensor veli palatini muscles. It also carries sensory information from the anterior two-thirds of the tongue, teeth, and mucosa, as well as the periosteum of the mandible and skin of the chin and lower lip. The mandibular nerve also carries sensory information from the skin over the mandible, except for that over the mandibular angle, the tragus and anterior part of the ear, and the skin over the posterior part of the temporalis muscle up to the scalp [16].

*7.2. Clinical Symptoms of Nerve Entrapment.* Trigeminal neuralgia is usually unilateral sharp, stabbing, or burning pain that typically radiates to the area innervated by one or more divisions of the trigeminal nerve (Figure 2(e)). Pain

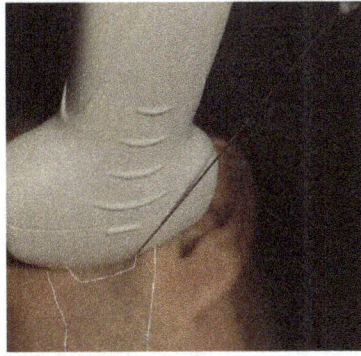

(a)

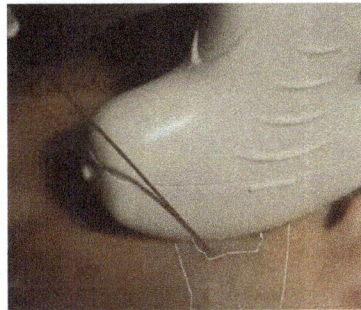

(b)

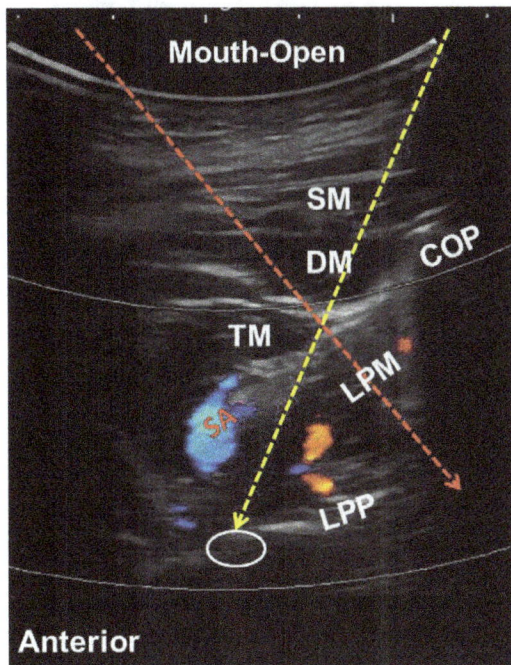

(c)

FIGURE 8: Ultrasound-guided injection technique for the maxillary and mandibular nerves: (a) the transducer position and required placement for the maxillary nerve, (b) the transducer position and required placement for the mandibular nerve, and (c) color Doppler image during mouth opening. The yellow dashed arrow represents the needle trajectory for injection of the maxillary nerve, while the red dashed arrow represents the needle trajectory for injection of the mandibular nerve. The empty white circle denotes the pterygopalatine fossa. COP: condylar process; DM: deep masseter; LPM: lateral pterygoid muscle; LPP: lateral pterygoid plate; TM: temporalis muscle; SM: superficial masseter; SA: sphenopalatine artery. All the pictures were obtained from the face of the first author.

can be triggered by irritation of the innervated skin or by activities such as eating, talking, washing the face, or cleaning the teeth. Between paroxysms, the patient is mostly asymptomatic. Imaging studies using magnetic resonance imaging and computed tomography are helpful in identifying causes, such as compression by the vessels adjacent to the nerve, mass lesions, or fractures of the skull bone [17].

*7.3. Sonoanatomy and Ultrasound-Guided Injection Technique.* During this procedure, the participant lies on his or her side with the affected side facing upward. Since the nerve is deeply situated, the use of a curvilinear transducer is preferred. The transducer is placed distal and parallel to the zygomatic arch to bridge the coronoid and condylar processes. The lateral pterygoid muscle can be seen originating from the condylar process and attaching to the lateral pterygoid plate. The power or color Doppler mode can be turned on to identify the sphenoid palatine artery, which is a branch of the maxillary artery, flowing to the pterygoid palatine fossa. The needle is introduced using an out-of-plane approach to target the pterygopalatine fossa (the area anterior to the lateral pterygoid plate) (Figures 8(a)–8(c); Table 1) [18, 19]. For the mandibular nerve block, the needle is introduced in the anterior-to-posterior direction to target the area posterior to the lateral pterygoid plate and between the medial and lateral pterygoid muscles (Figures 8(b) and 8(c)). Electrostimulation can be used to confirm the needle position for the deep block of the mandibular nerve. The technique of electrostimulation requires a 22 G, 10 cm insulated short beveled needle with a guard piece at 6 cm connected to a peripheral nerve simulator. The needle is inserted posterior to the lateral pterygoid plate under ultrasound guidance. The ground electrode should be placed on the anterior border of the ipsilateral masseter. The initial stimulating current should be set at 1.3 mA, with a frequency of 2 Hz. A motor response from the temporalis and masseter muscles results in a jaw jerk, and then, the current should be reduced to a threshold of 0.6 mA [20].

## 8. Conclusion

Using high-resolution ultrasound, pain interventionists can easily target the superficial branches of the trigeminal nerve and its deep branches by recognizing the adjacent muscular and bony structures. Most importantly, since the facial area is hypervascular, power Doppler imaging should be routinely turned on before intervention to avoid collateral injury to surrounding vessels. Accordingly, ultrasound-guided interventions for trigeminal neuralgia provide a safe effective solution for patients who are not responsive to or cannot tolerate oral medications and who are not appropriate candidates for surgery.

## Authors' Contributions

All authors contributed to data analysis and drafting and critically revising the paper, gave final approval to the version to be published, and agreed to be accountable for all aspects of the work.

## Acknowledgments

The current research project was supported by the National Taiwan University Hospital Bei-Hu Branch, the Ministry of Science and Technology (MOST 106-2314-B-002-180-MY3), and the Taiwan Society of Ultrasound in Medicine. The authors appreciate Dr. Manar Allam for drawing the pictures used in the review.

## References

[1] D. Spinner and J. S. Kirschner, "Accuracy of ultrasound-guided superficial trigeminal nerve blocks using methylene blue in cadavers," *Pain Medicine*, vol. 13, no. 11, pp. 1469–1473, 2012.

[2] C. Y. Hung, M. Y. Hsiao, L. Ozcakar et al., "Sonographic tracking of the lower limb peripheral nerves: a pictorial essay and video demonstration," *American Journal of Physical Medicine & Rehabilitation*, vol. 95, no. 9, pp. 698–708, 2016.

[3] U. Krishnan and A. Moule, "Mental nerve paraesthesia: a review of causes and two endodontically related cases," *Saudi Endodontic Journal*, vol. 5, no. 2, pp. 138–145, 2015.

[4] C. Tijssen, K. Schoemaker, and L. Visser, "Supraorbital neuralgia caused by nerve entrapment visualized on ultrasonography," *Headache*, vol. 53, no. 2, pp. 376-377, 2013.

[5] J. Stuginski-Barbosa, R. A. Murayama, P. C. Conti, and J. G. Speciali, "Refractory facial pain attributed to auriculotemporal neuralgia," *Journal of Headache and Pain*, vol. 13, no. 5, pp. 415–417, 2012.

[6] P. A. Lone, R. K. Singh, and U. S. Pal, "Treatment of traumatic infra orbital nerve paresthesia," *National Journal of Maxillofacial Surgery*, vol. 3, no. 2, pp. 218-219, 2012.

[7] D. Jankovic and P. Pesng, *Regional Nerve Blocks in Anesthesia and Pain Therapy*, Springer, Cham, Switzerland, 2015.

[8] E. J. Choi, Y. M. Choi, E. J. Jang, J. Y. Kim, T. K. Kim, and K. H. Kim, "Neural ablation and regeneration in pain practice," *Korean Journal of Pain*, vol. 29, no. 1, pp. 3–11, 2016.

[9] R. C. Webster, J. M. Gaunt, U. S. Hamdan, N. S. Fuleihan, P. R. Giandello, and R. C. Smith, "Supraorbital and supratrochlear notches and foramina: anatomical variations and surgical relevance," *Laryngoscope*, vol. 96, no. 3, pp. 311–315, 1986.

[10] D. N. Liu, J. L. Guo, Q. Luo et al., "Location of supraorbital foramen/notch and infraorbital foramen with reference to soft- and hard-tissue landmarks," *Journal of Craniofacial Surgery*, vol. 22, no. 1, pp. 293–296, 2011.

[11] J. A. Pareja and A. B. Caminero, "Supraorbital neuralgia," *Current Pain and Headache Reports*, vol. 10, no. 4, pp. 302–305, 2006.

[12] O. Y. Cok, S. Deniz, H. E. Eker, L. Oguzkurt, and A. Aribogan, "Management of isolated infraorbital neuralgia by ultrasound-guided infraorbital nerve block with combination of steroid and local anesthetic," *Journal of Clinical Anesthesia*, vol. 37, pp. 146–148, 2017.

[13] G. Greenstein and D. Tarnow, "The mental foramen and nerve: clinical and anatomical factors related to dental implant placement: a literature review," *Journal of Periodontology*, vol. 77, no. 12, pp. 1933–1943, 2006.

[14] J. E. Janis, D. A. Hatef, I. Ducic et al., "Anatomy of the auriculotemporal nerve: variations in its relationship to the superficial temporal artery and implications for the treatment of migraine headaches," *Plastic and Reconstructive Surgery*, vol. 125, no. 5, pp. 1422–1428, 2010.

[15] H. A. Kamel and J. Toland, "Trigeminal nerve anatomy: illustrated using examples of abnormalities," *American Journal of Roentgenology*, vol. 176, no. 1, pp. 247–251, 2001.

[16] M. Piagkou, T. Demesticha, P. Skandalakis, and E. O. Johnson, "Functional anatomy of the mandibular nerve: consequences of nerve injury and entrapment," *Clinical Anatomy*, vol. 24, no. 2, pp. 143–150, 2011.

[17] J. M. Zakrzewska, "Facial pain: neurological and non-neurological," *Journal of Neurology, Neurosurgery, and Psychiatry*, vol. 72, no. 2, pp. ii27–ii32, 2002.

[18] K. V. Chang, C. S. Lin, C. P. Lin, W. T. Wu, and L. Ozcakar, "Recognition of the lateral pterygoid muscle and plate during ultrasound-guided trigeminal nerve block," *Journal of Clinical and Diagnostic Research*, vol. 11, no. 5, pp. UL01–UL02, 2017.

[19] Y. J. Chen, P. H. Chang, K. V. Chang, W. T. Wu, and L. Özçakar, "Ultrasound guided injection for medial and lateral pterygoid muscles: a novel treatment for orofacial pain," *Medical Ultrasonography*, vol. 1, no. 1, pp. 115-116, 2018.

[20] N. Kumar, S. Shashni, R. Singh, and A. Jain, "Mandibular nerve block for peri-operative pain relief using a peripheral nerve stimulator," *Anaesthesia*, vol. 67, no. 1, pp. 77-78, 2012.

# 23

# Subjective Experiences and Sensitivities in Women with Fibromyalgia: A Quantitative and Comparative Study

P. De Roa,[1] P. Paris,[2] J. L. Poindessous,[3] O. Maillet,[4] and A. Héron ⓘ[4,5]

[1]*Pain Unit, Dreux Hospital, GHT28, France*
[2]*Department of Mental Health, Dreux Hospital, GHT28, France*
[3]*Center of Treatment and Pain Evaluation, Ambroise Paré Hospital, Paris, France*
[4]*Clinical Research Unit URC28, Dreux Hospital, GHT28, France*
[5]*Department of Human Physiology, Paris Descartes University, Paris, France*

Correspondence should be addressed to A. Héron; anne.heron@parisdescartes.fr

Academic Editor: Jacob Ablin

Fibromyalgia is a chronic widespread pain syndrome associated with chronic fatigue. Its pathogenesis is not clearly understood. This study presents subjective experiences and sensitivities reported by fibromyalgia patients, which should be considered in primary care to avoid medical nomadism, as well as stigmatization of the patients. The prevalence of significant characteristics was compared with others patients consulting at the same pain unit who suffer from rebel and disabling form of chronic migraine. Psychometric tests were anonymously completed by 78 patients of the Pain Unit (44 fibromyalgia patients and 34 migraine patients). Tests evaluated pain (Visual Analog scale), childhood traumas (Childhood Trauma Questionnaire), lack of parental affection, stressful life events (Holmes and Rahe Scale), anxiety and depression (Hospital Anxiety and Depression Scale), perceived hypersensitivity to 10 stimuli, and hyperactivity before illness. However, pain scores were comparable in the two groups, and the prevalence was significantly higher in fibromyalgia patients than in migraine patients for anxiety (81.8% versus 51.5%) and depression (57.1% versus 8.8%). Childhood physical abuses were more frequently reported in fibromyalgia than in migraine cases (25% versus 3%). Similarly, the feeling of lack of parental affection, subjective hypersensitivity to stress and stimuli (cold, moisture, heat, full moon, and flavors) or hyperactivity (ergomania), appeared as prominent features of fibromyalgia patients. Fibromyalgia patients considered themselves as being hypersensitive (mentally and physically) compared to migraine patients. They also have higher depression levels. Beyond somatic symptoms, precociously taking account of psychosocial and behavioral strategies would highly improve treatment efficiency of the fibromyalgia syndrome.

## 1. Introduction

Fibromyalgia is a chronic widespread pain syndrome associated with chronic fatigue. It affects 2–4% of the adult population, with a higher incidence in women [1, 2]. Considering the musculoskeletal pain symptoms, the World Health Organization quoted fibromyalgia as a rheumatologic disease (M79.7). If the reality of fibromyalgia syndrome is recognized, at least in its severe form, its causes and pathophysiology remain poorly understood and controversial. In 1990, the American College of Rheumatology specified diagnostic criteria of fibromyalgia [3]. In 2010, new criteria appeared taking into account nonrestorative sleep, cognitive impairment, and variable somatic symptoms associated with chronic pain [4].

Recent studies reported that interaction between genetic predispositions [5, 6], biochemical factors, psychological profiles [7], and triggering events which sensitize the central nervous system [8–10], could contribute to the etiology of the fibromyalgia syndrome.

During the clinical examination of painful patients at the Chronic Pain Unit, we used a semistructured interview. The consultation usually lasted 90 minutes and focused on the life history. The attentive listening of fibromyalgia patients revealed life adversity, especially during childhood. Patients usually reported lack of affection, indifference, neglect, or abuse from their family, in accordance with a recent meta-analysis which suggested that childhood traumas could be associated with fibromyalgia syndrome [11, 12]. In addition, patients often mentioned other life's traumas: bereavements, abandon, rapes, severe illness, or accidents. They also reported high sensitivity to stimuli and professional harassment.

The present cross-sectional study aimed to characterize childhood experiences, perceived lack of parental affection, hypersensitivity to stimuli, life stressors, anxio-depression, and ergomania mentioned by French fibromyalgia patients. The prevalence of these parameters was quantified using self-report questionnaires and was compared to that assessed in migraine patients treated in the same Pain Unit (as a control group). Indeed, fibromyalgia and migraine both preferentially affected women and resulted in a comparable pain score on the Visual Analogic Scale. They both represented chronic, rebels, and disabling forms of the pathologies, justifying the orientation of the patients to the Pain Unit [4, 13, 14].

## 2. Methods

*2.1. Study Population.* Subjects included in the study were adult women who consulted for fibromyalgia or migraine at the Pain Unit of Dreux Hospital. These patients were generally addressed by a neurologist or a rheumatologist, most often at the tertiary level after medical nomadism. Migraine patients were sent to the Pain Unit because of their resistance to treatments and daily chronic headaches.

In the case of fibromyalgia, the diagnosis was confirmed in the Pain Unit using the criteria of the American College of Rheumatology from 1990 to 2010 in case of fibromyalgia [3, 4]. The pain was chronic, that is, present for more than 3 months and resistant to usual drugs. It was associated with abnormal tenderness, fatigue, stiffness, sleep disturbance, depression, anxiety, and cognitive impairment. The presence of widespread chronic pain was reported on at least 7 of 19 possible tender points of the body and associated with 4 groups of symptoms whose patient quoted the discomfort from 0 to 3 (sum $\geq 6/12$): chronic fatigue (more than 3 months), sleep disorders, cognitive disorders, and functional disorders. Additional examinations were normal.

In the case of migraine, the diagnosis had used the criteria of the International Headache Society [13] in case of migraine diagnosis mentioned at least 5 headache attacks lasting 4–72 hours (untreated or unsuccessfully treated). Headache had at least two of the following characteristics: unilateral location, pulsating quality, moderate or severe pain intensity, and aggravation by or causing avoidance of routine physical activity (e.g., walking or climbing stairs), and during headache at least one of the following had occurred: nausea and/or vomiting, photophobia, and phonophobia, not attributed to another disorder. Additional clinical examinations were normal out of crises.

Patients with serious organic pathology evidenced by biological or imagery analysis (inflammatory arthritis and thyroid pathologies), sleep apnea, psychosis, or delirium, were excluded from the study. Fibromyalgia patients with migraine were also excluded from the study to avoid intergroup interferences that may reduce the visibility of the effects.

*2.2. Evaluation Tools.* A set of 6 self-report questionnaires were sent by post to the patients. Questionnaires should be returned anonymously completed, within two months. The set of questionnaires contained the following:

(i) The Visual Analogue Scale (VAS) to assess subjective perception of global pain on a 10 cm line (0, *no pain*, to 10, *pain as bad it could be*) [15].

(ii) The Childhood Trauma Questionnaire (CTQ) (French version), a 70-item self-administered inventory providing reliable and valid retrospective assessment of child abuse and neglect [16, 17]. Items asked about experiences in childhood and adolescence and were rated on a 5 point Likert-type scale with response options ranging from *Never True* to *Very Often True*. The CTQ had five clinical scales measuring physical and psychological maltreatments: physical, sexual, and emotional abuse, and physical and emotional neglect.

(iii) The Hospital Anxiety and Depression Scale (HADS), determining a score of anxiety and a score of depression [18]. These two scores varied from 0 to 21.

(iv) The Holmes and Rahe stress scale, measuring the level of stress associated with 43 life events that could contribute to illness if occurring in the past 2 years [19]. Events were scored from 11 to 100. If global score >150, the stress level is high or very high (if $150 <$ total score $\leq 300$) with a risk of illness. When total score $\leq 150$, the stress was considered as moderate with a slight risk of illness.

(v) One questionnaire concerned the sensitivity of the patient to ten different stimuli (light, noise, cold, warm, humidity, flavors, odors, full moon, allergies, and drugs). It allowed evaluation of the subjective sensitivity perceived by the patients. The question was, *"Would you say that you are very sensitive to the following stimuli?"* Possible answers for each stimulus were *"yes"* or *"no."*

(vi) Three further questions were added two regarding the lack of affection perceived during childhood (*"I have missed affection from my mother/father"*) and another one evaluating the subjective activity level before illness (*"Before my illness, I was a very active person"*). The possible answers were *"Never true,"* *"Rarely true,"* *"Sometimes true,"* *"Often true,"* and *"Very often true,"* respectively, quoted from 1 to 5.

After reception of the filled questionnaires, data analysis was realized on Excel by the Clinical Research Unit. The results were expressed in average $\pm$ standard deviation for scores or in percentage for frequencies. The statistic tests comparing fibromyalgia to migraine patients were realized with Student's $t$-test or the test of $\chi_2$ of Pearson. A value of $p < 0.05$ was considered as statistically significant.

## 3. Results

The analysis focused on 78 questionnaires returned by the patients to the Clinical Research Unit (44 from fibromyalgia

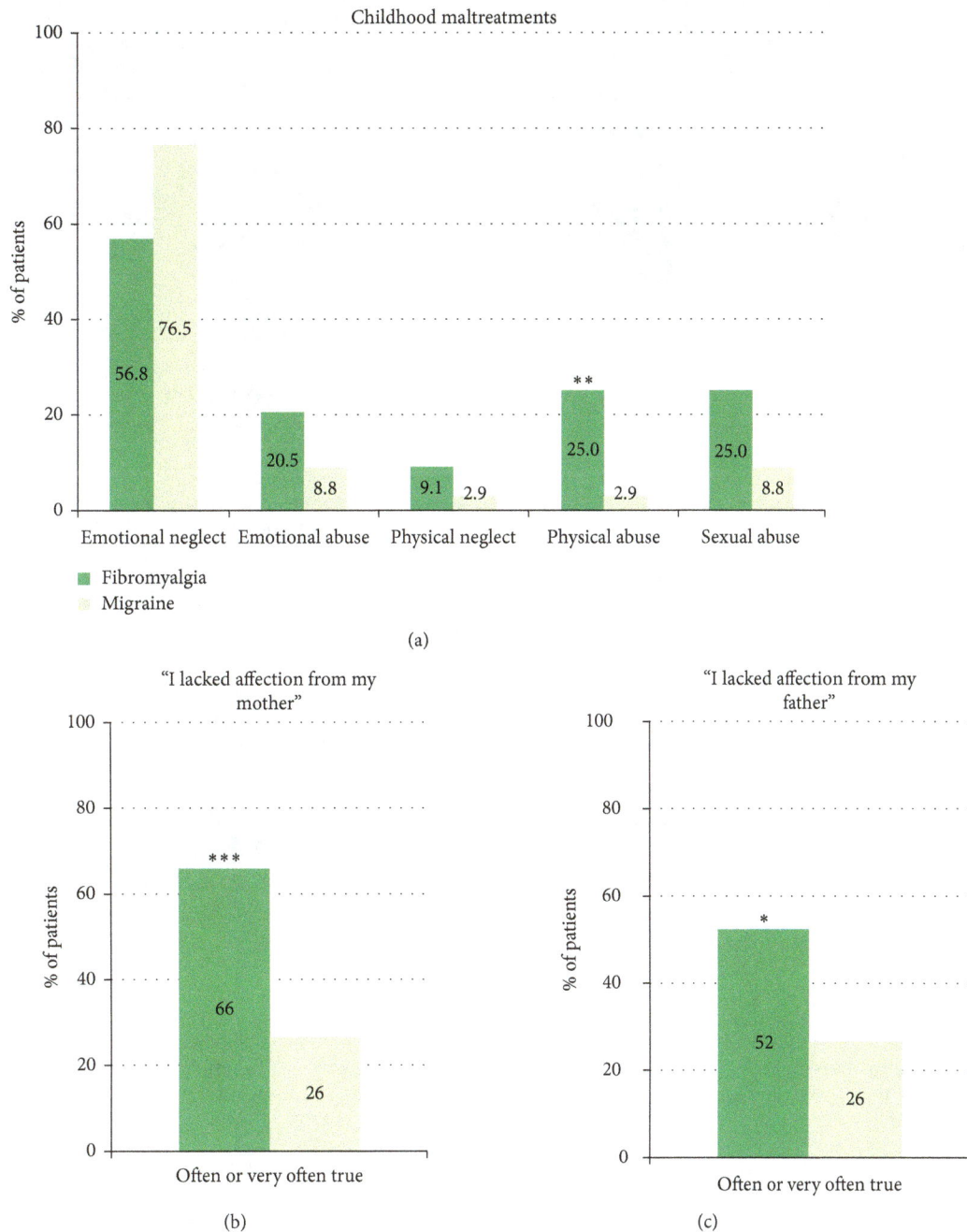

FIGURE 1: Childhood trauma evaluation. (a) Results of the Childhood Trauma Questionnaire (CTQ) assessing maltreatments of children from their familial environment: percentage of adult fibromyalgia and migraine patients who reported childhood abuses and neglects. (b, c) Percentage of patients who declared having often or very often suffered from maternal (b) or paternal (c) affective deprivation during childhood. Statistical significances between the two groups: $^{*}p < 0.05$, $^{**}p < 0.01$, and $^{***}p < 0.001$.

patients F and 34 from migraine patients M). Main characteristics of the two groups of women were comparable with mean age of $45 \pm 12$ years and mean pathology duration of $12 \pm 10$ years.

The Visual Analogic Scores (VASs) evaluating pain during the best moments, the worst moments, and at present (i.e., when patients completed the questionnaire). In the fibromyalgia group, mean VAS varied from $3.3 \pm 1.9$ during the best moments to $8.9 \pm 1.4$ during the worst moments. Scores were comparable and not statistically significant in the migraine group (resp. $1.8 \pm 2.3$ and $8.7 \pm 1.2$, data not shown).

Concerning maltreatments retrospectively evaluated by the Childhood Trauma Questionnaire (CTQ), emotional neglect was the most frequently maltreatment reported by fibromyalgia patients (56.8%), followed by physical and sexual abuses (25% of patients), emotional abuse (20.5%), and physical neglect (9.1%) (Figure 1(a)). History of physical abuse was more frequently reported in the fibromyalgia group (25%) than in the migraine group (2.9%) ($p < 0.01$). Physical abuse was defined as bodily assaults on a child by an older person that could lead to or had resulted in injuries.

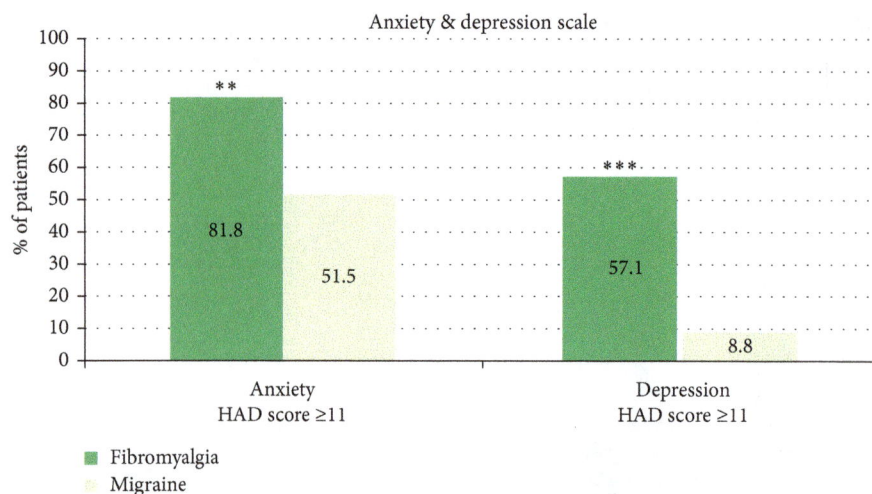

FIGURE 2: Results of the Hospital Anxiety and Depression (HAD) scale (scores varied from 0 to 21 and score ≥11 was considered as pathological). Percentage of fibromyalgia and migraine patients with pathological anxiety and/or depression. Statistical significances between the two groups: ** $p < 0.01$ and *** $p < 0.001$.

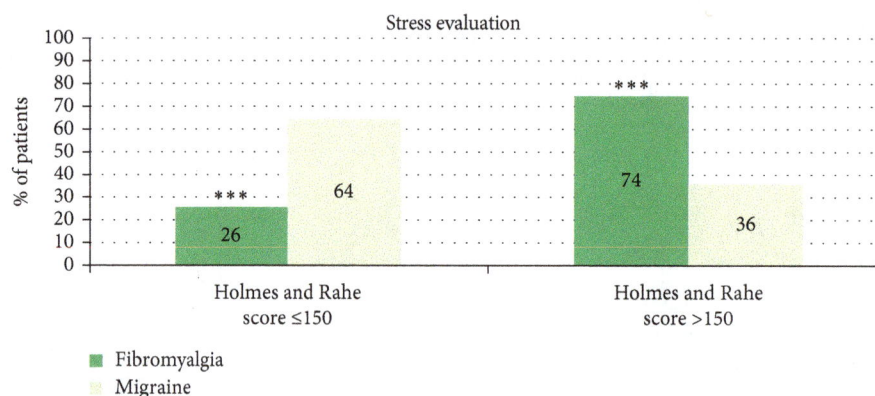

FIGURE 3: Results of the Holmes and Rahe stress scale measuring the level of stress associated with life events occurred in the past 2 years. Events were scored from 11 to 100. If global score>150, the stress level is high or very high and could contribute to the illness. When total score ≤150, the stress was considered as moderate to low. Results show the percentage of fibromyalgia and migraine patients with low (on the left) or high (on the right) score of stress. Statistical significances between the two groups *** $p < 0.001$.

The percentage of patients reporting other maltreatments, emotional maltreatments (humiliation, deamination, and failure of caretakers to provide emotional and psychological needs), physical neglects, or sexual abuses, did not statistically differ between the two groups. However, 52–66% of fibromyalgia patients reported lacks of parental affection versus 26% of migraine patients ($p < 0.001$ for lacks of maternal affection and $p < 0.05$ for lacks of paternal affection) (Figures 1(b) and 1(c)).

Prevalence of anxiety and depression was higher in fibromyalgia than in migraine (81.8% versus 51.5%, $p < 0.01$ and 57.1% versus 8.8%, $p < 0.001$, resp.) (Figure 2).

Stress evaluation by the Holmes and Rahe test showed that 74% of fibromyalgia patients (versus 36% for migraine patients, $p < 0.001$) reported major life stressors (score >150) to have occurred during the 2 years preceding the test (Figure 3).

In addition to stress sensitivity, fibromyalgia patients reported being particularly sensitive to external stimuli, with a significant difference for 5 of them in comparison with migraine patients cold, moisture, heat, full moon, and flavors

(Figure 4). The difference was not statistically significant for noise, light, odors, and drugs sensitivity.

Considering professional activity, 89% of fibromyalgia patients (versus 67% of migraine patients, $p < 0.05$) considered to have been very active people before illness (Figure 5).

## 4. Discussion

This quantitative and comparative study showed that despite a comparable level of pain score and invalidating impact of the disease in the two groups (fibromyalgia and migraine), the prevalence of abuses and deprivations (during infancy) reported by fibromyalgia women, as well as their current subjective sensitivity to stress and stimuli, was higher than in the migraine group. In addition, the fibromyalgia patients considered themselves to have been hyperactive women before their illness. Anxiety and depression were also significantly more frequent than in migraine patients.

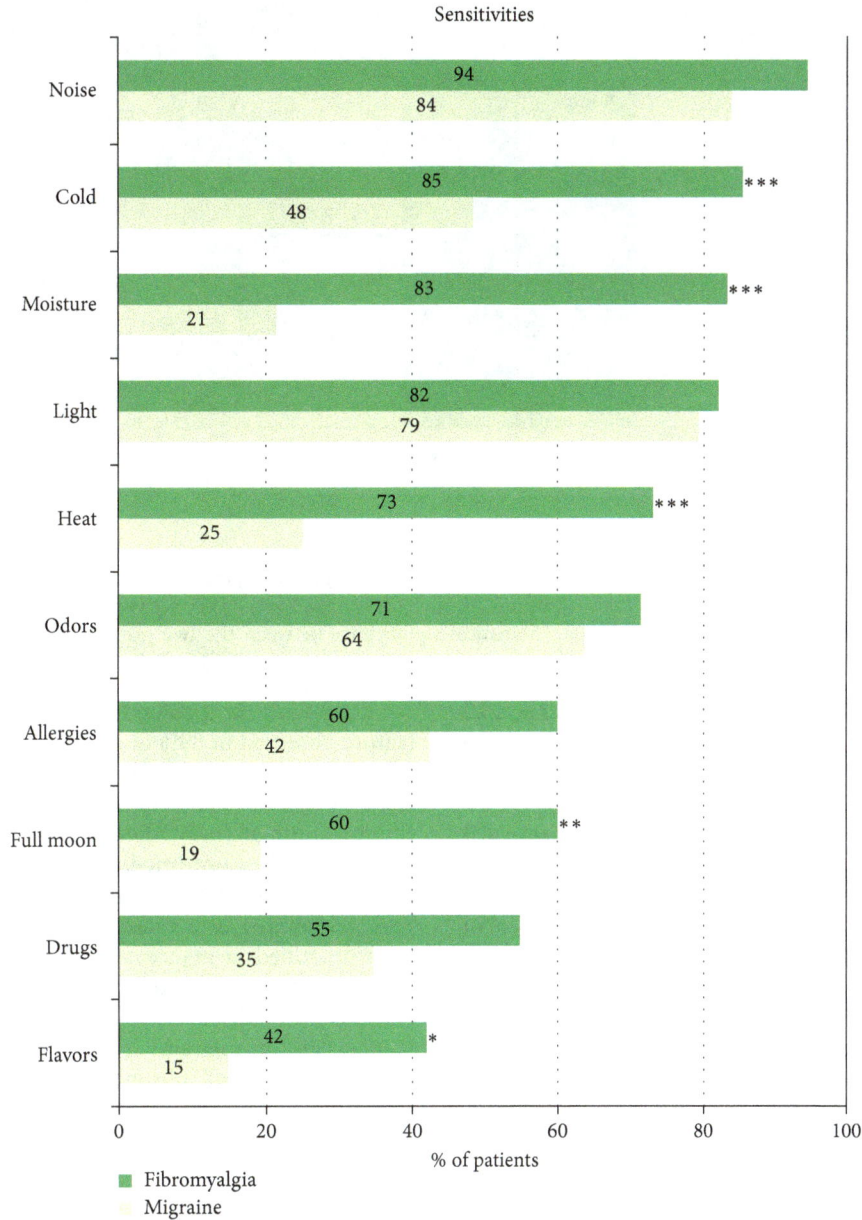

FIGURE 4: Evaluation of the subjective hypersensitivity perceived by the patients. Questionnaire concerned sensitivity to 10 different stimuli. Results show percentage of fibromyalgia and migraine patients who answered "yes" to the question, "would you say that you are very sensitive to the following stimuli?" Statistical significances between the two groups $^*p < 0.05$, $^{**}p < 0.01$, and $^{***}p < 0.001$.

In our study, physical abuses in childhood were retrospectively reported by 25% of adult fibromyalgia women. This prevalence was significantly higher than that measured in the migraine group or for the general female population [17]. Even if the causes of fibromyalgia are currently unknown, several studies suggested that physical traumas occurring during childhood could contribute to the physiopathology of this syndrome [7, 20, 21]. This etiology would differ from that of migraine: while the genetic and neurovascular origin of migraine is frequently reported [22], the fibromyalgia syndrome rather would be associated with psychic and environmental events occurring along a traumatic life history. The psycho-affective impact of traumatic experiences would contribute to their illness.

Moreover, the fibromyalgia patients declared more affective deficiencies than did migraine women. A lack of attention or of parental presence was more frequent and could have durably affected these patients [23, 24]. Some recent studies showed that a premature birth, a maternal deprivation or a kind of insecure affection could be associated with chronic pain and foster the pain sensitivity (for review, cf. [21]). This was confirmed by the high "emotional neglect" score measured by CTQ in fibromyalgia patients. This score was also very high in migraine patients, and the difference between the two groups was not significant. This may seem inconsistent with the precedent differences mentioned for affective deprivation. However, this apparent inconsistency could be explained by the fact that whereas the

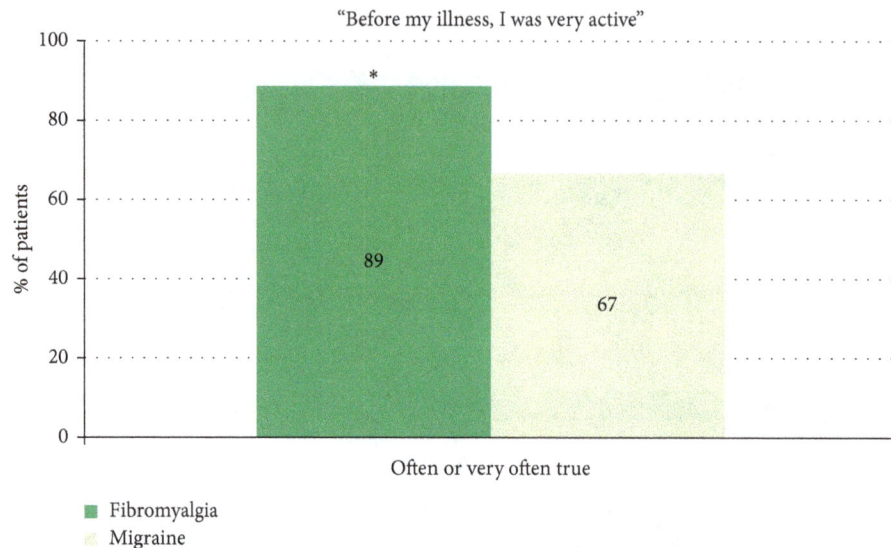

FIGURE 5: Evaluation of the subjective hyperactivity reported by the patients. Results show percentage of fibromyalgia and migraine patients who answered "Often true" or "Very often true" to the question, "Before my illness, I was a very active person". The other possible answers were "Never true," "Rarely true," and "Sometimes true." Statistical significance between the two groups: $*p < 0.05$.

CTQ referred to the relationships between the child and all the members of the family, concerning lack of affection, the child stated directly father and mother affection, so referred to the primordial attachment [23].

In addition to our observations, a recent study revealed that other childhood adversities could be associated with fibromyalgia: financial difficulties, conflicts in the family, parental divorce, chronic illnesses in the family, or alcohol problems [25]. These types of adversities could be at the origin of parental difficulties predisposing to a familial climate with lack of affection, emotional deprivation, or physical abuse of the patients during childhood.

The sensitivity to stimuli reported by patients and the results of the Holmes and Rahe test showed a multimodal hypersensitivity (cold, moisture, heat, full moon, and flavors), as well as increased sensitivity to stress, in fibromyalgia patients compared to those with migraine. Hypersensitivity in fibromyalgia has recently been shown to be correlated with neurophysiological events and depression [26].

Early traumatic events and affective deprivations during childhood could have disturbed the development of neurotransmitter systems, the pain processing, and the hypothalamic pituitary adrenal axis involved in stress management [7, 27, 28]. In fibromyalgia patients, early physical abuse could then have increased responsiveness of the central nervous system to a variety of stimuli. This central sensitization would occur because of decreased functional connectivity in the descending pain-modulating system [8] and augmented responses in sensory integration [26]. Moreover, modification of diurnal cortisol level associated with childhood maltreatment has been described in fibromyalgia and could contribute to great emotional distress and high catastrophism observed in these patients [29, 30]. Increased sympathetic activity has been suggested in fibromyalgia [31] and could explain the high sensitivity to stress.

Ergomania or professional hyperactivity was another feature observed in 89% of cases of fibromyalgia patients, as already described [32, 33]. Although in our study the declarative questionnaire could have been tainted by idealization, another study showed that the entourage of the patients usually confirmed this singularity [33]. Ergomania could be the expression of a low self-esteem associated with parental failures, or a strategy to escape depression as it has been described in maltreated children [32, 34].

Moreover, it should be noted that, in our study, depression was still observed in 57% of fibromyalgia patients (versus 9% of migraine patients, $p < 0.001$). The higher depressive rate of fibromyalgia patients could explain multimodal hypersensitivity [26] as well as their painful memory, catastrophism, and sleep alteration characteristic of the syndrome [35–37].

Finally, the nonrestorative awake sleep, associated with depression, anxiety, and multimodal hypersensitivity, could induce a permanent state of hypervigilance in fibromyalgia patients. Initially, this state would have been induced by insecure environment of fibromyalgia patients during childhood [21, 38]. All senses were maintained in alarm. Patients would then become more sensitive to stressful events (separation, layoff, financial problems, accident, disease, bereavement, etc.), with exacerbated physic or psychic stress related to daily life events [21, 30]. All these parameters associated with defensive hyperactivity and sleep deprivation would constitute a fertile field for the development of fibromyalgia. With time, sleep deprivation, natural decline of performances, and resistance with age would amplify symptoms. Hypervigilance and hyperactivity would result in overactivity, depression, and chronic fatigue, which ultimately lead to state of breakdown and exhaustion or "burn out" (professional, parental, conjugal, domestic, and social). The occurrence of musculoskeletal diseases such as osteoarthritis, hypothyroidism, inflammatory rheumatism, or other painful diseases would switch the patient from ergomania to invalidity. This would generate misunderstanding from relatives and medical team. Only personal positive adaptive and coping strategies could delay the switchover [39]. Patients with chronic migraine are frequently affected by diffuse pain, framed in fibromyalgia diagnosis. This comorbidity could be supported by common pathophysiological mechanisms [40].

This study has several strengths including the relatively large sample with clear diagnoses and the use of validated psychometric tests in order to objectivize psycho-affective parameters. However, it also includes some limitations. Bias is possible because it is a retrospective study based on self-reports. Patient memories may not be accurate and not objective. Moreover, the recruitment from the same unit and, a fortiori, from the same region and country, may limit generalizability of the findings. Results need to be confirmed by a multicenter international study. Further studies might also examine the role of emotional neglect in migraine patients.

Nevertheless, the results corroborate and objectivize our clinical experience and conform with the existing literature. The study invites to more attention to psycho-affective aspects in the treatment of fibromyalgia patients.

# 5. Conclusion

Our results confirm that life history and sensitivities of fibromyalgia patients should be more systematically taken into consideration in clinical practice. Fibromyalgia patients considered themselves as being more sensitive mentally and physically compared to migraine patients. They also have higher depression levels. Treatment of fibromyalgia syndrome taking account of psycho-affective impact of life experiences, stress management, behavioral, and coping strategies, should limit further examinations, medical nomadism, and stigmatization of fibromyalgia patients.

# Acknowledgments

The authors thank Professor Yves Gruel (CHU Tours, France) and Dr. Zelda Sense for the proofreading of the manuscript.

# References

[1] F. Wolfe, K. Ross, J. Anderson, I. Jon Russell, and L. Hebert, "The prevalence and characteristics of fibromyalgia in the general population," *Arthritis & Rheumatism*, vol. 38, no. 1, pp. 19–28, 1995.

[2] D. J. Clauw, "Fibromyalgia: a clinical review," *Journal of the American Medical Association-Journals*, vol. 311, no. 15, pp. 1547–1555, 2014.

[3] F. Wolfe, H. A. Smythe, M. B. Yunus et al., "The American College of Rheumatology criteria for the classification of fibromyalgia. Report of the multicenter criteria committee," *Arthritis & Rheumatism*, vol. 33, no. 2, pp. 160–172, 1990.

[4] F. Wolfe, D. J. Clauw, M. A. Fitzcharles et al., "The American College of Rhumatology: preliminary diagnostic criteria for fibromyalgia and measurement of symptom severity," *Arthritis Care & Research*, vol. 62, no. 5, pp. 600–610, 2010.

[5] Y. H. Lee, S. J. Choi, J. D. Ji, and G. G. Song, "Candidate gene studies of fibromyalgia: a systematic review and meta-analysis," *Rheumatology International*, vol. 32, no. 2, pp. 417–426, 2012.

[6] J. N. Ablin and D. Buskila, "Update on the genetics of the fibromyalgia syndrome," *Best Practice & Research Clinical Rheumatology*, vol. 29, no. 1, pp. 20–28, 2015.

[7] B. L. Loevinger, E. A. Shirtcliff, D. Muller et al., "Delineating psychological and biomedical profiles in a heterogeneous fibromyalgia population using cluster analysis," *Clinical Rheumatology*, vol. 31, no. 4, pp. 677–685, 2012.

[8] B. Cagnie, I. Coppieters, S. Denecker, J. Six, L. Danneels, and M. Meeus, "Central sensitization in fibromyalgia? A systematic review on structural and functional brain MRI," *Seminars in Arthritis and Rheumatism*, vol. 44, no. 1, pp. 68–75, 2014.

[9] T. Schmidt-Wilcke, E. Ichesco, J. P. Hampson et al., "Resting state connectivity correlates with drug and placebo response in fibromyalgia patients," *NeuroImage: Clinical*, vol. 6, pp. 252–261, 2014.

[10] J. Ablin, L. Neumann, and D. Buskila, "Pathogenesis of fibromyalgia-a review," *Joint Bone Spine*, vol. 75, no. 3, pp. 273–279, 2008.

[11] W. Häuser, M. Kosseva, N. Uceyler et al., "Emotional, physical and sexual abuse in fibromyalgia syndrome: a systematic review with meta-analysis," *Arthritis Care & Research*, vol. 63, no. 6, pp. 808–820, 2011.

[12] R. Hellou, W. Häuser, I. Brenner et al., "Self-reported childhood maltreatment and traumatic events among Israeli patients suffering from fibromyalgia and rheumatoid arthritis," *Pain Research and Management*, vol. 2017, Article ID 3865249, 8 pages, 2017.

[13] Headache Classification Committee, "The international classification of headache disorders, cranial neuralgia and facial pain," *Cephalalgia*, vol. 24, no. 1, pp. 1–160, 2004.

[14] Headache Classification Committee of the International Headache Society (IHS), "The international classification of headache disorders, 3rd edition (beta version)," *Cephalalgia*, vol. 33, no. 9, pp. 629–808, 2013.

[15] E. C. Huskisson, "Visual analogue scale," in *Pain Measurement and Assessment*, R. Melzack, Ed., pp. 33–37, Raven Press, New York, NY, USA, 1983.

[16] D. P. Bernstein, L. Fink, L. Handelsman et al., "Initial reliability and validity of a new retrospective measure of child abuse and neglect," *American Journal of Psychiatry*, vol. 151, no. 8, pp. 1132–1136, 1994.

[17] D. Paquette, L. Laporte, M. Bigras, and M. Zoccolillo, "Validation de la version française du CTQ et prévalence de l'histoire de maltraitance," *Santé mentale au Québec*, vol. 29, no. 1, pp. 201–220, 2004.

[18] A. S. Zigmond and R. P. Snaith, "The hospital anxiety and depression scale," *Acta Psychiatrica Scandinavica*, vol. 67, no. 6, pp. 361–370, 1983.

[19] T. H. Holmes and R. H. Rahe, "The social readjustment rating scale," *Journal of Psychosomatic Research*, vol. 11, no. 2, pp. 213–218, 1967.

[20] M. G. Haviland, K. R. Morton, K. Oda, and G. E. Fraser, "Traumatic experiences, major life stressors, and self-reporting a physician-given fibromyalgia diagnosis," *Psychiatry Research*, vol. 177, no. 3, pp. 335–341, 2010.

[21] L. Low and P. Schweinhardt, "Early life adversity as a risk factor for fibromyalgia in later life," *Pain Research and Treatment*, vol. 2012, Article ID 140832, 15 pages, 2012.

[22] V. Anttila, H. Stefansson, M. Kallela et al., "Genome-wide association study of migraine implicates a common susceptibility variant on 8q22.1," *Nature Genetics*, vol. 42, no. 10, pp. 869–873, 2010.

[23] J. Bowlby, "Attachment theory and its therapeutic implications," *Adolescent Psychiatry*, vol. 6, pp. 5–33, 1978.

[24] A. Main, K. Kaplan, and J. Cassidy, "Security in infancy, childhood, and adulthood: a move to the level of representation," in *Growing Points in Attachment Theory and Research. Monographs of the Society for Research in Child Development*, I. Bretherton and E. Waters, Eds., vol. 50, pp. 66–106, 1985.

[25] A. Varinen, E. Kosunen, K. Mattila, T. Koskela, and M. Sumanen, "The relationship between childhood adversities and fibromyalgia in the general population," *Journal of Psychosomatic Research*, vol. 99, pp. 137–142, 2017.

[26] M. López-Solà, C. W. Woo, J. Pujol et al., "Towards a neurophysiological signature for fibromyalgia," *Pain*, vol. 158, no. 1, pp. 34–47, 2017.

[27] C. J. Vierck, "Mechanisms underlying development of spatially distributed chronic pain (fibromyalgia)," *Pain*, vol. 124, no. 3, pp. 242–263, 2006.

[28] J. Desmeules, J. Chabert, M. Rebsamen et al., "Central pain sensitization, COMT Val158Met polymorphism, and emotional factors in fibromyalgia," *Journal of Pain*, vol. 15, no. 2, pp. 129–135, 2014.

[29] N. A. Nicolson, M. C. Davis, D. Kruszewski et al., "Childhood maltreatment and diurnal cortisol patterns in women with chronic pain," *Psychosomatic Medicine*, vol. 72, no. 5, pp. 471–480, 2010.

[30] R. R. Edwards, C. Cahalan, G. Mensing, M. Smith, and J. A. Haythornthwaite, "Pain, catastrophizing, and depression in the rheumatic diseases," *Nature Reviews Rheumatology*, vol. 7, no. 4, pp. 216–224, 2011.

[31] R. D. Chervin, M. Teodorescu, R. Kushwaha et al., "Objective measures of disordered sleep in fibromyalgia," *Journal of Rheumatology*, vol. 36, no. 9, pp. 2009–2016, 2009.

[32] B. Van Houdenhove and E. Neerinckx, "Is "ergomania" a predisposing factor to chronic pain and fatigue?," *Psychosomatics*, vol. 40, no. 6, pp. 529–530, 1999.

[33] B. Van Houdenhove, E. Neerinckx, P. Onghena, R. Lysens, and H. Vertommen, "Premorbid "overactive" lifestyle in chronic fatigue syndrome and fibromyalgia. An etiological factor or proof of good citizenship?," *Journal of Psychosomatic Research*, vol. 51, no. 4, pp. 571–576, 2001.

[34] B. Cyrulnik, "Ethology and the biological correlates of mood," *Dialogues in Clinical Neuroscience*, vol. 7, no. 3, pp. 217–221, 2005.

[35] J. L. Poindessous and A. Héron, "A study of sleeping problems in patients with fibromyalgia," *La Lettre de Médecine Physique et de Réadaptation*, vol. 28, no. 2, pp. 110–115, 2012.

[36] C. Diaz-Piedra, L. L. Di Stasi, C. M. Baldwin et al., "Sleep disturbances of adult women suffering from fibromyalgia: a systematic review of observational studies," *Sleep Medicine Reviews*, vol. 21, pp. 86–99, 2015.

[37] I. Yalcin and M. Barrot, "The anxiodepressive comorbidity in chronic pain," *Current Opinion in Anaesthesiology*, vol. 27, no. 5, pp. 520–527, 2014.

[38] C. Cedraschi, E. Girard, C. Luthy, M. Kossovsky, J. Desmeules, and A.-F. Allaz, "Primary attributions in women suffering fibromyalgia emphasize the perception of a disruptive onset for a long-lasting pain problem," *Journal of Psychosomatic Research*, vol. 74, no. 3, pp. 265–269, 2013.

[39] M. De Tommaso, A. Federici, A. Loiacono, M. Delussi, and O. Todarello, "Personality profiles and coping styles in migraine patients with fibromyalgia comorbidity," *Comprehensive Psychiatry*, vol. 55, no. 1, pp. 80–86, 2014.

[40] M. De Tommaso and V. Sciruicchio, "Migraine and central sensitization: clinical features, main comorbidities and therapeutic perspectives," *Current Rheumatology Reviews*, vol. 12, no. 2, pp. 113–126, 2016.

# 24

# Efficacy and Safety of Botulinum Toxin Type A in Treating Patients of Advanced Age with Idiopathic Trigeminal Neuralgia

**Jing Liu** [ID],[1,2] **Ying-Ying Xu,**[1,2] **Qi-Lin Zhang,**[1,2] **and Wei-Feng Luo** [ID][1,2]

[1]*Department of Neurology and Suzhou Clinical Research Center of Neurological Disease,*
*The Second Affiliated Hospital of Soochow University, Suzhou 215004, China*
[2]*Jiangsu Key Laboratory of Translational Research and Therapy for Neuro-Psychiatric-Diseases,*
*Soochow University, Suzhou, Jiangsu 215123, China*

Correspondence should be addressed to Wei-Feng Luo; lwfwxx@126.com

Academic Editor: Alberto Baldini

*Objective.* To assess the therapeutic efficacy and safety of botulinum toxin type A (BTX-A) for treating idiopathic trigeminal neuralgia (ITN) in patients ≥80 years old. *Methods.* Selected patients ($n = 43$) with ITN, recruited from the neurology clinic and inpatient department of the Second Affiliated Hospital of Soochow University between August 2008 and February 2014, were grouped by age, one subset ($n = 14$) ≥80 years old and another ($n = 29$) <60 years old. Each group scored similarly in degrees of pain registered by the visual analogue scale (VAS). Dosing, efficacy, and safety of BTX-A injections were compared by group. *Results.* Mean dosages of BTX-A were $91.3 \pm 25.6$ U and $71.8 \pm 33.1$ U in older and younger patients, respectively ($t = 1.930$, $p = 0.061$). The median of the VAS score in older patients at baseline (8.5) declined significantly at 1 month after treatment (4.5) ($p = 0.007$), as did that of younger patients (8.0 and 5.0, resp.) ($p = 0.001$). The median of the D values of the VAS scores did not differ significantly by group (older, 2.5; younger, 0; $Z = -1.073$, $p = 0.283$). Two patients in each group developed minor transient side effects ($p = 0.825$). Adverse reactions in both groups were mild, resolving spontaneously within 3 weeks. *Conclusions.* BTX-A is effective and safe in treating patients of advanced age (≥80 years old) with ITN, at dosages comparable to those used in much younger counterparts (<60 years old).

## 1. Introduction

Trigeminal neuralgia (TN) is characterized by paroxysms of intense, stabbing pain in the distribution of mandibular and maxillary divisions (rarely, the ophthalmic division) of the fifth cranial nerve. TN is one of the most common neurological pains involving the orofacial region, which generally has the most intensive type of pain [1]. According to epidemiologic studies, approximately 4–28.9/100,000 persons worldwide have experienced TN. It typically affects the elderly (1 in 25,000 of the population), with the most frequently reported cause being neurovascular compression [2, 3]. The morbidity of idiopathic trigeminal neuralgia increases with age, patients ≥80 years old account for a large proportion of TN sufferers [4]. Usually, TN patients are first treated with pharmacological agents [5]. The pain can be readily managed with medication in approximately 80% of patients. The first-line treatment is carbamazepine, which can relieve most of the observed symptoms. Other drugs, including oxcarbazepine, phenytoin, baclofen, lamotrigine, gabapentin, and sodium valproate, are also efficient in reducing the signs-symptoms of TN in most patients. Many drugs used in the treatment of TN are associated with several side effects, such as dizziness, lethargy, lack of fatigue, nausea, vomiting, occasional granulocyte reduction, reversible thrombocytopenia, and even induced aplastic anemia and toxic hepatitis. Considering insufficient effect or unacceptable side effects of pharmacological treatment, surgical treatment becomes an option. Several surgical approaches used to relieve the pain due to TN include neurectomy of the trigeminal nerve branches outside the skull, percutaneous radiofrequency thermal rhizotomy, percutaneous ablation that creates the trigeminal nerve or trigeminal ganglion lesions with heat, percutaneous retrogasserian glycerol rhizotomy, injection of glycerol into the trigeminal cistern, physical compression, trigeminal ganglion balloon microcompression, alcohol injections, botulinum toxin injection, cryotherapy, and gamma-knife radiosurgery (GKRS). Some of the surgical procedures may contribute to some complications [5], such as hearing loss, facial paresthesia, hypoesthesia, masseter weakness and paralysis, keratitis, transient paralysis of cranial nerves III and VI including diminished corneal reflex, dysesthesia, and anesthesia dolorosa, even an immediate complete loss of vision in one eye after trigeminal radiofrequency rhizotomy due to acute traumatic optic neuropathy.

In 2002, Micheli et al. first reported that BTX-A injection can relieve TN [4], supported by subsequent positive reports [6], and many studies have shown that botulinum toxin type A (BTX-A) may be effective and safe as treatment of TN [7–10]. The common side effects of botulinum toxin treatment on TN are dema/hematoma and facial asymmetry which include the muscle relaxation, distortion of commissure, and the ptosis of the eyelids at the site of injection. All these side effects were mild and automatically disappeared without any further treatment. No systemic side effects were observed [11, 12]. In February 2008, the U.S. Food and Drug Administration notified the public that Botox and Botox Cosmetic (botulinum toxin type A) and Myobloc (botulinum toxin type B) have been linked in some cases to adverse reactions, including respiratory failure and death, following treatment of a variety of conditions using a wide range of doses. The adverse reactions appear to be related to the spread of the toxin to areas distant from the site of injection, and mimic symptoms of botulism, which may include difficulty swallowing, weakness, and breathing problems. So the general fragility and often coexistent diseases of older patients imply perhaps greater susceptibility to side effects and needed reduction of BTX-A dosage. This research objective was to assess the therapeutic efficacy and safety of BTX-A in treating patients of advanced age (≥80 years old) with idiopathic trigeminal neuralgia (ITN).

## 2. Materials and Methods

*2.1. Subjects.* Eligible patents were recruited between August 2008 and February 2014 from the neurology clinic and the inpatient department of the Second Affiliated Hospital of Soochow University and were approved by the hospital ethic committee. Inclusion criteria were as follows: (i) diagnosis of classic ITN, as stipulated in the current version of the International Classification of Headache Disorders (ICHD-II); (ii) no prior exposure to BTX-A treatment; and (iii) failure of accepted medical and surgical interventions. Any conditions potentially heightening the risk of patient exposure to BTX-A (e.g., myasthenia gravis and motor neuron disease) or lack of pertinent medical information were grounds for exclusion.

*2.2. General Information and Grouping.* The study choose two groups of trigeminal neuralgia patients, one comprised

of patients ≥80 years old ($n = 14$) and another of patients <60 years old ($n = 29$). At baseline (prior to treatment), the median pain scores by the visual analogue scale (VAS) in both older and younger patient groups were 8.5 and 8.0, respectively, showing no significant difference ($Z = -1.411$, $p = 0.158$). In the older patient group (male, 4; female, 10), each patient suffered from hypertension, diabetes mellitus, and cardiac insufficiency, and two displayed hepatic compromise. The age range was 80–90 years (average, $82.6 \pm 2.9$ years). In the younger group of patients (male, 10; female, 19), one suffered from hypertension. Ages ranged from 34 to 59 years (average, $49.5 \pm 6.3$ years). Gender ratios of the two groups were similar ($p = 0.968$), but the incidence of coexistent diseases in the older (versus younger) age group was significantly higher ($p = 0.005$) (Table 1).

*2.3. Treatment.* BTX-A (100 U clostridium botulinum type A neurotoxin complex, 5 mg gelatin, 25 mg dextran, and 25 mg saccharose) was commercially procured (Lanzhou Institute of Biological Products, Lanzhou, China) and diluted to 25 U/mL for treatments, drawing 1-2 mL from vials for injection. Administration was guided by each patient's perceived pain and trigger zones, delivering BTX-A intradermally and/or submucosally via 1 mL syringe. The total dosages delivered varied, ranging from 30 to 200 U.

*2.4. Measures.* Pain severity was assessed through patient input (interview or telephone), using the visual analogue scale (VAS). Patient examinations were conducted at baseline and at 1 month after treatment, recording related side effects.

## 3. Statistical Analysis

All analytics assumed an intent-to-treat basis, using two-sided testing. If obeying normal distribution, data were assessed using mean ± SD. And between-group comparisons were evaluated by means of $t$-test, comparing incidences via the chi-square test. If not, data were assessed using median values and the rank sum test was used. Standard software (SPSS v17.0; SPSS Inc. (IBM), Chicago, IL, USA) was engaged for statistical computations, setting significance at $p < 0.05$.

## 4. Results

The dosages of BTX-A were 45 to 150 U in the older group and 30 to 200 U in the younger group. Mean BTX-A dosages of $91.3 \pm 25.6$ U and $71.8 \pm 33.1$ U were administered in older and younger patient groups, respectively ($t = 1.930$, $p = 0.061$). Median VAS scores 1 month after treatment in older (4.5) and in younger (4) patients were significantly lower than corresponding baseline values; and D values of VAS scores did not differ significantly by group (older, 2.5; younger, 0; $Z = -1.073$, $p = 0.283$), reflecting similar group therapeutic outcomes. Transient minor side effects developed in two older patients (whole-body discomfort in one, mild left eye ptosis, and slight oral deviation/drooling in

TABLE 1: Comparison of patient parameters in older (≥80 years old) and younger (<60 years old) BTX-A therapeutic groups.

| Clinical index | Older group ($n = 14$) | Younger group ($n = 29$) | $p$ value |
|---|---|---|---|
| Average age (years) | $82.6 \pm 2.9$ | $49.5 \pm 6.3$ | 0.000 |
| Gender (male/female) | 4/10 | 10/19 | 0.968 |
| Coexistent diseases (with/without) | 6/8 | 1/28 | 0.005 |
| Therapeutic doses (U) | $91.3 \pm 25.6$ | $71.8 \pm 33.1$ | 0.061 |
| D value of VAS (media, before and after treatment) | 2.5 | 0 | 0.283 |
| Side effect (total count) | $2^a$ | $2^b$ | 0.825 |

[a]Whole-body discomfort in one; mild left eye ptosis and slight oral deviation/drooling in the other; [b]Mild facial paralysis in one; moderate facial paralysis in the other; BTX-A: botulinum toxin type A; VAS: visual analogue scale.

TABLE 2: Comparison of VAS scores in older (≥80 years old) and younger (<60 years old) BTX-A therapeutic groups.

| | VAS score before treatment (median) | VAS score after treatment (median) | $Z$ | $p_1$ value |
|---|---|---|---|---|
| Older group ($n = 14$) | 8.5 | 4.5 | $-2.680$ | 0.007 |
| Younger group ($n = 29$) | 8.0 | 5.0 | $-3.360$ | 0.001 |
| $Z$ | $-1.411$ | $-0.040$ | — | — |
| $p_2$ value | 0.158 | 0.968 | — | — |

$p_1$: comparison of VAS scores between before treatment and after treatment; $p_2$: comparison of VAS scores between older group and younger group.

the other) and in two younger patients (mild facial paralysis comes in one and moderate facial paralysis comes in the other). Thus, the incidences of side effects did not differ significantly in these groups ($p = 0.825$), and all events resolved spontaneously within 3 weeks (Tables 1 and 2).

## 5. Discussion

TN is further categorized as idiopathic (ITN) or secondary type. ITN occurs in the absence of neurologic signs or organic lesions, whereas secondary TN is due to tumors, multiple sclerosis, small infarcts, or angiomas arising in the pons or medulla. In the patients of this study recruited, secondary TN was excluded, given a lack of clinical symptoms, physical evidence, and imaging abnormalities.

Although the mechanisms involved in TN remain unclear, there are three major hypotheses for its development [13, 14]: (1) the trigeminal nerve compression, (2) irritative lesions impacting the thalamic corticospinal nucleus of the trigeminal nerve, and (3) short-circuiting of the trigeminal nerve. Many treatments available for TN include medical agents, nerve blocks, surgical interventions, and stereotactic radiotherapy. Antiepileptic drugs, especially carbamazepine, are still the first-line medical treatment, and long-term antiepileptic medication is often required. However, the risk of side effects, such as nausea, dizziness, dystaxia, hepatic insufficiency, and leukopenia, increases with prolonged use [15]. Microvascular decompression is the most widely adopted surgical treatment worldwide, but the recurrence rate is 20–30%, and a host of potential complications may develop during and after surgery [16]. In light of current evidence, it seems fair to argue for a safer, better tolerated, and more efficacious treatment.

BTX-A is one of the most potent neurotoxins, whether natural or synthetic. It prevents axonal release of acetylcholine (Ach), thus blocking neuromuscular transmission and producing muscle relaxation. Common clinical uses include blepharospasm, hemifacial spasm, dystonia, and cosmetic imperfections [17]. BTX-A also readily blocks cholinergic synapses in salivary and sweat glands and is therefore useful in suppressing glandular hyperactivity. In 2002, Micheli et al. was the first to identify BTX-A as an agent for TN relief [4]. Subsequent studies also have shown the benefits of BTX-A in treatment of pain (including TN) [18]. BTX-A offers an effective means of treating TN that is increasingly gaining attention, rather than confronting the side effects of medical or surgical treatments.

The precise mechanism of action for BTX-A in pain relief is not well defined but may be multifactorial. When injected directly into contracting muscles, BTX-A binds to presynaptic nerve terminals and becomes internalized, preventing exocytosis of the neurotransmitter acetylcholine (Ach) at neuromuscular junctions. BTX-A may also exert peripheral neurovascular activity by inhibiting release of various neurotransmitters, such as substance P, neurokinin A, calcitonin gene related peptide (CGRP), and enteral polypeptide [18]. These transmitters act on blood vessels and glutamate, relieving pain by inhibiting neurogenic inflammation and reducing afferent nerve impulses [19, 20]. What is more, BTX-A exerts an antinociceptive function, directly modulating central sensitization by inhibiting excessive expression of TRPA1, TRPV1, and TRPV2 in the spinal trigeminal nucleus [21, 22]. Finally, BTX-A or its metabolite likely reduces sympathetic nerve transmissions to curb suppression of Renshaw cells within inhibitory intermediate neurons, acting upon the spinal cord indirectly to alleviate pain [23]. A new study has just revealed that the antinociceptive effects of BTX-A are conferred by inhibiting Nav1.7 upregulation in the trigeminal ganglion [24]. Thus, such effects are not confined to the neuromuscular junction, acting as well on central nerve structures (i.e., trigeminal ganglion, trigeminal nerve ridge nucleus, or spinal cord). Further research is needed to explore the pathways by which BTX-A relieves the pain of TN.

A recently published meta-analysis has concluded that BTX-A may be an effective and safe treatment option for patients with TN, yielding on average a 29.8% reduction in paroxysms per day [11]. In our preliminary study, it was found that pain relief peaked 1 month after local injection of BTX-A [10]. Hence, this study established a 1-month monitoring interval. In this study, VAS scores were performed again in patients with primary trigeminal neuralgia after injection of BTX-A for 1 month. The study found VAS scores had significantly lowered than those before treatment in both groups, and this suggested that BTX-A was effective for both younger and elderly. Meanwhile, the D values of VAS scores did not differ significantly between the two groups, indicating the similar curative effect for both groups.

In addition to the volumes of injected BTX-A, routes of injection, injection frequencies, and injection sites have varied among studies. As little as 25 U of BTX-A was administered according to Zhang et al. [7], compared with a maximum of 100 U given by Shehata et al. [9]. Generally, BTX-A is delivered via subcutaneous or intradermal route [11]. In patients of advanced age, heart disease and compromised respiratory function often coexisted, but the need for reduced dosages of BTX in older patients or their vulnerability to its side effects has not been addressed. The injection sites selected in this study were perceived pain and trigger zones. The injection dosage was determined according to the range of pain, and a multipoint injection method was adopted. In this study, the volumes of injected BTX-A ranged from 30 to 200 U, delivered through intradermal and/or submucosal routes. The dosage of BTX-A is 45 to 150 U in the older group and 30 to 200 U in the younger group. Though the mean BTX-A dosages of the older group was little higher than those of the younger group, no significant between-group difference in BTX-A dosage materialized, and the corresponding incidences of side effects did not differ significantly. Two groups improved pain fairly, prompts that both small dose and large dose may have obvious curative effects. This finding is consistent with the conclusion of Zhang et al. [7], which suggested that BTX-A injection in TN was safe and efficient, and low dose (25 U) and high dose (75 U) were similar in efficacy in short term.

In terms of safety, the two reported side effects of BTX-A injection have been facial asymmetry and injection-site edema/hematoma, both of which prove tolerable and transitory in nature [11]. In total, occurrences of facial asymmetry and edema/hematoma following BTX-A injection have ranged from 2 to 5% and 1-2%, respectively. Facial asymmetry typically requires 5–7 weeks for resolution, whereas edema/hematoma persists for just 5-6 days. Rates of coexistent diseases, in this study, such as hypertension, diabetes mellitus, renal insufficiency, and cardiac insufficiency, were significantly higher in the older patient group by comparison, but as in the younger group, only two patients developed transient minor side effects (i.e., whole-body discomfort, mild ptosis, and oral deviation/drooling). All resolved within 3 weeks and without serious adverse reactions. Consequently, in extremely older patients afflicted with various medical conditions dose reductions seem unwarranted. Of course, it also seemed that the dosages of BTX-A in advanced age patients with side effects were 100 U and 150 U and in the younger patients were 30 U and 75 U.

It seemed that the more the dosage in the older group, the greater the likelihood of side effects is. Therefore, it is suggested that it should be more carefully followed to see whether the patients have side effects after the treatment of elderly patients using a large dose of BTX-A.

Overall, BTX-A is an effective and safe treatment for ITN in patients of advanced age (≥80 years old), at dosages similar to those used in much younger counterparts (<60 years old). However, this study was limited to 14 older subjects, with no placebo group as reference, calling for more extensive randomized controlled trials.

## Abbreviations

BTX-A: Botulinum toxin type A
ITN:    Idiopathic trigeminal neuralgia
VAS:    Visual analogue scale
TN:     Trigeminal neuralgia
Ach:    Acetylcholine
CGRP:   Calcitonin gene related peptide
TRP:    Transient receptor potential
Nav:    Voltage gate sodium channel.

## Ethical Approval

This study was approved by the ethics committee of the national drug clinical trial institution of the Second Affiliated Hospital of Soochow University. Research project number: LK2008022.

## Disclosure

The authors alone are responsible for the content and drafting of this paper.

## Authors' Contributions

Jing Liu and Ying-Ying Xu contributed equally to this work.

## Acknowledgments

This work was funded by the National Natural Science Foundation (no. 81671270), the Youth Science and Technology Project of the Health Bureau of Suzhou City (KJXW2014012), the Second Affiliated Hospital of Soochow University Preponderant Clinic Discipline Group Project Funding (XKQ2015002), the Young Worker's Pre-research Foundation of the Second Affiliated Hospital of Soochow University (SDFEYQN1715), and this was also partly supported by the Suzhou Clinical Research Center of Neurological Disease (SZZX201503) and the Natural Science Foundation of Jiangsu Province of China (BK2011294).

# References

[1] A. M. Hegarty and J. M. Zakrzewska, "Differential diagnosis for orofacial pain, including sinusitis, TMD, trigeminal neuralgia," *Dental Update*, vol. 38, no. 6, pp. 396–400, 2011.

[2] P. J. Hamlyn and T. T. King, "Neurovascular compression in trigeminal neuralgia: a clinical and anatomical study," *Journal of Neurosurgery*, vol. 76, no. 6, pp. 948–954, 1992.

[3] D. A. Crooks and J. B. Miles, "Trigeminal neuralgia due to vascular compression in multiple sclerosis–Post-mortem findings," *British Journal of Neurosurgery*, vol. 10, no. 1, pp. 85–88, 1996.

[4] F. Micheli, M. C. Scorticati, and G. Raina, "Beneficial effects of botulinum toxin type a for patients with painful tic convulsif," *Clinical Neuropharmacology*, vol. 25, no. 5, pp. 260–262, 2002.

[5] M. Khan, S. E. Nishi, S. N. Hassan, M. A. Islam, and S. H. Gan, "Trigeminal neuralgia, glossopharyngeal neuralgia, and myofascial pain dysfunction syndrome: an update," *Pain Research and Management*, vol. 2017, Article ID 7438326, 18 pages, 2017.

[6] E. Piovesan, H. Teive, P. Kowacs, M. V. Della Coletta, L. C. Werneck, and S. D. Silberstein, "An open study of botulinum-A toxin treatment of trigeminal neuralgia," *Neurology*, vol. 65, no. 8, pp. 1306–1308, 2005.

[7] H. Zhang, Y. Lian, Y. Ma et al., "Two doses of botulinum toxin type a for the treatment of trigeminal neuralgia: observation of therapeutic effect from a randomized, double-blind, placebo-controlled trial," *Journal of Headache and Pain*, vol. 15, no. 1, p. 65, 2014.

[8] S. Li, Y. J. Lian, Y. Chen et al., "Therapeutic effect of botulinum toxin-A in 88 patients with trigeminal neuralgia with 14-month follow-up," *Journal of Headache and Pain*, vol. 15, no. 1, p. 43, 2014.

[9] H. S. Shehata, M. S. El-Tamawy, N. M. Shalaby, and G. Ramzy, "Botulinum toxin-type a: could it be an effective treatment option in intractable trigeminal neuralgia?," *Journal of Headache and Pain*, vol. 14, no. 1, p. 92, 2013.

[10] J. F. Shao, Q. L. Zhang, W. F. Luo et al., "Efficacy observation of botulinum toxin type A in elderly patients with primary intractable trigeminal neuralgia," *Chinese Journal of Geriatrics*, vol. 33, no. 1, pp. 44–46, 2012.

[11] M. E. Morra, A. Elgebaly, A. Elmaraezy et al., "Therapeutic efficacy and safety of botulinum toxin a therapyintrigeminal neuralgia: a systematic review and meta-analysis of randomized controlled trials," *Journal of Headache and Pain*, vol. 17, no. 1, p. 63, 2016.

[12] J. H. Xia, C. H. He, H. F. Zhang et al., "Botulinum toxin A in the treatment of trigeminal neuralgia," *International Journal of Neuroscience*, vol. 126, no. 4, pp. 348–353, 2016.

[13] P. J. Jannetta, "Arterial compression of the trigeminal nerve at the pons in patients with trigeminal neuralgia, 1967," *Journal of Neurosurgery*, vol. 107, no. 1, pp. 216–219, 2007.

[14] M. Devor, R. Govrin-Lippmann, and Z. H. Rappaport, "Mechanism of trigeminal neuralgia: an ultrastructural analysis of trigeminal root specimens obtained during microvascular decompression surgery," *Journal of Neurosurgery*, vol. 96, no. 3, pp. 532–543, 2002.

[15] T. P. Jorns and J. M. Zakrzewska, "Evidence-based approach to the medical management of trigeminal neuralgia," *British Journal of Neurosurgery*, vol. 21, no. 3, pp. 253–261, 2007.

[16] A. E. Bond, G. Zada, A. A. Gonzalez, C. Hansen, and S. L. Giannotta, "Operative strategies for minimizing hearing loss and other major complications associated with microvascular decompression for trigeminal neuralgia," *World Neurosurgery*, vol. 74, no. 1, pp. 172–177, 2010.

[17] C. J. Wu, J. H. Shen, Y. Chen, and Y. J. Lian, "Comparison of two different formulations of botulinum toxin a for the treatment of blepharospasm and hemifacial spasm," *Turkish Neurosurgery*, vol. 21, no. 4, pp. 625–629, 2011.

[18] G. Sandrini, R. De Icco, C. Tassorelli, N. Smania, and S. Tamburin, "Botulinum neurotoxin type a for the treatment of pain: not just in migraine and trigeminal neuralgia," *Journal of Headache and Pain*, vol. 18, no. 1, p. 38, 2017.

[19] K. R. Aoki, "Evidence for antinociceptive activity of botulinum toxin type a in pain management," *Headache: The Journal of Head & Face Pain*, vol. 43, no. 1, pp. S9–S15, 2003.

[20] R. Mazzocchio and M. Caleo, "More than at the neuromuscular synapse: actions of botulinum neurotoxin a in the central nervous system," *Neuroscientist*, vol. 21, no. 1, pp. 44–61, 2015.

[21] C. Ferrandiz-Huertas, S. Mathivanan, C. J. Wolf, I. Devesa, and A. Ferrer-Montiel, "Trafficking of thermoTRP channels," *Membranes*, vol. 4, no. 3, pp. 525–564, 2014.

[22] T. Shimizu, M. Shibata, H. Toriumi et al., "Reduction of TRPV1 expression in the trigeminal system by botulinum neurotoxin type-A," *Neurobiology of Disease*, vol. 48, no. 3, pp. 367–378, 2012.

[23] B. M. Guyer, "Mechanism of botulinum toxin in the relief of chronic pain," *Current Review of Pain*, vol. 3, no. 6, pp. 427–431, 1999.

[24] K. Y. Yang, M. J. Kim, J. S. Ju et al., "Antinociceptive effects of botulinum toxin type a on trigeminal neuropathic pain," *Journal of Dental Research*, vol. 95, no. 10, pp. 1183–1190, 2016.

# 25

# Ultrasound-Guided Prolotherapy with Polydeoxyribonucleotide for Painful Rotator Cuff Tendinopathy

**Kyoungho Ryu,**[1] **Dongchan Ko,**[1] **Goeun Lim,**[1] **Eugene Kim,**[2] **and Sung Hyun Lee** ⓘ[1]

[1]*Department of Anesthesiology and Pain Medicine, Kangbuk Samsung Hospital, Sungkyunkwan University School of Medicine, Seoul, Republic of Korea*
[2]*Department of Orthopedic Surgery, Kangbuk Samsung Hospital, Sungkyunkwan University School of Medicine, Seoul, Republic of Korea*

Correspondence should be addressed to Sung Hyun Lee; 4321hoho@naver.com

Academic Editor: Parisa Gazerani

*Background.* Rotator cuff tendinopathy is a primary cause of shoulder pain and dysfunction. Several effective nonsurgical treatment methods have been described for chronic rotator cuff tendinopathy. Prolotherapy with polydeoxyribonucleotide (PDRN), which consists of active deoxyribonucleotide polymers that stimulate tissue repair, is a nonsurgical regenerative injection that may be a viable treatment option. The objective of this study was to assess the efficacy of PDRN in the treatment of chronic rotator cuff tendinopathy. *Method.* The records of patients with chronic rotator cuff tendinopathy ($n = 131$) were reviewed retrospectively, and the patients treated with PDRN prolotherapy ($n = 32$) were selected. We measured the main outcome of the shoulder pain and disability index score on a numerical rating scale of average shoulder pain. *Results.* Compared with baseline data, significant improvements in the shoulder pain and disability index and pain visual analog scale scores were demonstrated at one week after the end of treatment, and at one month and three months later. *Conclusions.* PDRN prolotherapy may improve the conservative treatment of painful rotator cuff tendinopathy for a specific subset of patients.

## 1. Introduction

Shoulder pain is very common and affects one in three individuals during their lifetime [1]. In many cases, the shoulder is a "prime mover" for daily movement; therefore, restrictions to the activities of daily living are severe when experiencing shoulder disorders. Rotator cuff tendinopathy (RCT) is a primary cause of shoulder pain and disability. Nonoperative conservative treatment is the first-line treatment for most RCT. Conventional treatment strategies consist of rest, activity modification, physical therapy, and pain medication [2–5]. Considering the pathophysiology of rotator cuff disorder, prolotherapy is considered to be a nonsurgical treatment [6, 7]. The pathophysiology of RCT is characterized by continuous, degenerative denaturation within the tendon. Acute and chronic tendon overload increases the volume of the limited subacromial space, which may promote inflammation and

trigger a cascade of inflammatory cytokines, neuropeptides, and other materials within the tendon and bursal tissue [1, 8].

Prolotherapy is a regenerative injection therapy that introduces small volumes of an irritant into the insertion sites of the damaged tendon, joints, adjacent joint spaces, and ligament, which promotes the growth of normal tissue. Although hypertonic glucose is primarily used as the irritant, polidocanol, manganese, zinc, human growth hormone, and autologous cellular solutions such as platelet-rich plasma are also used. The mechanism of dextrose prolotherapy is not completely understood. However, the current hypothesis holds that the injected substance mimics the natural healing processes by facilitating a local inflammatory cascade, which triggers the release of growth factors and collagen deposition [9]. Considering this mechanism of prolotherapy, the use of polydeoxyribonucleotide (PDRN) as an injected proliferant may be a viable treatment agent.

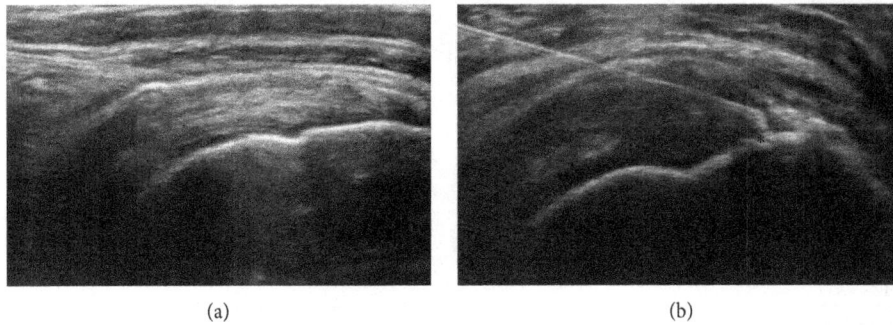

(a)                                                    (b)

FIGURE 1: (a) Ultrasound-guided injection into (a) the subacromial bursa and (b) the supraspinatus tendon. *The tear site of the supraspinatus tendon.

PDRN is obtained from the sperm of raised trout as a mixture of deoxyribonucleotide polymers with a chain length of 50–2000 base pairs. Several previous studies have reported that PDRN administration reduced inflammation by lowering proinflammatory mediators such as tumor necrosis factor-alpha, interleukin-6, and high mobility group box chromosomal protein 1 (HMGB 1) [10, 11]. In other studies, PDRN stimulated tissue repair and wound healing by inducing the expression of vascular endothelial growth factor during pathological conditions of low tissue perfusion [12, 13]. Some clinical studies have reported its effectiveness in treating several types of tendinopathy, such as achilles tendinopathy, plantar fasciitis, tibial tendon, and hip adductor tendinopathy [14–16]. However, only one study has reported the efficacy of PDRN injection in RCT [17]. The aim of this study, therefore, was to evaluate the efficacy of prolotherapy with PDRN as a therapeutic option for chronic RCT.

## 2. Materials and Methods

*2.1. Patients.* The protocol for this retrospective study was approved by the Institutional Review Board of Kang Buk Samsung Hospital, Seoul, Korea, a retrospective review of the medical records of patients who were diagnosed with chronic rotator cuff disease (tendinosis, partial- and full-thickness tears) between March 2016 and May 2017 was conducted. All subjects were outpatients at a pain clinic of this hospital. All patients underwent a standardized history collection, physical test, and ultrasonographic examination. Patients from 30 to 75 years of age with symptoms that had persisted for at least 3 months were refractory to other conservative methods such as physical therapy and exercise therapy, and rotator cuff lesions in the form of tendinosis, partial tear (<50% of involved tendon) on ultrasonography or magnetic resonance imaging (MRI), were included. Patients with rheumatic disease or other systemic inflammatory disease, osteomyelitis, active or chronic infection signs in the treatment area, previous shoulder or neck surgery, a full-thickness tear of the involved tendon, trauma history at the shoulder (within 3 months), bleeding tendency (hereditary or acquired), or pregnancy were excluded from this study.

All ultrasound- (Sonosite® X-porte-) guided PDRN injections were performed by the same physician (lead author).

The injection points were the subacromial bursa, peritendon space of the supraspinatus tendon, and the partial-thickness tear lesion of the supraspinatus tendon. If there is only tendinosis without tear was present, needling was performed once and the drug was applied to the peritendon area and the bursa above. If there was a tear, the tear area was targeted first, and the remaining drug was applied to the bursa. When the angle of the needle did not satisfactorily emerge from the bursa, the needle was withdrawn and needling was performed again. The probe was placed parallel to the long axis of the supraspinatus tendon, and the needle was inserted via the lateral approach (Figure 1) [18]. A 3 mL aliquot of PDRN (Placentex® Integro, Mastelli S.r.l., San Remo, Italy) mixed with 1 mL of 1% lidocaine was injected. The injections were repeated at weekly intervals. Injections were discontinued if the pain score decreased to at least one-quarter of preinjection levels, if the patient received the maximum of 5 injections, or if decided to withdraw from treatment.

*2.2. Evaluation.* The outcomes of interest were the pain visual analog scale (VAS) score, shoulder pain and disability index (SPADI), single assessment numeric evaluation (SANE), and adverse effects. The SPADI, which was designed to measure current shoulder pain and function of daily tasks in an outpatient setting, was investigated. The single assessment numeric evaluation (SANE), which was designed as a simple one-question, patient-based shoulder function assessment tool was investigated. The question of SANE is, "how would you rate your shoulder today as a percentage of normal (0% to 100%, with 100% being normal)?" Pain was measured using a VAS; a score of 0 indicated no pain and a score of 10 indicated the most severe pain. The administration of the SPADI, SANE questionnaires, and pain scoring was performed before each injection and 1 week, 1 month, and 3 months after the final injection. Any adverse effects were noted at each procedure.

*2.3. Statistical Analysis.* The data are presented as mean ± SEM. Statistical analyses were performed using SPSS version 24.0 (IBM Corp., Armonk, NY, USA) for Windows (Microsoft Corporation, Redmond, WA, USA). A two-way repeated measure analysis of variance (ANOVA) was

TABLE 1: Baseline characteristics of patients ($n = 32$).

| Characteristic | Treatment patient ($n = 32$) |
|---|---|
| Age ($y$) | $53.4 \pm 10.0$ |
| Pain score (VAS) | $5.3 \pm 1.1$ |
| Duration (month) | $6.6 \pm 6.3$ |
| Sex: man/woman | 17/15 |
| Shoulder affected: Rt/Lt | 19/13 |
| Ultrasonographic finding of rotator cuff lesion | |
|   Tendinosis | 23 |
|   Partial thickness tear | 9 |

Data presented as mean ± SEM unless otherwise indicated.

TABLE 2: Outcome measurements after treatment.

| | Before treatment | 1 week | 1 month | 3 months |
|---|---|---|---|---|
| VAS score | $5.3 \pm 1.2$ | $1.8 \pm 0.9^*$ | $1.7 \pm 1.1^*$ | $1.7 \pm 1.3^*$ |
| SANE | $46.6 \pm 11.2$ | $80.3 \pm 7.8^*$ | $84.0 \pm 10.4^*$ | $85.7 \pm 12.8^*$ |
| SPADI | $45.8 \pm 16.9$ | $20.1 \pm 12.04^*$ | $16.9 \pm 12.0^*$ | $12.6 \pm 13.0^*$ |

VAS = pain visual analog scale; SANE = single assessment numeric evaluation; SPADI = shoulder pain and disability index. $^*P < 0.001$ compared with before treatment.

performed to identify the effect of the injections at each time point, followed by Bonferroni post hoc tests. ANOVA in the repeated measurements was also used for intragroup analyses between the tendinosis group and partial tear group. A $P$ value $< 0.05$ was considered to be statistically significant.

## 3. Results

Patients with chronic RCT ($n = 131$) were reviewed retrospectively. Among them, patients who met the inclusion criteria and had received prolotherapy with PDRN were selected ($n = 32$). After the final analysis of 32 patients with refractory rotator cuff disease, the average number of injections was $3.9 \pm 0.7$. In total, 11 patients received 3 injections, 12 received 4, and 9 received 5. Table 1 summarizes the demographics data of the treated patients. Patients receiving prolotherapy with PDRN reported a significant reduction in pain as according to the VAS score, which resulted in a decrease in pain at 1 week, 1 month, and 3 months after the completion of treatment. Function assessed according to the SANE questionnaire demonstrated noticeable improvement. Disability measured using the SPADI was significantly decreased. Changes and significance of the VAS score, SANE, and SPADI are presented in Table 2. One week after treatment, the VAS score was significantly lower than before treatment and remained similar at 1 month and 3 months after treatment. In other words, there was no significant difference in pain score at 1 week, 1 month, and 3 months after the end of treatment. Functional fraction measured using SANE over a one-week period after treatment was more improved at 1 month and 3 months after treatment. Disability assessed with using SPADI after 1 month and 3 months also decreased more than that at 1 week. The pain was initially improved and relief lasted for at least three months. It could be concluded that improvement in function and reduction in disability was sustained up to one month after treatment and was maintained for at least

three months. During the treatment procedure, no complications such as infection, allergic reaction, or post-injection pain occurred.

## 4. Discussion

Prolotherapy with PDRN is an effective treatment for refractory chronic RCT because it reduces pain, improves function, and decreases disability in performing the activities of daily life. In this study, the meaningful increase in SANE, the significant decrease in pain score, and SPADI lasted for 3 months after the final treatment. Considering the presumed mechanism of PDRN, it is possible to consider superimposing prolotherapy instead of injection. The mechanism of PDRN treatment, demonstrated in previous studies, induced an anti-inflammatory reaction. Treatment with PDRN reduces the early inflammatory factors, including tumor necrosis factor-alpha, interleukin-1, and interleukin-6, and, later, the proinflammatory factor HMGB 1. PDRN also enhances the expression of anti-inflammatory factor interleukin-10. These effects have been showed to stimulate the wound healing process and reduce arthritis in animal experiments and clinical trials [10, 11]. Previous studies have demonstrated that PDRN enhanced the production of several growth factors, such as vascular endothelial growth factor (VEGF) and fibroblast growth factor (FGF), which resulted in stimulation of angiogenesis and wound healing in genetically induced diabetic mice and models of peripheral artery occlusive disease [12, 13, 19]. Based on the fact that PDRN promotes VEGF generation in a low-perfusion state, a mouse model of kidney transplantation demonstrated that PDRN was effective in preventing ischemia-reperfusion-induced acute kidney injury [20]. In the clinical trials comparing tissue regeneration after skin graft to the subject of diabetes mellitus foot ulcer patients, increase in tissue oxygenation and angiogenesis were demonstrated [21, 22]. In an in vivo study on an animal study investigating the musculoskeletal system, the level of FGF and VEGF involved in recovery after PDRN injections were increased in rats with injured achilles tendon, and tendon collagen type II level were increased after 4 weeks [23]. All of these positive effects of PDRN result from stimulation of the adenosine ($A_{2A}$) receptor. Concomitant administration of PDRN and 3,7-dimethyl-propargylxanthine, a specific antagonist of the purinergic $A_{2A}$ receptor, reflected the PDRN pathway. This information is supportive evidence that PDRN can be used as prolotherapy for regeneration purposes.

PDRN prolotherapy can confer several advantages compared with conventional therapies. First, it can be seen compared with steroid injection, which is the most commonly used method to treat RCT. Steroid injections are helpful for short-term pain relief; however, there are several adverse effects. In particular, repetitive steroid injections enhance the possibility of causing side effects such as focal inflammation, necrosis, tendon/ligament weakening or rupture, skin atrophy and depigmentation, elevation of serum glucose levels, and vaginal bleeding [24, 25]. PDRN injection can also be compared with prolotherapy, a treatment recently used for musculoskeletal systems. The most common prolotherapy agent is dextrose, which is used clinically at concentrations between 12.5% and 25%.

Although, the mechanism is not completely understood, the injected proliferant resembles the natural healing process in the body according to the three phases of the healing response: inflammatory, proliferative phase, and remodeling and maturation phase [9]. Through these presumed mechanisms, dextrose prolotherapy injections stimulate the production of extracellular matrix, which enhances the strength of ligaments, tendons, and joints, which in turn improve the durability and functionality of these structures. Several previous studies reported that dextrose prolotherapy had beneficial effects in the treatment of painful RCT; however, in some respects, PDRN prolotherapy is superior. The selection of analgesics is not restricted during prolotherapy with PDRN. However, anti-inflammatory agents such as nonsteroidal anti-inflammatory medications and steroids cannot be prescribed concomitantly with dextrose prolotherapy. The initial phase of dextrose prolotherapy, inflammatory phase is inhibited by steroid and nonsteroidal anti-inflammatory medications. When PDRN prolotherapy is performed, there are no drug restrictions because PDRN promotes proliferation without an inflammatory phase. Patients often complain of flare-up pain for several days after prolotherapy with dextrose, which promotes healing initially through an inflammatory reaction [26, 27]. However, pain is rarely exacerbated after PDRN injection. In our study, no side effects such as flare-up pain were observed. Prolotherapy with dextrose is administered at intervals of at least 3 weeks, the treatment interval is long, and time is required to complete the treatment course. In contrast, PDRN injections are usually performed at weekly intervals, which is an advantage of PDRN over dextrose. The duration of PDRN prolotherapy is 3 to 5 weeks, whereas dextrose prolotherapy may take form at least 9 weeks to as long as 20 weeks.

Limitations of this present study included its retrospective design and lack of a control group for comparison.

Determination of the clinical utility of PDRN for RCT will require assessment in larger randomized controlled trials, ideally in comparison with conventional therapy. In particular, a comparative study of PDRN prolotherapy and corticosteroid injection or dextrose prolotherapy is needed. An additional limitation was the lack of follow-up of the imaging changes in the supraspinatus tendon. At the end of the treatment period and follow-ups, ultrasound findings were not precisely recorded. Nevertheless, our study revealed significant differences in the VAS, SANE, and SPADI scores at the 3-month follow-up, indicating improved pain and function in patients with chronic RCT without any other complications.

## 5. Conclusions

Among the participants with RCT, prolotherapy with PDRN resulted in safe, meaningful, and sustained improvements in validated pain and function measures over a 3 month period. PDRN prolotherapy appeared to be effective for at least 3 months after therapy in most patients with chronic RCT who were refractory to conservative care. Additional randomized multidisciplinary effectiveness trials that include imaging outcomes such as ultrasound are required to verify the effect of PDRN for chronic RCT compared with current therapies, including prolotherapy with PDRN.

## References

[1] J. S. Lewis, "Rotator cuff tendinopathy," *British Journal of Sports Medicine*, vol. 43, no. 4, pp. 236–241, 2009.

[2] A. H. Gomoll, J. N. Katz, J. J. Warner, and P. J. Millett, "Rotator cuff disorders: recognition and management among patients with shoulder pain," *Arthritis & Rheumatism*, vol. 50, no. 12, pp. 3751–3761, 2004.

[3] W. Li, S. X. Zhang, Q. Yang, B.-L. Li, Q.-G. Meng, and Z.-G. Guo, "Effect of extracorporeal shock-wave therapy for treating patients with chronic rotator cuff tendonitis," *Medicine*, vol. 96, no. 35, p. e7940, 2017.

[4] K. M. Shin, "Partial-thickness rotator cuff tears," *Korean Journal of Pain*, vol. 24, no. 2, pp. 69–73, 2011.

[5] G. Matthewson, C. J. Beach, A. A. Nelson et al., "Partial thickness rotator cuff tears: current concepts," *Advances in Orthopedics*, vol. 2015, Article ID 458786, 11 pages, 2015.

[6] M. M. Seven, O. Ersen, S. Akpancar et al., "Effectiveness of prolotherapy in the treatment of chronic rotator cuff lesions," *Orthopaedics & Traumatology: Surgery & Research*, vol. 103, no. 3, pp. 427–433, 2017.

[7] H. Bertrand, K. D. Reeves, C. J. Bennett, S. Bicknell, and A. L. Cheng, "Dextrose prolotherapy versus control injections in painful rotator cuff tendinopathy," *Archives of Physical Medicine and Rehabilitation*, vol. 97, no. 1, pp. 17–25, 2016.

[8] J. Y. Ko, F. S. Wang, H. Y. Huang et al., "Increased IL-1β expression and myofibroblast recruitment in subacromial bursa is associated with rotator cuff lesions with shoulder stiffness," *Journal of Orthopaedic Research*, vol. 26, no. 8, pp. 1090–1097, 2008.

[9] R. A. Hauser, J. B. Lackner, D. Steilen-Matias, and D. K. Harris, "A systematic review of dextrose prolotherapy for chronic musculoskeletal pain," *Clinical Medicine Insights: Arthritis and Musculoskeletal Disorders*, vol. 9, pp. 139–159, 2016.

[10] W. Jeong, C. E. Yang, T. S. Roh, J. H. Kim, J. H. Lee, and W. J. Lee, "Scar prevention and enhanced wound healing induced by polydeoxyribonucleotide in a rat incisional wound-healing model," *International Journal of Molecular Sciences*, vol. 18, no. 12, p. 1698, 2017.

[11] A. Bitto, F. Polito, N. Irrera et al., "Polydeoxyribonucleotide reduces cytokine production and the severity of collagen-induced arthritis by stimulation of adenosine A2A receptor," *Arthritis & Rheumatism*, vol. 63, no. 11, pp. 3364–3371, 2011.

[12] A. Bitto, M. Galeano, F. Squadrito et al., "Polydeoxyribonucleotide improves angiogenesis and wound healing in experimental thermal injury," *Critical Care Medicine*, vol. 36, no. 5, pp. 1594–1602, 2008.

[13] A. Bitto, F. Polito, D. Altavilla, L. Minutoli, A. Migliorato, and F. Squadrito, "Polydeoxyribonucleotide (PDRN) restores blood flow in an experimental model of peripheral artery occlusive disease," *Journal of Vascular Surgery*, vol. 48, no. 5, pp. 1292–1300, 2008.

[14] J. K. Kim and J. Y. Chung, "Effectiveness of polydeoxyribonucleotide injection versus normal saline injection for treatment of chronic plantar fasciitis: a prospective randomised clinical trial," *International Orthopaedics*, vol. 39, no. 7, pp. 1329–1334, 2015.

[15] T. H. Lim, H. R. Cho, K. N. Kang et al., "The effect of polydeoxyribonucleotide prolotherapy on posterior tibial tendon dysfunction after ankle syndesmotic surgery: a case report," *Medicine*, vol. 95, no. 51, p. e5346, 2016.

[16] W. J. Kim, H. Y. Shin, G. H. Koo et al., "Ultrasound-guided prolotherapy with polydeoxyribonucleotide sodium in ischiofemoral impingement syndrome," *Pain Practice*, vol. 14, no. 7, pp. 649–655, 2014.

[17] Y. C. Yoon, D. H. Lee, M. Y. Lee, and S. H. Yoon, "Polydeoxyribonucleotide injection in the treatment of chronic supraspinatus tendinopathy: a case-controlled, retrospective, comparative study with 6-month follow-up," *Archives of Physical Medicine and Rehabilitation*, vol. 98, no. 5, pp. 874–880, 2017.

[18] L. Molini, S. Mariacher, and S. Bianchi, "US guided corticosteroid injection into the subacromial-subdeltoid bursa: technique and approach," *Journal of Ultrasound*, vol. 15, no. 1, pp. 61–68, 2012.

[19] M. Galeano, A. Bitto, D. Altavilla et al., "Polydeoxyribonucleotide stimulates angiogenesis and wound healing in the genetically diabetic mouse," *Wound Repair and Regeneration*, vol. 16, no. 2, pp. 208–217, 2008.

[20] E. K. Jeong, H. J. Jang, S. S. Kim et al., "Protective effect of polydeoxyribonucleotide against renal ischemia-reperfusion injury in mice," *Transplantation Proceedings*, vol. 48, no. 4, pp. 1251–1257, 2016.

[21] S. Kim, J. Kim, J. Choi, W. Jeong, and S. Kwon, "Polydeoxyribonucleotide improves peripheral tissue oxygenation and accelerates angiogenesis in diabetic foot ulcers," *Archives of Plastic Surgery*, vol. 44, no. 6, pp. 482–489, 2017.

[22] F. Squadrito, A. Bitto, D. Altavilla et al., "The effect of PDRN, an adenosine receptor A2A agonist, on the healing of chronic diabetic foot ulcers: results of a clinical trial," *Journal of Clinical Endocrinology & Metabolism*, vol. 99, no. 5, pp. E746–E753, 2014.

[23] S. H. Kang, M. S. Choi, H. K. Kim et al., "Polydeoxyribonucleotide improves tendon healing following achilles tendon injury in rats," *Journal of Orthopaedic Research*, 2017.

[24] B. K. Coombes, L. Bisset, and B. Vicenzino, "Efficacy and safety of corticosteroid injections and other injections for management of tendinopathy: a systematic review of randomised controlled trials," *The Lancet*, vol. 376, no. 9754, pp. 1751–1767, 2010.

[25] H. Tempfer, R. Gehwolf, C. Lehner et al., "Effects of crystalline glucocorticoid triamcinolone acetonide on cultured human supraspinatus tendon cells," *Acta Orthopaedica*, vol. 80, no. 3, pp. 357–362, 2009.

[26] D. Rabago, A. Slattengren, and A. Zgierska, "Prolotherapy in primary care practice," *Primary Care: Clinics in Office Practice*, vol. 37, no. 1, pp. 65–80, 2010.

[27] L. M. Distel and T. M. Best, "Prolotherapy: a clinical review of its role in treating chronic musculoskeletal pain," *PM&R*, vol. 3, no. 6, pp. S78–S81, 2011.

# 26

# Elevated Levels of Eotaxin-2 in Serum of Fibromyalgia Patients

Victoria Furer [ORCID],[1] Eyal Hazan,[2] Adi Mor,[3] Michal Segal,[3] Avi Katav,[3] Valerie Aloush,[1] Ori Elkayam,[1] Jacob George,[3,4] and Jacob N. Ablin[2]

[1]Tel Aviv Sourasky Medical Center and the Sackler Faculty of Medicine, Tel Aviv University, Tel Aviv, Israel
[2]Tel Aviv Sourasky Medical Center, Tel Aviv, Israel
[3]ChemomAb Ltd., Tel Aviv, Israel
[4]Kaplan Medical Center, Rehovot, Israel

Correspondence should be addressed to Victoria Furer; furer.rheum@gmail.com

Academic Editor: Manfred Harth

FMS patients demonstrate an altered profile of chemokines relative to healthy controls (HC). Eotaxin-2 is a potent chemoattractant distributed in a variety of tissues. The aim of the study was to compare serum levels of eotaxin-2 between FMS patients and HC and to examine a potential correlation between eotaxin-2 levels and clinical parameters of FMS. *Methods.* 50 patients with FMS and 15 HC were recruited. Data on the severity of FMS symptoms and depression were collected. Serum levels of eotaxin-2 (ELISA) were determined in all participants. High-sensitive CRP (hs-CRP) was measured in the FMS group. *Results.* The FMS cohort included predominantly females (84%), mean age of 49, and mean disease duration of 6 years. FMS patients exhibited significantly higher eotaxin-2 levels (pg/ml) versus HC: 833 ($\pm$384) versus 622 ($\pm$149), $p = 0.04$. Mean hs-CRP level among FMS patients was $4.8 \pm 6$ mg/l, a value not indicative of acute inflammation. No correlation was found between eotaxin-2 and hs-CRP levels. No correlation was found between eotaxin-2 and severity measures of FMS or depression. *Conclusion.* Eotaxin-2 does not appear to be a candidate for a disease activity biomarker in FMS. Further research is warranted into the role of this chemokine in the pathophysiology of the FMS.

## 1. Introduction

Fibromyalgia syndrome (FMS) is a highly prevalent chronic pain syndrome characterized by widespread pain and other somatic symptoms, including fatigue, sleep disturbances, cognitive dysfunction, and depression [1]. The diagnosis of FMS is based on clinical grounds [2], and despite many attempts to identify objective biomarkers for FMS, no such well-validated biochemical marker for either diagnosis or severity has emerged. While the pathogenesis of FMS remains incompletely understood, one leading paradigm is that of pain centralization, an increase of the processing of pain within the central nervous system (CNS) [3].

Recent studies suggest that cytokines may play a role in the pathogenesis of FMS, in particular, chemotactic cytokines referred as chemokines [4]. Chemokines are a family of small (8–10 kDa) proteins that induce chemotaxis of inflammatory cells. Emerging evidence reveals that chemokines play a role in the physiology of the nervous system, including neuronal migration, cell proliferation, and synaptic activity [5]. Chemokines and their receptors are among the key players responsible for communication between neurons and inflammatory cells, and this crosstalk is crucial for normal neurological functioning [5]. Furthermore, chemokines seem to contribute to a reciprocal interaction between neurons, glia, and microglia in a so-called "gliopathy," that is, activation of glial cells and neuroglial interactions as a basis for chronic pain [6–8]. Chemokines participate in synaptic transmission and in the formation of second-messenger systems in neurons and glial cells, favoring the noxious process. Chemokines enhance sensitivity to pain by direct action on chemokine receptors expressed in the entire pain pathway, from peripheral nerves to the dorsal ganglia and spinal cord. Simultaneously, they regulate the inflammatory response by acting on elements of the nervous system [5].

Since pain is the salient symptom of FMS, one may consider that, as modulators of nociception, certain chemokines may be involved in the pathophysiology of this syndrome. Increased levels of inflammatory cytokines and chemokines in serum [4, 9, 10] and cerebral spinal fluid [11] have been recently reported in cross-sectional studies in FMS cohorts. Subsequently, a prospective study by Wang et al. has not only confirmed the finding of increased circulating levels of cytokines in FMS, but also suggested a potential cytokine response to a therapeutic intervention [12, 13]. After 6 months of multidisciplinary pain therapy, baseline serum level of interleukin-8 (IL-8) reduced nearly to the normal range in correlation with a reduction in pain intensity. Ang et al. have further demonstrated that the level of pain in FMS corresponds to circulating chemokines levels, with uptrending levels of monocyte chemotactic protein-1 (MCP-1) and IL-8 in parallel with increasing pain severity over time [14].

Nonetheless, the relationship between the chemokine-cytokine network and FMS has yet to be clarified. Eotaxin-2 (CCL24), a member of the CC chemokine family, is a potent chemoattractant for eosinophils, basophils, and lymphocytes, distributed in a variety of tissues, including human brain [15]. To our best knowledge, no studies previously examined the eotaxin-2 profile in FMS patients. Thus, we conducted a case-control study to determine levels of circulating eotaxin-2 and high-sensitive C-reactive protein (hs-CRP) in FMS patients compared to healthy controls (HC). We further examined the relationship between these potential biomarkers and FMS severity.

## 2. Methods

50 patients suffering from primary FMS were consecutively recruited through the Rheumatology Clinic at the Tel Aviv Sourasky Medical Center. 15 healthy subjects were recruited as healthy controls (HC). Upon recruitment, patients were examined by a physician to verify the diagnosis of FMS and screened for alternative diagnoses such as inflammatory joint disease. Patients with a known diagnosis of inflammatory joint disease/chronic kidney disease/chronic liver disease/heart failure/diabetes mellitus/active malignancy were excluded from the study. Patients currently treated with immune-suppressive medications, including steroids, were excluded from the study. The diagnosis of FMS was verified according to the American College of Rheumatology (ACR) updated diagnostic criteria [2]. Patients subsequently filled out questionnaires to asses and document the severity of FMS symptoms. Questionnaires included basic demographic data (age, sex, smoking status, weight, height, use of medications, comorbidities, and previous medical history), widespread pain index (WPI), documenting extent of widespread pain, symptoms severity score (SSS), documenting severity of associated symptoms, Fibromyalgia Impact Questionnaire (FIQ), and Beck Depression Inventory (BDI) for evaluation of depression. Blood specimens for Eotaxin-2 and hs-CRP were drawn, separated, aliquoted, and stored frozen at $-20°C$ until analysis. Eotaxin-2 was measured using ELISA. The study was approved by the Institutional Review Board of the Hospital, and all patients provided written informed consent.

## 3. Statistical Analysis and Data Processing

Data were statistically analyzed with SPSS (version 20; IBM, Armonk, New York, NY, USA). Before analysis, residuals were tested for normal distribution (Shapiro–Wilk test) and equality of variance (Levene's test). Nonparametric tests were used where appropriate. Group comparisons were calculated using Student's independent $t$-test (parametric), Kruskal–Wallis test (nonparametric) or Pearson's chi test for categorical variables. According to the underlying hypotheses, a two-tailed test was performed. The significance level was set to $p = 0.05$. Values are given as means ± standard deviations (SD).

## 4. Results

Fifty-four patients suffering from FMS and 15 HC were enrolled in the study. Four patients were excluded due to impaired glucose tolerance treated pharmacologically ($n = 2$) or due to missing data ($n = 2$). The FMS cohort included predominantly females (84%) of $49 ± 14.6$ years of age, body mass index (BMI) of $26.8 ± 5.1$, and disease duration of $6 ± 5.5$ years. Thirty percent of FMS patients were smokers. Half of the patients were unemployed. Thirty-two percent of patients stated incapability to work due to FMS. HC cohort included subjects of $37.5 ± 12.6$ years of age, with a similar gender representation (53% females and 47% males) and BMI 22.6 (±3.3).

The levels of the mediators along with indices of disease activity in FMS are summarized in Table 1. FMS patients exhibited significantly higher eotaxin-2 levels as compared to healthy controls, 833 (±384) versus 622 (±149), $p = 0.04$, respectively, as presented in Figure 1. No significant gender-based difference was found in the mediators' levels or disease severity indices.

When examining the correlation between FMS severity indices and levels of eotaxin-2, no significant correlation was found. There was also no significant correlation between the parameters of FMS severity and hs-CRP. The lack of correlation between eotaxin-2 and hs-CRP is noteworthy. The majority of FMS patients had normal range of hs-CRP levels; however, the average level of hs-CRP was slightly elevated in FMS patients (4.81 mg/l). As expected, a positive correlation was found between hs-CRP and BMI ($r = 0.44$, $p = 0.02$), but not for eotaxin-2 levels and BMI ($r = 0.06$, $p = 0.8$). Smoking was not found to correlate neither with eotaxin-2/hs-CRP levels nor with disease severity indices.

## 5. Discussion

The present pilot study is the first one to report significantly increased circulating levels of eotaxin-2 in serum of FMS patients, compared with healthy controls, with no direct association between eotaxin-2 levels and FMS severity indices. This finding is consistent with the accumulating evidence regarding a distinct cytokine profile in FMS patients, further supporting the hypothesis of cytokines playing an important role in FMS pathophysiology [4, 10, 12–14].

TABLE 1: Levels of the mediators and indices of disease activity in FMS cohort ($N = 50$).

|  | Mean | Std. deviation |
| --- | --- | --- |
| Eotaxin-2 (pg/ml) | 833.82 | 384.67 |
| hs-CRP (mg/l) | 4.81 | 6.02 |
| WPI | 12.5 | 4.21 |
| SSS | 9.08 | 1.98 |
| FIQ | 63.88 | 16.81 |
| BDI | 20.00 | 11.05 |

hs-CRP, high sensitivity C-reactive protein; WPI, widespread pain index; SSS, symptoms severity score; FIQ, fibromyalgia impact questionnaire; BDI, beck depression inventory.

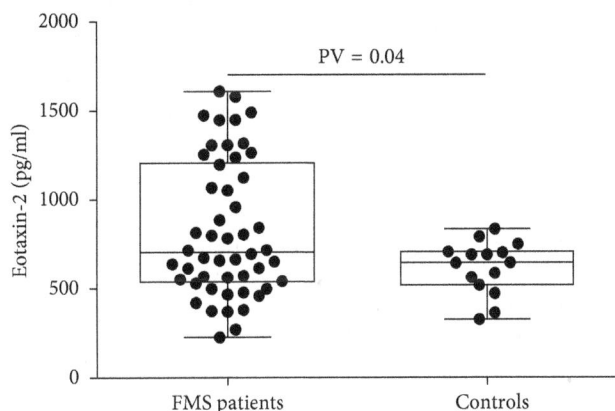

FIGURE 1: Eotaxin-2 levels in serum of patients with FMS and healthy controls.

Eotaxins are C-C motif chemokines first identified as potent eosinophil chemoattractants. They facilitate eosinophil recruitment to sites of inflammation in response to parasitic infections, as well as in allergic and autoimmune diseases such as asthma, atopic dermatitis, and inflammatory bowel disease [16]. The eotaxin family currently includes three members: eotaxin-1 (CCL11), eotaxin-2 (CCL24), and eotaxin-3 (CCL26). Despite having only ~30% sequence homology to one another, each was identified based on its ability to bind the chemokine receptor, CCR3. Increased serum eotaxin-1 levels have been reported in FMS patients [4, 10] and in patients with neurodegenerative diseases, including Alzheimer's disease, amyotrophic lateral sclerosis, Huntington's disease, and secondary progressive multiple sclerosis [17]. Since eotaxin-1 is capable of crossing the blood-brain barrier of normal mice, it is plausible that eotaxins generated in the periphery may exert physiological and pathological actions in the CNS.

Eotaxin-2 is a potent chemoattractant that binds to CCR3 for intracellular messaging. A variety of cells including respiratory epithelial cells, bronchial smooth muscle cells, vascular endothelial cells, fibroblasts, monocytes, helper T cells, and basophils express CCR3 and respond to eotaxin-2 stimulation [18], implicating a role in cellular communication. Interestingly, inhibition of eotaxin-2 by antibodies conveys an efficient protective effect in experimental arthritis [19] although the pathogenic mechanism is still unclear. While no data on the levels of eotaxin-2 in the

FMS are available in the literature, patients with the related chronic fatigue syndrome demonstrate a distinct cytokine/chemokine plasma profile, including elevated levels of eotaxin-2 compared to healthy controls [20].

In order to address the inflammatory status of the FMS cohort and to rule out the possibility that eotaxin-2 levels might represent a nonspecific acute phase reactant, hs-CRP levels were tested. The majority of the FMS cohort had indeed normal levels of hs-CRP. Yet, the mean level of hs-CRP was slightly elevated among the FMS patients, a value considered to represent an increased cardiovascular risk but not a state of acute inflammation. hs-CRP levels did not correlate with eotaxin-2 levels. Consistently, no correlation between hs-CRP and eotaxin-2 levels was found in a healthy and overweight Japanese cohort [21].

In the present study, there was no correlation between hs-CRP and FMS severity measures. Interestingly, a number of studies reported elevated CRP levels in FMS patients [9, 12, 22] though these studies did not examine the hs-CRP levels. In our study, there was a moderately positive correlation between hs-CRP and BMI. In the general population, a positive correlation between elevated BMI, visceral and abdominal subcutaneous adipose tissue, and waist circumference in respect to hs-CRP levels has previously been reported [23]. Thus, increased BMI among the FMS cohort in our study may explain the slightly elevated levels of mean hs-CRP.

No association between eotaxin-2 levels and measures of disease severity were found in the present study, thus not supporting a role for eotaxin-2 as a biomarker of disease severity.

A number of limitations of the current study should be pointed out. While our study focused on eotaxin-2, this chemokine acts in close interaction with a large number of additional mediators, which has not been investigated in the present cohort. Further, hs-CRP levels were measured only in the FMS and not healthy cohort. In view of our findings, it would be intriguing to further scrutinize additional chemokines and to sketch a more extensive map of chemokine aberrations in FMS. Identifying such individual patterns of chemokines expression might eventually lead to more precise characterization of individual patients, ultimately aiding in therapeutically targeting specific chemokines, as a strategy for individualized treatment. Another limitation of the study lies in the relatively limited sample size of patients and controls. Going back to the proposed hypothesis regarding the role of chemokines in a chronic pain related gliopathy, future research may be directed at cross-correlating alterations in chemokine levels (such as found in the current study) with advanced functional imaging techniques which may become available in order to study such a gliopathy [24].

In conclusion, in the current study, serum eotaxin-2 levels were investigated for the first time in FMS patients and found to be significantly increased compared to healthy controls. While eotaxin-2 levels did not correlate with FMS disease severity, this finding calls to search new pathogenetic mechanisms of the syndrome. A study of eotaxin-2 levels in the cerebrospinal fluid in relation to the level of sleep interruption and fatigue intensity may be of interest. Further studies of additional cytokines and especially chemokines are indicated in order to pinpoint a biochemical marker for FMS disease severity, while additional research is also necessary in order to uncover a possible pathogenetic role of eotaxin-2 in FMS and in order to evaluate its potential role as a therapeutic target.

## Authors' Contributions

Victoria Furer and Eyal Hazan equally contributed to this work.

## Acknowledgments

The present article was accepted and published as an abstract at the 2017 American College of Rheumatology Annual Meeting: http://acrabstracts.org/abstract/elevated-levels-of-eotaxin-2-in-serum-of-fibromyalgia-patients/

## References

[1] D. J. Clauw, "Fibromyalgia: a clinical review," *JAMA*, vol. 311, no. 15, pp. 1547–1555, 2014.

[2] F. Wolfe, D. J. Clauw, M. A. Fitzcharles et al., "The American College of Rheumatology preliminary diagnostic criteria for fibromyalgia and measurement of symptom severity," *Arthritis Care and Research*, vol. 62, no. 5, pp. 600–610, 2010.

[3] M. B. Yunus, "Fibromyalgia and overlapping disorders: the unifying concept of central sensitivity syndromes," *Seminars in Arthritis and Rheumatism*, vol. 36, no. 6, pp. 339–356, 2007.

[4] J. J. Garcia, A. Cidoncha, M. E. Bote, M. D. Hinchado, and E. Ortega, "Altered profile of chemokines in fibromyalgia patients," *Annals of Clinical Biochemistry*, vol. 51, no. 5, pp. 576–581, 2014.

[5] G. Ramesh, A. G. MacLean, and M. T. Philipp, "Cytokines and chemokines at the crossroads of neuroinflammation, neurodegeneration, and neuropathic pain," *Mediators of Inflammation*, vol. 2013, Article ID 480739, 20 pages, 2013.

[6] R. J. Miller, H. Jung, S. K. Bhangoo, and F. A. White, "Cytokine and chemokine regulation of sensory neuron function," *Handbook of Experimental Pharmacology*, vol. 194, pp. 417–449, 2009.

[7] E. D. Milligan and L. R. Watkins, "Pathological and protective roles of glia in chronic pain," *Nature Reviews Neuroscience*, vol. 10, no. 1, pp. 23–36, 2009.

[8] R. R. Ji, T. Berta, and M. Nedergaard, "Glia and pain: is chronic pain a gliopathy?," *Pain*, vol. 154, no. 1, pp. S10–S28, 2013.

[9] M. E. Bote, J. J. Garcia, M. D. Hinchado, and E. Ortega, "Inflammatory/stress feedback dysregulation in women with fibromyalgia," *Neuroimmunomodulation*, vol. 19, no. 6, pp. 343–351, 2012.

[10] Z. Zhang, G. Cherryholmes, A. Mao et al., "High plasma levels of MCP-1 and eotaxin provide evidence for an immunological basis of fibromyalgia," *Experimental Biology and Medicine*, vol. 233, no. 9, pp. 1171–1180, 2008.

[11] E. Kosek, R. Altawil, D. Kadetoff et al., "Evidence of different mediators of central inflammation in dysfunctional and inflammatory pain–interleukin-8 in fibromyalgia and interleukin-1 beta in rheumatoid arthritis," *Journal of Neuroimmunology*, vol. 280, pp. 49–55, 2015.

[12] H. Wang, M. Moser, M. Schiltenwolf, and M. Buchner, "Circulating cytokine levels compared to pain in patients with fibromyalgia—a prospective longitudinal study over 6 months," *Journal of Rheumatology*, vol. 35, no. 7, pp. 1366–1370, 2008.

[13] H. Wang, M. Buchner, M. T. Moser, V. Daniel, and M. Schiltenwolf, "The role of IL-8 in patients with fibromyalgia: a prospective longitudinal study of 6 months," *Clinical Journal of Pain*, vol. 25, no. 1, pp. 1–4, 2009.

[14] D. C. Ang, M. N. Moore, J. Hilligoss, and R. Tabbey, "MCP-1 and IL-8 as pain biomarkers in fibromyalgia: a pilot study," *Pain Medicine*, vol. 12, no. 8, pp. 1154–1161, 2011.

[15] M. Kitaura, T. Nakajima, T. Imai et al., "Molecular cloning of human eotaxin, an eosinophil-selective CC chemokine, and identification of a specific eosinophil eotaxin receptor, CC chemokine receptor 3," *Journal of Biological Chemistry*, vol. 271, no. 13, pp. 7725–7730, 1996.

[16] T. Adar, S. Shteingart, A. Ben Ya'acov, A. Bar-Gil Shitrit, and E. Goldin, "From airway inflammation to inflammatory bowel disease: eotaxin-1, a key regulator of intestinal inflammation," *Clinical Immunology*, vol. 153, no. 1, pp. 199–208, 2014.

[17] A. K. Huber, D. A. Giles, B. M. Segal, and D. N. Irani, "An emerging role for eotaxins in neurodegenerative disease," *Clinical Immunology*, vol. 189, pp. 29–33, 2016.

[18] U. Forssmann, M. Uguccioni, P. Loetscher et al., "Eotaxin-2, a novel CC chemokine that is selective for the chemokine receptor CCR3, and acts like eotaxin on human eosinophil and basophil leukocytes," *Journal of Experimental Medicine*, vol. 185, no. 12, pp. 2171–2176, 1997.

[19] J. N. Ablin, M. Entin-Meer, V. Aloush et al., "Protective effect of eotaxin-2 inhibition in adjuvant-induced arthritis," *Clinical and Experimental Rheumatology*, vol. 161, no. 2, pp. 276–283, 2010.

[20] A. Landi, D. Broadhurst, S. D. Vernon, D. L. Tyrrell, and M. Houghton, "Reductions in circulating levels of IL-16, IL-7 and VEGF-A in myalgic encephalomyelitis/chronic fatigue syndrome," *Cytokine*, vol. 78, pp. 27–36, 2016.

[21] I. Hashimoto, J. Wada, A. Hida et al., "Elevated serum monocyte chemoattractant protein-4 and chronic inflammation in overweight subjects," *Obesity*, vol. 14, no. 5, pp. 799–811, 2006.

[22] L. Bazzichi, A. Rossi, G. Massimetti et al., "Cytokine patterns in fibromyalgia and their correlation with clinical manifestations," *Clinical and Experimental Rheumatology*, vol. 25, no. 2, pp. 225–230, 2007.

[23] I. Schlecht, B. Fischer, G. Behrens, and M. F. Leitzmann, "Relations of visceral and abdominal subcutaneous adipose tissue, body mass index, and waist circumference to serum concentrations of parameters of chronic inflammation," *Obesity Facts*, vol. 9, no. 3, pp. 144–157, 2016.

[24] Y. Nakatomi, K. Mizuno, A. Ishii et al., "Neuroinflammation in patients with chronic fatigue syndrome/myalgic encephalomyelitis: an (1)(1)C-(R)-PK11195 PET study," *Journal of Nuclear Medicine*, vol. 55, no. 6, pp. 945–950, 2014.

# 27

# Assessment of the Short-Term Effectiveness of Kinesiotaping and Trigger Points Release Used in Functional Disorders of the Masticatory Muscles

**Danuta Lietz-Kijak,**[1] **Łukasz Kopacz,**[2] **Roman Ardan** ⓘ**,**[3] **Marta Grzegocka,**[2] **and Edward Kijak** ⓘ[4]

[1]*Independent Unit of Propaedeutic and Dental Physical Diagnostics, Faculty of Medicine and Dentistry, Pomeranian Medical University, Rybacka 1, 70-204 Szczecin, Poland*
[2]*Pomeranian Medical University, Rybacka 1, 70-204 Szczecin, Poland*
[3]*Department of Econometrics, Faculty of Economic Sciences, Koszalin University of Technology, Kwiatkowskiego 6e, 75-343 Koszalin, Poland*
[4]*Scientific Unit of Dysfunction of the Masticatory System, Chair and Department of Prosthodontics, Faculty of Medicine and Dentistry, Pomeranian Medical University, Rybacka 1, 70-204 Szczecin, Poland*

Correspondence should be addressed to Edward Kijak; edward.kijak@pum.edu.pl

Academic Editor: Mieszko Wieckiewicz

Chronic face pain syndrome is a diagnostic and therapeutic problem for many specialists, and this proves the interdisciplinary and complex nature of this ailment. Physiotherapy is of particular importance in the treatment of pain syndrome in the course of temporomandibular joint functional disorders. In patients with long-term dysfunction of masticatory muscles, the palpation examination can localize trigger points, that is, thickening in the form of nodules in the size of rice grains or peas. Latent trigger points located in the muscles can interfere with muscular movement patterns, cause cramps, and reduce muscle strength. Because hidden trigger points can spontaneously activate, they should be found and released to prevent further escalation of the discomfort. Kinesiotaping (KT) is considered as an intervention that can be used to release latent myofascial trigger points. It is a method that involves applying specific tapes to the patient's skin in order to take advantage of the natural self-healing processes of the body. The aim of the study was to evaluate the effect of the kinesiotaping method and trigger points inactivation on the nonpharmacological elimination of pain in patients with temporomandibular disorders. The study was conducted in 60 patients (18 to 35 years old). The subjects were randomly divided into two subgroups of 30 people each. Group KT (15 women and 15 men) were subjected to active kinesiotaping application. Group TrP, composed of 16 women and 14 men, was subjected to physiotherapy with the release of trigger points by the ischemic compression method. The results show that the KT method and TrP inactivation brought significant therapeutic analgesic effects in the course of pain-related functional disorders of the muscles of mastication. The more beneficial outcomes of the therapy were observed after using the KT method, which increased the analgesic effect in dysfunctional patients.

## 1. Introduction

Chronic myofascial pain syndrome is a diagnostic and therapeutic problem for many specialists, such as dentists, laryngologists, neurologists, neurosurgeons, general surgeons, anesthetists, psychiatrists, and oncologists [1]. This indicates the interdisciplinary and complex nature of these diseases. The prevalence of dysfunctional pain syndrome is estimated at around 12% of the adult population and 50% of the elderly population; it is more frequent in women between 20 and 40 years of age [2]. The percentage of women with headache associated with temporomandibular dysfunctions reaches up to 15%, and 10% in men [3]. Pain intensity varies from dull to acute. In people gnashing their teeth at night (occlusal parafunction, bruxism), morning pain in the joint and muscles is characteristic; it intensifies while eating and disappears during the day. In people clenching their teeth during the day, the pain may be most intense in the evening [4]. Signs and symptoms associated with temporomandibular dysfunctions include the pathological wear of the teeth as a result of bruxism, increased muscle tone in the masticatory muscles, overgrowth of the masseter, tinnitus, and changes in the psychological profile [5]. Differential diagnosis of pain in the course of temporomandibular dysfunction should exclude other pathologies of the temporomandibular joint, as well as tumours of the zygomatic bone, neoplasms of the nose, mandible, and parapharyngeal area, systemic connective tissue diseases, giant cell arteritis (mandible claudication), cluster headache, and reflex sympathetic dystrophy of the face [6].

The role of occlusal and nonocclusal parafunctions is emphasized potential etiological factors, along with malocclusion, missing teeth in the lateral areas, macro- and microinjuries of the joint, stress leading to hyperactivity of the masticatory muscles, the activation of masticatory muscles by the route descending from the limbic system and reticular formation, the lack of effective contraction of both lateral pterygoid muscles, and rheumatic diseases [7].

The multiple manifestations of the symptoms lead to a multitude of treatment methods and indicate that there is still no consensus in understanding the pathophysiology of the underlying TMD mechanisms. Because of the heterogeneity of the causes, the treatment of pain syndrome in the course of temporomandibular dysfunction should have a multiprofile character [8, 9].

Temporary pain relief can be obtained by pharmacological treatment with nonsteroidal anti-inflammatory drugs. Drugs that reduce muscle tone, antidepressants, and intra-articular steroids are also used. Dental treatment includes the use of, among others, flexible or hard occlusal splints [10–12]. Physiotherapy is of particular importance in the treatment of pain syndrome in the course of temporomandibular joint functional disorders. Positive therapeutic effects are obtained using botuline, laser therapy, heat therapy, light therapy, electrotherapy, electromagnetic field, manual therapy, proprioceptive neuromuscular motion paving, kinesiotherapy, relaxation techniques, autogenic training, and biofeedback to change of parafunctional behaviors [13, 14].

In patients with long-term dysfunction of masticatory muscles, the palpation examination can localize trigger points, that is, thickening in the form of nodules in the size of rice grains or peas. These are muscle fibres with increased tension, felt as thickening in the course of the muscle fibres. Latent trigger points located in the muscles can interfere with muscular movement patterns, cause cramps, and reduce muscle strength. Because hidden trigger points can spontaneously activate, they should be found and released to prevent further escalation of the discomfort [15]. Physiotherapeutic treatment is primarily based on the inactivation of trigger points by various techniques, such as compressive

mobilization, positional release, myofascial relaxation, active relaxation technique, postisometric relaxation technique, or integrated neuromuscular inhibition technique (INIT) [16, 17]. Among the commonly used methods, we should also mention deep tissue massage and passive stretching of the muscles. Kinesiotaping is considered an intervention that can be used to release latent myofascial trigger points. This method involves the use of specific tapes applied to the patient's skin in order to take advantage of the natural self-healing processes of the body. It is very often applied as an element supportive of the therapeutic effect. The action of the method is mainly based on normalizing muscle tension, supporting the work of joints, improving the function of weakened muscles, and increasing microcirculation at the application site [18–20].

## 2. Study Objective

The aim of the study was to evaluate the effect of the kinesiotaping method and trigger points inactivation on the nonpharmacological elimination of pain in patients with temporomandibular disorders.

## 3. Materials and Methods

*3.1. Material: Inclusion and Exclusion Criteria.* The study was conducted during the years 2015-2016 in 60 patients (18 to 35 years old). All qualified patients suffered from painful functional disorders within the masticatory muscles of myofascial characteristic. Patients were also tested by the research diagnostic criteria for temporomandibular disorders (RDC/TMD) introduced by Dworkin and LeResche in 1992 [21]. This enables the standardization of the procedures of epidemiological studies, the unification of TMD diagnostic and exploratory criteria, and the comparison of results of other similar studies. The results of the study were based on the RDC/TMD Axis I diagnostic criteria. All researchers have been trained and calibrated in accordance with the adopted norms presented on the official website of the International RDC/TMD Consortium [22].

The exclusion criteria were as follows: regular drug therapy, mental illness, coagulopathy, diabetes, or chronic infections. The subjects were not addicted to nicotine, alcohol, or drugs. The participants with joint clicking and a clinical diagnosis of disc displacement were also excluded, and they were asked to refrain or not to use self-treatment during the therapy.

The study was approved by the Bioethics Committee of the Pomeranian Medical University in Szczecin (KB–0012/36/15). It is in accordance with ethical standards; all participants signed written informed consent and were acquainted with the technique and the course of the research.

*3.2. Method.* The subjects were randomly divided into two subgroups of 30 people each. Group KT (15 female and 15 male) were subjected to active kinesiotaping application (K-Active Tape Classic, 50 mm × 17 m; Nitto Denko Corporation, Japan) (Figure 1). Subjects undergoing therapy were

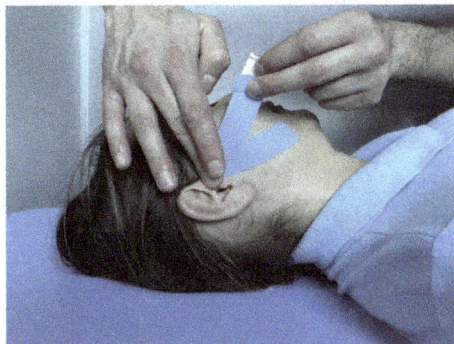

FIGURE 1: The muscular application of KT to the area of the masseter.

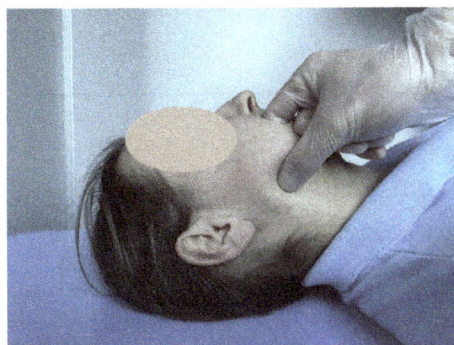

FIGURE 2: The release of TrP by the ischemic compression method.

diagnosed with excessive strain of masseter muscles and muscular pain, without limitations in the movements of the mandible and without disc derangement and joint pain. The muscular application was used for the region of the masseter with a tape (5 cm wide) cut into 2 parts, called tails, which covered the treatment sites without tension. The base was located in the region of the temporomandibular joint. The upper tail ran across the buccal surface of the face towards the nose, while the lower tail was directed towards the chin and thus included the masseter. This type of application raised the surface of the skin, which was translated into a decrease in the tension of the affected area. All participants of the study were obliged to wear the kinesiology tape for a period of 5 days and were advised to carry out everyday activities without unnecessary care.

Group TrP, composed of 16 women and 14 men, was subjected to physiotherapy with the release of trigger points by the ischemic compression method, which was based on applying pressure to the active trigger point until it was switched off, that is, the pain disappeared (Figure 2). Subjects undergoing therapy were diagnosed with excessive strain of masseter muscles and muscular pain, without limitations in the movements of the mandible and without disc derangement and joint pain. The localization of the trigger points, on average 4 on the right and on the left side, was done palpably with the dental arches clenched, using a pliers grip covering the dense tissue inside and outside the cheek with the thumb and index finger. Trigger point therapy was

performed within the upper and lower attachment of the masseter, on the right and left sides. The procedure of de-activation of trigger points was performed three times, on the first, third, and fifth days of therapy.

Before performing the physiotherapeutic procedures in groups KT and TrP and after their application, all patients were subjected to diagnostic actions, including the measurement of pain intensity using the visual analogue scale (VAS). Two dentists were involved in the selection of participants. Only one physiotherapist performed KT applications and TrP therapies. The therapeutic effectiveness of the two methods was verified by comparing the mean values of pain intensity before and after performing the physiotherapeutic procedures. Changes in pain intensity were considered as dependent variable, while the therapy used and patients' gender and age were considered as independent variables.

Prior to the examination, each patient gave written consent to participate in the therapy and was provided with information about the technique and the course of the tests. The protocol was developed in accordance with the latest version of the World Medical Declaration of the Helsinki Association [23]. The patients were also informed about the principle of anonymity of the tests.

## 4. Statistical Analysis

The statistical analysis included determining the physiotherapeutic effects, examining the influence of gender and patient's age on the outcomes, and comparing the analgesic efficacy of the treatment methods. In order to check the efficacy of the therapy, mean pain values were compared before and after performing the procedures. The statistical significance of the change in mean values was verified using the paired sample Welch $t$-test. The linear regression models were also used to examine the influence of gender and age on treatment efficacy.

The hypothesis about greater analgesic efficacy of KT compared to TrP was additionally tested. For this purpose, the mean values of absolute and relative pain intensity changes obtained from two groups of patients were compared using the unpaired sample Welch t-test. (The Welch $t$-test is a generalization of Student's $t$-test for populations with different variances. Significant differences in the value of variance were observed in the measurements taken before and after the treatment, as well as in the comparison of changes after the use of both therapeutic methods.)

## 5. Results

5.1. Physiotherapeutic Effects. The basic statistics of patients' age and measurements for the methods applied in particular groups of patients are summarized in Table 1.

The $t$-test confirms the statistical significance of both therapeutic methods in reducing pain symptoms (Table 2.)

5.2. Comparison of the Analgesic Effect of KT and TrP. In order to compare the analgesic effect of KT and TrP, absolute change in pain level AbsCh was calculated for each

TABLE 1: The basic statistics of patients' age and pain intensity measurements before and after the application of both methods.

| | Method of therapy | | | | | |
|---|---|---|---|---|---|---|
| Characteristic | KT | | | TrP | | |
| | Age (years) | Pain (VAS units) | | Age (years) | Pain (VAS units) | |
| Measurement | | Before | After | | Before | After |
| *All patients* | | | | | | |
| Minimum | 18 | 3 | 1 | 18 | 4 | 2 |
| Maximum | 35 | 10 | 6 | 35 | 9 | 7 |
| Mean | 25.87 | 6.50 | 3.10 | 27.37 | 6.27 | 4.17 |
| SD | 4.86 | 1.74 | 1.35 | 5.08 | 1.41 | 1.36 |
| *Male patients* | | | | | | |
| Minimum | 18 | 4 | 1 | 18 | 4 | 3 |
| Maximum | 32 | 8 | 5 | 35 | 9 | 7 |
| Mean | 26.07 | 5.93 | 2.93 | 28.93 | 6.57 | 4.50 |
| SD | 4.92 | 1.44 | 1.10 | 5.36 | 1.55 | 1.30 |
| *Female patients* | | | | | | |
| Minimum | 19 | 3 | 1 | 19 | 4 | 2 |
| Maximum | 35 | 10 | 6 | 34 | 8 | 6 |
| Mean | 25.67 | 7.06 | 3.27 | 26.00 | 6.00 | 3.88 |
| SD | 4.97 | 1.87 | 1.58 | 4.51 | 1.25 | 1.37 |

KT, kinesiotaping; TrP, trigger point therapy.

TABLE 2: The significance of therapeutic methods' test results.

| Method | Pain (VAS units, mean ± SD) | | $t$-statistic | $p$ value |
|---|---|---|---|---|
| | Before | After | | |
| KT | 6.50 ± 1.74 | 3.10 ± 1.35 | 14.92 | <0.001 |
| TrP | 6.27 ± 1.41 | 4.17 ± 1.36 | 8.23 | <0.001 |

TABLE 3: Comparison of the analgesic effect of KT and TrP results.

| Characteristic | KT Mean ± SD | TrP Mean ± SD | $t$-statistic | $p$ value |
|---|---|---|---|---|
| AbsCh | −3.40 ± 1.24 | −2.10 ± 1.40 | −3.80 | <0.001 |
| RelCh | −0.53 ± 0.15 | −0.32 ± 0.21 | −4.31 | <0.001 |

patient as the difference of measurement after and before treatment. In addition, to account for the different levels of initial pain in the two groups of patients entering therapy, relative change RelCh was also calculated:

$$\text{AbsCh} = \text{pain after} - \text{pain before,}$$

$$\text{RelCh} = \frac{\text{AbsCh}}{\text{pain before}}. \tag{1}$$

Relative change shows what fraction of patient's initial pain was eliminated during treatment.

Although both methods proved to be efficacious, the mean values of the changes after KT and TrP suggest that the KT method gives greater improvement in the reduction of pain. The unpaired sample Welch $t$-test confirms this (Table 3).

*5.3. Study of the Influence of Gender and Patient's Age on Therapeutic Outcomes.* The therapeutic outcomes obtained by using both methods (KT and TrP) in the group of male and female patients were compared by analyzing the mean values of changes using the $t$-test. For both methods, no significant differences were found in the treatment effects between male and female patients.

In the linear regression models, the absolute change in pain intensity was a dependent variable. For both therapy methods, the models with age, gender, and their cross-factor as independent variables were examined. There were no significant variables in any model ($t$-statistic values less than 1).

## 6. Discussion

Face and oral pain syndromes lasting longer than 6 months are a multidisciplinary issue. Close cooperation between neurologists, laryngologist, physiotherapists, psychiatrists, and dentists can help in identifying the causes of these ailments and avoiding the misdiagnosis or false causal relationship. The diagnostic and therapeutic management of facial pain depends on the suspected cause of pain and the accompanying symptoms. It is important to remember that every chronic condition, including pain, causes an impact on the psychological and social status of patients and reduces the quality of life [24].

The study presents cooperation between physiotherapists and dentists by investigating the impact of kinesiotaping and inactivation of trigger points applied to the area of the masseter in the course of functional disorders of the muscles of mastication, with particular emphasis on pain. The original research revealed a significant reduction of pain. The results of the study confirm the observations of other authors who have given special attention to the influence of the kinesiotaping method on the human body.

Youngsook identified changes in myofascial pain and examined the range of movement in the temporomandibular joint after the application of the kinesiotaping method in patients with latent myofascial trigger points within the sternocleidomastoid muscle [25]. He concluded that pain intensity significantly decreased, and the range of motion in the temporomandibular joint considerably increased. Wei-Ting et al. suggest that the KT method can be used as a regular therapy or as a complement to the treatment of myofascial pain [26]. The therapeutic value of the kinesiotaping method in the muscular application is emphasized in the publications of other authors who include this method in the algorithm for treating pain originating from different muscles. Öztürk et al., who used the application of active tapes in patients with myofascial pain syndrome, demonstrated a statistically significant improvement in pain intensity and strength of the upper trapezius muscle [27].

Kalichman et al. described the case of a patient suffering from meralgia paresthetica with symptoms of numbness, paresthesia, and pain in the anterolateral part of the thigh. After using the KT method for 4 weeks, the symptoms significantly regressed and the quality of life improved [28]. Using KT in patients with an acute cervical spine injury, Osterhues showed an immediate decrease in pain intensity in the study group [29].

There are also critical opinions about the use of the kinesiotaping method which we have to take into consideration. Montalvo et al. conducted a meta-analysis of the available literature on KT to assess its efficacy in pain management therapy in patients with musculoskeletal injuries. Articles published between 2003 and 2013 were selected by searching SPORTDiscus, Scopus, ScienceDirect, CINAHL, Cochrane Library, PubMed, and PEDro databases with the terms kinesio tap*, kinesiology tap*, kinesiotap*, and pain. Thirteen articles investigating the effects of kinesiology tape application on pain with at least level II evidence were selected. Combined results of this meta-analysis indicate that KT may have a limited potential to reduce pain in individuals with musculoskeletal injury. The authors suggest using KT in conjunction with or instead of more conventional therapies. However, further research that compares KT to other clinical interventions is needed to evaluate its efficacy [30].

Morris et al. conducted a systematic review of RCTs investigating the use of KT in the management of clinical conditions. A systematic literature search was performed in the following databases: CINAHL, MEDLINE, OVID, AMED, ScienceDirect, PEDro, www.internurse.com, SPORTDiscus, British Nursing Index, www.kinesiotaping.co.uk, www.kinesiotaping.com, Cochrane Central Register of Clinical Trials, and ProQuest.

The review included articles published until April 2012. Evaluation of the risk of bias and the quality of evidence was conducted in accordance with the Cochrane methodology. Eight RCTs met the full inclusion criteria. Six of these included patients with musculoskeletal conditions. There was limited to moderate evidence that KT is no more clinically effective than sham or usual care tape/bandage. There was limited evidence from one moderate quality RCT that KT in conjunction with physiotherapy was clinically beneficial for plantar fasciitis-related pain in the short term. There are, however, serious concerns about the internal validity of this RCT. There is currently insufficient evidence to support the use of KT over other clinical interventions [31].

Parreira et al. conducted a systematic review comparing KT to sham KT. Twelve randomized trials with 495 participants in total were included in the review. The efficacy of KT was assessed in patients with shoulder pain in two trials, knee pain in three trials, chronic low back pain in two trials, neck pain in three trials, plantar fasciitis in one trial, and multiple musculoskeletal conditions in one trial. The methodological quality of the studies that met the inclusion criteria was moderate, with a mean score of 6.1 points on the 10-point PEDro scale. The study found that KT was better than sham KT/placebo and active comparison groups. However, the effect sizes were small and probably not clinically significant or of low quality [32].

In their research, Tremblay and Karam concluded that the application of KT had little effect at the neuromuscular level. The changes in sensory feedback assigned to an elastic tape are probably insufficient to modulate corticospinal excitability in the functional sense [33]. Therefore, more research should be carried out to explain the effectiveness of the KT method in the elimination of TMD-related ailments, which is very difficult due to the need to perform random configurations and double-blind tests. The cosmetic defect caused by sticking active tapes to the skin of the face is also important. Therefore, the analgesic action is local, and its main goal is to enlarge the space between the skin and soft tissues in order to expand the movement space, facilitate the circulation of blood and lymph, and increase the rate of tissue healing, as suggested by Skirven et al. [34].

The pain associated with TMD often reduces the activity of the masticatory muscles. The implementation of the appropriate set of exercises significantly improves the action of analgesic methods and all physical fitness parameters [35]. Because of the multidimensional nature of the problem, patients with musculoskeletal pain of the face should be treated by an interdisciplinary team. There is increasing evidence that psychosocial factors have a significant impact on therapeutic outcomes and may also affect the symptoms reported by patients. Taiminen et al. found that many patients complaining of chronic headache are also diagnosed with a psychiatric or personality disorder that blurs the manifestation of the disease, which considerably affects the treatment [36]. Because a few health care workers believe that they are able to help them on their own and that these people require multidisciplinary treatment, Hals et al. indicate that these patients are often marked as "difficult" [37].

## 7. Conclusions

(1) The methods of kinesiotaping (KT) and TrP inactivation have brought significant analgesic effects to the treatment of painful forms of functional disorders of the masticatory muscles.

(2) The more beneficial results were observed after using the KT method, which increased the analgesic effect in dysfunctional patients.

(3) No influence of gender or patient's age on the treatment results was reported.

(4) There is also a need to develop algorithms for the diagnosis and treatment of oral and facial pain syndromes with a strict definition of the role of dentists and physiotherapists.

# References

[1] M. Pihut, M. Szuta, E. Ferendiuk, and D. Zeńczak-Więckiewicz, "Differential diagnostics of pain in the course of trigeminal neuralgia and temporomandibular joint dysfunction," *BioMed Research International*, vol. 2014, Article ID 563786, 7 pages, 2014.

[2] G. Madland and C. Feinmann, "Chronic facial pain: a multidisciplinary problem," *Journal of Neurology, Neurosurgery, and Psychiatry*, vol. 71, no. 6, pp. 716–719, 2001.

[3] M. N. Janal, K. G. Raphael, S. Nayak, and J. Klausner, "Prevalence of myofascial temporomandibular disorder in US community women," *Journal of Oral Rehabilitation*, vol. 14, no. 11, pp. 801–809, 2008.

[4] M. Więckiewicz, N. Grychowska, K. Wojciechowski et al., "Prevalence and correlation between TMD based on RDC/TMD diagnoses, oral parafunctions and psychoemotional stress in Polish University students," *BioMed Research International*, vol. 2014, Article ID 472346, 7 pages, 2014.

[5] M. Więckiewicz, A. Paradowska-Stolarz, and W. Więckiewicz, "Psychosocial aspects of bruxism: the most paramount factor influencing teeth grinding," *BioMed Research International*, vol. 2014, Article ID 469187, 7 pages, 2014.

[6] W. Więckiewicz, A. Bieniek, M. Więckiewicz, and Ł. Sroczyk, "Interdisciplinary treatment of basal cell carcinoma located on the nose–review of literature," *Advances in Clinical and Experimental Medicine*, vol. 22, no. 2, pp. 289–293, 2013.

[7] R. Ohrbach, R. B. Fillingim, F. Mulkey et al., "Clinical findings and pain symptoms as potential risk factors for chronic TMD: descriptive data and empirically identified domains from the OPPERA case–control study," *Journal of Pain*, vol. 14, no. 11, pp. T27–T45, 2011.

[8] J. C. Nobrega, S. R. Tesseroli de Siquera, and J. T. Tesseroli de Siquera, "Diferential diagnosis in atypical pain: a clinical study," *Arquivos de Neuro-Psiquiatria*, vol. 65, no. 2, pp. 256–261, 2007.

[9] G. Meyer, U. Lotzmann, and B. Koeck, *Pharmacological Treatment and Physiotherapeutic Methods of Muscle Relaxation and Biofeedback*, Urban and Partner, Wrocław, Poland, 1997.

[10] J. C. Türp, F. Komine, and A. Hugger, "Efficacy of stabilization splints for the management of patients with masticatory muscle pain: a qualitative systematic review," *Clinical Oral Investigations*, vol. 8, no. 4, pp. 179–195, 2004.

[11] F. J. Alencar and A. Becker, "Evaluation of different occlusal splints and counselling in the management of myofascial pain dysfunction," *Journal of Oral Rehabilitation*, vol. 36, no. 2, pp. 79–85, 2009.

[12] A. Nekora, G. Evlioglu, A. Ceyhan et al., "Patient responses to vacuum formed splints compared to heat cured acrylic splints: pilot study," *Journal of Maxillofacial and Oral Surgery*, vol. 8, no. 1, pp. 31–33, 2009.

[13] M. Wieckiewicz, K. Boening, P. Wiland, Y. Shiau, and A. Paradowska-Stolarz, "Reported concepts for the treatment modalities and pain management of temporomandibular disorders," *Journal Headache and Pain*, vol. 16, p. 106, 2015.

[14] M. Pihut, E. Ferendiuk, M. Szewczyk, K. Kasprzyk, and M. Wieckiewicz, "The efficiency of botulinum toxin type A for the treatment of masseter muscle pain in patients with temporomandibular joint dysfunction and tension-type headache," *Journal of Headache and Pain*, vol. 17, no. 1, 2016.

[15] M. Mohamadi, S. Piroozi, I. Rashidi, and S. Hosseinifard, "Friction massage versus kinesiotaping for short-term management of latent trigger points in the upper trapezius: a randomized controlled trial," *Chiropractic and Manual Therapies*, vol. 25, no. 1, p. 25, 2017.

[16] R. La Touche, C. Fernandez-De-Las-Penas, J. Fernandez Cornero et al., "The effects of manual therapy and exercise directed at the cervical spine on pain and pressure pain sensitivity in patients with myofascial temporomandibular disorders," *Journal of Oral Rehabilitation*, vol. 36, no. 9, pp. 644–652, 2009.

[17] V. K. Capellini, G. S. de Souza, and C. R. de Faria, "Massage therapy in the management of myogenic TMD: a pilot study," *Journal of Applied Oral Science*, vol. 14, no. 1, pp. 21–26, 2006.

[18] M. Mostafavifar, J. Wertz, and J. Borchers, "A systemic review of the effectiveness of Kinesio taping for musculoskeletal injury," *Physician and Sportsmedicine*, vol. 40, no. 4, pp. 33–40, 2012.

[19] E. Kaya, M. Zinnuroglu, and I. Tugcu, "Kinesio taping compared to physical therapy modalities for the treatment shoulder impingement syndrome," *Clinical Rheumatology*, vol. 30, no. 2, pp. 201–207, 2011.

[20] K. Kase, J. Wallis, and T. Kase, *Clinical Therapeutic Applications of the Kinesio Taping Method*, Kinesio Taping Association International, Albuquerque, NM, USA, 2013.

[21] S. F. Dworkin and L. LeResche, "Research diagnostic criteria for temporomandibular disorders: review, criteria, examinations and specifications, critique," *Journal of Craniomandibular and Sleep Practice*, vol. 6, no. 4, pp. 301–355, 1992.

[22] E. Schiffman, R. Ohrbach, E. Truelove et al., "Diagnostic criteria for temporomandibular disorders (DC/TMD) for clinical and research applications: recommendations of the International RDC/TMD Consortium Network and Orofacial Pain Special Interest," *Journal Oral Facial Pain Headache*, vol. 28, no. 1, pp. 6–27, 2014.

[23] World Medical Association (WMA), "World Medical Association Declaration of Helsinki: ethical principles for medical research involving human subjects," *Journal of the American Dental Association*, vol. 310, pp. 2191–2194, 2013.

[24] C. Tassorelli, M. Tramontano, M. Berlangieri et al., "Assessing and treating primary headaches and cranio-facial pain in patients undergoing rehabilitation for neurological diseases," *Journal of Headache and Pain*, vol. 18, no. 1, p. 99, 2017.

[25] B. Youngsook, "Change the myofascial pain and range of motion of the temporomandibular joint following kinesio taping of latent myofascial trigger points in the sternocleidomastoid muscle," *Journal of Physical Therapy Science*, vol. 26, no. 9, pp. 1321–1324, 2014.

[26] W. Wei-Ting, H. Chang-Zern, and C. Li-Wei, "The kinesio taping method for myofascial pain control," *Evidence-Based Complementary and Alternative Medicine*, vol. 2015, Article ID 950519, 9 pages, 2015.

[27] G. Öztürk, D. G. Külcü, N. Mesci, A. D. Şilte, and E. Aydog, "Efficacy of kinesio tape application on pain and muscle strength in patients with myofascial pain syndrome: a placebo-controlled trial," *Journal of Physical Therapy Science*, vol. 28, no. 4, pp. 1074–1079, 2016.

[28] L. Kalichman, E. Vered, and L. Volchek, "Relieving symptoms of meralgia paresthetica using kinesio taping: a pilot study," *Archives of Physical Medicine and Rehabilitation*, vol. 91, no. 7, pp. 1137–1139, 2010.

[29] D. J. Osterhues, "The use of Kinesio Taping in the management of traumatic patella dislocation. A case study," *Physiotherapy Theory and Practice*, vol. 20, no. 4, pp. 267–270, 2004.

[30] A. M. Montalvo, E. L. Cara, and G. D. Myer, "Effect of kinesiology taping on pain in individuals with musculoskeletal injuries: systematic review and meta-analysis," *Physician and Sports Medicine*, vol. 42, no. 2, pp. 48–57, 2014.

[31] D. Morris, D. Jones, H. Ryan, and C. G. Ryan, "The clinical effects of Kinesio Tex taping: a systematic review," *Physiotherapy theory and practice*, vol. 29, no. 4, pp. 259–70, 2013.

[32] P. do Carmo Silva Parreira, L. da Cunha Menezes Costa, L. C. Hespanhol, A. D. Lopes, and L. O. P. Costa, "Current evidence does not support the use of Kinesio Taping in clinical practice: a systematic review," *Journal of Physiotherapy*, vol. 60, no. 1, pp. 31–39, 2014.

[33] F. Tremblay and S. Karam, "Kinesio-taping application and corticospinal excitability at the ankle joint," *Journal of Athletic Training*, vol. 50, no. 8, pp. 840–846, 2015.

[34] T. M. Skirven, A. L. Osterman, J. M. Fedorczyk, and P. C. Amadio, "Rehabilitation of the hand and upper extremity," *Elastic Taping*, vol. 6, pp. 1529–1538, 2011.

[35] E. Kijak, D. Lietz-Kijak, Z. Śliwiński, and B. Frączak, "Muscle activity in the course of rehabilitation of masticatory motor system functional disorders," *Advances in Hygiene and Experimental Medicine*, vol. 67, pp. 507–516, 2013.

[36] T. Taiminen, L. Kuusalo, L. Lehtinen et al., "Psychiatric (axis 1) and personality (axis 11) disorders in patients with burning mouth syndrome or atypical facial pain," *Scandinavian Journal of Pain*, vol. 2, no. 4, pp. 155–160, 2011.

[37] E. K. B. Hals and A. Stubhaug, "Mental and somatic comorbidities in chronic orofacial pain conditions: pain patients in need of multiprofessional team approach," *Scandinavian Journal of Pain*, vol. 14, no. 4, pp. 153-154, 2011.

# 28

# The Influence of Expectation on Nondeceptive Placebo and Nocebo Effects

Hua Wei [iD],[1,2,3] Lili Zhou [iD],[1,2] Huijuan Zhang [iD],[1,2,3] Jie Chen [iD],[4] Xuejing Lu [iD],[1,2] and Li Hu [iD][1,2,3,4]

[1]CAS Key Laboratory of Mental Health, Institute of Psychology, Beijing, China
[2]Department of Psychology, University of Chinese Academy of Sciences, Beijing, China
[3]Faculty of Psychology, Southwest University, Chongqing, China
[4]Cognition and Human Behavior Key Laboratory of Hunan Province, Hunan Normal University, Changsha, Hunan, China

Correspondence should be addressed to Jie Chen; xlxchen@163.com and Xuejing Lu; luxj@psych.ac.cn

Hua Wei and Lili Zhou contributed equally to this work.

Academic Editor: Filippo Brighina

Nondeceptive placebo has demonstrated its efficiency in clinical practice. Although the underlying mechanisms are still unclear, nondeceptive placebo effect and nondeceptive nocebo effect may be mediated by expectation. To examine the extent to which expectation influences these effects, the present study compared nondeceptive placebo and nocebo effects with different expectation levels. Seventy-two healthy female participants underwent a standard conditioning procedure to establish placebo and nocebo effects. Sequentially, participants were randomized to one of the four experimental groups—baseline (BL), no expectation intervention (NoEI), expectation increasing (EI), and expectation decreasing (ED) groups, to receive either no intervention or interventions through different verbal suggestions that modulated their expectation. Placebo and nocebo effects were established in all four groups after the conditioning phase. However, after disclosing the placebo and nocebo, the analgesic and the hyperalgesic effects only persisted in the EI group, when compared with the BL group. Our results provide evidence highlighting the critical role of increased expectation in nondeceptive placebo and nocebo effects. The finding suggests that open-label placebo or nocebo per se might be insufficient to induce strong analgesic or hyperalgesic response and sheds insights into administrating open-label placebo and avoiding open-label nocebo in clinical practice.

## 1. Introduction

Placebo effect is a psychobiological effect that occurs following the administration of a placebo, that is, an inert treatment [1]. In most studies, a sham substance or sham equipment was administrated deceptively to induce individual's expectation of placebo, promoting the treatments for pain, motor disorders, anxiety, depression, and other diseases [1–6]. Given that disclosing the placebo may reduce the individuals' expectation on positive treatments or interventions, deceptively administrating placebo is considered as a standard approach to ensure that the positive expectation can be established [7]. On the other hand, open-label placebo is being paid close attention to in practice, given its nondeceptive nature [8, 9]. It has been demonstrated that open-label placebo accompanied with positive verbal suggestion and/or a context of supportive patient-practitioner relationship alters pain perception in patients with irritable bowel syndrome (IBS) or chronic low back pain [10, 11]. In addition, once individuals have experienced the pain reduction after receiving a placebo, the disclosure of the placebo would not lead to a failure of the placebo effect [12, 13].

Why placebo treatment is still effective even when the people have known that the treatment is inert? One plausible explanation is that verbal suggestion, supportive patient-practitioner relationship, and conditioning procedure induce additional expectation on the efficacy of the placebo, therefore mediating the effect [2, 4, 14, 15]. However, the extent to which expectation influences the nondeceptive placebo effect is still unclear. If one's expectation underlies the efficacy of placebos, one would expect a reduction or even an elimination of the placebo effect after revealing the nature of the placebo without increased expectation intervention. In other words, an increased expectation of open-label placebo may contribute to the placebo effect, while a decreased expectation may further reduce the effect.

To test this hypothesis, in the present study, different expectation interventions (i.e., no expectation, increasing expectation, and decreasing expectation) were administrated accompanied with the disclosure of the placebo after the participants have experienced the placebo effect. In addition, given that an administration of placebos may not be only lead to placebo effect but also result in nocebo effect [16, 17], a negative response to the treatment [4, 17, 18], the examinations on how expectation interventions influence the nocebo effect were also included to provide insights into the avoidance of the nocebo effect via expectation modulation.

## 2. Methods

*2.1. Participants.* A total of 76 healthy (mean age = 20.89 ± 1.34 years; ranging from 18 to 24 years) volunteers were recruited from the Southwest University, China. Only right-handed female volunteers were recruited in the present study to rule out the possible confounding factors of handedness and gender [19, 20]. None reported with cardiovascular or neurological diseases, family or personal history of psychiatric disorders, acute or chronic pain, color blindness, current use of any medication, or contraindications of electrical stimulation. To avoid confounding effects on pain perception, they were further instructed not to consume products containing caffeine, nicotine, or alcohol 24 h before the experiment [21, 22]. Four participants who were unable to discriminate the distinct levels of electrical pain stimuli used in the conditioning phase were excluded from further investigation. Upon arrival, the Chinese versions of the State-Trait Anxiety Inventory (STAI) [23] were adopted to assess the anxiety state (STAI-S) and anxiety trait (STAI-T), respectively, in all participants. All participants gave their written consents and were informed of their rights to discontinue participation at any time. They were informed that the study aimed at examining the effect of *subliminal electric stimulus equipment* for pain modulation. The experiment procedure was approved by the Ethics Committee of the Southwest University and carried out in accordance with the approved guidelines. This trial is registered with ChiCTR1800014737.

*2.2. Pain Induction.* The painful stimuli were delivered to the inner side of the left forearm through three stainless steel concentric bipolar needle electrodes connected to a constant current stimulator (model DS7A, Digitimer Ltd, Hertfordshire, UK). Each electrode consisted of a needle cathode (length: 0.1 mm, diameter: 0.2 mm) surrounded by a cylindrical anode (diameter: 1.4 mm). All electrodes were located according to

an equilateral triangle shape on the inner side of the left forearm, which has been proved to preferentially activate Aδ nociceptive fibers in the superficial skin layers [24–27]. The method of limits (an ascending series of stimuli in steps of 0.1 mA were delivered starting from subtactile threshold until pain sensation was induced) was used to identify the stimulus intensity that would elicit individual pain experience [28]. Each stimulus (mean intensity = 1.21 ± 0.50 mA across all participants) consisted of several succeeding constant current, square wave pulses (2 pulses for low pain, 10 pulses for moderate pain, and 20 pulses for high pain, resp.), with 50 Hz frequency. Before the formal experiment, participants were familiarized with a series of electrical pain stimuli.

*2.3. Procedures.* The experiment consisted of two phases: a conditioning phase and a test phase, with a 10 min break set between the two phases. During the whole procedure, participants wore a sham subliminal electric stimulus equipment on the middle finger of their left hand.

Participants were sitting approximately 60 cm from a 19-inch monitor (display resolution: $1440 \times 900$ pixels). As shown in Figure 1, in the conditioning phase, each trial started with a 3 s white fixation cross centered on the screen with black background. Sequentially, a solid circle (diameter: 2 cm), which was red, white, or green in color, was presented on the screen for 1 s. All participants were told that the visual cue in a certain color was associated with a certain effect (hyperalgesic effect, no effect, or analgesic effect) caused by the equipment. To rule out possible confounding effect related to color itself, half of the participants for each group were informed that the green cue was associated with an analgesic effect of the equipment with low-frequency current, the red cue was linked to a hyperalgesic effect of the equipment with high-frequency current, and white cue suggested a deactivation of the equipment. The other half were told the associations between the green cue and a hyperalgesic effect and between the red cue and an analgesic effect. Two seconds after the visual cue disappeared from the screen, a pain stimulus was delivered to the left forearm at low, moderate, or high level to ensure the analgesic and the hyperalgesic effects were established accordingly. Participants were required to verbally rate the perceived pain intensity 2 s later on a 11-point numeric rating scale (0 = no pain at all; 10 = unbearable pain) within 6 s. The interval between trials varied from 8 s to 12 s. This phase consisted of two sessions, Conditioning 1 and Conditioning 2, separated by a 3 min interval. There were 30 trials for each session, with 10 trials for each association between the visual cue and pain stimulus. The sequence of visual cues (red, white, or green) paired with different pain levels (defined as low/moderate/high pain cues, resp.) were counterbalanced across all participants.

For the test phase, the procedure was identical to that in the conditioning phase, except that the intensity of pain stimulus was set at the moderate level (i.e., the intensity associated with the white cue in the conditioning phase) in accordance with a previously described paradigm [29]. To reduce the possible effect of habituation/sensory adaption on placebo/nocebo responses [30, 31], two sessions of 24 trials

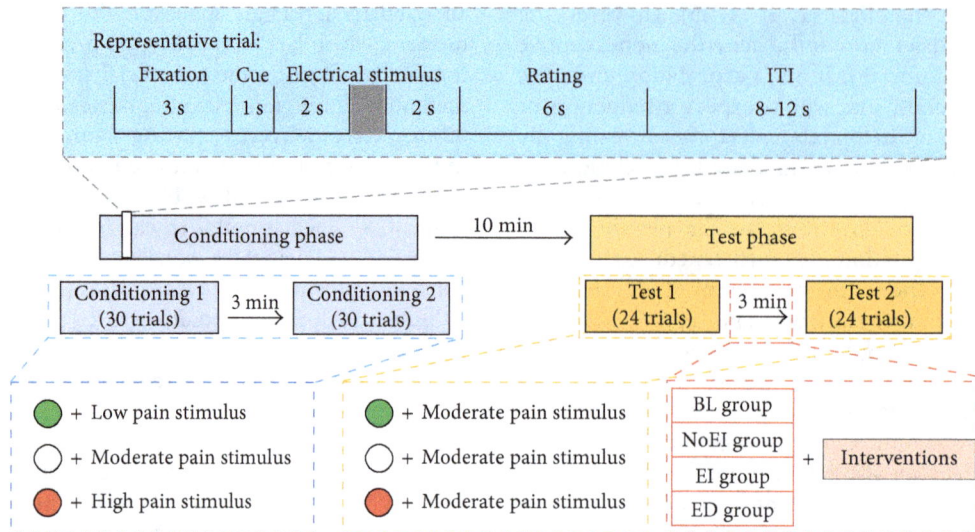

FIGURE 1: Experimental design. The experiment consisted of two phases: conditioning phase and test phase, separated by a 10 min break. In the conditioning phase, each trial started with a 3 s fixation. Sequentially, a 1 s visual cue was displayed. All participants were told that the visual cue in a certain color was associated with a certain effect (hyperalgesic effect, no effect, or analgesic effect) caused by the equipment. Two seconds after the disappearance of the visual cue, an electrical stimulus was delivered to the participants. Following by a 2 s gap, participants were asked to rate the perceived pain intensity within 6 s. The interval between trials varied from 8 to 12 s. Two sessions of 30 trials were included in the conditioning phase, separately by 3 min blank. In the test phase, the procedure was identical to that in the conditioning phase, except that (1) each session consisted of 24 trials and (2) all visual cues were associated with a moderate pain stimulus. After Test 1, different interventions were given to the four groups.

for each (rather than 30 trials) were included in the test phase, with eight trials for each color of visual cues.

After Test 1, each participant was randomized into one of the four different experimental groups: baseline (BL) group ($N = 18$), no expectation intervention (NoEI) group ($N = 18$), expectation increasing (EI) group ($N = 18$), and expectation decreasing (ED) group ($N = 18$) to receive different interventions as follows:

(1) Participants in the BL group were given no intervention.

(2) Participants in the NoEI group were told that the subliminal electric stimulus equipment had been closed in Test 1, and the change of pain ratings reflected their placebo and nocebo responses. In the following Test 2, the subliminal electric stimulation equipment would still be closed.

(3) Participants in the EI group were told the same instruction as those in the NoEI group, except that they were further told that previous studies indicate that the nondeceptive placebo/nocebo can also change the pain perception.

(4) Participants in the ED group were told the same instruction as those in the NoEI group, except that they were further told that previous studies indicated that the placebo/nocebo responses would vanish after the placebo/nocebo has been disclosed.

*2.4. Statistical Analysis.* To compare the characteristics of participants in different experimental groups, we performed one-way analysis of variance (ANOVA) on (1) age, (2) anxiety state (STAI-S), and (3) anxiety trait (STAI-T) using "Group" (BL, NoEI, EI, and ED) as a between-subject factor.

To exclude the difference of pain ratings among groups in the conditioning phase, a two-way repeated measures ANOVA was conducted on the pain ratings, using "Cue type" (low, moderate, and high pain cues) as a within-subject factor and "Group" (BL, NoEI, EI, and ED) as a between-subject factor. To correct the violation of the assumption of sphericity, either the Huynh–Feldt correction (when epsilon > 0.75) or Greenhouse–Geisse correction was applied (when epsilon < 0.75) [32]. Multiple comparisons were adjusted by using the Bonferroni correction, when necessary (the same hereinafter).

To assess whether placebo and nocebo effects were induced successfully, a two-way repeated measures ANOVA was conducted on the pain ratings for Test 1, using "Cue type" (low, moderate, and high pain cues) as a within-subject factor and "Group" (BL, NoEI, EI, and ED) as a between-subject factor.

The decrease of perceived pain intensity, an index of the placebo effect, was obtained by subtracting the ratings paired with low pain cue from those paired with moderate pain cue; the increase of perceived pain intensity, an index of the nocebo effect, was obtained by subtracting the ratings paired with moderate pain cue from those paired with high pain cue. To assess the influence of different interventions on placebo and nocebo effects, we performed two-way repeated measures ANOVA on the placebo effect and nocebo effect, respectively, using "Test" (Test 1 and

Test 2) as a within-subject factor and "Group" as a between-subject factor.

In addition, paired-sample $t$ tests were performed across groups in Test 1 and Test 2, respectively, to verify the difference between the placebo effect and the nocebo effect.

## 3. Results

*3.1. Participant Characteristics.* Participant characteristics for each experimental group are summarized in Table 1. Results of one-way ANOVA indicated that participant characteristics were not significantly different across groups (age: $F(3, 68) = 1.96$, $P = 0.13$, $\eta_p^2 = 0.08$; STAI-S: $F(3, 68) = 0.64$, $P = 0.59$, $\eta_p^2 = 0.03$; STAI-T: $F(3, 68) = 0.03$, $P = 0.99$, $\eta_p^2 = 0.001$), thus avoiding possible bias due to individual differences when assessing the placebo and nocebo effects.

*3.2. No Difference of Pain Ratings in the Conditioning Phase.* Two-way repeated measures ANOVA revealed that pain ratings in the conditioning phase were significantly modulated by the main effect of "Cue type" ($F(1.65, 112.02) = 1171.98$, $P < 0.001$, $\eta_p^2 = 0.95$) but not by the main effect of "Group" ($F(3, 68) = 0.23$, $P = 0.88$, $\eta_p^2 = 0.01$), and the interaction of the two factors ($F(6, 136) = 0.68$, $P = 0.66$, $\eta_p^2 = 0.006$) (Table 2). This observation indicated that there was no difference in pain ratings among groups in the conditioning phase.

*3.3. The Induction of Placebo and Nocebo Effects.* To ensure successful inductions of placebo and nocebo effects, a two-way repeated measures ANOVA was conducted on the pain ratings for Test 1. A significant main effect of "Cue type" was found ($F(1.13, 76.76) = 126.23$, $P < 0.001$, $\eta_p^2 = 0.65$) with nonsignificant interaction between "Cue type" and "Group" ($F(6, 136) = 0.15$, $P = 0.99$, $\eta_p^2 = 0.006$). As shown in Table 3, participants reported highest pain scores when the stimuli were presented with high pain cues and lowest pain scores when the stimuli were presented with low pain cues (all $P < 0.001$), indicating the placebo and nocebo effects were induced successfully. This pattern was consistent across groups, as no significant main effect of "Group" was found ($F(3, 68) = 2.11$, $P = 0.11$, $\eta_p^2 = 0.09$).

*3.4. The Influence of Expectation on Nondeceptive Placebo and Nocebo Effects.* A two-way repeated measures ANOVA on the placebo effect showed that a significant main effect of "Test" ($F(1, 68) = 46.74$, $P < 0.001$, $\eta_p^2 = 0.41$) and a significant interaction between "Test" and "Group" ($F(3, 68) = 3.04$, $P = 0.04$, $\eta_p^2 = 0.12$). As can be seen in Figure 2 and Table 4, post hoc analyses showed that participants who underwent no intervention (i.e., BL group) showed comparable placebo effect in Test 1 and Test 2 ($P = 0.22$). Participants in the NoEI, EI, and ED groups, on the other hand, showed smaller placebo effect (but still significant when compared with "0" to demonstrate the existence of the placebo effect; all $T(17) > 2.79$ and all $P < 0.05$) in Test 2 when compared with Test 1

TABLE 1: Characteristics of participants in each experimental group.

| Group | N | Age | STAI-S | STAI-T |
|---|---|---|---|---|
| BL | 18 | $21.06 \pm 1.83$ | $39.72 \pm 9.43$ | $41.72 \pm 5.80$ |
| NoEI | 18 | $21.00 \pm 1.45$ | $37.72 \pm 8.01$ | $42.33 \pm 8.04$ |
| EI | 18 | $21.50 \pm 1.62$ | $36.28 \pm 3.98$ | $42.17 \pm 6.34$ |
| ED | 18 | $21.28 \pm 1.60$ | $37.83 \pm 7.46$ | $42.28 \pm 6.73$ |

Data are expressed as mean ± standard deviation. N: number of participants; STAI-S: state subscale of State-Trait Anxiety Inventory; STAI-T: trait subscale of State-Trait Anxiety Inventory.

TABLE 2: Pain ratings of each experimental group in the conditioning phase.

| Group | Pain ratings in conditioning phase | | |
|---|---|---|---|
| | Low pain cue | Moderate pain cue | High pain cue |
| BL | $1.18 \pm 0.66$ | $4.38 \pm 1.15$ | $7.22 \pm 1.27$ |
| NoEI | $1.10 \pm 0.77$ | $3.83 \pm 0.93$ | $7.26 \pm 1.23$ |
| EI | $1.07 \pm 0.55$ | $4.07 \pm 0.93$ | $7.23 \pm 1.06$ |
| ED | $1.17 \pm 0.51$ | $4.16 \pm 0.97$ | $7.05 \pm 1.11$ |

Data are expressed as mean ± standard deviation.

TABLE 3: Pain ratings of each experimental group in Test 1.

| Group | Pain ratings in Test 1 | | |
|---|---|---|---|
| | Low pain cue | Moderate pain cue | High pain cue |
| BL | $4.43 \pm 1.59$ | $5.65 \pm 1.36$ | $6.86 \pm 1.62$ |
| NoEI | $3.43 \pm 1.47$ | $4.62 \pm 1.29$ | $5.77 \pm 1.77$ |
| EI | $3.48 \pm 1.37$ | $4.93 \pm 1.38$ | $6.14 \pm 1.74$ |
| ED | $3.27 \pm 1.88$ | $4.63 \pm 1.75$ | $5.92 \pm 2.16$ |

Data are expressed as mean ± standard deviation.

(all $P < 0.003$). More importantly, NoEI and ED interventions but not EI interventions were more likely to reduce the placebo effect established in Test 1 when compared to the baseline (both $P < 0.05$). No other significant effects were found.

Similar to the results of the placebo effect, the analysis of the nocebo effect showed a significant main effect of "Test" ($F(1, 68) = 40.37$, $P < 0.001$, $\eta_p^2 = 0.37$), along with a significant interaction between "Test" and "Group" ($F(3, 68) = 7.93$, $P < 0.001$, $\eta_p^2 = 0.26$). As can be seen in Figure 2 and Table 4, post hoc pairwise comparisons showed that the nocebo effect was smaller for the NoEI group (but still significant when compared with "0" to demonstrate the existence of the nocebo effect, $T(17) = 2.96$, $P = 0.009$) and disappeared for the ED group (not significant when compared with "0" to show the disappearance of the nocebo effect, $T(17) = -0.18$, $P = 0.86$) in Test 2 in comparison to Test 1 (all $P < 0.001$). Furthermore, the nocebo effect was less affected in the BL and EI groups than in the NoEI and ED groups in Test 2 (all $P < 0.05$, except the $P$ value for the comparison between the BL and NoEI groups was 0.06). No other significant effects were found.

*3.5. The Comparison between Placebo and Nocebo Effects.* There were no significant difference between the placebo effect and nocebo effect for each group in Test 1 (BL

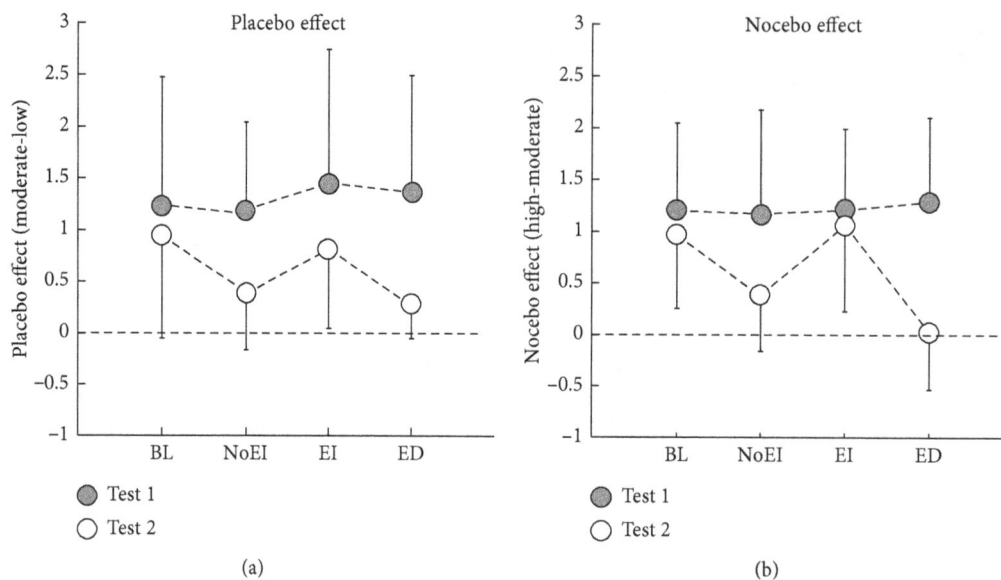

FIGURE 2: Placebo effect (a) and nocebo effect (b) in Test 1 and Test 2. Error bars indicate one standard deviation, and data from participants in Test 1 and Test 2 are marked in solid and hollow circles, respectively.

group: $T(17) = 0.02$, $P = 0.99$; NoEI group: $T(17) = 0.22$, $P = 0.83$; EI group: $T(17) = 1.12$, $P = 0.28$; ED group: $T(17) = 0.44$, $P = 0.67$) and in Test 2 (BL group: $T(17) = -0.07$, $P = 0.95$; NoEI group: $T(17) = -0.35$, $P = 0.73$; EI group: $T(17) = -1.94$, $P = 0.07$; ED group: $T(17) = 1.53$, $P = 0.14$).

## 4. Discussion

The aim of the present study was to investigate the extent to which expectation affects nondeceptive placebo and nocebo effects. To this end, all participants first underwent a conditioning phase, where after associations between pain stimuli and visual cues were established, as reflected by the placebo and nocebo effects in Test 1. Sequentially, participants were assigned to one of the four experimental groups (i.e., BL, NoEI, EI, and ED) to receive no intervention or different verbal interventions that modulated their expectation of the upcoming pain stimuli in Test 2.

Three main findings emerged in the present study. First, when revealing that the treatment in Test 1 was a placebo, the placebo effect persisted only in the group with increased expectation on the placebo, when compared with the baseline. In contrast, the placebo effect was significantly reduced in groups with decreased or no expectation in compared to that in the BL group. Second, results on the nocebo effect yielded to similar pattern, where the disclosure of the nocebo has neither hindered nor reduced the nocebo effect if expectation increasing intervention was introduced, but it reduced when no expectation was administered and disappeared when decreasing expectation intervention was administered. Third, no difference on effect size between nondeceptive placebo and nocebo effects was found for all groups.

One major finding of the present study is that non-deceptive placebo effect only persisted when individuals

TABLE 4: Placebo and nocebo effects of each experimental group in the test phase.

| Group | Test 1 | | Test 2 | |
|---|---|---|---|---|
| | Placebo effect | Nocebo effect | Placebo effect | Nocebo effect |
| BL | $1.22 \pm 1.25$ | $1.22 \pm 0.83$ | $0.96 \pm 1.02$ | $0.98 \pm 0.73$ |
| NoEI | $1.18 \pm 0.85$ | $1.15 \pm 1.02$ | $0.33 \pm 0.50$ | $0.38 \pm 0.54$ |
| EI | $1.45 \pm 1.29$ | $1.20 \pm 0.78$ | $0.81 \pm 0.77$ | $1.08 \pm 0.86$ |
| ED | $1.36 \pm 1.13$ | $1.29 \pm 0.81$ | $0.23 \pm 0.28$ | $-0.02 \pm 0.51$ |

Data are expressed as mean $\pm$ standard deviation.

were administered with expectation increasing intervention. This observation is partly inconsistent with previous studies showing that nondeceptive placebo treatments could lower participants' disease symptoms and pain perception [10–12], as reduced nondeceptive placebo effects were found in groups with decreased and no expectation intervention when compared with the baseline. It is possible because the claim on effectiveness of nondeceptive placebo is usually based on the manipulations that only positive verbal suggestion was given to participants as open-label placebo (e.g., Carvalho et al.'s study) or the disclosure of placebo just happens after participants have experienced the analgesic effect (e.g., Schafer et al.'s study), which contributes to the placebo effect [33–35]. In other words, different from the present study, the previous studies did not compare situations with increased, decreased, and/or no expectation of placebo effect. From this perspective, our finding extends our current understanding of nondeceptive placebo effect by emphasizing the important role of expectation in the process.

Indeed, it has been proved that expectation is one of the main underlying psychological mechanisms of the placebo effect [3, 4, 36–39]. To evaluate the relationship between expectation and nondeceptive placebo effect, we altered participants' expectation on the effectiveness of placebo by administrating different verbal suggestions. Verbal suggestion is widely used as an approach of expectation modulation. For example, healthy individuals' pain tolerance is increased after receiving suggestion of analgesic placebo given verbally [4]. Verbal suggestion can also change patients' expectations and mediate placebo effects in many diseases [1], such as Parkinson's disease [40], and clinical pain [41, 42].

The modulation of expectation can also affect nondeceptive nocebo effect. For our sample, the disclosure of the nocebo eliminated the established nocebo effect for those receiving decreased intervention and reduced the nondeceptive nocebo effect for those with no expectation intervention but not for those with expectation increasing intervention. It is possible because increased expectation of the upcoming treatments not only leads to the placebo effect but also leads to perceived side effects [4]. In other words, the manipulation on expectation increased group made those participants to believe that they would experience similar placebo and nocebo effects as in deceptive condition (i.e., Test 1). This finding is in good agreement with a recent study suggesting that individuals with higher-priced treatment (usually leads to higher expectation) tend to exhibit stronger nocebo effect [43]. In contrast, for those participants with no or decreased expectation on the nocebo, the disclosure of nocebo may arouse their suspicions of the treatment, thus reducing participants' expectation of nocebo. In brief, compared with nondeceptive placebo effect, nondeceptive nocebo effect might be more susceptible to verbal suggestion.

Deceptive placebo and nocebo are widely administrated in double-blinded experimental settings to evaluate the effectiveness of the target manipulation (e.g., administration of inert substance or sham treatment) without conscious deception [7, 44]. Typically, individuals are induced to believe that the inert substance or sham treatment is effective [44, 45]. Although such a placebo has been widely used in clinical practice [8, 9], giving a placebo intervention deceptively as a treatment is totally unacceptable in some cases [44, 46]. From this perspective, open-label placebos should be used when individuals have positive expectation of the treatment [8, 9, 47]. However, as the efficacy of the placebo may decrease after disclosure, how to maintain or improve the effectiveness of placebos without deception in various clinical situations needs to be further studied.

In addition, side effects caused by nondeceptive placebo and nocebo should be taken into consideration seriously in clinical practice. As previous findings suggested, individuals with increased expectation of the treatment may also show increased nocebo effect [16, 43, 48]. Therefore, when disclosing of pharmacological properties of the drug and possible side effect in the informed consent, there is a risk that it may cause patient's suspicion of the drug effectiveness, resulting in negative response to the treatment [17, 49, 50]. To avoid it, sufficient and rational explanation of the potential side effects is needed.

## 5. Conclusion

The present study provides experimental evidence showing that deception is not necessary to achieve a placebo response [9]. Open-label placebo with positive verbal intervention (i.e., increased expectation) can also alter one's pain perception. In addition, to our knowledge, it is the first study to demonstrate that the modulation of expectation can also affect nondeceptive nocebo effect, which provides an alternative way to avoid side effects of placebo treatment or medical therapy. Overall, our study demonstrated that expectation plays a vital role in nondeceptive placebo and nocebo effects, which calls for future studies focusing on translating the present experimental findings into clinical practice settings.

## Authors' Contributions

Hua Wei, Huijuan Zhang, and Li Hu conceived and designed the experiments. Hua Wei performed the experiments. Hua Wei, Lili Zhou, Xuejing Lu, and Li Hu analysed the data. Hua Wei, Lili Zhou, Jie Chen, Xuejing Lu, and Li Hu wrote the paper. Hua Wei and Lili Zhou contributed equally to this work.

## Acknowledgments

This work was supported by the National Natural Science Foundation of China (nos 31471082, 31671141, 31701000, and 31771240), Chongqing Research Program of Basic Research and Frontier Technology (no. cstc2015jcyjBX0050), the Scientific Foundation Project of Institute of Psychology, Chinese Academy of Sciences (nos Y6CX021008 and Y6CX281007), and Cognition and Human Behavior Key Laboratory of Hunan Province, Hunan Normal University (CBL201605). The funders had no role in study design, data collection and analysis, decision to publish, or preparation of the manuscript.

## References

[1] F. Benedetti, "Mechanisms of placebo and placebo-related effects across diseases and treatments," *Annual Review of Pharmacology and Toxicology*, vol. 48, no. 1, pp. 33–60, 2008.

[2] P. Enck, U. Bingel, M. Schedlowski, and W. Rief, "The placebo response in medicine: minimize, maximize or personalize?," *Nature Reviews Drug Discovery*, vol. 12, no. 3, pp. 191–204, 2013.

[3] U. Bingel, V. Wanigasekera, K. Wiech et al., "The effect of treatment expectation on drug efficacy: imaging the analgesic benefit of the opioid remifentanil," *Science Translational Medicine*, vol. 3, no. 70, p. 70ra14, 2011.

[4] F. Benedetti, A. Pollo, L. Lopiano, M. Lanotte, S. Vighetti, and I. Rainero, "Conscious expectation and unconscious conditioning in analgesic, motor, and hormonal placebo/nocebo responses," *Journal of Neuroscience*, vol. 23, no. 10, pp. 4315–4323, 2003.

[5] P. Petrovic, T. Dietrich, P. Fransson, J. Andersson, K. Carlsson, and M. Ingvar, "Placebo in emotional processing—induced expectations of anxiety relief activate a generalized modulatory network," *Neuron*, vol. 46, no. 6, pp. 957–969, 2005.

[6] H. Zhang, L. Zhou, H. Wei, X. Lu, and L. Hu, "The sustained influence of prior experience induced by social observation on placebo and nocebo responses," *Journal of Pain Research*, vol. 10, pp. 2769–2780, 2017.

[7] F. G. Miller, D. Wendler, and L. C. Swartzman, "Deception in research on the placebo effect," *PLoS Medicine*, vol. 2, no. 9, p. e262, 2005.

[8] J. M. Mundt, D. Roditi, and M. E. Robinson, "A comparison of deceptive and non-deceptive placebo analgesia: efficacy and ethical consequences," *Annals of Behavioral Medicine*, vol. 51, no. 2, pp. 307–315, 2017.

[9] J. E. Charlesworth, G. Petkovic, J. M. Kelley et al., "Effects of placebos without deception compared with no treatment: a systematic review and meta-analysis," *Journal of Evidence-Based Medicine*, vol. 10, no. 2, pp. 97–107, 2017.

[10] T. J. Kaptchuk, E. Friedlander, J. M. Kelley et al., "Placebos without deception: a randomized controlled trial in irritable bowel syndrome," *PLoS One*, vol. 5, no. 12, article e15591, 2010.

[11] C. Carvalho, J. M. Caetano, L. Cunha, P. Rebouta, T. J. Kaptchuk, and I. Kirsch, "Open-label placebo treatment in chronic low back pain: a randomized controlled trial," *Pain*, vol. 157, no. 12, pp. 2766–2772, 2016.

[12] S. K. Chung, D. D. Price, N. G. Verne, and M. E. Robinson, "Revelation of a personal placebo response: its effects on mood, attitudes and future placebo responding," *Pain*, vol. 132, no. 3, pp. 281–288, 2007.

[13] S. M. Schafer, L. Colloca, and T. D. Wager, "Conditioned placebo analgesia persists when subjects know they are receiving a placebo," *Journal of Pain*, vol. 16, no. 5, pp. 412–420, 2015.

[14] T. J. Kaptchuk, J. M. Kelley, L. A. Conboy et al., "Components of placebo effect: randomised controlled trial in patients with irritable bowel syndrome," *BMJ*, vol. 336, no. 7651, pp. 999–1003, 2008.

[15] C. Locher, A. F. Nascimento, I. Kirsch, J. Kossowsky, A. Meyer, and J. Gaab, "Is the rationale more important than deception? A randomized controlled trial of open-label placebo analgesia," *Pain*, vol. 158, no. 12, pp. 2320–2328, 2017.

[16] A. J. Barsky, R. Saintfort, M. P. Rogers, and J. F. Borus, "Nonspecific medication side effects and the nocebo phenomenon," *JAMA*, vol. 287, no. 5, pp. 622–627, 2002.

[17] L. Colloca and F. G. Miller, "The nocebo effect and its relevance for clinical practice," *Psychosomatic Medicine*, vol. 73, no. 7, pp. 598–603, 2011.

[18] J. Kong, R. L. Gollub, G. Polich et al., "A functional magnetic resonance imaging study on the neural mechanisms of hyperalgesic nocebo effect," *Journal of Neuroscience*, vol. 28, no. 49, pp. 13354–13362, 2008.

[19] D. Pud, Y. Golan, and R. Pesta, "Hand dominancy—a feature affecting sensitivity to pain," *Neuroscience Letters*, vol. 467, no. 3, pp. 237–240, 2009.

[20] P. Hjemdahl, S. Borg, A. J. Hiltunen, and L. Saxon, "Gender-related differences in response to placebo in benzodiazepine withdrawal: a single-blind pilot study," *Psychopharmacology*, vol. 153, no. 2, pp. 231–237, 2001.

[21] C. Horn-Hofmann, P. Büscher, S. Lautenbacher, and J. Wolstein, "The effect of nonrecurring alcohol administration on pain perception in humans: a systematic review," *Journal of Pain Research*, vol. 8, pp. 175–187, 2015.

[22] D. Holle, A. Heber, S. Naegel, H.-C. Diener, Z. Katsarava, and M. Obermann, "Influences of smoking and caffeine consumption on trigeminal pain processing," *Journal of Headache and Pain*, vol. 15, no. 1, p. 39, 2014.

[23] D. T. Shek, "Reliability and factorial structure of the Chinese version of the State-Trait Anxiety Inventory," *Journal of Psychopathology and Behavioral Assessment*, vol. 10, no. 4, pp. 303–317, 1988.

[24] K. Inui, T. D. Tran, M. Hoshiyama, and R. Kakigi, "Preferential stimulation of Aδ fibers by intra-epidermal needle electrode in humans," *Pain*, vol. 96, no. 3, pp. 247–252, 2002.

[25] R. Kakigi, K. Inui, and Y. Tamura, "Electrophysiological studies on human pain perception," *Clinical Neurophysiology*, vol. 116, no. 4, pp. 743–63, 2005.

[26] L. Hu, L. Zhang, R. Chen, H. Yu, H. Li, and A. Mouraux, "The primary somatosensory cortex and the insula contribute differently to the processing of transient and sustained nociceptive and non-nociceptive somatosensory inputs," *Human Brain Mapping*, vol. 36, no. 11, pp. 4346–4360, 2015.

[27] C. Zhao, E. Valentini, and L. Hu, "Functional features of crossmodal mismatch responses," *Experimental Brain Research*, vol. 233, no. 2, pp. 617–629, 2015.

[28] R. H. Gracely, "Studies of pain in normal man," in *Textbook of Pain*, P. Wall and R. Melzack, Eds., pp. 315–336, Churchill Livingstone, New York, NY, USA, 3rd edition, 1994.

[29] L. Colloca, P. Petrovic, T. D. Wager, M. Ingvar, and F. Benedetti, "How the number of learning trials affects placebo and nocebo responses," *Pain*, vol. 151, no. 2, pp. 430–9, 2010.

[30] C. H. Rankin, T. Abrams, R. J. Barry et al., "Habituation revisited: an updated and revised description of the behavioral characteristics of habituation," *Neurobiology of Learning and Memory*, vol. 92, no. 2, pp. 135–138, 2009.

[31] R. F. Thompson and W. A. Spencer, "Habituation: a model phenomenon for the study of neuronal substrates of behavior," *Psychological Review*, vol. 73, no. 1, pp. 16–43, 1966.

[32] E. R. Girden, *ANOVA: Repeated Measures*, Sage, Newbury Park, CA, USA, 1992.

[33] L. Colloca and F. Benedetti, "How prior experience shapes placebo analgesia," *Pain*, vol. 124, no. 1-2, pp. 126–133, 2006.

[34] S. Kessner, K. Wiech, K. Forkmann, M. Ploner, and U. Bingel, "The effect of treatment history on therapeutic outcome: an experimental approach," *JAMA Internal Medicine*, vol. 173, no. 15, pp. 1468-1469, 2013.

[35] S. Kessner, K. Forkmann, C. Ritter, K. Wiech, M. Ploner, and U. Bingel, "The effect of treatment history on therapeutic outcome: psychological and neurobiological underpinnings," *PLoS One*, vol. 9, no. 10, article e109014, 2014.

[36] G. H. Montgomery and I. Kirsch, "Classical conditioning and the placebo effect," *Pain*, vol. 72, no. 1-2, pp. 107–113, 1997.

[37] T. D. Wager, J. K. Rilling, E. E. Smith et al., "Placebo-induced changes in FMRI in the anticipation and experience of pain," *Science*, vol. 303, no. 5661, pp. 1162–1167, 2004.

[38] J. K. Zubieta, J. A. Bueller, L. R. Jackson et al., "Placebo effects mediated by endogenous opioid activity on mu-opioid receptors," *Journal of Neuroscience*, vol. 25, no. 34, pp. 7754–7762, 2005.

[39] J. Kong, R. L. Gollub, I. S. Rosman et al., "Brain activity associated with expectancy-enhanced placebo analgesia as measured by functional magnetic resonance imaging," *Journal of Neuroscience*, vol. 26, no. 2, pp. 381–388, 2006.

[40] A. Pollo, E. Torre, L. Lopiano et al., "Expectation modulates the response to subthalamic nucleus stimulation in Parkinsonian patients," *Neuroreport*, vol. 13, no. 11, pp. 1383–1386, 2002.

[41] L. Vase, M. E. Robinson, N. G. Verne, and D. D. Price, "The contributions of suggestion, desire, and expectation to

placebo effects in irritable bowel syndrome patients: an empirical investigation," *Pain*, vol. 105, no. 1-2, pp. 17–25, 2003.

[42] D. D. Price, J. Craggs, G. Nicholas Verne, W. M. Perlstein, and M. E. Robinson, "Placebo analgesia is accompanied by large reductions in pain-related brain activity in irritable bowel syndrome patients," *Pain*, vol. 127, no. 1-2, pp. 63–72, 2007.

[43] A. Tinnermann, S. Geuter, C. Sprenger, J. Finsterbusch, and C. Büchel, "Interactions between brain and spinal cord mediate value effects in nocebo hyperalgesia," *Science*, vol. 358, no. 6359, pp. 105–108, 2017.

[44] D. G. Finniss, T. J. Kaptchuk, F. Miller, and F. Benedetti, "Biological, clinical, and ethical advances of placebo effects," *The Lancet*, vol. 375, no. 9715, pp. 686–695, 2010.

[45] R. Klinger and L. Colloca, "Placebo effects: basic mechanisms and clinical applications," *Zeitschrift für Psychologie*, vol. 222, no. 3, pp. 121–123, 2014.

[46] C. Blease, L. Colloca, and T. J. Kaptchuk, "Are open-label placebos ethical? Informed consent and ethical equivocations," *Bioethics*, vol. 30, no. 6, pp. 407–414, 2016.

[47] G. Petkovic, J. E. G. Charlesworth, J. Kelley, F. Miller, N. Roberts, and J. Howick, "Effects of placebos without deception compared with no treatment: protocol for a systematic review and meta-analysis," *BMJ Open*, vol. 5, no. 11, p. e009428, 2015.

[48] L. Colloca and F. Benedetti, "Nocebo hyperalgesia: how anxiety is turned into pain," *Current Opinion in Anaesthesiology*, vol. 20, no. 5, pp. 435–439, 2007.

[49] S. Cohen, "The nocebo effect of informed consent," *Bioethics*, vol. 28, no. 3, pp. 147–154, 2014.

[50] R. E. Wells and T. J. Kaptchuk, "To tell the truth, the whole truth, may do patients harm: the problem of the nocebo effect for informed consent," *American Journal of Bioethics*, vol. 12, no. 3, pp. 22–29, 2012.

# 29

# Intranasal Pharmacokinetics of Morphine ARER, a Novel Abuse-Deterrent Formulation: Results from a Randomized, Double-Blind, Four-Way Crossover Study in Nondependent, Opioid-Experienced Subjects

**Lynn R. Webster ⓘ,[1] Carmela Pantaleon,[2] Matthew Iverson,[2] Michael D. Smith,[1] Eric R. Kinzler,[2] and Stefan Aigner[2]**

[1]*PRA Health Sciences, Salt Lake City, UT, USA*
[2]*Inspirion Delivery Sciences LLC, Morristown, NJ, USA*

Correspondence should be addressed to Lynn R. Webster; lrwebstermd@gmail.com

Academic Editor: Shinya Kasai

*Objective.* To investigate the pharmacokinetics (PK) of Morphine ARER, an extended-release (ER), abuse-deterrent formulation of morphine sulfate after oral and intranasal administration. *Methods.* This randomized, double-blind, double-dummy, placebo-controlled, four-way crossover study assessed the PK of morphine and its active metabolite, M6G, from crushed intranasal Morphine ARER and intact oral Morphine ARER compared with crushed intranasal ER morphine following administration to nondependent, recreational opioid users. The correlation between morphine PK and the pharmacodynamic parameter of drug liking, a measure of abuse potential, was also evaluated. *Results.* Mean maximum observed plasma concentration ($C_{max}$) for morphine was lower with crushed intranasal Morphine ARER (26.2 ng/mL) and intact oral Morphine ARER (18.6 ng/mL), compared with crushed intranasal ER morphine (49.5 ng/mL). The time to $C_{max}$ ($T_{max}$) was the same for intact oral and crushed intranasal Morphine ARER (1.6 hours) and longer for crushed intranasal morphine ER (1.1 hours). Higher mean maximum morphine $C_{max}$, $T_{max}$, and abuse quotient ($C_{max}/T_{max}$) were positively correlated with maximum effect for drug liking ($R^2 \geq 0.9795$). *Conclusion.* These data suggest that Morphine ARER maintains its ER profile despite physical manipulation and intranasal administration, which may be predictive of a lower intranasal abuse potential compared with ER morphine.

## 1. Introduction

Despite implementation of opioid risk management plans (including efforts to increase public awareness, guidelines for safe prescribing, clinical assessment tools, prescription drug monitoring programs, etc.), abuse of prescription opioids remains a serious public health concern. In 2016, an estimated 11.5 million individuals aged 12 years or older reported current abuse or misuse of prescription pain relievers in the United States [1]. In 2015, there were more than 15,000 deaths associated with prescription opioids (not including illicitly manufactured fentanyl or heroin) [2].

Controlled- or extended-release (ER) formulations of opioids were developed to provide patients who experience chronic pain severe enough to warrant around-the-clock opioid therapy with a consistent and sustained plasma levels of analgesic opioid. When intact tablets are taken whole, ER formulations have less appeal to abusers than their immediate-release (IR) counterparts [3]. However, because of their higher drug content per dose, ER formulations are often manipulated and administered through unintended routes. In particular, ER formulations of morphine, oxymorphone, and hydromorphone are more likely to be abused through injection because of their low oral bioavailability [4, 5]. Based on abuse rates, one study modeled the likelihood of abusing ER morphine through different routes of abuse and found that with the exception of hydromorphone, ER morphine is more likely to be abused through injection than all other opioids [4]. Manipulation of ER opioids often accelerates the release of the active opioid, essentially converting the ER opioid to an IR opioid, providing a higher blood concentration and more rapid onset of psychotropic effects compared with oral delivery as intended [6].

Abuse-deterrent formulations (ADFs) are designed to provide pain relief while deterring common methods of manipulation and reducing the potential for nonoral abuse and misuse. These formulations have properties that make nonoral abuse more difficult, less appealing, or less rewarding for one or more routes of abuse. However, these formulations are not abuse-proof, and abuse of opioid ADFs by the oral, intranasal, and intravenous routes is still possible. Clinical trials of several abuse-deterrent opioids have reported lower ratings of drug liking and positive subjective effects following manipulation compared with manipulation of nonabuse-deterrent formulations [7–9]. Furthermore, these clinical studies appear to successfully predict real-world reductions in abuse; after introduction of abuse-deterrent ER oxycodone (OxyContin, Purdue Pharma LP, Stamford, CT, USA), postmarketing data showed a decrease in rates of ER oxycodone abuse ranging from 30% to 85%, a decrease of 66% in doctor shopping for ER oxycodone, and an 85% decrease in overdose fatalities associated with ER oxycodone [10]. However, after introduction of abuse-deterrent ER oxycodone, many abusers found methods to circumvent the tamper-resistant properties or switched to other non-ADF opioids or heroin [11–14]. These data highlight the fact that opioid ADFs are one component of a comprehensive opioid risk management plan.

A novel oral ADF of ER morphine sulfate tablets (Morphine ARER, MorphaBond ER, Daiichi Sankyo, Inc., Basking Ridge, NJ, USA) resists physical and chemical manipulation, forms a viscous material if crushed and placed in liquid to prepare for injection, and retains its ER characteristics despite manipulation [15–17]. Previously published data suggest that Morphine ARER has a lower abuse potential through the intranasal route of administration when compared with ER morphine [18]. Here, we describe and compare the pharmacokinetic (PK) profile of morphine and its main metabolite morphine 6-glucuronide (M6G) for crushed intranasal Morphine ARER, intact oral Morphine ARER, and crushed intranasal ER morphine (MS Contin, Purdue Pharma, LP, Stamford, CT, USA) following administration to nondependent, recreational opioid users. Additionally, we evaluated the correlation between PK of Morphine ARER and drug liking.

## 2. Methods

### 2.1. Subjects.
The selection of subjects has been detailed in a previous publication [18]. In brief, the study enrolled healthy male and female subjects aged 18 to 55 years who were nondependent, recreational users of opioids. Recreational use was defined as nonmedical use of opioids on at least 10 occasions in the past year and at least once in the preceding 12 weeks. Additionally, subjects had to have insufflated drugs at least three times in the past year. Subjects being treated for substance abuse disorder or with a history of drug or alcohol dependence were excluded.

### 2.2. Study Design and Treatment.
Details of the study design have been previously reported [18]. Subjects meeting enrollment criteria first entered a qualification phase that consisted of a naloxone challenge test to exclude opioid-dependent subjects and a drug discrimination test to exclude subjects who could not distinguish the positive subjective effects of morphine from those of placebo and those who were unable to insufflate the combined volume of a 30 mg tablet of crushed morphine sulfate IR plus a crushed placebo tablet.

Qualified subjects entered a double-blind treatment period during which they were randomized to one of four treatment sequences in a four-way crossover double-dummy design, with each treatment period separated by a 7-day washout period. The following treatments were administered: crushed intranasal placebo plus oral placebo (referred to as placebo), crushed intranasal ER morphine (MS Contin) 60 mg with crushed placebo tablet added for volume plus intact oral placebo (referred to as crushed intranasal ER morphine), crushed intranasal Morphine ARER 60 mg plus oral placebo (referred to as crushed intranasal Morphine ARER), and crushed intranasal placebo plus intact oral Morphine ARER 60 mg (referred to as intact oral Morphine ARER).

The study was conducted in accord with the Good Clinical Practice Guideline (US Code of Federal Regulations, 21 CFR parts, 50, 56, and 312), the International Conference on Harmonisation (ICH), the Declaration of Helsinki, and all applicable federal and local regulation and institutional review board requirements, as appropriate. All subjects provided written informed consent to participate in the study.

### 2.3. Assessments

#### 2.3.1. Pharmacokinetics.
During each treatment period, blood samples for PK assessments were obtained predose and at 0.25, 0.5, 1, 1.5, 2, 3, 4, 6, 8, 10, 12, and 24 hours postdose. A validated liquid chromatography-tandem mass spectrometry method was used to assay morphine and M6G in plasma. The calibration ranges were from 0.725 to 145 ng/mL for morphine and from 2.50 to 500 ng/mL for M6G; the lower limit of quantification for morphine was 0.725 ng/mL and for M6G was 2.50 ng/mL. Values below the lower limit of quantification were reported as 0 ng/mL.

Pharmacokinetic parameters were calculated with Phoenix WinNonlin 6.3 (Certara, Princeton, NJ, USA) using the noncompartmental model. For the PK evaluation, the following parameters were calculated using actual elapsed sampling times: maximum observed plasma concentration ($C_{max}$); time associated with $C_{max}$ ($T_{max}$); area under the plasma concentration-time curve from 0 to 0.5, 1, 2, 8, 12, or 24 hours ($AUC_{0-0.5}$, $AUC_{0-1}$, $AUC_{0-2}$, $AUC_{0-8}$, $AUC_{0-12}$, and AUC$_{0-24}$); AUC from 0 to the last measurable concentration (AUC$_{0-t}$); AUC from 0 extrapolated to infinity (AUC$_{0-\infty}$); elimination rate constant ($k_e$); and apparent first-order terminal elimination half-life ($t_{1/2}$). The abuse quotient (AQ; $C_{max}/T_{max}$), a PK parameter associated with drug liking and abuse potential [6, 19], was also calculated.

*2.3.2. Drug-Liking Bipolar Visual Analog Scale.* A bipolar visual analog scale (VAS) was used to assess drug liking, the primary pharmacodynamic (PD) parameter of interest (0 = strong disliking, 50 = neither like nor dislike, 100 = strong liking). At 0.5, 1, 1.5, 2, 3, 4, 6, 8, 10, 12, and 24 hours postdose, subjects recorded their response to the question, "Do you like the drug effect you are feeling now?" by marking a single line on the VAS. The mean maximum effect ($E_{max}$) and area under the drug-liking curve (AUE) for 0-1, 2, 8, 12, and 24 hours (AUE$_{0-1}$, AUE$_{0-2}$, AUE$_{0-8}$, AUE$_{0-12}$, and AUE$_{0-24}$) were calculated [18].

*2.4. Statistical Analysis*

*2.4.1. Pharmacokinetic Analyses.* The PK analysis population consisted of all subjects with any available $C_{max}$ and AUC data. The PD population consisted of all subjects who completed all four treatment periods with at least one PD assessment in each treatment period. Sample size calculations have been described previously and were determined based on the primary PD endpoint [18].

Morphine and M6G PK parameters for each treatment were summarized for the PK population using descriptive statistics. Additionally, relative bioavailability was calculated for $C_{max}$, partial AUCs (AUC$_{0-0.5}$, AUC$_{0-1}$, AUC$_{0-2}$, AUC$_{0-8}$, AUC$_{0-12}$, and AUC$_{0-24}$), AUC$_{0-\infty}$, and AUC$_{0-t}$ using the ratio (and 90% confidence interval (CI)) of geometric means for morphine and M6G. The SAS statistical software (Version 9.2 or higher; SAS Institute, Cary, NC, USA) mixed-effect linear model procedure (PROC MIXED) was used to construct the analysis of variance models of log$_e$-transformed values for each PK parameter. The model included terms for sequence, period, and treatment as fixed effects and subjects nested within sequences as a random effect. Ninety percent CIs for the difference (test minus reference) in the mean between treatments were constructed for the log$_e$ scale values of each parameter. Confidence intervals were based on the least squares (LS) means estimation using the mean square error from the analysis of variance models. Least squares geometric means and 90% CIs were provided for each treatment and treatment comparison.

*2.4.2. Pharmacokinetic/Pharmacodynamic Analyses.* Pharmacokinetic/pharmacodynamic analyses dose-response curve plots for drug liking that showed the logarithmic regression lines and coefficient of determination ($R^2$) using logarithmic regression and the means of each parameter and treatment were created for the following: $E_{max}$ versus $C_{max}$ and $T_{max}$ and AQ; all AUE parameters versus $C_{max}$, $T_{max}$, and

AQ; AUE$_{0-1}$ versus AUC$_{0-1}$; AUE$_{0-2}$ versus AUC$_{0-2}$; AUE$_{0-8}$ versus AUC$_{0-8}$; AUE$_{0-12}$ versus AUC$_{0-12}$; and AUE$_{0-24}$ versus AUC$_{0-24}$.

# 3. Results

*3.1. Subjects.* Forty-eight subjects entered and passed the naloxone challenge; of these, 27 passed the drug discrimination test and entered the treatment phase. Twenty-five subjects completed the treatment phase [18]. PK data for intact oral Morphine ARER, crushed intranasal Morphine ARER, and crushed intranasal ER morphine, were available for 26, 26, and 27 subjects, respectively. All intranasal doses were 100% insufflated as confirmed by intranasal check.

The demographics profile of the subjects has been described previously [18]. The mean age was 25.4 years, and a majority were male (85.2%), white (96.3%), alcohol users (88.9%), and tobacco users (74.1%). All subjects had used opioids recreationally in the past 12 weeks (mean of 12.1 times for men and 9.0 times for women).

*3.2. Intranasal Pharmacokinetics*

*3.2.1. Morphine.* The mean maximum plasma morphine concentration ($C_{max}$) was lower for crushed intranasal Morphine ARER (26.2 ng/mL) and intact oral Morphine ARER (18.6 ng/mL) compared with crushed intranasal ER morphine (49.5 ng/mL) (Figure 1(a) and Table 1). Based on LS means, morphine $C_{max}$ was 49% lower for crushed intranasal Morphine ARER than for crushed intranasal ER morphine ($P$ value < 0.0001). Exposure to morphine at early sampling times was also lower with crushed intranasal Morphine ARER and intact oral Morphine ARER than with crushed intranasal ER morphine (Table 1). Exposure in the first 30 min (AUC$_{0-0.5h}$) was 75% lower for crushed intranasal Morphine ARER compared with crushed intranasal ER morphine ($P$ value < 0.0001). The median $T_{max}$ for morphine was 46% longer ($P$ value < 0.0001) for crushed intranasal Morphine ARER (1.6 hours) than for crushed intranasal ER morphine (1.1 hours).

*3.2.2. M6G Metabolite.* As with morphine, the mean $C_{max}$ for M6G was lower with crushed intranasal Morphine ARER (58.2 ng/mL) and intact oral Morphine ARER (108.2 ng/mL) compared with crushed intranasal ER morphine (169.0 ng/mL (Figure 1(b) and Table 2)). Based on LS means, M6G $C_{max}$ was 68% lower ($P$ value < 0.0001) for crushed intranasal Morphine ARER than for crushed intranasal ER morphine. Early exposure to M6G (AUC$_{0-0.5h}$) was 68% lower ($P$ value < 0.0001) with crushed intranasal Morphine ARER compared with crushed intranasal ER morphine. Median $T_{max}$ for M6G was 94% longer for crushed intranasal Morphine ARER (3.1 hours) than for crushed intranasal ER morphine (1.6 hours).

*3.2.3. Morphine ARER: Intranasal versus Intact Oral Pharmacokinetics.* Intranasal administration of crushed Morphine ARER resulted in slightly higher mean $C_{max}$,

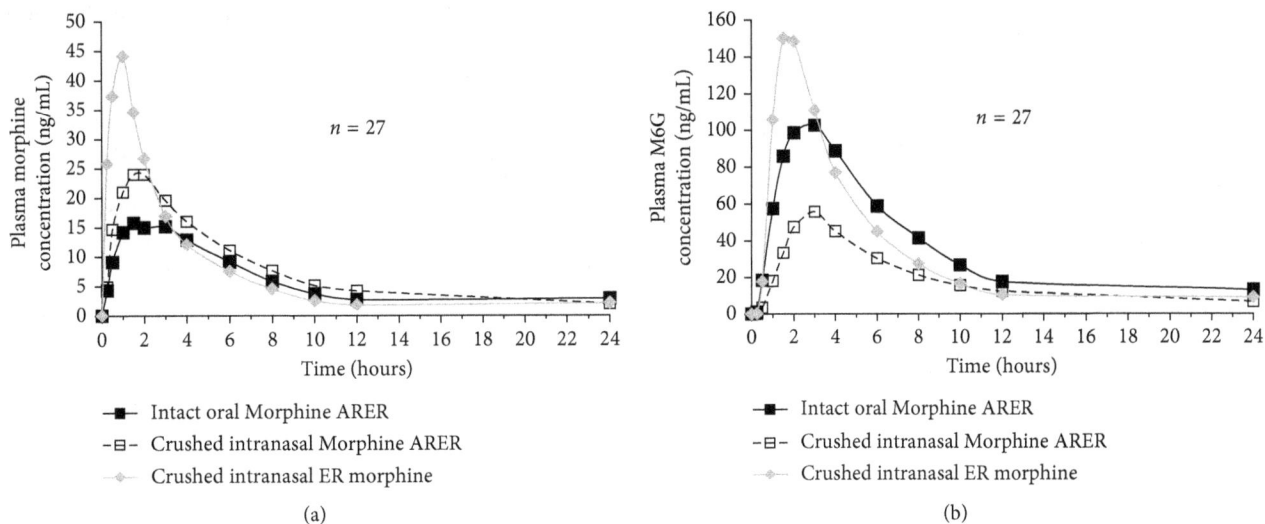

FIGURE 1: Mean plasma concentration-time profile of (a) morphine and (b) M6G by treatment (PK population, $n = 27$).

TABLE 1: Pharmacokinetic parameters for morphine after administration of crushed intranasal Morphine ARER, crushed intranasal ER morphine, or intact oral Morphine ARER (PK population, $n = 27$).

| Parameter | Mean (SD) | | |
|---|---|---|---|
| | Intact oral Morphine ARER | Crushed intranasal Morphine ARER | Crushed intranasal ER morphine |
| $C_{max}$ (ng/mL) | 18.6 (5.7) | 26.2 (11.2) | 49.5 (17.3) |
| $T_{max}$ (hr) | 1.6 (0.5–3.1) | 1.6 (1.0–3.1) | 1.1 (0.2–1.6) |
| $AUC_{0-t}$ (ng·hr/mL) | 139.4 (40.1) | 178.5 (77.7) | 171.6 (55.2) |
| $AUC_{0-\infty}$ (ng·hr/mL) | 158.0 (21.9)* | 219.8 (97.4)† | 188.0 (51.5)‡ |
| $k_e$ (hr$^{-1}$) | 0.0688 (0.0399)§ | 0.0997 (0.0649)‖ | 0.0684 (0.0583)* |
| $t_{1/2}$ (hr) | 18.4 (20.0)§ | 10.8 (8.3)‖ | 21.0 (20.9)* |
| $AUC_{0-0.5h}$ (ng·hr/mL) | 2.1 (1.3) | 2.8 (1.2) | 10.9 (5.2) |
| $AUC_{0-1}$ (ng·hr/mL) | 7.5 (3.2) | 11.2 (4.8) | 30.8 (12.1) |
| $AUC_{0-2h}$ (ng·hr/mL) | 22.6 (7.5) | 34.2 (13.7) | 67.0 (22.9) |
| $AUC_{0-8h}$ (ng·hr/mL) | 89.3 (25.4) | 120.9 (48.2) | 136.5 (43.4) |
| $AUC_{0-12h}$ (ng·hr/mL) | 105.6 (29.5) | 143.2 (57.8) | 148.1 (47.4) |
| $AUC_{0-24h}$ (ng·hr/mL) | 139.4 (40.1) | 181.1 (75.9) | 171.6 (55.2) |

$n = 27$ for crushed intranasal ER morphine and $n = 26$ for both Morphine ARER treatments, except as noted: *$n = 5$, †$n = 19$, ‡$n = 4$, §$n = 7$, ‖$n = 22$; $AUC_{0-0.5, 0-1, 0-2, 0-8, 0-12, 0-24}$ = area under the plasma concentration-time curve from 0 h to 0.5 h, 1 h, 2 h, 8 h, 12 h, and 24 h; $AUC_{0-t}$ = area under the plasma concentration-time curve from 0 h to the last measurable concentration above the lower limit of quantification; $AUC_{0-\infty}$ = area under the plasma concentration-time curve from 0 h to infinity; $C_{max}$ = maximum observed plasma concentration; ER = extended release; $h$ = hour; $k_e$ = elimination rate constant; PK = pharmacokinetic; $T_{max}$ = time associated with $C_{max}$; $t_{1/2}$ = half-life; values for $T_{max}$ are medians and ranges.

$AUC_{0-5}$, and $AUC_{0-t}$ values for morphine compared with intact oral Morphine ARER, with similar $T_{max}$ values (Table 1). However, the parameters for M6G were lower with crushed intranasal Morphine ARER, and $T_{max}$ was longer compared with intact oral Morphine ARER (Table 2). Least-squares means data showed that morphine $C_{max}$ was 35% higher and M6G $C_{max}$ was 54% lower for crushed intranasal Morphine ARER compared with intact oral Morphine ARER. Similarly, $AUC_{0-0.5h}$ for morphine was 43% higher and $AUC_{0-0.5h}$ for M6G was 74% lower with crushed intranasal Morphine ARER compared with intact oral Morphine ARER. These data indicate that less morphine was metabolized to M6G within the first 30 minutes following intranasal administration of Morphine ARER. Notably, overall exposure to morphine and M6G (defined as $AUC_{0-t}$ for morphine combined with $AUC_{0-t}$ for M6G) was

approximately 37% lower for crushed intranasal Morphine ARER compared with intact oral Morphine ARER (620.3 versus 983.8 ng·hr/mL).

3.3. Abuse Quotient. The AQ for crushed intranasal and intact oral Morphine ARER was 77% and 84% lower than that for crushed intranasal ER morphine, respectively (Figure 2). There was a large variability in the $T_{max}$ for ER morphine, resulting in a wide range for AQ (15.9 to 298.7 ng/mL/hr); this variability was likely caused by the additional filler material added to blind the volumes.

3.4. Pharmacokinetic/Pharmacodynamic Relationships. A strong association across all active treatments was observed between mean morphine PK parameters and drug liking.

Table 2: Pharmacokinetic parameters for morphine 6-glucuronide (M6G) after administration of crushed intranasal Morphine ARER, crushed intranasal ER morphine, or intact oral Morphine ARER (PK population, $n = 27$).

| Parameter | Mean (SD) | | |
| --- | --- | --- | --- |
| | Intact oral Morphine ARER | Crushed intranasal Morphine ARER | Crushed intranasal ER morphine |
| $C_{max}$ (ng/mL) | 108.2 (18.2) | 58.2 (30.7) | 169.0 (55.0) |
| $T_{max}$ (hr) | 2.1 (1.6–4.1) | 3.1 (2.1–10.0) | 1.6 (1.1–10.1) |
| $AUC_{0-t}$ (ng·hr/mL) | 844.4 (146.5) | 441.8 (202.0) | 777.9 (156.9) |
| $AUC_{0-\infty}$ (ng·hr/mL) | 1054.7 (154.5)* | 575.1 (263.5)† | 907.7 (158.6)‡ |
| $k_e$ (hr$^{-1}$) | 0.0720 (0.0365)§ | 0.0768 (0.0448)‖ | 0.0761 (0.0384)‡ |
| $t_{1/2}$ (hr) | 14.0 (11.4)§ | 11.9 (6.1)‖ | 11.5 (6.2)‡ |
| $AUC_{0-0.5h}$ (ng·hr/mL) | 2.2 (1.3) | 0.4 (0.5) | 1.9 (1.3) |
| $AUC_{0-1}$ (ng·hr/mL) | 18.3 (6.5) | 4.8 (3.1) | 26.9 (13.3) |
| $AUC_{0-2h}$ (ng·hr/mL) | 96.6 (20.3) | 35.8 (18.9) | 161.4 (68.5) |
| $AUC_{0-8h}$ (ng·hr/mL) | 545.2 (90.1) | 266.6 (124.2) | 588.3 (151.5) |
| $AUC_{0-12h}$ (ng·hr/mL) | 659.7 (116.5) | 331.8 (149.8) | 660.3 (145.7) |
| $AUC_{0-24h}$ (ng·hr/mL) | 844.4 (146.5) | 446.8 (196.5) | 777.9 (156.9) |

$n = 27$ for crushed intranasal ER morphine and $n = 26$ for both Morphine ARER treatments, except as noted: *$n = 11$, †$n = 14$, ‡$n = 6$, §$n = 13$, ‖$n = 19$; $AUC_{0-0.5, 0-1, 0-2, 0-8, 0-12, 0-24}$ = area under the plasma concentration-time curve from 0 h to 0.5 h, 1 h, 2 h, 8 h, 12 h, and 24 h; $AUC_{0-t}$ = area under the plasma concentration-time curve from 0 h to the last measurable concentration above the lower limit of quantification; $AUC_{0-\infty}$ = area under the plasma concentration-time curve from 0 h to infinity; $C_{max}$ = maximum observed plasma concentration; ER = extended release; $h$ = hour; $k_e$ = elimination rate constant; PK = pharmacokinetic; $T_{max}$ = time associated with $C_{max}$; $t_{1/2}$ = half-life; values for $T_{max}$ are medians and ranges.

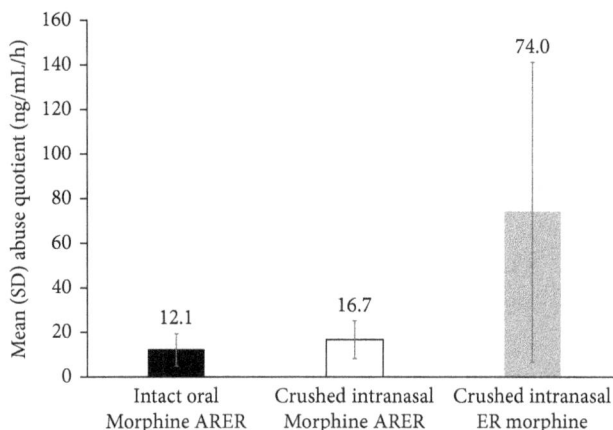

Figure 2: Mean (SD) abuse quotient. SD = standard deviation.

$E_{max}$ was well correlated with $C_{max}$, $T_{max}$, and AQ (Figures 3(a)–3(c)) with an $R^2 \geq 0.9795$ for all comparisons. A good correlation was also observed between partial AUEs and $C_{max}$, $T_{max}$, and AQ ($R^2$ values $\geq 0.9911$, $\geq 0.9052$, and $\geq 0.9454$, resp.) (Figures 4(a)–4(c)). There was strong correlation between $AUC_{0-1}$ and $AUE_{0-1}$ ($R^2$ value = 0.9944) and between $AUC_{0-2}$ and $AUE_{0-2}$ ($R^2$ value = 0.9816); however, the correlations became weaker over time with $R^2$ value of 0.4684 over a 24-hour period (Figure 4(d)).

## 4. Discussion

To attain more intense euphoric effects, nonmedical users of opioids often begin abusing prescription opioids by excessive consumption of intact tablets. Abusers may progress to inhaling, injecting, or smoking the drug. Injection and insufflation are common routes of abuse for morphine [5, 20], likely because they avoid the large amount of first-pass metabolism of morphine. Data from RADARS (Researched Abuse, Diversion, and Addiction-Related Surveillance)

System indicate high rates of abuse of ER morphine (both oral and nonoral) [21]. Abuse of morphine by injection and insufflation are associated with a greater risk of death or major event than ingestion by the oral route [22]. In accord with FDA guidance for evaluating abuse-deterrent opioid formulations [23], this study investigated the PK of intact oral or crushed intranasal Morphine ARER, an ER abuse-deterrent formulation of morphine, in comparison with the PK of crushed intranasal ER morphine in recreational drug abusers.

Short-term exposures to morphine and its pharmacologically active metabolite M6G were substantially lower for crushed intranasal Morphine ARER than for crushed intranasal ER morphine. Intranasal administration of crushed Morphine ARER was associated with a 49% and 68% reduction in $C_{max}$ for morphine and M6G, respectively, and a 75% and 68% reduction in $AUC_{0-0.5}$ for morphine and M6G, respectively, compared with crushed intranasal ER morphine. Crushing defeated the extended-release mechanism of ER morphine so that its PK resembled that of an IR formulation.

Crushed intranasal Morphine ARER and intact oral Morphine ARER exhibited similar PK profiles, indicating that Morphine ARER maintained its ER properties, despite physical manipulation and intranasal administration. Early exposure to morphine was slightly higher and early exposure to M6G was lower for crushed intranasal Morphine ARER than for intact oral Morphine ARER, which may be because of both the route of administration and an apparent reduction in overall bioavailability of intranasally administered Morphine ARER. At early time points, the increase in plasma morphine concentrations and the reduction in M6G concentrations compared with oral administration of intact tablets indicate that a portion of crushed intranasal Morphine ARER was directly absorbed through the nasal passage into the circulation without first-pass metabolism. Importantly, overall exposure to active morphine and M6G was reduced when Morphine ARER was crushed and insufflated compared with intact oral Morphine ARER. This reduction

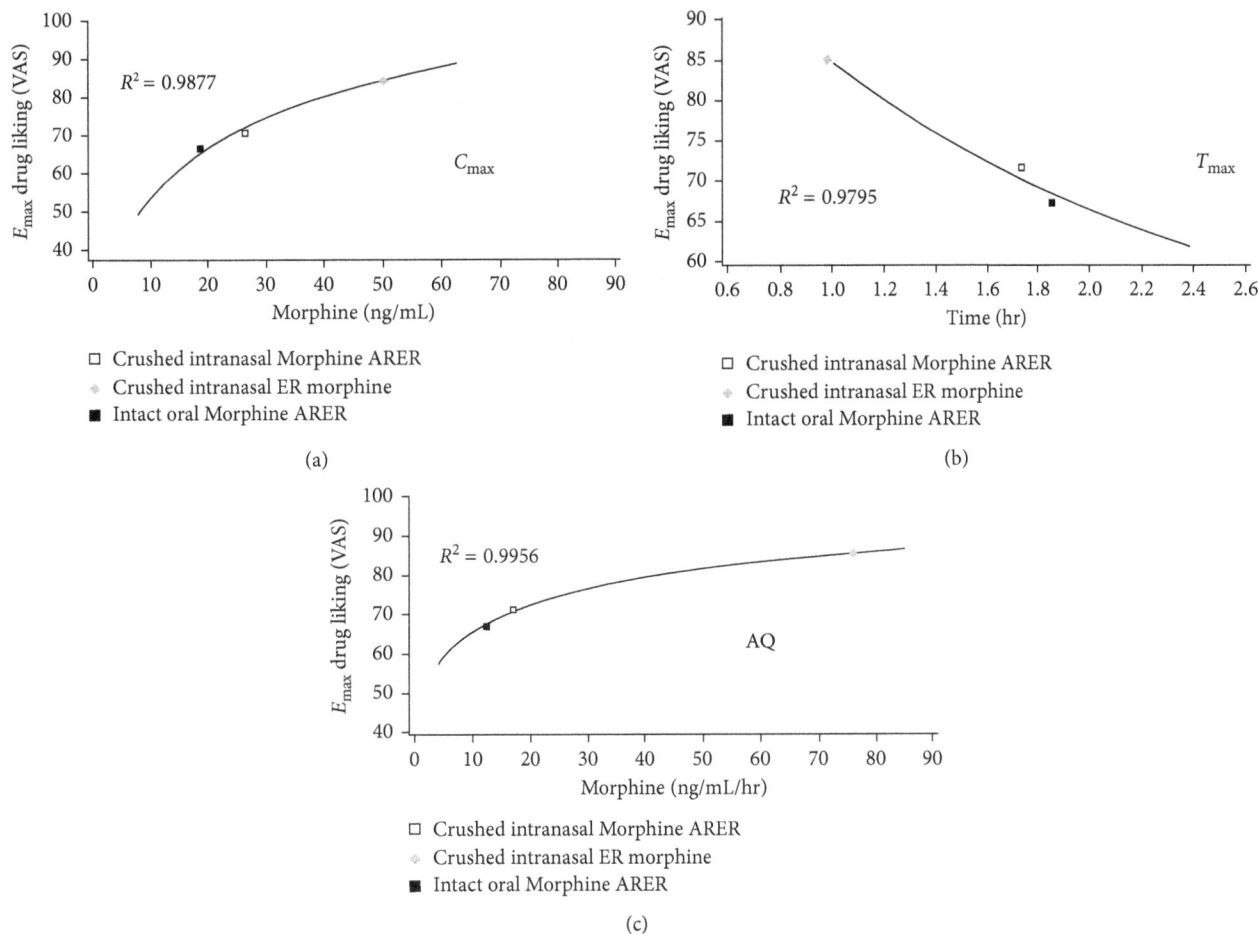

FIGURE 3: Average time-curve plots of $E_{max}$ for drug liking (a) VAS versus $C_{max}$, (b) $E_{max}$ for drug-liking VAS versus $T_{max}$, and (c) $E_{max}$ for drug-liking VAS versus AQ (PD population, $N = 25$). AQ = abuse quotient, $C_{max}$ = maximum observed plasma concentration, $E_{max}$ = mean maximum effect for drug liking, $T_{max}$ = time to $C_{max}$, VAS = visual analog scale.

in overall bioavailability was likely the result of the physicochemical abuse-deterrent properties of Morphine ARER.

This study extends previous findings of reduced drug liking with Morphine ARER [18] to show strong associations between morphine PK parameters and drug liking, suggesting that the PKs of morphine from Morphine ARER are predictive of reduced drug liking and hence, of lower intranasal abuse potential. As previously reported, both crushed intranasal and intact oral Morphine ARER are associated with significantly less drug liking relative to crushed intranasal ER morphine [18]. The maximum drug-liking placebo-adjusted VAS score was 40% lower for crushed intranasal Morphine ARER compared with crushed intranasal ER morphine, and early drug-liking AUE values (over the first hour and first 2 hours) were significantly ($P$ value < 0.0001) reduced for crushed intranasal Morphine ARER versus crushed intranasal ER morphine. The current PK results support these PD results, with substantially higher peak plasma concentrations in the crushed intranasal ER morphine arm, whereas crushed intranasal Morphine ARER maintained an ER PK profile that was similar to that of intact oral Morphine ARER. The lower $C_{max}$ and longer $T_{max}$ for morphine and M6G suggest that Morphine ARER may reduce drug liking relative to ER

morphine and may be less desirable for recreational drug abusers. The AQ is a calculated parameter that captures the extent and rate of increase in plasma drug concentration as determined by $C_{max}$ and $T_{max}$ [6, 19, 24]. The strong correlations between AQ and drug liking support the use of AQ as a surrogate measure for drug liking. The use of AQ comparisons may be one measure to determine if a manipulated non-abuse-deterrent medication has the same abuse potential as an ADF.

Studies assessing the public health impact of an ADF of ER oxycodone (OxyContin) reported lower rates of oral and nonoral abuse for the reformulated product following its introduction [10, 12, 13, 25–27]. Across 10 studies that assessed different measures of abuse and associated consequences, the introduction of reformulated abuse-deterrent oxycodone resulted in reductions in associated oral and nonoral abuse rates, opioid use disorder, overdose, doctor shopping, and diversion [10]. However, the data also show that many users switch to other non-abuse-deterrent opioids or heroin or find methods to circumvent the tamper-resistant properties [11–14, 28]. Another ER opioid with purported abuse-deterrent properties, Opana ER, was removed from the market at the request of the FDA because of dangerous shifts

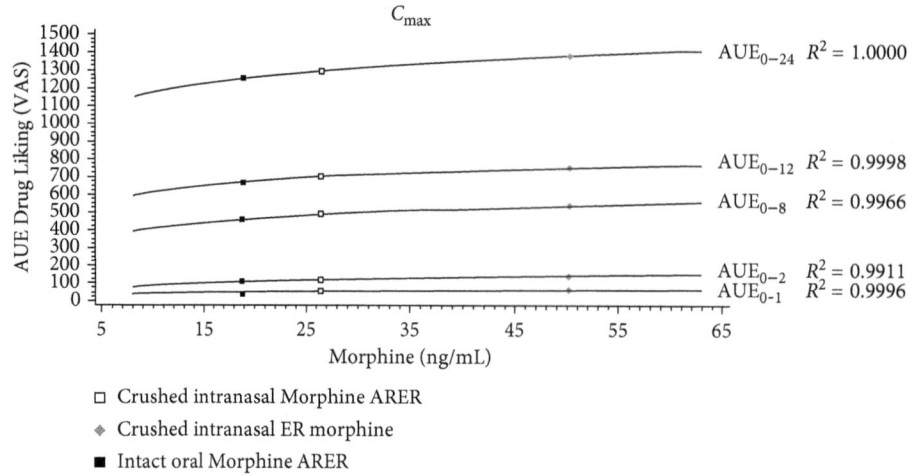

**(a)**

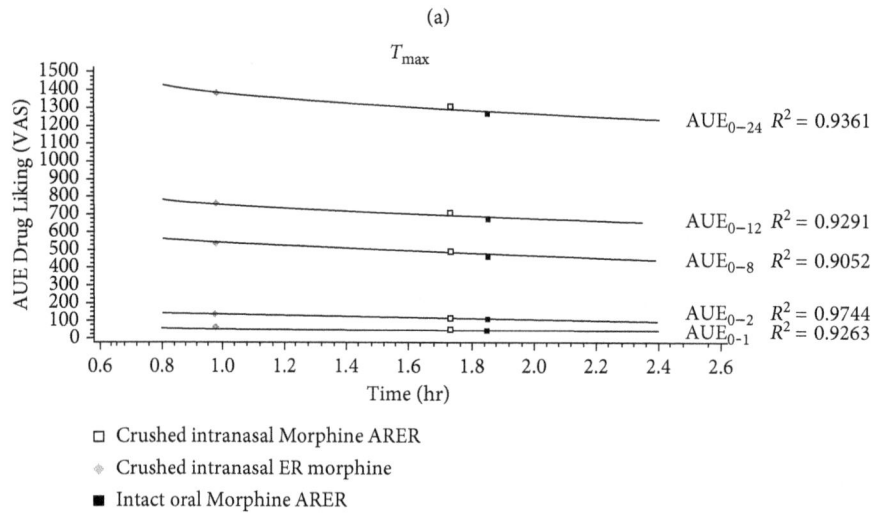

**(b)**

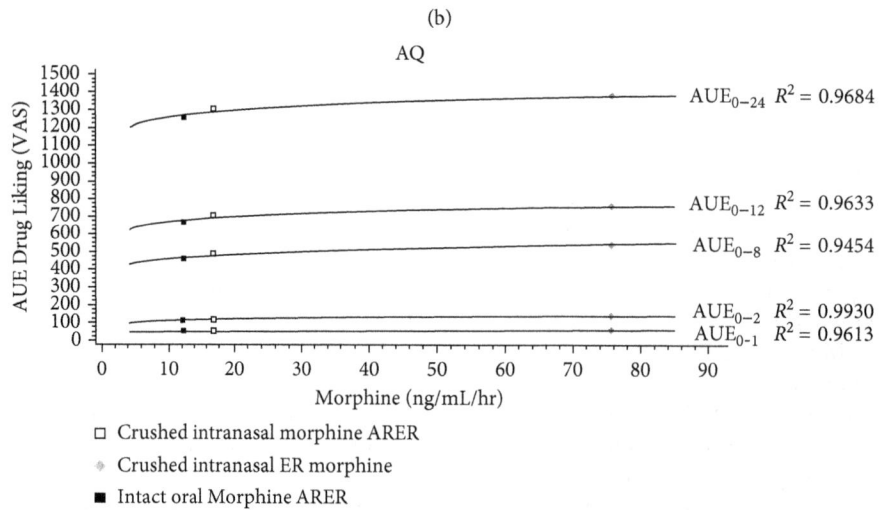

**(c)**

FIGURE 4: Continued.

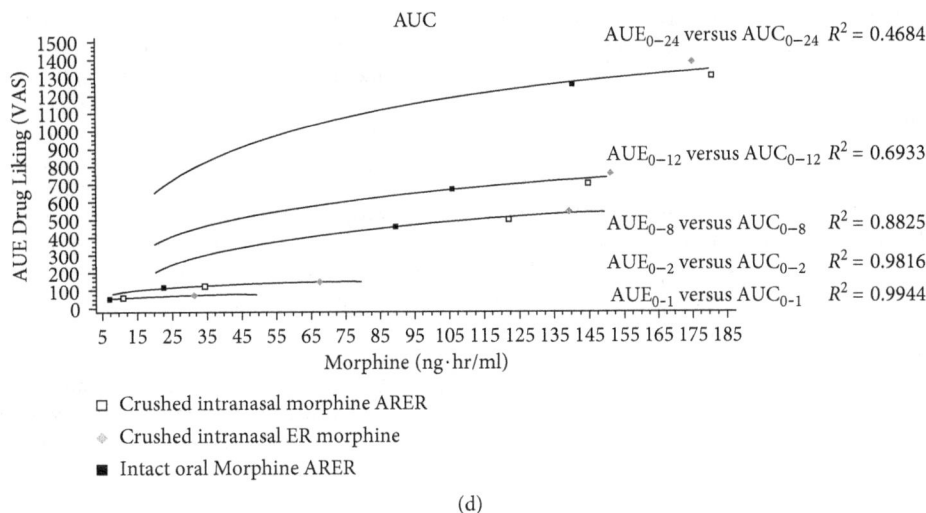

FIGURE 4: Average time-curve plot of AUE (0-1 h, 0–2 h, 0–8 h, 0–12 h, and 0–24 h) for drug-liking VAS versus (a) $C_{max}$, (b) $T_{max}$, (c) AQ, and (d) AUC (0-1 h, 0–2 h, 0–8 h, 0–12 h, and 0–24 h) (PD population, $N = 25$). AQ = abuse quotient, AUE = area under the drug-liking curve, AUC = area under the plasma concentration-time curve, $C_{max}$ = maximum observed plasma concentration, $h$ = hour, $T_{max}$ = time to $C_{max}$, and VAS = visual analog scale.

in the route of abuse from intranasal to intravenous abuse [29]. This shift in route of abuse highlights the need to assess the abuse potential of opioid ADFs by all routes of abuse in both pre- and postmarketing studies. As always, it is important to remember that the currently available opioid ADFs are not abuse-proof and that abuse by the oral, intranasal, and intravenous routes is still possible.

Widespread availability and adoption of opioid ADFs by prescribers, combined with significantly reduced availability or even elimination of non-ADFs of opioids could potentially temper the rates of abusers switching to non-ADFs of opioids. Collecting real-world data on the value of ADFs has been challenging because of physicians' reluctance to prescribe opioids over concerns of possible misuse and abuse and lack of awareness of abuse patterns and impact of ADFs, underscoring the need to disseminate knowledge about prescription drug abuse [20, 30, 31].

Because of the higher cost of branded or innovator products, insurance coverage may also be limited, creating another initial barrier to uptake of abuse-deterrent opioids [20]. The results from a recent health economic analysis model indicate that converting all opioids to ADFs would reduce abuse-related costs by $266 million and improve outcomes when considering the impact on patients and rates of diversion [32].

The overall impact of ADFs on the medical system is not well understood; some studies have predicted that ADFs would increase overall health-care costs by $533 million [32], whereas others have reported potential annual medical costs savings of $429 million in the United States [33] and $4.3 billion in Canada [34]. As more opioids are developed with abuse-deterrent properties, studies assessing the impact on societal cost and outcomes are essential for determining the real-world value of opioid ADFs.

Balancing the needs of patients who have chronic pain while minimizing the diversion and abuse of prescription opioids remains a health-care challenge. Because ER opioid formulations are twice as likely to result in an overdose when compared with IR formulations [35], the reductions in drug liking seen with ADFs including Morphine ARER suggest that Morphine ARER should demonstrate a real-world benefit. Ultimately, opioid ADFs represent one component of an overall public health strategy to reduce abuse and misuse while maintaining access to pain relief [36].

## 5. Conclusions

This study demonstrates that when Morphine ARER was crushed and administered intranasally or taken orally intact, exposure to morphine and its active metabolite early after administration was significantly lower compared with crushed intranasal ER morphine. Importantly, the PK profile of Morphine ARER is similar between crushed intranasal and intact oral administration indicating that the ER characteristics of Morphine ARER were maintained after manipulation and intranasal administration. A strong and consistent association was noted between morphine PK parameters and the PD endpoint of drug liking. The results of this PK study reinforce previous findings that Morphine ARER has lower potential for intranasal abuse than non-abuse-deterrent ER morphine and support the use of AQ as a surrogate measure for drug liking.

## Authors' Contributions

All authors assisted in the design of the study, interpreted the data, critically reviewed the manuscript, and approved the final version for submission. Lynn R. Webster and Michael D. Smith also collected the data for the study. All authors accept responsibility for the accuracy of the data, analysis of the data, and development of this report.

## Acknowledgments

This study was supported by Inspirion Delivery Sciences LLC, Morristown, NJ, USA. The authors acknowledge Manish Shah and Ray DiFalco of Cerovene, for their role in the study. Medical writing assistance (funded by Daiichi Sankyo, Inc.) was provided by Kelly M Cameron, Ph.D, ISMPP Certified Medical Publications Professional, of JB Ashtin who developed the first draft based on an author-approved outline and assisted in implementing author revisions throughout the editorial process.

## References

[1] Center for Behavioral Health Statistics and Quality, *Behavioral Health Trends in the United States: Results from the 2014 National Survey on Drug Use and Health*, HHS Publication No. SMA 15–4927, NSDUH Series H–50, 2015.

[2] Centers for Disease Control and Prevention, *Opioid Data Analysis*, October 2017.

[3] L. R. Webster, B. Bath, R. A. Medve, T. Marmon, and G. J. Stoddard, "Randomized, double-blind, placebo-controlled study of the abuse potential of different formulations of oral oxycodone," *Pain Medicine*, vol. 13, no. 6, pp. 790–801, 2012.

[4] S. F. Butler, R. A. Black, T. A. Cassidy, T. M. Dailey, and S. H. Budman, "Abuse risks and routes of administration of different prescription opioid compounds and formulations," *Harm Reduction Journal*, vol. 8, no. 1, p. 29, 2011.

[5] N. Katz, R. C. Dart, E. Bailey, J. Trudeau, E. Osgood, and F. Paillard, "Tampering with prescription opioids: nature and extent of the problem, health consequences, and solutions," *American Journal of Drug and Alcohol Abuse*, vol. 37, no. 4, pp. 205–217, 2011.

[6] R. Moorman-Li, C. A. Motycka, L. D. Inge, J. M. Congdon, S. Hobson, and B. Pokropski, "A review of abuse-deterrent opioids for chronic nonmalignant pain," *Pharmacy and Therapeutics*, vol. 37, no. 7, pp. 412–418, 2012.

[7] S. C. Harris, P. J. Perrino, I. Smith et al., "Abuse potential, pharmacokinetics, pharmacodynamics, and safety of intranasally administered crushed oxycodone HCl abuse-deterrent controlled-release tablets in recreational opioid users," *Journal of Clinical Pharmacology*, vol. 54, no. 4, pp. 468–477, 2014.

[8] B. Setnik, V. Goli, N. Levy-Cooperman, C. Mills, M. Shram, and I. Smith, "Assessing the subjective and physiological effects of intranasally administered crushed extended-release morphine formulations with and without a sequestered naltrexone core in recreational opioid users," *Pain Research and Management*, vol. 18, no. 4, pp. e55–e62, 2013.

[9] L. R. Webster, M. D. Smith, J. Lawler, K. Lindhardt, and J. M. Dayno, "Human abuse potential of an abuse-deterrent (AD), extended-release (ER) morphine product candidate (morphine-ADER injection-molded tablets) vs. extended-release morphine administered intranasally in nondependent recreational opioid users," *Pain Medicine*, vol. 18, no. 9, pp. 1695–1705, 2017.

[10] P. M. Coplan, H. D. Chilcoat, S. F. Butler et al., "The effect of an abuse-deterrent opioid formulation (OxyContin) on opioid abuse-related outcomes in the postmarketing setting," *Clinical Pharmacology & Therapeutics*, vol. 100, no. 3, pp. 275–286, 2016.

[11] T. A. Cassidy, P. Dasmahapatra, R. A. Black, M. S. Wieman, and S. F. Butler, "Changes in prevalence of prescription opioid abuse after introduction of an abuse-deterrent opioid formulation," *Pain Medicine*, vol. 15, no. 3, pp. 440–451, 2014.

[12] T. J. Cicero and M. S. Ellis, "Abuse-deterrent formulations and the prescription opioid abuse epidemic in the united states: lessons learned from OxyContin," *JAMA Psychiatry*, vol. 72, no. 5, pp. 424–430, 2015.

[13] P. M. Coplan, H. Kale, L. Sandstrom, C. Landau, and H. D. Chilcoat, "Changes in oxycodone and heroin exposures in the National Poison Data System after introduction of extended-release oxycodone with abuse-deterrent characteristics," *Pharmacoepidemiology and Drug Safety*, vol. 22, no. 12, pp. 1274–1282, 2013.

[14] E. C. Mcnaughton, P. M. Coplan, R. A. Black, S. E. Weber, H. D. Chilcoat, and S. F. Butler, "Monitoring of internet forums to evaluate reactions to the introduction of reformulated OxyContin to deter abuse," *Journal of Medical Internet Research*, vol. 16, no. 5, p. e119, 2014.

[15] R. P. Bianchi, E. R. Kinzler, R. Difalco, M. S. Shah, and S. Aigner, "Extraction testing of a novel extended-release, abuse-deterrent formulation of morphine, Morphine ARER, in common solvents," in *Proceedings of the 33rd Annual Scientific Meeting of the American Pain Society*, Tampa, FL, USA, April 2014.

[16] R. Difalco, E. R. Kinzler, C. Pantaleon, and S. Aigner, "Abuse-resistant, extended-release morphine is resistant to physical manipulation techniques commonly used by opioid abusers," in *Proceedings of the PAINWeek*, Las Vegas, NV, USA, September 2014.

[17] E. R. Kinzler, R. Difalco, C. Pantaleon, and S. Aigner, "In vitro evaluation of Morphine ARER potential for abuse via injection," in *Proceedings of the PAINWeek*, Las Vegas, NV, USA, September 2014.

[18] L. R. Webster, C. Pantaleon, M. S. Shah et al., "A randomized, double-blind, double-dummy, placebo-controlled, intranasal drug liking study on a novel abuse-deterrent formulation of morphine-Morphine ARER," *Pain Medicine*, vol. 18, no. 7, pp. 1303–1313, 2017.

[19] L. R. Webster, B. Bath, and R. A. Medve, "Opioid formulations in development designed to curtail abuse: who is the target?," *Expert Opinion on Investigational Drugs*, vol. 18, no. 3, pp. 255–263, 2009.

[20] M. Gasior, M. Bond, and R. Malamut, "Routes of abuse of prescription opioid analgesics: a review and assessment of the potential impact of abuse-deterrent formulations," *Postgraduate Medicine*, vol. 128, no. 1, pp. 85–96, 2016.

[21] R. Raffa, J. Pergolizzi, R. Taylor, and E. R. Kinzler, "Trends and characteristics of individuals who abuse ER morphine: data from the RADARS system," in *Proceedings of the 33rd Annual Scientific Meeting of the American Pain Society*, Tampa, FL, USA, April-May 2014.

[22] S. H. Budman, J. M. Grimes Serrano, and S. F. Butler, "Can abuse deterrent formulations make a difference? Expectation and speculation," *Harm Reduction Journal*, vol. 6, no. 1, p. 8, 2009.

[23] Food and Drug Administration, *Guidance for Industry: Abuse-Deterrent Opioids-Evaluation and Labeling*, 2015.

[24] P. J. Perrino, S. V. Colucci, G. Apseloff, and S. C. Harris, "Pharmacokinetics, tolerability, and safety of intranasal administration of reformulated OxyContin® tablets compared with original OxyContin® tablets in healthy adults," *Clinical Drug Investigation*, vol. 33, no. 6, pp. 441–449, 2013.

[25] S. F. Butler, T. A. Cassidy, H. Chilcoat et al., "Abuse rates and routes of administration of reformulated extended-release oxycodone: initial findings from a sentinel surveillance sample of individuals assessed for substance abuse treatment," *Journal of Pain*, vol. 14, no. 4, pp. 351–358, 2013.

[26] M. R. Larochelle, F. Zhang, D. Ross-Degnan, and J. F. Wharam, "Rates of opioid dispensing and overdose after introduction of abuse-deterrent extended-release oxycodone and withdrawal of propoxyphene," *JAMA Internal Medicine*, vol. 175, no. 6, pp. 978–987, 2015.

[27] S. G. Severtson, M. S. Ellis, S. P. Kurtz et al., "Sustained reduction of diversion and abuse after introduction of an abuse deterrent formulation of extended release oxycodone," *Drug and Alcohol Dependence*, vol. 168, pp. 219–229, 2016.

[28] T. J. Cicero, M. S. Ellis, and H. L. Surratt, "Effect of abuse-deterrent formulation of OxyContin," *New England Journal of Medicine*, vol. 367, no. 2, pp. 187–189, 2012.

[29] S. Gottlieb and J. Woodcock, "Marshaling FDA benefit-risk expertise to address the current opioid abuse epidemic," *JAMA*, vol. 318, no. 5, pp. 421-422, 2017.

[30] J. Pergolizzi, R. Taylor, R. Raffa, and E. R. Kinzler, "Practitioner's knowledge, attitudes, and practices regarding opioid abuse-deterrent formulations, abstract 488," *Journal of Pain*, vol. 15, no. 4, p. S88, 2014.

[31] D. C. Turk, E. J. Dansie, H. D. Wilson, B. Moskovitz, and M. Kim, "Physicians' beliefs and likelihood of prescribing opioid tamper-resistant formulations for chronic noncancer pain patients," *Pain Medicine*, vol. 15, no. 4, pp. 625–636, 2014.

[32] Institute for Clinical and Economic Review, *Abuse-Deterrent Opioids: Final Evidence Report*, 2017.

[33] L. F. Rossiter, N. Y. Kirson, A. Shei et al., "Medical cost savings associated with an extended-release opioid with abuse-deterrent technology in the US," *Journal of Medical Economics*, vol. 17, no. 4, pp. 279–287, 2014.

[34] B. J. Skinner, *Societal Cost Savings from Abuse Deterrent Formulations for Prescription Opioids in Canada*, Canadian Health Policy, Toronto, Canada, 2017.

[35] M. Miller, C. W. Barber, S. Leatherman et al., "Prescription opioid duration of action and the risk of unintentional overdose among patients receiving opioid therapy," *JAMA Internal Medicine*, vol. 175, no. 4, pp. 608–615, 2015.

[36] H. V. Kunins, "Abuse-deterrent opioid formulations: part of a public health strategy to reverse the opioid epidemic," *JAMA Internal Medicine*, vol. 175, no. 6, pp. 987-988, 2015.

# Permissions

# List of Contributors

**Aldric Hama, Takahiro Natsume, Shin'ya Ogawa and Hiroyuki Takamatsu**
Hamamatsu Pharma Research, Inc., Hamamatsu, Shizuoka 431-2103, Japan

**Noriyuki Higo**
Human Informatics Research Institute, National Institute of Advanced Industrial Science and Technology (AIST), Tsukuba, Ibaraki 305-8568, Japan

**Ikuo Hayashi**
Hamamatsu Pharma Research USA, Inc., San Diego, CA 92122, USA

**Kathryn Schopmeyer**
Department of Veterans Affairs, San Francisco VA Healthcare System, 4150 Clement Street, San Francisco, CA, USA

**Nidhi S. Anamkath, Sarah A. Palyo, Sara C. Jacobs, Alain Lartigue and Irina A. Strigo**
Department of Veterans Affairs, San Francisco VA Healthcare System, 4150 Clement Street, San Francisco, CA, USA
University of California, San Francisco, CA, USA

**Dang Huy Quoc Thinh**
Department of Radiation Oncology, HCMC Oncology Hospital, Ho Chi Minh City, Vietnam

**Wimonrat Sriraj**
Department of Anesthesiology, Faculty of Medicine, Srinagarind Hospital, Khon Kaen University, Khon Kaen, Thailand

**Marzida Mansor**
Department of Anesthesiology, Faculty of Medicine, University of Malaya, Kuala Lumpur, Malaysia

**Kian Hian Tan**
Department of Anaesthesiology, Singapore General Hospital, Singapore

**Cosphiadi Irawan**
Department of Internal Medicine, Cipto Mangunkusumo General Hospital (RSCM), University of Indonesia, Jakarta Pusat, Indonesia

**Johan Kurnianda**
Department of Internal Medicine, Dr. Sardjito General Hospital, Gadjah Mada University, Yogyakarta, Indonesia

**Yen Phi Nguyen**
Department of Palliative Care and Pain Management, K Hospital, Vietnam National Cancer Hospital, Hanoi, Vietnam

**Annielyn Ong-Cornel**
Veterans Memorial Medical Centre, Quezon City, Philippines

**Yacine Hadjiat and Hanlim Moon**
APAC LATAM MEA, Mundipharma, Singapore

**Francis O. Javier**
Pain Management Center, St. Luke's Medical Center, Quezon City, Philippines

**Marceline C. Willekens**
Health Center "het Wantveld", Noordwijk, Netherlands

**Don Postel and Martin D. M. Keesenberg**
Corpus Mentis, Center for Physical Therapy and Science, Leiden, Netherlands

**Robert Lindeboom**
Academic Medical Center, Department of Clinical Epidemiology and Biostatistics, University of Amsterdam, Amsterdam, Netherlands

**Fausto Salaffi, Marco Di Carlo and Sonia Farah**
Rheumatological Clinic, Università Politecnica delle Marche, Jesi, Ancona, Italy

**Marina Carotti**
Department of Radiology, Università Politecnica delle Marche, Ancona, Italy

**Nathalie Bitar and Stéphane Potvin**
Centre de recherche de l'Institut Universitaire en Santé Mentale de Montréal, Montreal, QC, Canada
Department of Psychiatry, Faculty of Medicine, Université de Montréal, Montréal, QC, Canada

**Serge Marchand**
Centre de recherche du Centre Hospitalier de l'Université de Sherbrooke, Sherbrooke, QC, Canada
Department of Surgery, Faculty of Medicine and Health Sciences, Université de Sherbrooke, Sherbrooke, QC, Canada

**Liliana Szyszka-Sommerfeld, Monika Machoy and Krzysztof Woźniak**
Department of Orthodontics, Pomeranian Medical University of Szczecin, Al. Powstańców Wlkp. 72, Szczecin 70111, Poland

**Teresa Matthews-Brzozowska**
Department and Clinic of Maxillofacial Orthopaedics and Orthodontics, Poznan University of Medical Sciences, 70 Bukowska Street, Poznań 60812, Poland

**Beata Kawala**
Department of Maxillofacial Orthopaedics and Orthodontics, Wroclaw Medical University, 26 Krakowska Street, Wrocław 50425, Poland

**Marcin Mikulewicz**
Department of Maxillofacial Orthopaedics and Orthodontics, Division of Facial Abnormalities, Wroclaw Medical University, 26 Krakowska Street, Wrocław 50425, Poland

**Włodzimierz Więckiewicz**
Department of Prosthetic Dentistry, Wroclaw Medical University, 26 Krakowska Street, Wrocław 50425, Poland

**Sang-Wook Song and Sung-Goo Kang**
Department of Family Medicine, St. Vincent's Hospital, College of Medicine, The Catholic University of Korea, Suwon, Republic of Korea

**Kyung-Soo Kim**
Department of Family Medicine, CMC Clinical Research Coordinating Center, Seoul St. Mary's Hospital, College of Medicine, The Catholic University of Korea, Seoul, Republic of Korea

**Moon-Jong Kim, Doo-Yeoun Cho and Young-Sang Kim**
Department of Family Medicine, CHA Bundang Medical Center, CHA Medical University, Seongnam, Republic of Korea

**Kwang-Min Kim, Nam-Seok Joo and Kyu-Nam Kim**
Department of Family Practice and Community Health, Ajou University School of Medicine, Suwon, Republic of Korea

**Doo-Hwan Kim, Sooyoung Kim, Chan Sik Kim, Sukyung Lee, In-Gyu Lee, Jong-Hyuk Lee, Sung-Moon Jeong and Kyu Taek Choi**
Department of Anesthesiology and Pain Medicine, Asan Medical Center, University of Ulsan College of Medicine, Seoul, Republic of Korea

**Hee Jeong Kim**
2Division of Breast and Endocrine Surgery, Department of Surgery, Asan Medical Center, University of Ulsan College of Medicine, Seoul, Republic of Korea

**Satomi Yoshida, Aki Kuwauchi and Koji Kawakami**
Department of Pharmacoepidemiology, Graduate School of Medicine and Public Health, Kyoto University, Yoshidakonoe-cho, Sakyo-ku, Kyoto 606-8501, Japan

**Mikito Hirakata**
Department of Pharmacoepidemiology, Graduate School of Medicine and Public Health, Kyoto University, Yoshidakonoe-cho, Sakyo-ku, Kyoto 606-8501, Japan
Toxicology and Pharmacokinetics Laboratories, Pharmaceutical Research Laboratories, Toray Industries, Inc., 10-1, Tebiro 6-chome, Kamakura, Kanagawa 248-8555, Japan

**Sachiko Tanaka-Mizuno**
Department of Pharmacoepidemiology, Graduate School of Medicine and Public Health, Kyoto University, Yoshidakonoe-cho, Sakyo-ku, Kyoto 606-8501, Japan
Department of Medical Statistics, Shiga University of Medical Science, Seta Tsukinowa-cho, Otsu, Shiga 520-2192, Japan

**Rogier J. Scherder, Evelien T. Wolf and Erik J. A. Scherder**
Department of Clinical Neuropsychology, Vrije Universiteit, Amsterdam, Netherlands

**Neeltje Kant**
Department of Neuropsychology, Reade, Amsterdam, Netherlands

**Bas C. M. Pijnenburg**
Acibadem International Medical Center, Amsterdam, Netherlands

**Frank Lobbezoo and Maurits K. A. van Selms**
Department of Oral Kinesiology, Academic Centre for Dentistry Amsterdam (ACTA), University of Amsterdam and Vrije Universiteit Amsterdam, Amsterdam, Netherlands

**Carolina Marpaung**
Department of Oral Kinesiology, Academic Centre for Dentistry Amsterdam (ACTA), University of Amsterdam and Vrije Universiteit Amsterdam, Amsterdam, Netherlands
Department of Prosthodontics, Faculty of Dentistry, Trisakti University, Jakarta, Indonesia

**Oznur Buyukturan, Buket Buyukturan, Caner Kararti and İsmail Ceylan**
School of Physical Therapy and Rehabilitation, Ahi Evran University, Kırşehir, Turkey

**Senem Sas**
Department of Physical Medicine and Rehabilitation, Ahi Evran University Training and Research Hospital, Kırşehir, Turkey

**Tatsuya Hirase, Shigeru Inokuchi, Jiro Nakano and Junya Sakamoto**
Department of Physical Therapy Science, Nagasaki University Graduate School of Biomedical Sciences, 1-7-1 Sakamoto, Nagasaki 852-8520, Japan

**Hideki Kataoka**
Department of Locomotive Rehabilitation Science, Nagasaki University Graduate School of Biomedical Sciences, 1-7-1 Sakamoto, Nagasaki 852-8520, Japan
Department of Rehabilitation, Nagasaki Memorial Hospital, 11-54 Fukahori, Nagasaki 851-0301, Japan

**Minoru Okita**
Department of Locomotive Rehabilitation Science, Nagasaki University Graduate School of Biomedical Sciences, 1-7-1 Sakamoto, Nagasaki 852-8520, Japan

**Richard King and Victoria Robinson**
The Pain Clinic, South Tees Hospitals NHS Foundation Trust, Middlesbrough TS3 4BW, UK

**Helene L. Elliott-Button, James A. Watson, Cormac G. Ryan and Denis J. Martin**
Health and Social Care Institute, Teesside University, Middlesbrough TS1 3BA, UK

**James Marcus and Yin Wan**
Pharmerit International, Bethesda, MD, USA

**Kathryn Lasch**
Pharmerit International, Boston, MA, USA

**Mei Yang and Ching Hsu**
Daiichi Sankyo, Inc., Basking Ridge, NJ, USA

**Domenico Merante**
Daiichi Sankyo Development Ltd., Gerrards Cross, Buckinghamshire, UK

**Chiara Angeletti and Martina Paesani**
Operative Unit of Anesthesiology, Intensive Care and Pain Medicine, Civil Hospital G. Mazzini of Teramo, Teramo, Italy

**Cristiana Guetti**
Struttura Operativa Dipartimentale Complessa, Cure Intensive per il Trauma e Supporti Extracorporei, Azienda Ospedaliero-Universitaria Careggi, Firenze, Italy

**Silvia Colavincenzo, Alessandra Ciccozzi and Paolo Matteo Angeletti**
Department of Life, Health and Environmental Sciences, University of L'Aquila, L'Aquila, Italy

**Aleksandra Nitecka-Buchta, Karolina Walczynska-Dragon and Jolanta Batko-Kapustecka**
Department of Temporomandibular Disorders, Unit SMDZ in Zabrze, Medical University of Silesia in Katowice, Traugutta Sq. 2, 41-800 Zabrze, Poland

**Mieszko Wieckiewicz**
Department of Experimental Dentistry, Faculty of Dentistry, Wroclaw Medical University, 26 Krakowska St., 50-425 Wroclaw, Poland

**Kordian Staniszewski, Siv Kvinnsland, Lisa Willassen and Espen Helgeland**
Department of Clinical Dentistry, University of Bergen, Bergen, Norway

**Henning Lygre**
Department of Clinical Dentistry, University of Bergen, Bergen, Norway
Oral Health Center of Expertise in Western Norway, Stavanger, Rogaland, Norway

**Ersilia Bifulco**
Department of Clinical Science, University of Bergen, Bergen, Norway

**Trond Berge and Annika Rosén**
Department of Clinical Dentistry, University of Bergen, Bergen, Norway
Department of Oral and Maxillofacial Surgery, Haukeland University Hospital, Bergen, Norway

**Zhiyou Peng, Yanfeng Zhang, Jianguo Guo, Xuejiao Guo and Zhiying Feng**
Department of Pain Medicine, First Affiliated Hospital, School of Medicine, Zhejiang University, Hangzhou 310003, China

**José Manuel Pérez-González, Ricardo Martínez-Rider and Miguel Ángel Noyola-Frías**
Department of Oral and Maxillofacial Surgery, Faculty of Dentistry, San Luis Potosi University, San Luis Potosí, SLP, Mexico

**Vicente Esparza-Villalpando**
Engineering and Materials Science Postgraduate Program, San Luis Potosi University, San Luis Potosí, SLP, Mexico

**Amaury Pozos-Guillén**
Basic Sciences Laboratory, Faculty of Dentistry, San Luis Potosi University, San Luis Potosí, SLP, Mexico

**Abdallah El-Sayed Allam**
Department of Physical Medicine, Rheumatology and Rehabilitation, Tanta University Hospitals, Faculty of Medicine, Tanta University, Tanta, Egypt

**Adham Aboul Fotouh Khalil**
New Kasr El-Aini Teaching Hospital, Cairo, Egypt

**Basma Aly Eltawab**
Department of Radiology, Tanta University Hospitals, Tanta, Egypt

**Wei-Ting Wu and Ke-Vin Chang**
Department of Physical Medicine and Rehabilitation, National Taiwan University Hospital Bei-Hu Branch, Taipei, Taiwan

**P. De Roa**
Pain Unit, Dreux Hospital, GHT28, France

**P. Paris**
Department of Mental Health, Dreux Hospital, GHT28, France

**J. L. Poindessous**
Center of Treatment and Pain Evaluation, Ambroise Par´e Hospital, Paris, France

**O. Maillet**
Clinical Research Unit URC28, Dreux Hospital, GHT28, France

**A. Héron**
Clinical Research Unit URC28, Dreux Hospital, GHT28, France
Department of Human Physiology, Paris Descartes University, Paris, France

**Jing Liu, Ying-Ying Xu, Qi-Lin Zhang and Wei-Feng Luo**
Department of Neurology and Suzhou Clinical Research Center of Neurological Disease,
The Second Affiliated Hospital of Soochow University, Suzhou 215004, China
Jiangsu Key Laboratory of Translational Research and Therapy for Neuro-Psychiatric-Diseases,
Soochow University, Suzhou, Jiangsu 215123, China

**Kyoungho Ryu, Dongchan Ko, Goeun Lim and Sung Hyun Lee**
Department of Anesthesiology and Pain Medicine, Kangbuk Samsung Hospital, Sungkyunkwan University School of Medicine, Seoul, Republic of Korea

**Eugene Kim**
Department of Orthopedic Surgery, Kangbuk Samsung Hospital, Sungkyunkwan University School of Medicine, Seoul, Republic of Korea

**Victoria Furer, Valerie Aloush and Ori Elkayam**
Tel Aviv Sourasky Medical Center and the Sackler Faculty of Medicine, Tel Aviv University, Tel Aviv, Israel

**Eyal Hazan and Jacob N. Ablin**
Tel Aviv Sourasky Medical Center, Tel Aviv, Israel

**Adi Mor, Michal Segal and Avi Katav**
ChemomAb Ltd., Tel Aviv, Israel

**Jacob George**
ChemomAb Ltd., Tel Aviv, Israel
Kaplan Medical Center, Rehovot, Israel

**Danuta Lietz-Kijak**
Independent Unit of Propaedeutic and Dental Physical Diagnostics, Faculty of Medicine and Dentistry, Pomeranian Medical University, Rybacka 1, 70-204 Szczecin, Poland

**Łukasz Kopacz and Marta Grzegocka**
Pomeranian Medical University, Rybacka 1, 70-204 Szczecin, Poland

**Roman Ardan**
Department of Econometrics, Faculty of Economic Sciences, Koszalin University of Technology, Kwiatkowskiego 6e, 75-343 Koszalin, Poland

**Edward Kijak**
Scientific Unit of Dysfunction of the Masticatory System, Chair and Department of Prosthodontics, Faculty of Medicine and Dentistry, Pomeranian Medical University, Rybacka 1, 70-204 Szczecin, Poland

**Lili Zhou and Xuejing Lu**
CAS Key Laboratory of Mental Health, Institute of Psychology, Beijing, China
Department of Psychology, University of Chinese Academy of Sciences, Beijing, China

**Hua Wei and Huijuan Zhang**
CAS Key Laboratory of Mental Health, Institute of Psychology, Beijing, China
Department of Psychology, University of Chinese Academy of Sciences, Beijing, China
Faculty of Psychology, Southwest University, Chongqing, China

**Jie Chen**
Cognition and Human Behavior Key Laboratory of Hunan Province, Hunan Normal University, Changsha, Hunan, China

**Li Hu**
CAS Key Laboratory of Mental Health, Institute of Psychology, Beijing, China
Department of Psychology, University of Chinese Academy of Sciences, Beijing, China
Faculty of Psychology, Southwest University, Chongqing, China
Cognition and Human Behavior Key Laboratory of Hunan Province, Hunan Normal University, Changsha, Hunan, China

**Lynn R. Webster and Michael D. Smith**
PRA Health Sciences, Salt Lake City, UT, USA

**Carmela Pantaleon, Matthew Iverson, Eric R. Kinzler and Stefan Aigner**
Inspirion Delivery Sciences LLC, Morristown, NJ, USA

# Index

www.ingramcontent.com/pod-product-compliance
Lightning Source LLC
Chambersburg PA
CBHW080513200326

41458CB00012B/4187